Oncology Nutrition *for* Clinical Practice

Second Edition

Oncology Nutrition Dietetic Practice Group

Editors: Anne Coble Voss, PhD, RDN, LDN, *and*
Valaree Williams, MS, RD, CSO, LDN, CNSC, FAND

eat right. Academy of Nutrition and Dietetics

Academy of Nutrition and Dietetics

120 S. Riverside Plaza, Suite 2190

Chicago, IL 60606

Oncology Nutrition for Clinical Practice, Second Edition

ISBN 978-0-88091-067-5 (print)

ISBN 978-0-88091-154-2 (eBook)

Catalog Number 527421 (print)

Catalog Number 527421e (eBook)

10   9   8   7   6   5   4   3   2

For more information on the Academy of Nutrition and Dietetics, visit www.eatright.org.

Library of Congress Cataloging-in-Publication Data

Names: Coble Voss, Anne, editor. | Williams, Valaree, editor. | Academy of Nutrition and Dietetics. Pediatric Nutrition Practice Group, publisher.
Title: Oncology nutrition for clinical practice / editors, Anne Coble Voss, PhD, RDN, LDN, and Valaree Williams, MS, RD, CSO, LDN, CNSC, FAND.
Description: Second edition. | Chicago : Academy of Nutrition and Dietetics, 2021. | Includes bibliographical references and index.
Identifiers: LCCN 2021007365 (print) | LCCN 2021007366 (ebook) | ISBN 9780880910675 (paperback) | ISBN 9780880911542 (ebook)
Subjects: LCSH: Cancer--Diet therapy. | Cancer--Patients--Nutrition.
Classification: LCC RC268.45 .O53 2021 (print) | LCC RC268.45 (ebook) | DDC 616.99/40654--dc23
LC record available at https://lccn.loc.gov/2021007365
LC ebook record available at https://lccn.loc.gov/2021007366

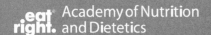

Oncology Nutrition *for* Clinical Practice

Second Edition

Oncology Nutrition Dietetic Practice Group

Editors: Anne Coble Voss, PhD, RDN, LDN, *and*
Valaree Williams, MS, RD, CSO, LDN, CNSC, FAND

Contents

Boxes, Tables, and Figures

Boxes

Tables

Figures

Contributors

Alice Bender, MS, RDN
*Consultant, American
Institute for Cancer Research
Washington, DC*

Michelle Bratton, RDN, CSO
*Clinical Nutritionist,
University of Arizona
Cancer Center
Tucson, AZ*

Laura Brown, MS, RD,
CSO, CNSC
*Oncology Dietitian, SCL
Health, Cancer Centers
of Colorado
Lafayette, CO*

Jennifer Caceres, MS, RD,
CSP, LDN
*Operations Manager,
Nicklaus Children's Hospital
Miami, FL*

Audrey Caspar-Clark, MA,
RDN, LDN
*Advanced Clinical Dietitian
Specialist, Hospital of
the University of
Pennsylvania, Department
of Radiation Oncology
Philadelphia, PA*

Karen Collins, MS, RDN, CDN,
FAND
*Consultant and Nutrition
Advisor, American Institute
for Cancer Research
Bemus Point, NY*

Tracy E. Crane, PhD,
MS, RDN
*Assistant Professor of
Nursing, Public Health and
Nutrition Science,
University of Arizona
Tucson, AZ*

Alison Donato, RDN, CSO, CD
*Registered Dietitian,
MultiCare Health System
Tacoma, WA*

Colleen Gill, MS, RDN, CSO
*Private Practice Dietitian,
Nutrition Foundations, LLC
Denver, CO*

Alicia Gilmore, MS, RD,
CSO, LD
*Clinical Instructor, School
of Health Professions at
University of
Texas Southwestern
Medical Center
Dallas, TX*

Ally F. Gottfried, MFN, RDN,
CSO, LD
*Clinical Dietitian,
Community Cancer Center
Roseburg, OR*

Barbara L. Grant, MS, RDN,
CSO, FAND
*Oncology Dietitian
Nutritionist, Saint Alphonsus
Cancer Institute
Boise, ID*

Gretchen B. Gruender, MS,
RDN, CSO, CD
*Clinical Dietitian
Seattle, WA*

Kathryn K. Hamilton, MA,
RDN, CSO, CDN, FAND
*Outpatient Oncology
Dietitian Nutritionist,
Morristown Medical Center,
Morristown, NJ*

Jill Hamilton-Reeves, PhD,
RDN, CSO, NSCA-CPT
*Associate Professor,
University of Kansas
Medical Center
Kansas City, KS*

Katie Harper, MS, RD,
CNSC, CSO
*Clinical Dietitian, University
of Colorado Hospital
Aurora, CO*

Rachel Hill, RD, CSO,
LD, CNSC
*Clinical Dietitian, Cook
Children's Medical Center
Fort Worth, TX*

Elizabeth A. Huddleston,
MS, RDN
*Registered Dietitian
Nutritionist, Compassus
Hospice and Palliative Care
Branson, MO*

Maki Inoue-Choi, PhD,
MS, RD
*Staff Scientist, Metabolic
Epidemiology Branch,
Division of Cancer
Epidemiology and
Genetics, National Cancer
Institute, National Institutes
of Health, HHS
Bethesda, MD*

Liz Isenring, PhD, AdvAPD
*Director of LINC Nutrition,
Adjunct Honorary Professor,
Master of Nutrition
and Dietetic Practice,
Bond University
Robina, QLD, Australia*

Sandeep (Anu) Kaur, MS,
RDN, RYT-500
*Nutrition Research
Consultant, Certified
WellCoach, Registered
Yoga Teacher, www
.ANuHealthyYou.com
Ashburn, VA*

Nicole Kiss, BSc, PhD,
MNutDiet
*Senior Clinical Research
Fellow, Institute for Physical
Activity and Nutrition,
Deakin University
Burwood, VIC, Australia*

Natalie Ledesma, MS,
RD, CSO
*Clinical Nutrition Specialist,
Smith Integrative Oncology
and UCSF Helen Diller
Family Comprehensive
Cancer Center
Corte Madera, CA*

Maureen S. Leser, MS,
RDN, LD
Leesburg, FL

Rhone M. Levin, MEd, RDN,
CSO, LDN, FAND
*Oncology Dietitian, Duke
University Hospital,
Adult Oncology
Durham, NC*

Greta Macaire, MA, RD, CSO
*Oncology Registered
Dietitian Nutritionist,
University of California
San Francisco Helen Diller
Family Comprehensive
Cancer Center
San Francisco, CA*

Kerry K. McMillen, MS, RD,
CSO, FAND
*Manager, Medical Nutrition
Therapy, Seattle Cancer
Care Alliance
Seattle, WA*

Kacie Merchand, MS, RD, CSO, LD
Clinical Oncology Dietitian, formerly at Norris Cotton Cancer Center, Dartmouth-Hitchcock Medical Center
Lebanon, NH

Kristen Miller, MS, RD, CSP, CLEC
Pediatric Clinical Dietitian, Oncology and Ketogenic Diet, Children's Hospital Orange County
Orange, CA

Jeannine B. Mills, MS, RDN, CSO, LD
Board Certified Specialist in Oncology Nutrition, Norris Cotton Cancer Center, Dartmouth-Hitchcock Medical Center
Lebanon, NH

Kelli Oldham, MS, RDN, CSO, LDN
Registered Dietitian, Vidant Medical Center
Greenville, NC

Amy Patton, RD, CSO, CNSC
Associate Director, Hospital Dietetics, The Ohio State University Wexner Medical Center and Arthur G. James Cancer Hospital
Columbus, Ohio

Maria Q.B. Petzel, RD, CSO, LD, CNSC, FAND
Senior Clinical Dietitian, The University of Texas MD Anderson Cancer Center
Houston, TX

Karen Ringwald-Smith, MS, RDN, LDN, FAND
Project Manager, St. Jude Children's Research Hospital
Memphis, TN

Kim Robien, PhD, RD, LD, CSO, FAND
Associate Professor, Department of Exercise and Nutrition Services, Milken Institute of Public Health, George Washington University
Washington, DC

Shayne Robinson, RD, CSO, CDN
Clinical Dietitian, Herbert Irving Comprehensive Center, New York Presbyterian, Columbia University Irving Medical Center
New York, NY

Lindsay Rypkema, RD, CSP, CLEC
Clinical Dietitian, Children's Hospital Orange County
Orange, CA

Nancy Sacks, MS, RD, LDN
Pediatric Oncology Nutritionist, Research Coordinator, The Children's Hospital of Philadelphia, Department of Nursing and Clinical Care Services and Center for Childhood Cancer Research and Division of Oncology
Philadelphia, PA

Megan Schoenfeld, RD
Clinical Research Dietitian,
National Institutes of Health
Clinical Center
Bethesda, MD

Cynthia A. Thomson, PhD,
RDN, FAND, FTOS
Professor, Health Promotions
Sciences, University
of Arizona, Mel & Enid
Zuckerman College of Public
Health, University of Arizona
Associate Director
Population Sciences,
University of Arizona
Cancer Center
Tucson, AZ

Cheryl D. Toner, MS, RDN
Director of Food Sector
Engagement, American
Heart Association
Washington, DC

Kelay E. Trentham, MS, RDN,
CSO, FAND
Lead Oncology Dietitian,
MultiCare Regional Cancer
Center
Tacoma, WA

Elaine B. Trujillo, MS, RDN
Nutritionist, National
Cancer Institute, National
Institutes of Health
Rockville, MD

Erin Williams, RD,
CSO, CNSC
Clinical Dietitian, University
of Colorado Cancer Center
Aurora, CO

Reviewers

Heather Bell-Temin, MS, RDN, CSO, FAND
American Oncology Network, LLC
Fort Myers, FL

Shanna B. Yang, MPH, RDN
Metabolic Research Dietitian, National Institutes of Health Clinical Center, Nutrition Department
Bethesda, MD

Katie Birks, RD, CSO
Contract Dietitian
Denver, CO

Janice Newell Bissex, MS, RDN, FAND
CEO, Jannabis Wellness Professor, John Patrick University School of Integrative and Functional Medicine
Melrose, MA

Michelle Bratton, RDN, CSO
Clinical Nutritionist, University of Arizona Cancer Center
Tucson, AZ

Tricia Cox, MS, RD, CNSC, LD
Oncology Dietitian, Baylor Scott and White Medical Center
Dallas, TX

Sharon Day, RD, CSO, CNSC, MBA
Director of Integrative Services and Chief of Nutrition, Cancer Treatment Centers of America
Goodyear, AZ

Heidi Ganzer DCN, RDN, CSO, LD
Allina Health Cancer Institute
Rochester, MN

Sommer Gaughan, RD, CSO
Registered Dietitian, University of Colorado School of Medicine, Department of Pediatrics
Aurora, CO

Kristy Gibbons, MS, RD, CSP, CSO, LDN
Lead Clinical Dietitian, St. Jude Children's Research Hospital
Memphis, TN

Alicia Gilmore, MS, RD, CSO, LD
Clinical Instructor, School of Health Professions at University of Texas Southwestern Medical Center
Dallas, TX

Jodie Greear, MS, RD, CSO, LDN
Clinical Dietitian, St Jude Children's Research Hospital
Memphis, TN

Lisa Heneghen, MPH, RD, CSO, CNSC
Clinical Dietitian, UCHealth
Aurora, CO

Melissa Kingery, MS, RD, CSO, LD/N
Clinical Oncology Nutritionist, Florida Cancer Specialists
Fort Myers, FL

Heather Lazarow, MS, RD, CSO, LDN
Advanced Practice Clinical Dietitian Specialist, Hospital of the University of Pennsylvania
Philadelphia, PA

Natalie Ledesma, MS, RD, CSO
Clinical Nutrition Specialist, Smith Integrative Oncology and UCSF Helen Diller Family Comprehensive Cancer Center
Corte Madera, CA

Paula Charuhas Macris, MS, RD, CSO, FAND, CD
Nutrition Education Coordinator, Seattle Cancer Care Alliance
Seattle, WA

Jeannine B. Mills, MS, RDN, CSO, LD
Board Certified Specialist in Oncology Nutrition, Norris Cotton Cancer Center, Dartmouth-Hitchcock Medical Center
Lebanon, NH

Samantha Peterson, MS, RD, CSO
Registered Dietitian, Simply Wellness LLC
Goodyear, AZ

Kim Robien, PhD, RD, LD, CSO, FAND
Associate Professor, Department of Exercise and Nutrition Services, Milken Institute of Public Health, George Washington University
Washington, DC

Sara Schumacher, MS, RD, CSO, CNSC
Clinical Oncology Dietitian, Cancer Treatment Centers of America
Goodyear, AZ

Renee Thornton, MS, RD, CSO, LDN
Clinical Oncology Dietitian, Cancer Treatment Centers of America
Philadelphia, PA

Preface

Anne Coble Voss, PhD, RDN, LDN
Valaree Williams, MS, RD, CSO, LDN, CNSC, FAND

Editors, *Oncology Nutrition for Clinical Practice*, Second Edition

Oncology Nutrition for Clinical Practice, first published in 2013 by the Oncology Nutrition Dietetic Practice Group, has served as a vital text for registered dietitian nutritionists (RDNs) providing nutrition care to patients with cancer. The intent of this fully updated second edition is to provide both evidence- and experienced-based information for application in clinical practice.

Written and reviewed by knowledgeable RDNs practicing in oncology, this comprehensive resource can be read cover to cover, especially by those new to oncology nutrition, or individual chapters can serve as a guide for clinical practice for both experienced oncology practitioners as well as those who may only work occasionally with patients with cancer. To complement this edition, the new *Oncology Nutrition: Educational Handouts and Resources*, also developed by the Oncology Nutrition Dietetic Practice Group, provides handouts and practical guidance for the nutrition professional to use when counseling their patients with cancer.

This second edition addresses nutrition through the cancer continuum—from carcinogenesis and prevention to treatment, survivorship, and palliative care. All steps of the Nutrition Care Process are addressed with chapters covering nutrition screening, assessment, diagnosis and treatment of nutrition impact symptoms, and intervention and monitoring through medical nutrition therapy. Thirteen chapters address medical nutrition therapy of specific cancer sites, with a new chapter covering hematological malignancies. New to this edition is a chapter that provides rationale and guidance for the use of medical cannabis in cancer treatment.

To direct readers to the most current cancer treatments, in light of the rapidly changing nature of treatment regimens, an overview of treatment modalities and their associated nutrition impact symptoms are discussed in Chapters 9 and 10, and within the medical nutrition therapy chapters, readers are directed to the National Comprehensive Cancer Network (NCCN) guidelines for treatment of cancer by site for regimens for each specific cancer site discussed. NCCN Guidelines are available at www.nccn.org/professionals (free access after registration).

To demonstrate the use of standardized language, sample cancer-specific nutrition diagnosis (PES) statements, developed through collaboration with the Oncology Nutrition Dietetic Practice Group and Academy of Nutrition and Dietetics Nutrition Care Process staff, are included at the end of each medical nutrition therapy chapter. These sample nutrition diagnostic statements support the efforts of the Oncology Nutrition Dietetic Practice Group to increase use of standardized language in documentation of patient care by the RDN to support nutrition outcome measures in the future. In addition to concise, uniform, and complete documentation of nutrition interventions and outcomes by the RDN, standardized language is also essential to the evaluation and coordination of care, determination of the type, level, and complexity of the nutrition intervention, and—most importantly—to the generation of new understanding of the effectiveness and outcomes of nutrition intervention provided by the oncology RDN.

Of special note is the use of the term *cancer survivor* in this edition. Although the National Cancer Institute and some other groups consider a patient to be a survivor from the time of diagnosis until the end of life, this book uses cancer survivor to describe the period posttreatment, and separate from diagnosis, treatment, and end-of-life care. This definition helps to differentiate the nutrition care provided to those living after cancer therapy who may be disease-free or who have stable disease and desire medical nutrition therapy to maintain or improve quality of life and institute measures to prevent future cancers (see Chapters 2 and 8).

We are grateful to the contributors for sharing their expertise and to the reviewers for providing thoughtful, thorough review. With the known impact of nutrition on the development, treatment, and outcomes of cancer, we hope that readers find this second edition to be an essential and useful professional resource to further their expertise and practice.

About the Editors and the Oncology Nutrition Dietetic Practice Group

Anne Coble Voss, PhD, RDN, LDN, writes, lectures and consults on oncology nutrition and oncology nutrition research design following a career as an associate research fellow in the Volwiler Society at Abbott Nutrition.

Dr Voss has experience in the creation of national and international oncology nutrition guidelines and has extensive experience in oncology nutrition research. She held leadership positions in local and state dietetic associations and the Oncology Nutrition Dietetic Practice Group and sat on the Council on Research for the Academy of Nutrition and Dietetics. Dr Voss worked for The Ohio State University College of Medicine, The Ohio State University Hospitals, and Johns Hopkins Hospital. She has published over 75 journal articles, monographs, and book chapters.

Dr Voss earned her undergraduate degree in medical dietetics and a PhD in nutritional biochemistry from The Ohio State University. She recently received the Academy of Nutrition and Dietetics Distinguished Practice Award, The Ohio State University Distinguished Alumni Award, a President's Award, and a Luminary Award from Abbott Laboratories.

Valaree Williams, MS, RD, CSO, LDN, CNSC, FAND is a clinical dietitian at the Hospital of the University of Pennsylvania of the University of Pennsylvania Health System in Philadelphia. Over the past 9 years, she has specialized in caring for patients with cancer, focusing on cancers of the gastrointestinal tract. She serves in several volunteer roles for the Academy of Nutrition and Dietetics and is a commissioner for the Commission on Dietetic Registration. Additionally, she has contributed to textbooks on nutrition for patients with cancer.

Valaree received a bachelor of science degree in dietetics from the Indiana University of Pennsylvania, completed her dietetic internship at the University of Pittsburgh Medical Center Presbyterian-Shadyside, and obtained her master of health sciences degree from Chatham University.

Oncology Nutrition Dietetic Practice Group (ON DPG) is a dietetic practice group of the Academy of Nutrition and Dietetics with the mission of empowering members as oncology nutrition leaders and experts through advocacy, education, and research. Efforts of the ON DPG focus on oncology nutrition practice in areas including research, prevention, treatment, recovery, palliative care, and hospice. The ON DPG provides oncology nutrition resources for the public in addition to supporting dietetic professionals with evidence-based tools and professional networking opportunities to assist with managing the complexities of oncology nutrition practice.

Chapter 1
Overview of Cancer, Carcinogenesis, and the Role of Nutrition

Maki Inoue-Choi, PhD, MS, RD
Kim Robien, PhD, RD, LD, CSO, FAND

The term *cancer* refers to a group of neoplastic diseases characterized by the uncontrollable growth and spread of abnormal cells, which if left untreated may result in death. There are more than 100 types of cancer, each with its own etiology, progression, recommended treatment, and prognosis.[1]

This chapter addresses the following:

- cancer statistics in the US adult population
- health care expenditures for cancer care
- cancer screening
- cancer classification (staging) methods
- the role of nutrition across the cancer continuum

Box 1.1 lists the five most common types of new cancer cases in the United States for men and women in order of most to least common.

Box 1.1
The Five Most Common Types of New Cancer Cases in the United States[2]

Men	Women
1. Prostate	1. Breast
2. Lung and bronchus	2. Lung and bronchus
3. Colorectal	3. Colorectal
4. Urinary (bladder)	4. Uterine
5. Melanoma (skin)	5. Thyroid

Cancer Statistics

Using data from the Surveillance, Epidemiology, and End Results Program of the National Cancer Institute (NCI), a premier source for cancer statistics in the United States, the American Cancer Society (ACS) estimated that approximately 1.8 million new cancer cases would be diagnosed in 2020.[1] Cancer is the second most common cause of death in the United States, after heart disease; it accounts for nearly one in every four US deaths and caused approximately 600,000 deaths in 2020.[2]

Approximately 40% of men and 38% of women in the United States will develop cancer during their lifetime.[1] Among all racial and ethnic groups in the nation, Blacks and non-Hispanic Whites have the highest cancer incidence rates.[3]

The 5-year survival rate for all cancers has improved from 49% for cancers diagnosed between 1975 and 1977 to 69% for cancers diagnosed between 2009 and 2015; yet it remains lower among Blacks (64%) than Whites (70%) (see Figure 1.1 on page 2).[2] Survival rates vary significantly by cancer type and stage at the time of diagnosis.

Cost of Cancer Care

The financial costs of cancer care are a burden for cancer patients, their families, and society. Individually, cancer survivors face not only direct costs related to health care expenses but also lost income due to illness, decreased productivity, and premature mortality.[4]

The NCI estimates that the cost of cancer care in 2010 was $157 billion. This figure was expected to reach $173 billion by 2020, given the growth and aging of the US population.[4,5] Additional costs will occur with the increase in cancer incidence expected with increased longevity.[6] Even if cancer incidence remains constant or decreases, the absolute number

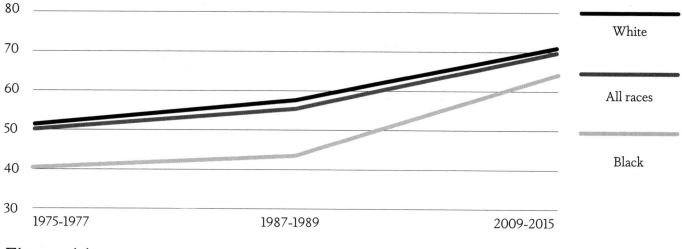

Figure 1.1
Trends in 5-year cancer survival rates by race

Adapted from American Cancer Society. Cancer Facts & Figures 2020. American Cancer Society; 2020. Accessed January 5, 2021. www.cancer.org/research/cancer-facts-statistics/all-cancer-facts-figures/cancer-facts-figures-2020.html. See reference 2.

of people treated for cancer will increase, as the overall population increases and ages. The largest projected increase in costs for 2020 was expected to result from long-term continuing care for survivors of breast cancer and prostate cancer, the most common cancers in women and men, respectively.[5]

Cancer Screening

Regular screening can result in early detection of precancerous lesions and diagnosis of cancer at an early stage, when it is most treatable. "Early" cancer detection is the identification of tumors before they become palpable; early detection is an active area of cancer research with the potential to significantly decrease cancer morbidity, mortality, and health care costs.[5] Over the last few decades, significant decreases in death rates from certain cancers, such as breast and colorectal, have been attributed largely to increased screening, as well as to advancements in treatment options.[2] There are several types of screening that can be employed:

- Palpation (physical examination) (eg breast or testicle self-examination or a skin examination)

is the most common type of screening; however, by the time a cancer is detected by palpation, it can be fairly advanced.

- Blood tests, such as prostate-specific antigen testing, are used to determine levels of circulating tumor cell metabolites.

- Imaging procedures, such as mammograms and colonoscopies, can detect cancers that are too small to feel by physical examination.

- Molecular techniques (for genetic biomarkers), such as genotyping or gene expression assays, look for certain genetic mutations that are linked to some types of cancer. Researchers are also exploring possible use in early cancer detection, as well as many radiographic techniques.

With all types of screening, false test results can occur. For example, test results might appear to be abnormal, even though there is no cancer. False-positive results can cause anxiety in patients and are usually followed by more invasive tests and procedures. Conversely, screening results might appear to be normal, even though a cancer is present. False-negative test results may delay appropriate medical care. The ACS publishes annual cancer screening guidelines on its website (www.cancer.org).[7]

Cancer Staging

Staging is a process for describing the severity of a cancer based on the extent of disease and whether the primary tumor has spread to other areas of the body (metastasized) at the time of diagnosis. Staging is essential to determining the appropriate treatment plan and estimating prognosis at the time of diagnosis. A number of different staging systems are used to classify cancer, but the tumor, (lymph) node, metastasis (TNM) classification system[8,9] is one of the most widely used tumor staging tools,

especially for solid tumors. Each tumor is assigned a grade for each letter: the T grade reflects the size and extent of the tumor; the N grade is for the extent of spread to local lymph nodes; and the M grade indicates the presence or absence of distant metastasis. The number added to each letter indicates the size or extent of the primary cancer and the extent of cancer spread (see Box 1.2).

For some cancers, the TNM classification is not the only system that determines the stage. For most cancers, a grading system is also used. Grade is a measure of how abnormal the cancer cells look under the microscope; this is called differentiation (see Box 1.3 on page 4). Grade can be important because cancers that look more abnormal, or that are more differentiated, tend to grow and spread faster. Each type of cancer has a unique grading

---

Box 1.2
Summary of the Tumor, Lymph Node, Metastasis (TNM) Classification System[9]

Primary tumor (T)

Grade	Definition
TX	Tumor cannot be evaluated
T0	No evidence of tumor
Tis	*Carcinoma in situ* (CIS): Abnormal cells are present but not spread to neighboring tissues Although not cancer, CIS may become cancer
T1	Tumor not palpable or visible by imaging
T2	Tumor confined to the primary cancer site
T3	Tumor extends to the neighboring tissue
T4	Metastatic disease

Lymph nodes (N)

Grade	Definition
NX	Regional lymph nodes cannot be evaluated
N0	No regional lymph node involvement
N1 N2 N3	Involvement of regional lymph nodes (number of lymph nodes indicates extent of spread)

Distant metastasis (M)

Grade	Definition
MX	Distant metastasis cannot be evaluated
M0	No distant metastasis
M1	Distant metastasis is present

---

system. Tumors also are described according to their nuclear grade, which describes the size and shape of the nucleus in the tumor cells and the percentage of tumor cells that are actively dividing.[8]

Carcinogenesis

Carcinogenesis is the process by which normal cells transform into cancer cells, usually as a result of accumulated genetic damage. Carcinogenesis is commonly described as a process consisting of three phases:

1. Initiation, during which normal cells develop some type of DNA damage

2. Promotion, during which initiated cells are stimulated to grow

3. Progression, when the tumor grows rapidly and invades neighboring tissues

In the initiation phase, normal cells develop genetic damage as a result of exposure to environmental factors, such as radiation, chemicals, or viruses. DNA damage also can result from chronic inflammation due to long-term disease. Some of these factors damage DNA directly. Others, especially some chemicals, attach to the DNA and prevent normal transcription and translation of the DNA.[10]

Under normal conditions, cellular processes involving DNA repair enzymes allow cells to repair individual instances of DNA damage. If the damage cannot be repaired, it can trigger what is called cell cycle arrest, which results in a process known as apoptosis (programmed cell death). However, if the initiated cell does not undergo cell cycle arrest and apoptosis, it could progress to become cancer. Damage that occurs within the DNA repair genes can lead to alterations in these normal repair processes and stimulate uncontrolled tumor growth.[10]

Although genetic susceptibility increases the risk for developing certain types of cancer, other factors commonly associated with cancer incidence and progression include:

- internal environmental factors, such as hormones and the immune system;

- external environmental factors, such as infections and exposure to environmental toxins; and

- unhealthy behaviors, such as smoking, excessive sunlight exposure, and unhealthy diet.[11,12]

These factors may act in combination to initiate or promote carcinogenesis. Estimates are that one-third of cancer deaths are smoking-related, and another third are related to overweight or obesity, physical inactivity, and poor diet.[13]

Nutrition and Carcinogenesis

Evidence, primarily from in vitro studies, suggests that nutrients can play a protective role during all stages of carcinogenesis (see Figure 1.2 on page 6).[10] Chapter 2 addresses the role of nutrition in cancer prevention in more detail. In general, mechanisms by which food components might have protective effects in preventing cancer incidence and progression include:

- promotion of detoxification of carcinogens;

- prevention of oxidative damage to DNA;

- inhibition of the cell cycle or induction of apoptosis in initiated cancer cells; and

- support of DNA repair, cell differentiation, hormone regulation, carcinogen metabolism, and anti-inflammatory responses.

The roles that energy balance and body weight play in cancer incidence and treatment outcomes are becoming better understood; however, the exact mechanisms are complex and not fully known. Higher levels of adiposity and lower lean body mass have consistently been associated with increased risk for many types of cancers, as well as for poor treatment outcomes.[14] Excess adipose tissue has been shown to alter the interactions between insulin, growth hormone, insulin-like growth factors, sex hormones, and adipocyte-derived cytokine levels to precipitate favorable environments for cancer incidence and progression.[15] See Chapter 3 for more details about the relationship between energy balance and cancer incidence.

Certain diet-related factors also might increase the risk for developing cancer. For example, cooking meats at high temperatures (eg, grilling over an open flame) can precipitate formation of heterocyclic amines and polycyclic aromatic hydrocarbons, which have been shown to form DNA adducts (a portion of DNA attached to a cancer-causing chemical).[15,16] Foods also can serve as a vehicle for exposure to environmental toxins, such as aflatoxins (a family of fungal toxins associated with peanuts and other agricultural crops), which form DNA adducts,[17] or the endocrine-disrupting chemical bisphenol A (BPA, found in plastic bottles and food containers), which can stimulate proliferation of estrogen-mediated cancers, such as breast or ovarian cancer.[18] Excessive doses of nutrients more than the Recommended Dietary Allowance also might enhance progression of initiated cancer cells.[11,12]

Role of Nutrition in Cancer Treatment

Primary treatments for cancer include surgery, radiation, chemotherapy, hormone therapy, immunotherapy, biological therapy, targeted therapy, transplantation, and various combinations of these modalities.[19] Treatment selection depends on the cancer type, stage of disease, and other factors, such as the patient's age and comorbid conditions. Supportive care with nutrition and physical activity interventions, as well as complementary and alternative medicine approaches, is increasingly being used.

As noted previously, nutrients can play different roles at different stages of carcinogenesis (see Figure 1.2 on page 6). For example, folate is a vital nutrient for maintaining accurate DNA synthesis and repair; thus, adequate folate intake is important for preventing many types of cancers. However, once carcinogenesis has been initiated, folate can facilitate DNA synthesis in cancer cells, leading to proliferation and expansion of the tumor.[20] Methotrexate, an antifolate chemotherapeutic agent, targets this metabolic process by inhibiting folate-mediated DNA synthesis, thus stopping cancer-cell proliferation. Folate in the form of leucovorin calcium may be used to "rescue" patients from methotrexate toxicity or, alternatively, to enhance the effectiveness of drugs, such as fluorouracil (5-FU), that target enzymes that use folate as a cofactor.[21]

Chemotherapeutic agents are designed to kill cancer cells, which often grow and divide more rapidly than normal cells. However, most chemotherapy drugs are indiscriminate and also damage normal cells, such as blood cells in the bone marrow, cells in the digestive tract (including the mouth, esophagus, stomach, and intestines), cells in the reproductive system, and hair follicles.[19] Common side effects of chemotherapy, such as loss of appetite, nausea, mucositis, and diarrhea, result from this

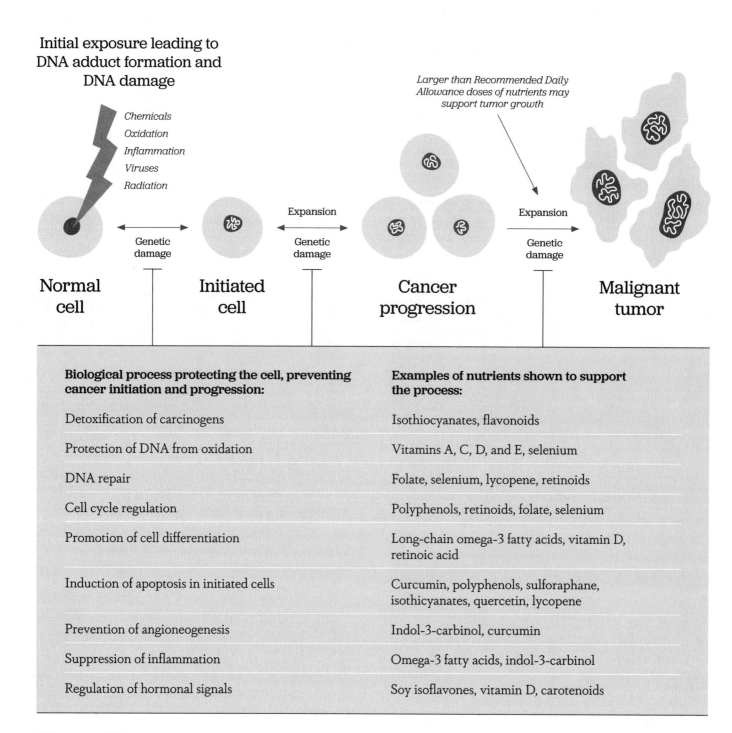

Figure 1.2

Possible effects of nutrients on various stages of carcinogenesis

Healthy cells can develop genetic damage from exposure to environmental factors, such as radiation, chemicals, or viruses. Nutrients can play a protective role in these early carcinogenetic processes.

Adapted from World Cancer Research Fund/American Institute for Cancer Research. The cancer process. In: *Diet, Nutrition, Physical Activity and Cancer: A Global Perspective. Continuous Update Project Expert Report 2018.* Accessed January 12, 2020. www.wcrf.org/dietandcancer/cancerprocess. See reference 10.

cellular damage. Radiation therapy can also cause side effects by damaging normal, healthy cells near the treatment site.[19] Nutrition and pharmacologic intervention can help prevent significant malnutrition and loss of muscle mass caused by treatment side effects. Studies suggest that nutrition intervention during cancer treatment is associated with fewer treatment-related side effects,[22-25] fewer hospitalizations,[24-26] and improved quality of life.[22,23,27] The role of nutrition interventions during site-specific cancer treatment is discussed in further detail in Chapters 13 through 25.

The Role of Posttreatment Nutrition

Nutrition remains a fundamental component of recovery after cancer treatment. Individuals who have completed cancer treatment might experience treatment-related late effects, such as changes in body composition, bone density, or cardiovascular complications. Cancer recurrence or second primary cancers also can be a concern. Healthy dietary choices are an important part of an overall strategy to prevent or manage these conditions. See Chapter 8 for further discussion of the role of nutrition after cancer treatment.

Summary

As shown in Box 1.4 on pages 8 and 9, nutrition plays a significant role across the cancer continuum. A healthy diet and lifestyle can help decrease the risk of cancer development and can improve cancer outcomes. More research is needed to gain a clearer understanding of the specific role nutrition plays in cancer biology, treatment regimens, and management of treatment side effects.

Box 1.4
Potential Nutrition-Related Concerns and Outcomes Across the Cancer Continuum

Stage in continuum	Cancer prevention	Diagnosis Initial treatment
Potential nutrition concerns	▪ Obesity, loss of muscle mass ▪ Energy-dense food intake ▪ Excessive micronutrient intake from dietary supplements ▪ Food contaminants (toxins, chemicals)	▪ Treatment side effects (eg, nausea, vomiting, diarrhea, mucositis, taste changes) ▪ Fatigue ▪ Pain ▪ Anorexia ▪ Treatment-related cachexia ▪ Immunosuppression ▪ Weight or body-composition changes ▪ Drug-nutrition interactions
Potential outcomes of nutrition interventions	▪ Improved weight and body composition ▪ Improved blood glucose control ▪ Improved immune surveillance	▪ Ability to adhere to scheduled treatment ▪ Fewer infectious complications ▪ Improved weight and body composition ▪ Delay or prevention of disease progression ▪ Improved chances of survival ▪ Improved quality of life

Adapted from Robien K, Demark-Wahnefried W, Rock CL. Evidence-based nutrition guidelines for cancer survivors: current guidelines, knowledge gaps, and future research directions. *J Am Diet Assoc*. 2011;111(3):368-375. See reference 28.

Early posttreatment	Long-term cancer survivorship
■ Fatigue	■ Weight loss or gain
■ Pain	■ Decreased bone density
■ Endocrine disorders	■ Endocrine disorders
■ Weight or body-composition changes	■ Cardiovascular complications
■ Cognitive deficits	■ Cognitive deficits
■ Dental caries or complications	■ Dental caries or complications
■ Decreased fatigue	■ Fewer late effects of treatment
■ Improved functional status	■ Improved functional status
■ More rapid recovery from treatment	■ Improved weight and body composition
■ Improved weight and body composition	■ Decreased risk of cancer recurrence and subsequent primary cancers
■ Decreased risk for cancer recurrence and subsequent primary cancers	■ Improved chances of survival
■ Improved chances of survival	■ Improved quality of life
■ Improved quality of life	■ Decreased health care costs

References

1. What is cancer? National Cancer Institute website. September 2020. Accessed January 5, 2021. www.cancer.gov/about-cancer/understanding/what-is-cancer

2. American Cancer Society. *Cancer Facts & Figures 2020*. American Cancer Society; 2020. Accessed January 5, 2021. www.cancer.org/research/cancer-facts-statistics/all-cancer-facts-figures/cancer-facts-figures-2020.html

3. Noone AM, Howlader N, Krapcho M, et al, eds. SEER cancer statistics review, 1975–2015, National Cancer Institute. Surveillance, Epidemiology, and End Results Program website. Posted April 2018. Accessed June 8, 2020. https://seer.cancer.gov/csr/1975_2015

4. National Cancer Institute. Cancer Prevalence and Cost of Care Projections website. Accessed June 8, 2020. https://costprojections.cancer.gov

5. Mariotto AB, Yabroff KR, Shao Y, Feuer EJ, Brown ML. Projections of the cost of cancer care in the United States: 2010–2020. *J Natl Cancer Inst*. 2011;103(2):117-128. doi:10.1093/jnci/djq495

6. Yabroff KR, Lamont EB, Mariotto A, et al. Cost of care for elderly cancer patients in the United States. *J Natl Cancer Inst*. 2008;100(9):630-641.

7. American Cancer Society Guidelines for the Early Detection of Cancer. American Cancer Society website. May 2018. Accessed June 8, 2020. www.cancer.org/healthy/find-cancer-early/cancer-screening-guidelines/american-cancer-society-guidelines-for-the-early-detection-of-cancer.html

8. Sobin LH, Wittekind C, International Union Against Cancer. *TNM: Classification of Malignant Tumors*. 6th ed. Wiley-Liss; 2002.

9. American Joint Committee on Cancer. *AJCC Cancer Staging Manual*. 8th ed. Springer; 2016.

10. World Cancer Research Fund/American Institute for Cancer Research. The cancer process. In: *Diet, Nutrition, Physical Activity and Cancer: A Global Perspective*. Continuous Update Project Expert Report 2018. Accessed January 12, 2020. www.wcrf.org/dietandcancer/cancer-process

11. World Cancer Research Fund/American Institute for Cancer Research. *Diet, Nutrition, Physical Activity and Cancer: A Global Perspective*. Continuous Update Project Expert Report 2018. Accessed April 30, 2020. www.wcrf.org/dietandcancer

12. Rock CL, Thomson C, Gansler T, et al. American Cancer Society guideline for diet and physical activity for cancer prevention. *CA A Cancer J Clin*. 2020;70:245-271. doi:10.3322/caac.21591

13. Willett WC. Balancing life-style and genomics research for disease prevention. *Science*. 2002;296(5568):695-698.

14. Demark-Wahnefried W, Schmitz KH, Alfano CM, et al. Weight management and physical activity throughout the cancer care continuum. *CA Cancer J Clin*. 2018;68(1):64-89.

15. Turesky RJ, Le Marchand L. Metabolism and biomarkers of heterocyclic aromatic amines in molecular epidemiology studies: lessons learned from aromatic amines. *Chem Res Toxicol*. 2011;24(8):1169-1214.

16. Turesky RJ. Formation and biochemistry of carcinogenic heterocyclic aromatic amines in cooked meats. *Toxicol Lett*. 2007;168(3):219-227.

17. De Ruyck K, De Boevre M, Huybrechts I, De Saeger S. Dietary mycotoxins, co-exposure, and carcinogenesis in humans: short review. *Mutat Res Rev Mutat Res*. 2015;766:32-41.

18. Shafei A, Ramzy MM, Hegazy AI, et al. The molecular mechanisms of action of the endocrine disrupting chemical bisphenol A in the development of cancer. *Gene*. 2018;647:235-243.

19. Treatments and side effects. American Cancer Society website. Accessed June 8, 2020. www.cancer.org/treatment/treatments-and-side-effects

20. Choi SW, Mason JB. Folate and carcinogenesis: an integrated scheme. *J Nutr.* 2000;130(2):129-132.

21. Robien K. Folate during antifolate chemotherapy: what we know . . . and do not know. *Nutr Clin Pract.* 2005;20(4):411-422.

22. Ravasco P, Monteiro-Grillo I, Vidal PM, Camilo ME. Dietary counseling improves patient outcomes: a prospective, randomized, controlled trial in colorectal cancer patients undergoing radiotherapy. *J Clin Oncol.* 2005;23(7):1431-1438.

23. Ravasco P, Monteiro-Grillo I, Marques Vidal P, Camilo ME. Impact of nutrition on outcome: a prospective randomized controlled trial in patients with head and neck cancer undergoing radiotherapy. *Head Neck.* 2005;27(8):659-668.

24. Odelli C, Burgess D, Bateman L, et al. Nutrition support improves patient outcomes, treatment tolerance and admission characteristics in oesophageal cancer. *Clin Oncol (R Coll Radiol).* 2005;17(8):639-645.

25. Paccagnella A, Morello M, Da Mosto MC, et al. Early nutritional intervention improves treatment tolerance and outcomes in head and neck cancer patients undergoing concurrent chemoradiotherapy. *Support Care Cancer.* 2010;18(7):837-845.

26. Hill A, Kiss N, Hodgson B, Crowe TC, Walsh AD. Associations between nutritional status, weight loss, radiotherapy treatment toxicity and treatment outcomes in gastrointestinal cancer patients. *Clin Nutr.* 2011;30(1):92-98.

27. Ollenschlager G, Thomas W, Konkol K, Diehl V, Roth E. Nutritional behaviour and quality of life during oncological polychemotherapy: results of a prospective study on the efficacy of oral nutrition therapy in patients with acute leukaemia. *Eur J Clin Invest.* 1992;22(8):546-553.

28. Robien K, Demark-Wahnefried W, Rock CL. Evidence-based nutrition guidelines for cancer survivors: current guidelines, knowledge gaps, and future research directions. *J Am Diet Assoc.* 2011;111(3):368-375.

Chapter 2
Nutrition and Cancer Prevention

Karen Collins, MS, RDN, CDN, FAND
Alice Bender, MS, RDN

A substantial proportion of cancer cases in the United States are preventable. An estimated 40% of cases could be prevented through healthful dietary patterns, regular physical activity, maintaining a healthy weight (low body mass index and low adiposity), avoiding tobacco and excess sun exposure, and getting certain vaccines and regular screenings.[1]

In 2018, the World Cancer Research Fund (WCRF) and the American Institute for Cancer Research (AICR) jointly established recommendations for cancer prevention based on a structured and systematic approach of analyses and review of the literature on food, nutrition, physical activity, and cancer by an expert panel. These recommendations and the science behind them are outlined in this chapter.[2] The chapter also includes a section on emerging food and nutrition topics of special interest. These topics are being actively studied, but currently there is limited or inconsistent evidence regarding the effects of the various foods and practices on cancer risk.

Recommendations for Cancer Prevention

The 2018 World Cancer Research Fund and American Institute for Cancer Research (WCRF/AICR) cancer prevention recommendations are aimed at the overall prevention of cancer and are compatible with the *2020–2025 Dietary Guidelines for Americans*, which focus on promoting overall health, reducing the prevalence of overweight and obesity, and preventing diet-related chronic diseases.[3] They also align with the American Cancer Society (ACS) guidelines on nutrition and physical activity for cancer prevention.[4] Box 2.1 on pages 14 and 15 summarizes the WCRF/AICR recommendations for cancer prevention. Appendix A compares cancer prevention diet and lifestyle recommendations from various organizations. Each section that follows addresses a WCRF/AICR recommendation and describes the link to specific cancers, the proposed mechanisms, and key practice points.

Adiposity and Weight Gain

Maintaining a healthy body weight throughout life may be the most important lifestyle factor in reducing cancer risk, second only to not using tobacco products.[5] There is convincing evidence that a greater degree of body fatness—or greater adiposity—is a cause of cancers of the esophagus (adenocarcinoma), pancreas, colorectum, breast (postmenopausal), endometrium, liver, and kidney. Greater body fatness is probably also a cause of cancers of the stomach (cardia), gallbladder, ovaries, and mouth, pharynx, and larynx; and it has also been implicated in advanced prostate cancers.[2]

Excess body fatness could influence cancer risk through several possible mechanisms:

- Excess body fat is associated with insulin resistance, resulting in elevated levels of insulin and increased bioavailable insulin-like growth factor 1 (IGF-1).[2,6] Insulin and IGF-1 can activate signaling pathways that promote growth and proliferation of cancer cells and inhibit apoptosis (programmed cell death).[7-9]

- Overweight and obesity can lead to chronic low-grade systemic inflammation, which can

Box 2.1
World Cancer Research Fund/American Institute for Cancer Research Cancer Prevention Recommendations[2]

Recommendation	Goal
Be a healthy weight. *Keep your weight within the healthy range and avoid weight gain in adult life.*	Ensure that body weight during childhood and adolescence projects toward the lower end of the healthy adult body mass index (BMI) range. Keep weight as low as possible within the healthy range (BMI of 18.5-24.9) throughout life. A slightly higher range is recommended for adults over 65 (BMI 25-27). Avoid weight gain (measured as body weight or waist circumference) throughout adulthood.
Be physically active. *Be physically active as part of everyday life—walk more and sit less.*	Be at least moderately physically active, and follow or exceed national guidelines. Limit sedentary habits.
Eat a diet rich in whole grains, vegetables, fruit, and beans. *Make whole grains, vegetables, fruit, and pulses (legumes), such as beans and lentils, a major part of your usual daily diet.*	Consume a diet that provides at least 30 g/d of fiber from food sources. Include in most meals foods containing whole grains, nonstarchy vegetables, fruit, and pulses (legumes), such as beans and lentils. Eat a diet high in all types of plant foods, including at least five portions or servings of a variety of nonstarchy vegetables and fruit every day. If you eat starchy roots and tubers as staple foods, eat nonstarchy vegetables, fruit, and pulses (legumes) regularly too, if possible.
Limit consumption of fast foods and other processed foods high in fat, starches, or sugars. *Limiting these foods helps control energy intake and maintain a healthy weight.*	Limit consumption of processed foods high in fat, starches, or sugars—including fast foods, many prepared dishes, snacks, bakery foods, and desserts; and confectionery (candy).
Limit consumption of red and processed meat. *Eat no more than moderate amounts of red meat, such as beef, pork, and lamb. Eat little, if any, processed meat.*	If red meat is consumed, limit consumption to no more than about three portions per week. Three portions are equivalent to about 350 to 500 grams (about 12 to 18 ounces) cooked weight of red meat. Consume very little, if any, processed meat.
Limit consumption of sugar-sweetened drinks. *Drink mostly water and unsweetened drinks.*	Do not consume sugar-sweetened drinks.
Limit alcohol consumption. *For cancer prevention, it's best not to drink alcohol.*	For cancer prevention, do not consume alcohol.

(continued)

Box 2.1
World Cancer Research Fund/American Institute for Cancer Research Cancer
Prevention Recommendations[2] *(continued)*

Recommendation	Goal
Do not use supplements for cancer prevention. *Aim to meet nutrition needs through diet alone.*	High-dose dietary supplements are not recommended for cancer prevention—aim to meet nutrition needs through diet alone.
For mothers: breastfeed your baby, if you can. *Breastfeeding is good for both mother and baby.*	This recommendation aligns with the advice of the World Health Organization, which recommends infants are exclusively breastfed for 6 months, and then up to 2 years of age or beyond alongside appropriate complementary foods.
After a cancer diagnosis: follow our recommendations, if you can. *Follow American Institute for Cancer/World Health Organization recommendations. Check with your health professional to learn what is right for you.*	All cancer survivors should receive nutritional care and guidance on physical activity from trained professionals. Unless otherwise advised, all cancer survivors are advised to follow the Cancer Prevention Recommendations as far as possible after the acute stage of treatment.

promote heightened local inflammation and cancer development. Inflammation-induced elevations in free radicals promote oxidative stress that can damage DNA.[2] White adipose cells engorged with stored fat secrete cytokines (signaling proteins) that stimulate growth and metastasis of cancer cells.[2,8,10]

■ Adipose tissue is the primary site of estrogen production in postmenopausal women. Obese women tend to have higher levels of bioavailable estrogen, which is associated with endometrial cancer and postmenopausal breast cancer.[2,8]

■ Increased levels of the hormone leptin are associated with obesity and appear to activate signaling that promotes cell proliferation and angiogenesis (the process of generating new blood vessels) while inhibiting apoptosis.[7] Leptin also induces the aromatase enzyme required for adipose estrogen production.[10]

■ Excess body fat is linked with decreased levels of adiponectin, which is a cancer-protective hormone that decreases insulin resistance and inflammation and promotes apoptosis.[2,8]

Other possible mechanisms include altered immune responses, obesity-linked changes in the gut microbiome, and various organ-specific effects.[2,11]

Evaluating Weight-Related Risk

Body mass index (BMI), although commonly used as a measure of excess body fatness, is imperfect for this purpose, especially in the elderly and certain other groups. See Box 2.2 on page 16 for key practice points for adiposity and weight gain. In addition to BMI, consider the following when evaluating weight-related risk of developing cancer:

■ Waist circumference is a measure of abdominal fatness, although it cannot differentiate subcutaneous versus the more metabolically active visceral fat stores, which are particularly linked to hyperinsulinemia and chronic low-grade inflammation. Increased waist circumference is associated with greater risk for cancers of the esophagus (adenocarcinoma), pancreas, colorectum, breast (postmenopausal), endometrium, kidney, and prostate

---

Box 2.2
Key Practice Points for Adiposity and Weight Gain[2,8,12-17]

Overweight and obesity in young adulthood (approximately age 18 to 30 years) probably reduces the risk of both premenopausal and postmenopausal breast cancer. However, having overweight or obesity later in life increases the risk of postmenopausal breast cancer, which is more common. Thus, any potential benefit of overweight and obesity is outweighed by the increased risk for postmenopausal breast cancer and for other chronic diseases.

For people already overweight or obese, even modest weight loss may reduce cancer risk. Data are limited, but current studies suggest that intentional weight loss is associated with clinically significant changes in biomarkers of cancer risk.

Adult weight gain and large waist size, even in those within the normal BMI range, are associated with unhealthy metabolic changes and increased risk for some cancers. For some people, an appropriate goal may be to stop a trend of weight gain.

Research is in progress on the potential for cancer-risk reduction through addressing obesity-related metabolic abnormalities using dietary strategies such as macronutrient proportions and intermittent fasting or energy restriction. Emerging evidence shows potential benefit but is not currently consistent or sufficient to support recommendations.

(advanced). Waist circumference should be no larger than 37 inches (94 cm) in men, and 31.5 inches (80 cm) in women; these circumferences are associated with lower BMIs than the respective targets of 40 inches (101.6 cm) and 35 inches (89 cm) commonly referenced in the United States.[2]

■ Based on differences in obesity-related biomarkers of risk, waist circumference thresholds are lower for people of Asian ethnicity.[2,18] Research is in progress on other ethnicity-related differences in body composition and fat distribution that might support additional ethnicity-specific thresholds for adiposity-related risk.

■ Regardless of how it is measured, adult weight gain may better reflect excess body fat than weight itself, and may be a valuable target. Adult weight gain is particularly linked with risk of postmenopausal breast cancer.[2]

Physical Activity

All forms of regular physical activity, including recreational and occupational, protect against cancers of the colon, breast (postmenopausal), and endometrium. Vigorous activity protects again premenopausal breast cancer.[2] Physical activity may also reduce the risk of developing other cancers indirectly by protecting against weight gain, overweight, and obesity. Box 2.3 contains key practice points for physical activity.

Recommendations for adults are to get at least 150 minutes of moderate activity or 75 minutes of vigorous activity each week.[2,4] As fitness improves, and for greater protection, this should be increased to 45 to 60 minutes of moderate or 30 minutes or more of vigorous physical activity every day. Children and adolescents should engage in at least 60 minutes of moderate to vigorous physical activity daily.[2,19]

An emerging body of research points to sedentary behavior, including sitting and television viewing, as a risk factor for cancer independent of physical activity. Mechanisms under investigation include effects on waist size, insulin levels, and inflammation.[20,21] Recommendations are to limit sedentary behavior, such as sitting, lying down, and watching television.[2,4]

Mechanisms through which physical activity can positively influence cancer risk include[2,19,20]:

- reduced weight gain and easier maintenance of a healthy level of body fat;

- improved insulin sensitivity and reduced insulin levels;

- decreased levels of bioavailable sex steroid hormones;

- more rapid gut transit time, which reduces colon cells' exposure to carcinogens; and

- improved immune function.

Research is needed to examine the potential for identifying critical life-course periods when physical activity is most beneficial or when sedentary behavior particularly affects cancer risk.

A Predominantly Plant-Based Diet

Whole grains, vegetables, fruits, and pulses (legumes) are consistent features of diets associated with a lower risk of cancer. Evidence for the association of the consumption of nonstarchy vegetables and fruits with reduced cancer risk is currently limited, but the WCRF/AICR expert panel concluded that a pattern of protective association is consistent. Nonstarchy vegetables and fruits probably protect against cancers of the mouth, pharynx, larynx, and esophagus. Limited evidence suggests that nonstarchy vegetables and fruits may also reduce the risk for cancers of the lung (in people

Box 2.3
Key Practice Points for Physical Activity

Physical activity, along with appropriate calorie reduction, plays a key role in weight and body-fat reduction and in maintaining intentional weight loss.

Increasing physical activity provides protective benefits against cancer regardless of body weight.

Emphasizing these and the numerous other health benefits of physical activity to patients can help them set appropriate goals and expectations.

Patients should be encouraged to take regular breaks from long periods of sitting, such as while working at a computer or watching television, to reduce sedentary time.

who smoke or used to smoke tobacco), breast (estrogen-receptor-negative type), and bladder. Limited evidence links a low intake of nonstarchy vegetables and fruits with increased risk of colorectal and stomach cancers. Foods that provide dietary fiber—and whole grains specifically—probably protect against colorectal cancer.[2]

Plant foods are rich in phytochemicals, vitamins, and minerals that, as part of the whole food, may protect against cancer in several ways. Limited evidence links foods that provide β-carotene and other carotenoids, vitamin C, and isoflavones with reduced risk of lung, breast, and colorectal cancers.[2]

Many nutrients and phytochemicals show an ability to inhibit phase I carcinogen-activating enzymes (such as cytochrome P-450) and promote activity of phase II carcinogen-detoxifying enzymes (such as glutathione S-transferase) in laboratory studies. In cell and animal studies, nutrients and phytochemicals found in plant foods show effects on cell cycle regulation, processes of angiogenesis, apoptosis, DNA repair, and inflammation.[2] These effects may be accomplished through several mechanisms:

- Epigenetic effects are changes in gene expression that occur without changing the genetic sequence itself. Laboratory studies have found that constituents in plant foods and their metabolites—including isothiocyanates and indole-3-carbinol formed from glucosinolates in cruciferous vegetables, allyl sulfides from vegetables in the garlic and onion family, genistein from soybeans and other legumes, folate from dark green vegetables, and stilbenes (eg, resveratrol from grapes and berries) can change histone acetylation, DNA methylation, and microRNAs that directly and indirectly regulate cancer progression. These epigenetic changes, in essence, may either silence or promote the expression of genes, such as tumor suppressor genes.[22-25]

- Consumption of plant foods may also affect hormones influential in the cancer process. For example, viscous dietary fiber slows glucose absorption, reducing insulin secretion and hyperinsulinemia that promotes cell proliferation, and may decrease circulating levels of estrogen due to decreased reabsorption from the digestive tract.[26,27]

- Vitamins and phytochemicals support antioxidant defenses that quench DNA-damaging free radicals. Some carotenoids and vitamins C and E may provide direct antioxidant protection. Other phytochemicals, such as flavonoids and other polyphenols and allyl sulfur compounds, appear to stimulate endogenous antioxidant systems. Carotenoids show potential to alter cell signaling to inhibit cancer cell growth and promote apoptosis.[2,28]

- The intestinal microbiota act on fermentable fiber and resistant starch to produce butyrate, a short-chain fatty acid that promotes normal

Box 2.4
Key Practice Points for a Predominately Plant-Based Diet[2,4,33-39]

Consumption of five or more standard servings of nonstarchy vegetables and fruits daily (a total of 2½ cups, though more when this includes raw leafy greens) meets recommendations for reducing cancer risk and has also been linked with cardiovascular health benefits.

Targeting a daily total of at least 30 g of dietary fiber from food sources is recommended in the WCRF/AICR report.

A high dietary glycemic load is linked to greater risk of endometrial cancer, probably due to effects on postprandial glucose and insulin levels. The actual glycemic effects of a food vary with how it is prepared and other foods consumed at the same time, and individual responses vary. Eating patterns focused on minimally processed plant foods with appropriate portion sizes tend to be lower in glycemic load than a typical Western diet.

Selecting a variety of vegetables and fruits provides a broad spectrum of protective compounds, which can act protectively through additive and perhaps synergistic effects. Starchy roots and tubers fit into a healthful diet if nonstarchy vegetables, fruits, and pulses are eaten regularly too.

The cancer-protective effect of whole grains likely extends beyond dietary fiber to differences in nutrient and phytochemical content. Although the fiber content of whole grains and refined grains with added fiber may be comparable, it is unlikely that their benefits are equivalent.

Legumes have not been strongly tied to direct associations with reduced cancer risk; however, they offer valuable nutrients and several forms of potential protective benefits. They provide high levels of viscous, fermentable, and insoluble types of dietary fiber that may reduce insulin resistance and support satiety and a healthy gut microbiome. They also provide a low-cost protein source that can help overcome the costs of a healthful diet.

colon cell development and may reduce inflammation. The microbiota also convert some phytochemicals to bioavailable, active forms.[23,29-32]

Growing evidence suggests that a predominantly plant-based dietary pattern, which can be implemented in a variety of ways, may provide greater protective effects against cancer than consumption of any particular nutrients, compounds, or individual foods.[2,33] See Box 2.4 for key practice points for a plant-based diet.

Foods That Promote Weight Gain

Research indicates that processed foods high in added sugars, fat, and refined grains promote weight gain, overweight, and obesity when consumed frequently or in large portions.[2,40,41] Limiting these choices supports a healthy body weight an, in doing so, helps protect against cancer. These foods provide concentrated energy (often in portions or forms that do not induce satiety) and negatively influence metabolic risk and tendency toward abdominal adiposity.[33,42] Evidence does not support avoidance of all high-fat foods for weight control or lower cancer risk, however.[2,33,42]

Steps for promoting weight management include reducing the frequency and portion of traditional "fast foods" and other processed foods high in fat, added sugars, and refined grains, and replacing them with vegetables, fruits, and relatively unprocessed grains.[33,42,43] These changes tend to enhance overall diet quality, which is associated with less weight gain.[44] See Box 2.5 for key practice points for promoting weight gain.

Red and Processed Meats

The WCRF/AICR recommendations for cancer prevention include limiting consumption of red meat (beef, lamb, and pork) and avoiding

consumption of processed meats. People who eat red meat should consume no more than 12 to 18 oz/wk and very little, if any, processed meat.[2]

The term *processed meat* refers to meat (usually, but not exclusively, red meat) that is preserved by smoking, curing, fermenting, or salting, or by the addition of chemical preservatives. Processed meats include ham, bacon, hot dogs, pastrami, salami, and other sausages prepared by these methods. There is strong evidence that red meat and processed meat are causes of colorectal cancer. The risk of developing colorectal cancer increases by an estimated 12% for every 100 g of red meat consumed daily, and by 16% for every 50 g of processed meat consumed daily.[2]

There are several plausible mechanisms that explain the association between consumption of red meat or processed meat and colorectal cancer:

■ Red meat contains heme iron, which can lead to the production of free radicals, resulting in oxidative damage to DNA, protein, and cell membranes. Heme iron promotes the formation of carcinogenic *N*-nitroso compounds (NOCs) within the gut.[2,4,48]

- NOCs also form when nitrites used to preserve meat combine with amines from amino acids; they can be created during the meat-curing process as well as in the digestive tract.[2,4,48]

- Cooking meat at high temperatures or over open flames causes production of heterocyclic amines and polycyclic aromatic hydrocarbons, both of which are carcinogenic in animals.[2,4,48]

- Emerging evidence suggests that the gut microbiota may convert protein residues and fat-stimulated bile acids from diets high in meat to substances that are carcinogenic or proinflammatory or both.[31,49]

Vegan and other vegetarian diets have been associated with reduced incidence of cancer in many studies.[50] Although observational studies adjust for known risk factors and lifestyle choices, vegetarians may differ from meat eaters in unknown and unmeasured ways that could influence cancer risk. Also, various vegetarian eating patterns may differ

---

Box 2.6
Key Practice Points for Red and Processed Meats

Because red meat provides heme iron, which seems to underlie its association with cancer risk, the message to limit consumption is distinct from messages aimed at lowering blood lipid levels, which focus on the fat content of meat to define its healthfulness.

Processed meat is produced by a variety of methods, yet because studies often classify all processed meats together, it is not clear whether some pose more risk than others, or whether antioxidant or other additives or changes in smoking, curing, or other procedures might lead to a type of processed meat that poses a lower risk for cancer. That is why, for now, it is recommended that consumption of all forms of processed meat be minimized.

---

in their overall effect on cancer risk. Thus a predominantly, but not exclusively, plant-based diet might provide similar reductions in cancer risk. Box 2.6 contains key practice points for red and processed meats.

Other Animal Foods

Not all animal foods are associated with cancer. Limited evidence links fish consumption with lower risk of liver and colorectal cancer, but the WCRF/AICR expert panel concluded that this evidence was not strong enough to support a specific recommendation. There is a lack of conclusive evidence that poultry and eggs are associated with either an increase or decrease in cancer risk. Available evidence on milk, cheese, and other dairy products is difficult to interpret due to contradictions regarding colorectal cancer (decreased risk) and prostate cancer (limited evidence for increased risk). Limited evidence suggests that dairy products are associated with reduced risk of premenopausal breast cancer, and diets high in calcium with reduced risk of both premenopausal and postmenopausal breast cancer. Evidence for dairy and ovarian cancer risk was judged to be too limited for any conclusion. The WCRF/AICR report does not include a recommendation regarding dairy products.[2]

Sugar-Sweetened Beverages

Drinking sugar-sweetened beverages is a cause of weight gain as well as overweight and obesity in both children and adults.[2,51] These beverages include sugar-sweetened soft drinks, tea, and coffee; energy drinks; and juice drinks. These beverages provide energy but may not provide satiety in the same way food does, leading to excess energy intake and weight gain, indirectly increasing risk for at least 12 types of cancer.[52] Research supports limiting

> *Box 2.7*
> ### Key Practice Points for Sugar-Sweetened Beverages[2,3,33,53]
>
> It is best to drink water and other unsweetened drinks, such as unsweetened tea or coffee.
>
> Fruit juice (100%) can add nutritional value to a diet, but most people should limit their intake to one serving a day. Fruit juice is likely to promote weight gain in a similar way to sugar-sweetened drinks.
>
> For patients and clients who consume large amounts of sugar-sweetened drinks, encourage gradual reduction and replacement with noncaloric beverages.
>
> Alternatives to sugar-sweetened beverages include many flavored waters without added sweeteners on the market, or tap or bottled water with herbs, fruit, or small amounts of juice added.
>
> Data on artificially sweetened drinks were assessed as being too few, too inconsistent, and too low-quality to reach conclusions on how these beverages may be linked to weight gain, overweight, obesity, and other health and disease outcomes in a published analysis and for inclusion in recent recommendations. Because the research findings are mixed, decisions about the use of artificially sweetened drinks are best made on an individual basis.

sugar-sweetened beverages to reduce energy intake and promote weight loss. key practice points for sugar-sweetened beverages are covered in Box 2.7.

Alcoholic Beverages

WCRF/AICR and ACS recommend limiting alcohol consumption. For cancer prevention, it is best to not drink alcohol. For those who do drink, amounts should be limited to no more than one standard drink daily for women and no more than two standard drinks daily for men. A standard drink is defined as 14 g of ethanol, which is the equivalent of 5 oz of wine, 12 oz of beer, or 1½ oz of liquor.[33]

There is strong evidence that drinking alcohol is a cause of cancers of the mouth, pharynx, larynx, esophagus (squamous cell carcinoma), liver, stomach, colorectum, and breast (both premenopausal and postmenopausal). The effect of alcoholic drinks is from ethanol, regardless of the type of drink. The extent to which alcohol increases cancer risk depends on the amount of alcohol consumed and the type of cancer.[2]

Alcohol increases cancer risk through several mechanisms[2,54]:

- Ethanol in alcoholic beverages is classified as a human carcinogen, and when it is metabolized, it forms acetaldehyde, another human carcinogen.

- Ethanol acts as a solvent, enhancing penetration of dietary carcinogens into cells.

- Alcohol metabolism generates reactive oxygen species that can damage DNA.

- Alcohol acts synergistically with tobacco, acting as a solvent for its carcinogens, multiplying the risk of mouth and throat cancers for people exposed to both substances.

- Alcohol may increase circulating levels of estrogen, which is an established risk factor for breast cancer.

Emerging research suggests that total lifetime alcohol intake, including during adolescence, affects breast cancer risk later in life.[55] Box 2.8 on page 22 contains key practice points for alcoholic beverages.

Dietary Supplements

Evidence indicates that dietary supplements can be protective against cancer or can cause cancer. The WCRF/AICR expert panel concluded that the overall body of evidence does not support the use of dietary supplements as an effective strategy for reducing cancer risk.[2] However, dietary

Box 2.8
Key Practice Points for Alcoholic Beverages[2,54,55-58]

A modest increase in breast cancer risk for women occurs even with intakes of the recommended maximum of one standard drink per day.

Although some studies indicate that small or moderate amounts of alcohol, particularly red wine, may protect against coronary heart disease, these studies involve multiple confounding factors, and alcohol consumption is not recommended as a heart-health strategy.

Resveratrol is a phytochemical found in red wine that laboratory studies link with anticarcinogenic effects. However, research in humans does not support red wine as different from other alcoholic beverages in relationship to cancer risk.

supplements may at times be beneficial for specific population groups, mainly for reasons not related to cancer.

Calcium supplements at a dose above 200 mg/d probably protect against colorectal cancer.[2] Limited evidence suggests that diets high in calcium (including supplements and food) increase risk for prostate cancer.[2] There is no strong evidence at this time that other dietary supplements protect against cancer.

Dietary supplements associated with increased risk for cancer include high-dose β-carotene and vitamin E. Based on results of six randomized controlled trials, smokers who take high-dose β-carotene supplements are at increased risk for lung cancer.[2,59,60]

Although limited evidence links low plasma levels of α-tocopherol with greater risk of prostate cancer, results of the Selenium and Vitamin E Cancer Prevention Trial (SELECT) suggest that high-dose vitamin E supplements may promote a modest increase in risk.[61,62] Current evidence is too

limited to support recommendations on vitamin E supplements.[2,63]

Limited evidence suggests that men with low body levels of selenium may have increased risk of prostate cancer. However, prostate cancer risk was not reduced by selenium supplements in the SELECT study,[62,64] and current evidence is too limited to support recommendations about supplementation.[2]

Vitamin D may act throughout the cancer process to reduce cancer risk,[65] and evidence is limited—but suggestive—that vitamin D, including from the diet and from supplements, may reduce risk for colorectal cancer.[2] Benefits of supplementation are not clear, however. For example, a large randomized controlled trial, the VITamin D and omegA-3 TriaL (VITAL), found no difference in incidence of invasive cancer overall or several specific cancers among the study groups.[66] Some observational studies suggest a benefit of higher blood levels of vitamin D, but results are inconsistent, especially regarding target blood levels and the level of intake that different people need

Box 2.9
Key Practice Points for Dietary Supplements[2,71,72]

Obtaining nutrients and other compounds from food rather than from dietary supplements provides the potential for beneficial and synergistic effects against carcinogenesis.

Research has shown that while supplementation with a particular nutrient in people with a low dietary intake or low body levels of that nutrient may be beneficial, supplements may have no effect or even be harmful in people who already have adequate amounts of that nutrient or if the nutrient is given to achieve super-physiologic levels. This stands in contrast to the common belief among the public regarding antioxidants and nutrients that if some is good, more is better.

to reach any given target.[67-70] See Box 2.9 for key practice points for dietary supplements.

As research moves forward, understanding the role of supplements as they relate to cancer risk and to overall optimal health requires addressing multiple factors. These include the effects of differences in dietary intake of particular supplements, other lifestyle factors, and environmental factors. In addition, genetic polymorphisms that affect nutrient metabolism need to be better understood, as does the dose, duration of exposure, and impact of timing of supplementation in the life cycle and within the stage of cancer development.

Lactation and Breastfeeding

There is strong evidence that lactation reduces a mother's risk of both premenopausal and postmenopausal breast cancer.[2] It is also well established that breastfeeding offers immune and other health benefits to babies. Infants who are breastfed gain protection against excess weight gain, overweight,

Box 2.10
Key Practice Points for Lactation and Breastfeeding

Exclusive breastfeeding for the first 6 months means giving babies no other nourishment, including water, except for vitamin drops when needed. After that, solid foods and other liquids are to be added at age-appropriate times.

The Centers for Disease Control and Prevention (CDC) collects data and promotes best practices in health care settings to support breastfeeding in the United States. To learn more about resources for your community and hospital or health care setting, visit the breastfeeding section of CDC website (www.cdc.gov/breastfeeding).

and obesity.[73] Excess body fatness during childhood tends to track into adulthood.[2]

In general, the longer women breastfeed their babies, the greater their protection against cancer. Mechanisms by which lactation may protect against breast cancer include[2]:

- During lactation, the associated period of amenorrhea reduces lifetime exposure to estrogen.

- Cells with potential DNA damage are eliminated through exfoliation of breast tissue during lactation and through a major apoptosis of epithelial cells at the end of lactation.

Box 2.10 includes key practice points for lactation and breastfeeding.

Cancer Survivors

WCRF/AICR defines the term *cancer survivor* as people who have been diagnosed with cancer, including those who have recovered, from the time of diagnosis onward. During cancer treatment and in cases in which the ability to consume or metabolize food has been altered by treatment, people may have special nutritional needs. Especially in these cases, survivors need nutritional counseling from an appropriately trained health professional. Registered dietitian nutritionists (RDNs) who are certified specialists in oncology nutrition (CSOs) have special expertise in oncology nutrition. Box 2.11 on page 24 covers key practice points for survivors of cancer.

Breast Cancer Survival

There is growing evidence that lifestyle, including physical activity and other steps to promote a healthy weight, may improve survival and other health outcomes after a breast cancer diagnosis. Although there is no strong evidence regarding diet, nutrition, physical activity, and breast cancer survival, WCRF/AICR found "limited but suggestive" evidence for factors affecting all-cause mortality.[2] Limited but suggestive means that the evidence indicates an effect but is not strong enough to make recommendations.

Evidence suggests that the following factors *reduce* the chance of dying early after a breast cancer diagnosis:

- being physically active before and after diagnosis;

- eating a diet higher in foods containing fiber, both before and after diagnosis; and

- eating foods containing soy in the year after diagnosis and beyond (see Emerging Topics).

Limited evidence suggests that the following factors *increase* the risk of dying early:

- body fatness (before and after diagnosis) and

- eating a diet high in total or saturated fatty acids (before diagnosis).

WCRF/AICR advises that, if possible, and unless otherwise advised by a qualified professional,

Box 2.11
Key Practice Points for Cancer Survivors[74-76]

The following national organizations, among others, have developed guidelines for cancer survivors, and all three support general lifestyle messages of achieving and maintaining a healthy weight, engaging in regular physical activity, and creating a dietary pattern that is high in vegetables, fruits, and whole grains:

- American Cancer Society
- American College of Sports Medicine
- National Comprehensive Cancer Network

Chapter 8 provides additional detailed information regarding research into early posttreatment and longer-term survivorship treatment.

the recommendations for cancer prevention be followed by cancer survivors after the acute stage of treatment. As cancer survivors live increasingly longer, they are at risk of developing new primary cancers, as well as other chronic diseases, and are likely to benefit from this guidance.[2]

Emerging Topics
Organic Foods

Organic foods are produced using approved cultural, biological, and mechanical methods. Synthetic pesticides and fertilizers, sewage sludge, irradiation, and genetic engineering cannot be used in their production.

Health-related interest in organic foods often relates to two primary factors, pesticide residue and protective contributions.

Pesticide residue The amount of pesticide residue is generally lower in organic than in conventional foods.[77] Yet a 2016 report from the US Department of Agriculture (USDA) Pesticide Data Program noted that only 22% of samples of organically grown foods had no detectable pesticide residue, and 0.46% had residue levels above US Environmental Protection Agency tolerances, which include a safety margin.[77] Some people may be unaware that organic crops can be raised with pesticides that include natural ingredients, some of which also pose concerns for mutagenicity.

Potentially protective contributions Potential benefits from polyphenol compounds and vitamins may be greater from organic plant foods than from their corresponding conventionally grown counterparts, according to some research.[78] However, some reviews conclude that these differences are relatively small and have not been associated with any difference in health-related biomarkers, so they may not be relevant to health outcomes in the context of a healthful diet.[79,80]

Selecting Foods Based on Pesticide Levels

A popular methodology for creating lists of fruits and vegetables that are the most and least likely to contain elevated levels of pesticides based on USDA tests has been criticized by some as inaccurately characterizing consumption-related risk.[81,82] However, others contend that, based on updated science, regulatory limits for some pesticides should be lowered.[83] One analysis concluded that the most commonly detected pesticides on produce pose negligible risks to consumers, and switching to organic forms does not result in any appreciable reduction of consumer risks.[82]

Washing to Reduce Exposure to Pesticides

Both organic and conventionally grown produce should be washed in running water. Outer leaves of leafy vegetables, such as lettuce and cabbage, should be thrown away.[84]

The US Food and Drug Administration does not recommend washing fruits and vegetables with soap, detergent, or commercial produce wash.[85] Specialty produce washes are reportedly no more effective in removing pesticide residues than water alone. Dish soap and bleach should not be used on produce, which often has pores that allow residues of these products to be trapped or absorbed, and their safety has not been evaluated.[86]

Genetically Engineered Foods

There is currently no substantiated evidence that foods from genetically engineered crops (such as genetically modified organisms, or GMOs) are less safe or increase cancer risk compared to crops that are not genetically engineered.[87]

Anti-Inflammatory Foods

Inflammation is a hallmark of cancer cells, and biomarkers of inflammation are associated with greater cancer risk.[2,10,28,88] Many factors can lead to chronic, low-grade inflammation, and there are multiple dietary approaches that may reduce it.

Foods Containing Antioxidant Nutrients

Vitamins C and E and some carotenoids provide direct antioxidant activity to reduce the development of reactive oxygen species that lead to inflammation.

Foods Containing Phytochemicals With Antioxidant and Anti-Inflammatory Potential

Polyphenol compounds in tea, berries, onions, nuts, grapes, and spices (eg, turmeric and ginger) are often referred to as antioxidant or anti-inflammatory agents. In laboratory studies, these compounds activate endogenous antioxidant defenses and reduce inflammatory cell signaling pathways. However, in the human gut, these phytochemicals are metabolized into smaller, more bioavailable compounds; therefore, though cell studies using intact phytochemicals can show potential, they cannot establish benefit in humans. And animal studies need to be interpreted cautiously because digestion, absorption, and half-life of phytochemicals in animals may differ from that in humans.

Randomized controlled trials in humans generally use isolates and extracts of phytochemicals. This enables consistency of the intervention but does not represent effects on bioavailability or metabolism of the whole food.

Phytochemical effects are likely dose-related. Interpretation of laboratory studies and randomized controlled trials in humans with isolated compounds needs to consider whether people can realistically achieve optimal effective dose and serum levels through food choices.

Foods Supporting a Protective Microbiome

Gut bacteria may provide anti-inflammatory effects within the colon and perhaps with broader effects on cancer risk.[29,32,89] Foods with inulin, inulin-type fructans, and other carbohydrates with demonstrated prebiotic effects include pulses and allium vegetables. In addition, gut microbes use fermentable dietary fiber, resistant starch, and β-glucans (found especially in pulses and whole grains, such as oats and barley) to produce butyrate, a short-chain fatty acid that shows potential anti-inflammatory and tumor-suppressive properties.[31,32,90] Microbes in the colon also break down polyphenols from a variety of plant foods, forming compounds that may have anti-inflammatory effects.[32,49]

Foods Supplying Omega-3 Fatty Acids

Eicosapentaenoic acid (EPA) and docosahexaenoic acid (DHA) are used to produce anti-inflammatory eicosanoid compounds. Observational studies in healthy adults suggest potential for a diet rich in omega-3 fatty acids to prevent and reduce inflammation, but intervention studies have yielded inconsistent results.[2,91,92] Evidence is inconclusive regarding an association of inflammation and α-linolenic acid (ALA), an omega-3 fatty acid found in plant foods.

Overall Dietary Patterns for Reducing Inflammation

Eating patterns that provide an abundance of foods with anti-inflammatory potential and that limit consumption of red and processed meats, refined grains, and sugar-sweetened beverages are linked to lower biomarkers of inflammation[93-96] and cancer risk.[97-99]

Soy Foods

Isoflavones in soy foods are often studied in relation to cancer risk. However, many soy foods are also good sources of dietary fiber and selenium, and some are fortified with calcium. Research suggests that soy foods do not increase cancer risk, and in some cases may lower it. The role of soy in an overall cancer-protective diet needs more study, as do individual differences that may modify its effects.[100,101]

Phytoestrogens

The soy isoflavones genistein and daidzein are classified as phytoestrogens based on their chemical structure, and they can bind to estrogen receptors. In cell and animal studies, these compounds have slowed the growth of cancer cells. Some early studies in rodents suggested that genistein increased the growth of estrogen-receptor-positive (ER+) breast cancer cells and promoted breast cancer growth. However, later research showed that rats and mice metabolize phytoestrogens (eg, genistein) differently than humans do.[102] The binding of soy isoflavones to β rather than α forms of estrogen receptors may be cancer-protective, but this needs further study.[103,104] Laboratory studies suggest that soy isoflavones may also provide protective antioxidant, antiangiogenesis, and epigenetic effects.[28]

Human Data on Soy Consumption

Observational studies in humans suggest that soy may protect against some forms of cancer. Soy consumption is associated with lower breast cancer risk in Asia, where throughout their lives, women consume moderate amounts of soy.[105] Protective effects of soy may stem from consumption in childhood and adolescence.[106]

Limited evidence suggests that foods containing isoflavones may lower risk of lung cancer in people who have never smoked.[2] Research in humans linking soy or total isoflavone consumption to lower risk of cancers of the prostate, stomach, and colon is too limited to support any recommendation.[2,107]

Breast Cancer Survivors and Soy

Analysis of observational studies in the WCRF/AICR report do not show any significant association of soy consumption with breast cancer–specific outcomes but found limited evidence that the consumption of soy foods a year or more after diagnosis may reduce the risk of all-cause mortality.[2] In a pooled analysis of breast cancer survivors in the United States and Asia, moderate soy food consumption was associated with decreased recurrence.[108] This was most significant in women with estrogen-receptor-negative (ER–) cancers, but there was no sign of increased risk among those with estrogen-receptor-positive (ER+) cancers. Further, these studies do not show any harmful interactions with tamoxifen, an antiestrogen medication. A link between lower breast-cancer mortality and higher soy consumption in another prospective study was especially significant among women with ER+ cancers.[109]

Dietary Soy Amounts

Moderate soy consumption is considered to be one to two standard servings daily of whole soy foods, such as tofu, soy milk, edamame, or soy nuts. (One serving averages about 7 g of protein and 25 mg of isoflavones.) Up to three servings a day of soy (up to 100 mg of isoflavones per day) have been consumed in Asian populations long-term without a link to increased breast cancer risk.[110] The health effects of consuming more than 100 mg of isoflavones daily and isoflavone supplements are not known.

Flaxseed

Most research on flaxseed has focused on lignans and ALA (the omega-3 fatty acid present in the seed), though flaxseed's high fiber content may also be pertinent. Evidence suggests that consuming 1 to 4 tablespoons of ground flaxseed daily appears to be safe and may contribute to a lower risk of breast or other cancers.[111,112] However, research is currently too limited to be conclusive or to support a recommendation.

Dietary lignans are converted by intestinal bacteria into enterolignans, which can be absorbed from the colon and circulated in the blood. The amount of these enterolignans produced and absorbed varies substantially from person to person. Human observational studies show mixed results regarding an association between lignan intake and overall breast cancer risk, though these studies generally do link higher lignan intake with reduced risk of postmenopausal breast cancer.[111] Studies may use serum or urinary levels of enterolactone (the main circulating enterolignan) as a biomarker of lignan consumption. Some meta-analyses of serum enterolignans and breast cancer risk show only nonsignificant trends, but one meta-analysis of 13 observational studies found that women with the highest serum enterolactone levels had a lower breast cancer risk than those with lowest levels.[111,113]

In some studies, lignan consumption seems to promote a shift in women's serum estrogen to a form less likely to promote cancer.[111] Some animal and human studies suggest that lignans may also decrease IGF-1 and other growth factors to decrease cell proliferation and the angiogenesis that enables tumors to grow.

The ALA present in flaxseed can be very slowly converted in the body to the long-chain omega-3 fatty acids EPA and DHA. This conversion is inefficient (up to 8% is converted to EPA and less than 1% to DHA), with some differences depending on sex, background diet, and genetics.[114,115] Research is inconsistent regarding the potential benefits of ALA independent of its conversion to EPA and DHA.

Flaxseed is high in viscous fiber, which can improve insulin sensitivity,[116] a mechanism that emerging data suggest could reduce the risk of some cancers.

Cancer Survivors and Flaxseed

Breast cancer survivors who want to use flaxseed on a regular basis should discuss it with their physicians. Only a few observational studies following breast cancer survivors for 6 to 10 years or longer are available, but they are relatively consistent in linking higher dietary or blood levels of lignans with fewer deaths.[111] In studies on animals, flaxseed did not interfere with the effectiveness of the breast cancer drug tamoxifen. Human clinical data are very limited but so far show no interference of flaxseed with tamoxifen. Limited data from human studies even suggest flaxseed's potential to enhance tamoxifen's effectiveness.[111] Studies in rodents show no interference of lignans with trastuzumab, a common treatment for HER2 receptor positive breast cancer.[111] More clinical studies are needed before recommendations can be made.

Limited cell and animal studies suggest flaxseed or enterolactone can inhibit the growth and metastasis of prostate cancer.[117,118] In very limited studies of men with prostate cancer, flaxseed has lowered tumor biomarkers or presurgery rates of cell proliferation.[112,119]

References

1. Islami F, Goding Sauer A, Miller KD, et al. Proportion and number of cancer cases and deaths attributable to potentially modifiable risk factors in the United States. *CA Cancer J Clin.* 2018;68(1):31-54.

2. World Cancer Research Fund/American Institute for Cancer Research. Diet, Nutrition, Physical Activity and Cancer: A Global Perspective. Continuous Update Project Expert Report 2018. Accessed January 9, 2020. www.wcrf.org/dietandcancer

3. US Department of Health and Human Services, US Department of Agriculture. *2020–2025 Dietary Guidelines for Americans.* 9th ed. US Department of Agriculture; 2020. Accessed January 6, 2021. https://dietaryguidelines.gov

4. Rock CL, Thomson C, Gansler T, et al. American Cancer Society guideline for diet and physical activity for cancer prevention. *CA A Cancer J Clin.* 2020;70: 245-271.

5. Ligibel JA, Alfano CM, Courneya KS, et al. American Society of Clinical Oncology position statement on obesity and cancer. *J Clin Oncol.* 2014;32(31):3568-3574.

6. Giovannucci E. A framework to understand diet, physical activity, body weight, and cancer risk. *Cancer Causes Control.* 2018;29(1):1-6.

7. Lashinger LM, Ford NA, Hursting SD. Interacting inflammatory and growth factor signals underlie the obesity-cancer link. *J Nutr.* 2014;144(2):109-113.

8. Smith LA, O'Flanagan CH, Bowers LW, Allott EH, Hursting SD. Translating mechanism-based strategies to break the obesity-cancer link: a narrative review. *J Acad Nutr Diet.* 2018;118(4): 652-667.

9. Klement RJ, Fink MK. Dietary and pharmacological modification of the insulin/IGF-1 system: exploiting the full repertoire against cancer. *Oncogenesis.* 2016;5:e193.

10. Iyengar NM, Gucalp A, Dannenberg AJ, Hudis CA. Obesity and cancer mechanisms: tumor microenvironment and inflammation. *J Clin Oncol.* 2016;34(35):4270-4276.

11. Gallagher EJ, LeRoith D. Obesity and diabetes: the increased risk of cancer and cancer-related mortality. *Physiol Rev.* 2015;95(3):727-748.

12. Harvie MN, Howell T. Could intermittent energy restriction and intermittent fasting reduce rates of cancer in obese, overweight, and normal-weight subjects? A summary of evidence. *Adv Nutr.* 2016;7(4):690-705.

13. Byers T, Sedjo RL. Does intentional weight loss reduce cancer risk? *Diabetes Obes Metab.* 2011;13(12):1063-1072.

14. van Gemert WA, Monninkhof EM, May AM, et al. Association between changes in fat distribution and biomarkers for breast cancer. *Endocr Relat Cancer.* 2017;24(6):297-305.

15. Fabian CJ, Kimler BF, Donnelly JE, et al. Favorable modulation of benign breast tissue and serum risk biomarkers is associated with >10 % weight loss in postmenopausal women. *Breast Cancer Res Treat.* 2013;142(1): 119-132.

16. Patterson RE, Marinac CR, Sears DD, et al. The effects of metformin and weight loss on biomarkers associated with breast cancer outcomes. *J Natl Cancer Inst.* 2018;110(11):1239-1247.

17. Oliveros E, Somers VK, Sochor O, Goel K, Lopez-Jimenez F. The concept of normal weight obesity. *Prog Cardiovasc Dis.* 2014;56(4):426-433.

18. Alberti KG, Eckel RH, Grundy SM, et al. Harmonizing the metabolic syndrome: a joint interim statement of the International Diabetes Federation Task Force on Epidemiology and Prevention; National Heart, Lung, and Blood Institute; American Heart Association; World Heart Federation; International Atherosclerosis Society; and International Association for the Study of Obesity. *Circulation.* 2009;120(16):1640-1645.

19. US Department of Health and Human Services. *Physical Activity Guidelines for Americans.* 2nd ed. US Department of Health and Human Services; 2018. Accessed January 10, 2020. https://health.gov/sites/default/files/2019-09/Physical_Activity_Guidelines_2nd_edition.pdf

20. Kerr J, Anderson C, Lippman SM. Physical activity, sedentary behaviour, diet, and cancer: an update and emerging new evidence. *Lancet Oncol.* 2017;18(8):e457-e471.

21. Schmid D, Leitzmann MF. Television viewing and time spent sedentary in relation to cancer risk: a meta-analysis. *J Natl Cancer Inst.* 2014;106(7). doi:10.1093/jnci/dju098

22. Gupta P, Kim B, Kim SH, Srivastava SK. Molecular targets of isothiocyanates in cancer: recent advances. *Mol Nutr Food Res.* 2014;58(8):1685-1707.

23. Paul B, Barnes S, Demark-Wahnefried W, et al. Influences of diet and the gut microbiome on epigenetic modulation in cancer and other diseases. *Clin Epigenetics.* 2015;7:112.

24. George VC, Dellaire G, Rupasinghe HPV. Plant flavonoids in cancer chemoprevention: role in genome stability. *J Nutr Biochem.* 2017;45:1-14.

25. Bishop KS, Ferguson LR. The interaction between epigenetics, nutrition and the development of cancer. *Nutrients.* 2015;7(2):922-947.

26. McRorie JW Jr, McKeown NM. Understanding the physics of functional fibers in the gastrointestinal tract: an evidence-based approach to resolving enduring misconceptions about insoluble and soluble fiber. *J Acad Nutr Diet.* 2017;117(2):251-264.

27. Aune D, Chan DS, Greenwood DC, et al. Dietary fiber and breast cancer risk: a systematic review and meta-analysis of prospective studies. *Ann Oncol.* 2012;23(6):1394-1402.

28. Li W, Guo Y, Zhang C, et al. Dietary phytochemicals and cancer chemoprevention: a perspective on oxidative stress, inflammation, and epigenetics. *Chem Res Toxicol.* 2016;29(12):2071-2095.

29. Bultman SJ. The microbiome and its potential as a cancer preventive intervention. *Semin Oncol.* 2016;43(1):97-106.

30. Slavin J. Fiber and prebiotics: mechanisms and health benefits. *Nutrients.* 2013;5(4):1417-1435.

31. O'Keefe SJ. Diet, microorganisms and their metabolites, and colon cancer. *Nat Rev Gastroenterol Hepatol.* 2016;13(12):691-706.

32. Sheflin AM, Melby CL, Carbonero F, Weir TL. Linking dietary patterns with gut microbial composition and function. *Gut Microbes.* 2017;8(2):113-129.

33. Dietary Guidelines Advisory Committee. *Scientific Report of the 2020 Dietary Guidelines Advisory Committee: Advisory Report to the Secretary of Agriculture and the Secretary of Health and Human Services.* US Department of Agriculture, Agricultural Research Service; 2020. Accessed January 6, 2021. www.dietaryguidelines.gov/2020-advisory-committee-report

34. Zeevi D, Korem T, Zmora N, et al. Personalized nutrition by prediction of glycemic responses. *Cell.* 2015;163(5):1079-1094.

35. Matthan NR, Ausman LM, Meng H, Tighiouart H, Lichtenstein AH. Estimating the reliability of glycemic index values and potential sources of methodological and biological variability. *Am J Clin Nutr.* 2016;104(4):1004-1013.

36. Meng H, Matthan NR, Ausman LM, Lichtenstein AH. Effect of macronutrients and fiber on postprandial glycemic responses and meal glycemic index and glycemic load value determinations. *Am J Clin Nutr.* 2017;105(4):842-853.

37. Jeurnink SM, Buchner FL, Bueno-de-Mesquita HB, et al. Variety in vegetable and fruit consumption and the risk of gastric and esophageal cancer in the European Prospective Investigation into Cancer and Nutrition. *Int J Cancer.* 2012;131(6):E963-973.

38. Liu RH. Health-promoting components of fruits and vegetables in the diet. *Adv Nutr.* 2013;4(3):384S-392S.

39. Rebello CJ, Greenway FL, Finley JW. Whole grains and pulses: a comparison of the nutritional and health benefits. *J Agric Food Chem.* 2014;62(29):7029-7049.

40. Perez-Escamilla R, Obbagy JE, Altman JM, et al. Dietary energy density and body weight in adults and children: a systematic review. *J Acad Nutr Diet.* 2012;112(5):671-684.

41. Rouhani MH, Haghighatdoost F, Surkan PJ, Azadbakht L. Associations between dietary energy density and obesity: a systematic review and meta-analysis of observational studies. *Nutrition.* 2016;32(10):1037-1047.

42. Mozaffarian D. Dietary and policy priorities for cardiovascular disease, diabetes, and obesity: a comprehensive review. *Circulation.* 2016;133(2):187-225.

43. Blatt AD, Roe LS, Rolls BJ. Hidden vegetables: an effective strategy to reduce energy intake and increase vegetable intake in adults. *Am J Clin Nutr.* 2011;93(4):756-763.

44. Fung TT, Pan A, Hou T, et al. Long-term change in diet quality is associated with body weight change in men and women. *J Nutr.* 2015;145(8):1850-1856.

45. Tan SY, Dhillon J, Mattes RD. A review of the effects of nuts on appetite, food intake, metabolism, and body weight. *Am J Clin Nutr.* 2014;100(suppl 1):412S-422S.

46. Saquib N, Natarajan L, Rock CL, et al. The impact of a long-term reduction in dietary energy density on body weight within a randomized diet trial. *Nutr Cancer.* 2008;60(1):31-38.

47. Stanton MV, Robinson JL, Kirkpatrick SM, et al. DIETFITS study (diet intervention examining the factors interacting with treatment success)—study design and methods. *Contemp Clin Trials.* 2017;53:151-161.

48. Hammerling U, Bergman Laurila J, Grafström R, Ilbäck N-G. Consumption of red/processed meat and colorectal carcinoma: possible mechanisms underlying the significant association. *Crit Rev Food Sci Nutr.* 2016;56(4):614-634.

49. Singh RK, Chang HW, Yan D, et al. Influence of diet on the gut microbiome and implications for human health. *J Transl Med.* 2017;15(1):73.

50. Melina V, Craig W, Levin S. Position of the Academy of Nutrition and Dietetics: vegetarian diets. *J Acad Nutr Diet.* 2016;116(12):1970-1980.

51. Luger M, Lafontan M, Bes-Rastrollo M, Winzer E, Yumuk V, Farpour-Lambert N. Sugar-sweetened beverages and weight gain in children and adults: a systematic review from 2013 to 2015 and a comparison with previous studies. *Obes Facts.* 2017;10(6):674-693.

52. Pan A, Hu FB. Effects of carbohydrates on satiety: differences between liquid and solid food. *Curr Opin Clin Nutr Metab Care.* 2011;14(4):385-390.

53. Lohner S, Toews I, Meerpohl JJ. Health outcomes of non-nutritive sweeteners: analysis of the research landscape. *Nutr J.* 2017;16(1):55.

54. International Agency for Research on Cancer. Consumption of alcoholic beverages. In *Personal Habits and Indoor Combustions: A Review of Human Carcinogens.* Vol 100E. International Agency for Research on Cancer; 2012.

55. Colditz GA, Bohlke K, Berkey CS. Breast cancer risk accumulation starts early: prevention must also. *Breast Cancer Res Treat.* 2014;145(3):567-579.

56. Shield KD, Soerjomataram I, Rehm J. Alcohol use and breast cancer: a critical review. *Alcohol Clin Exp Res.* 2016;40(6):1166-1181.

57. Allen NE, Beral V, Casabonne D, et al. Moderate alcohol intake and cancer incidence in women. *J Natl Cancer Inst.* 2009;101(5):296-305.

58. LoConte NK, Brewster AM, Kaur JS, Merrill JK, Alberg AJ. Alcohol and cancer: a statement of the American Society of Clinical Oncology. *J Clin Oncol.* 2018;36(1):83-93.

59. Omenn GS, Goodman GE, Thornquist MD, et al. Effects of a combination of beta carotene and vitamin A on lung cancer and cardiovascular disease. *N Engl J Med.* 1996;334(18):1150-1155.

60. Alpha-Tocopherol, Beta Carotene Cancer Prevention Study Group. The effect of vitamin E and beta carotene on the incidence of lung cancer and other cancers in male smokers. *N Engl J Med.* 1994;330(15):1029-1035.

61. Klein EA, Thompson IM Jr, Tangen CM, et al. Vitamin E and the risk of prostate cancer: the Selenium and Vitamin E Cancer Prevention Trial (SELECT). *JAMA.* 2011;306(14):1549-1556.

62. Kristal AR, Darke AK, Morris JS, et al. Baseline selenium status and effects of selenium and vitamin E supplementation on prostate cancer risk. *J Natl Cancer Inst.* 2014;106(3):djt456. doi:10.1093/jnci/djt456

63. Final recommendation statement: vitamin supplementation to prevent cancer and CVD: preventive medication. US Preventive Services Task Force website. September 2017. Accessed January 10, 2020. www.uspreventiveservicestask force.org/Page/Document /RecommendationStatementFinal /vitamin-supplementation -to-prevent-cancer-and-cvd -counseling

64. Lippman SM, Klein EA, Goodman PJ, et al. Effect of selenium and vitamin E on risk of prostate cancer and other cancers: the Selenium and Vitamin E Cancer Prevention Trial (SELECT). *JAMA.* 2009;301(1):39-51.

65. Feldman D, Krishnan AV, Swami S, Giovannucci E, Feldman BJ. The role of vitamin D in reducing cancer risk and progression. *Nat Rev Cancer.* 2014;14(5):342-357.

66. Manson JE, Cook NR, Lee I-M, et al. Vitamin D supplements and prevention of cancer and cardiovascular disease. *New Engl J Med.* 2019;380(1):33-44.

67. Gandini S, Boniol M, Haukka J, et al. Meta-analysis of observational studies of serum 25-hydroxyvitamin D levels and colorectal, breast and prostate cancer and colorectal adenoma. *Int J Cancer.* 2011;128(6):1414-1424.

68. Chung M, Lee J, Terasawa T, Lau J, Trikalinos TA. Vitamin D with or without calcium supplementation for prevention of cancer and fractures: an updated meta-analysis for the U.S. Preventive Services Task Force. *Ann Intern Med.* 2011;155(12):827-838.

69. Pilz S, Kienreich K, Tomaschitz A, et al. Vitamin D and cancer mortality: systematic review of prospective epidemiological studies. *Anticancer Agents Med Chem.* 2013;13(1):107-117.

70. Touvier M, Chan DS, Lau R, et al. Meta-analyses of vitamin D intake, 25-hydroxyvitamin D status, vitamin D receptor polymorphisms, and colorectal cancer risk. *Cancer Epidemiol Biomarkers Prev.* 2011;20(5):1003-1016.

71. Mayne ST, Playdon MC, Rock CL. Diet, nutrition, and cancer: past, present and future. *Nat Rev Clin Oncol.* 2016;13(8):504-515.

72. Yang CS, Chen JX, Wang H, Lim J. Lessons learned from cancer prevention studies with nutrients and non-nutritive dietary constituents. *Mol Nutr Food Res.* 2016;60(6):1239-1250.

73. Victora CG, Bahl R, Barros AJ, et al. Breastfeeding in the 21st century: epidemiology, mechanisms, and lifelong effect. *Lancet.* 2016;387(10017):475-490.

74. Rock CL, Doyle C, Demark-Wahnefried W, et al. Nutrition and physical activity guidelines for cancer survivors. *CA Cancer J Clin.* 2012;62(4):243-274.

75. Schmitz KH, Courneya KS, Matthews C, et al. American College of Sports Medicine roundtable on exercise guidelines for cancer survivors. *Med Sci Sports Exerc.* 2010;42(7): 1409-1426.

76. Denlinger CS, Sanft T, Baker KS, et al. Survivorship, version 2.2017, National Comprehensive Cancer Network Clinical Practice Guidelines. *J Natl Compr Canc Netw.* 2017;15(9):1140-1163. doi:10 .6004/jnccn.2017.0146

77. US Department of Agriculture. *Pesticide Data Program Annual Summary, Calendar Year 2016.* Washington, DC: US Department of Agriculture, Agricultural Marketing Program; 2018.

78. Baranski M, Srednicka-Tober D, Volakakis N, et al. Higher antioxidant and lower cadmium concentrations and lower incidence of pesticide residues in organically grown crops: a systematic literature review and meta-analyses. *Br J Nutr.* 2014;112(5):794-811.

79. Norwegian Scientific Committee for Food Safety. *Comparison of Organic and Conventional Food and Food Production. Overall Summary: Impact on Plant Health, Animal Health and Welfare, and Human Health.* 2014. Accessed January 10, 2020. https://vkm.no/download/18 .13735ab315cffecbb513 8642/1501774854136/7852b1a 164.pdf

80. Smith-Spangler C, Brandeau ML, Hunter GE, et al. Are organic foods safer or healthier than conventional alternatives? A systematic review. *Ann Intern Med.* 2012;157(5):348-366.

81. Winter CK. Chronic dietary exposure to pesticide residues in the United States. *International Journal of Food Contamination.* 2015;2(1):11.

82. Winter CK, Katz JM. Dietary exposure to pesticide residues from commodities alleged to contain the highest contamination levels. *J Toxicol.* 2011;2011. doi:10 .1155/2011/589674

83. Myers JP, Antoniou MN, Blumberg B, et al. Concerns over use of glyphosate-based herbicides and risks associated with exposures: a consensus statement. *Environ Health.* 2016;15:19.

84. Alliance for Food and Farming. Just wash it. Safe Fruits and Vegetables website. Accessed May 30, 2018. www .safefruitsandveggies.com/just -wash-it

85. Selecting and serving produce safely. US Food and Drug Administration website. February 2018. Accessed June 8, 2020. www.fda.gov/Food /ResourcesForYou/Consumers /ucm114299.htm

86. How can I wash pesticides from fruit and veggies? National Pesticide Information Center website. Accessed June 8, 2020. http://npic.orst.edu/capro /fruitwash.html

87. National Academies of Sciences, Engineering, and Medicine. *Genetically Engineered Crops: Experiences and Prospects.* National Academies Press; 2016. Accessed January 10, 2020. doi:10.17226/23395

88. Hanahan D, Weinberg RA. Hallmarks of cancer: the next generation. *Cell.* 2011;144(5): 646-674.

89. Bhatt AP, Redinbo MR, Bultman SJ. The role of the microbiome in cancer development and therapy. *CA Cancer J Clin.* 2017;67(4): 326-344.

90. Lockyer S, Nugent AP. Health effects of resistant starch. *Nutrition Bulletin.* 2017;42(1):10-41. doi:10.1111/nbu.12244

91. Mozaffarian D, Wu JHY. Omega-3 fatty acids and cardiovascular disease: effects on risk factors, molecular pathways, and clinical events. *J Am Coll Cardiol.* 2011;58(20):2047-2067.

92. Robinson LE, Mazurak VC. N-3 polyunsaturated fatty acids: relationship to inflammation in healthy adults and adults exhibiting features of metabolic syndrome. *Lipids.* 2013;48(4): 319-332.

93. Shivappa N, Steck SE, Hurley TG, et al. A population-based dietary inflammatory index predicts levels of C-reactive protein in the Seasonal Variation of Blood Cholesterol Study (SEASONS). *Public Health Nutr.* 2014;17(8):1825-1833.

94. Tabung FK, Smith-Warner SA, Chavarro JE, et al. An empirical dietary inflammatory pattern score enhances prediction of circulating inflammatory biomarkers in adults. *J Nutr.* 2017;147(8):1567-1577.

95. Wirth MD, Hebert JR, Shivappa N, et al. Anti-inflammatory Dietary Inflammatory Index scores are associated with healthier scores on other dietary indices. *Nutr Res.* 2016;36(3):214-219.

96. Huang T, Tobias DK, Hruby A, Rifai N, Tworoger SS, Hu FB. An increase in dietary quality is associated with favorable plasma biomarkers of the brain-adipose axis in apparently healthy US women. *J Nutr.* 2016;146(5): 1101-1108.

97. Shivappa N, Godos J, Hebert JR, et al. Dietary Inflammatory Index and colorectal cancer risk—a meta-analysis. *Nutrients.* 2017;9(9). pii: E1043. doi:10.3390 /nu9091043

98. Fowler ME, Akinyemiju TF. Meta-analysis of the association between dietary inflammatory index (DII) and cancer outcomes. *Int J Cancer.* 2017;141(11): 2215-2227.

99. Liu L, Nishihara R, Qian ZR, et al. Association between inflammatory diet pattern and risk of colorectal carcinoma subtypes classified by immune responses to tumor. *Gastroenterology.* 2017;153(6):1517-1530.

100. Lampe JW. Emerging research on equol and cancer. *J Nutr.* 2010;140(7):1369S-1372S.

101. Nagata C. Factors to consider in the association between soy isoflavone intake and breast cancer risk. *J Epidemiol.* 2010;20(2):83-89.

102. Setchell KD, Brown NM, Zhao X, et al. Soy isoflavone phase II metabolism differs between rodents and humans: implications for the effect on breast cancer risk. *Am J Clin Nutr.* 2011;94(5):1284-1294.

103. Shanle EK, Xu W. Selectively targeting estrogen receptors for cancer treatment. *Adv Drug Deliv Rev.* 2010;62(13):1265-1276.

104. Spagnuolo C, Russo GL, Orhan IE, et al. Genistein and cancer: current status, challenges, and future directions. *Adv Nutr.* 2015;6(4):408-419.

105. Chen M, Rao Y, Zheng Y, et al. Association between soy isoflavone intake and breast cancer risk for pre- and post-menopausal women: a meta-analysis of epidemiological studies. *PLoS One.* 2014;9(2):e89288.

106. Messina M, Rogero MM, Fisberg M, Waitzberg D. Health impact of childhood and adolescent soy consumption. *Nutr Rev.* 2017;75(7):500-515.

107. Jiang R, Botma A, Rudolph A, Husing A, Chang-Claude J. Phyto-oestrogens and colorectal cancer risk: a systematic review and dose-response meta-analysis of observational studies. *Br J Nutr.* 2016;116(12):2115-2128.

108. Nechuta SJ, Caan BJ, Chen WY, et al. Soy food intake after diagnosis of breast cancer and survival: an in-depth analysis of combined evidence from cohort studies of US and Chinese women. *Am J Clin Nutr.* 2012;96(1):123-132.

109. Zhang YF, Kang HB, Li BL, Zhang RM. Positive effects of soy isoflavone food on survival of breast cancer patients in China. *Asian Pac J Cancer Prev.* 2012;13(2):479-482.

110. Shu XO, Zheng Y, Cai H, et al. Soy food intake and breast cancer survival. *JAMA.* 2009;302(22):2437-2443.

111. Mason JK, Thompson LU. Flaxseed and its lignan and oil components: can they play a role in reducing the risk of and improving the treatment of breast cancer? *Appl Physiol Nutr Metab.* 2014;39(6):663-678.

112. Azrad M, Vollmer RT, Madden J, et al. Flaxseed-derived enterolactone is inversely associated with tumor cell proliferation in men with localized prostate cancer. *J Med Food.* 2013;16(4):357-360.

113. Zaineddin AK, Vrieling A, Buck K, et al. Serum enterolactone and postmenopausal breast cancer risk by estrogen, progesterone and herceptin 2 receptor status. *Int J Cancer.* 2012;130(6): 1401-1410.

114. Fleming JA, Kris-Etherton PM. The evidence for α-linolenic acid and cardiovascular disease benefits: comparisons with eicosapentaenoic acid and docosahexaenoic acid. *Adv Nutr.* 2014;5(6):863S-876S.

115. Baker EJ, Miles EA, Burdge GC, Yaqoob P, Calder PC. Metabolism and functional effects of plant-derived omega-3 fatty acids in humans. *Prog Lipid Res.* 2016;64:30-56.

116. Brahe LK, Le Chatelier E, Prifti E, et al. Dietary modulation of the gut microbiota—a randomised controlled trial in obese postmenopausal women. *Br J Nutr.* 2015;114(3):406-417.

117. Chen LH, Fang J, Sun Z, et al. Enterolactone inhibits insulin-like growth factor-1 receptor signaling in human prostatic carcinoma PC-3 cells. *J Nutr.* 2009;139(4):653-659.

118. Saarinen NM, Tuominen J, Pylkkanen L, Santti R. Assessment of information to substantiate a health claim on the prevention of prostate cancer by lignans. *Nutrients.* 2010;2(2):99-115.

119. Demark-Wahnefried W, Polascik TJ, George SL, et al. Flaxseed supplementation (not dietary fat restriction) reduces prostate cancer proliferation rates in men presurgery. *Cancer Epidemiol Biomarkers Prev.* 2008;17(12):3577-3587.

Chapter 3
Energy Balance, Body Composition, and Physical Activity for Cancer Prevention, Treatment, and Survivorship

Elaine B. Trujillo, MS, RDN
Jill Hamilton-Reeves, PhD, RDN, CSO, NSCA-CPT

Overweight and obesity are conditions characterized by the excessive accumulation of body fat that presents a risk to health. Body fatness and weight gain throughout life are largely determined by modifiable risk factors, such as excess energy intake from food and beverages and, to a lesser extent, physical inactivity.[1] More than 70% of adults are overweight or obese—32.5% are considered overweight, and 37.7% are considered obese—and about 17% of children and adolescents are obese.[2]

Obesity is associated with morbidity from type 2 diabetes, coronary heart disease, stroke, osteoarthritis, and several cancers.[2]

Physical activity lowers the risk of 13 cancers,[3] and physical activity after a cancer diagnosis is associated with a reduced risk of cancer recurrence and improved overall survival.[4] Physical activity provides health benefits beyond the effects on energy balance and preventing body fat and weight gain. Health benefits vary by the type of regular physical activity undertaken. Generally, both aerobic training and anaerobic training (ie, short duration and high intensity, like sprinting or jumping) lead to cardiovascular and respiratory conditioning. Resistance training (ie, squats, push-ups, weight lifting) increases muscular strength, improves muscle tone, and retains muscle mass. Stretching leads to greater flexibility. Balance exercises help prevent falls. Physical activity also leads to improvement in overall health-related quality of life.[5,6] Time spent engaged in sedentary activities is distinct from physical activity and has been shown to be a health risk that increases the likelihood of cancer and other chronic diseases.[7]

Energetics and Cancer Risk

Obesity, Weight Gain, and Cancer Risk

There is consistent evidence that a high body mass index (BMI) is associated with cancer risk. The evidence that excess body weight is a risk factor for many cancers has strengthened over the last decade.[8] Reports by the International Agency for Research on Cancer (IARC) Handbook Working Group[1] and the World Cancer Research Fund (WCRF) and American Institute for Cancer Research (AICR)[8] identified the strength of the evidence for the increased risks associated with excess body fatness on cancer type, and their findings are summarized in Figure 3.1 on page 38. In the 10-year period from 2005 to 2014, more than 630,000 people received a cancer diagnosis that was associated with overweight and obesity, and these cancers comprised more than 55% of all cancers diagnosed among women and 24% of all cancers diagnosed among men. Interestingly, cancers related to overweight and obesity were increasingly diagnosed among younger people; there was a 1.4% annual increase in cancers related to overweight and obesity among individuals aged 20 to 49 years and a 0.4% increase in these cancers among individuals aged 50 to 64 years.[9,10]

Only about half of US residents are aware that adults who are overweight or obese are at increased risk for cancer.[11] Americans should be aware that just an 11-lb (5-kg) increase in weight beginning in early adulthood can increase their risk for cancers related to overweight and obesity[12] and that maintaining a healthy weight throughout life may reduce their risk of these cancers.[1,10]

Weight gain during adult life, and especially following menopause, increases breast cancer risk

Chapter 3 *Energy Balance, Body Composition, and Physical Activity for Cancer Prevention, Treatment, and Survivorship*

37

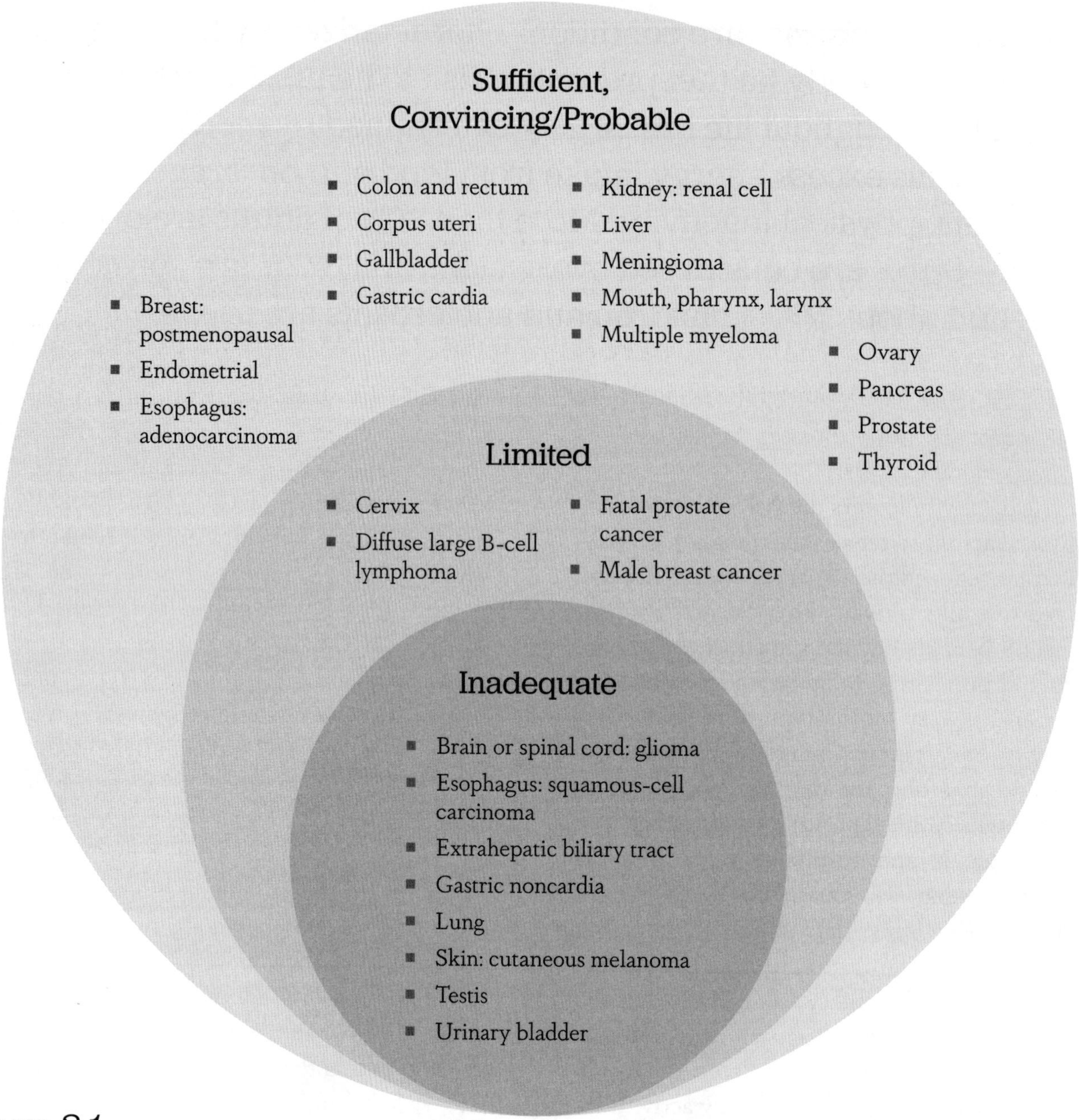

Sufficient, Convincing/Probable

- Colon and rectum
- Corpus uteri
- Gallbladder
- Gastric cardia
- Kidney: renal cell
- Liver
- Meningioma
- Mouth, pharynx, larynx
- Multiple myeloma
- Breast: postmenopausal
- Endometrial
- Esophagus: adenocarcinoma
- Ovary
- Pancreas
- Prostate
- Thyroid

Limited

- Cervix
- Diffuse large B-cell lymphoma
- Fatal prostate cancer
- Male breast cancer

Inadequate

- Brain or spinal cord: glioma
- Esophagus: squamous-cell carcinoma
- Extrahepatic biliary tract
- Gastric noncardia
- Lung
- Skin: cutaneous melanoma
- Testis
- Urinary bladder

Figure 3.1

Strength of the evidence for excess body fatness and increased cancer risk

Of the more than 1,000 epidemiologic studies assessed by the International Agency for Research on Cancer Handbook Working Group, most were observational, based on adult body mass index, and the evidence was assessed as sufficient, limited, or inadequate. In the World Cancer Research Fund/American Institute for Cancer Research report, systematic reviews and meta-analyses were analyzed by an international independent panel of experts to assess whether the evidence was convincing, probable, or limited with respect to greater body fatness and increased cancer risk.

Adapted from:

- Lauby-Secretan B, Scoccianti C, Loomis D, Grosse Y, Bianchini F, Straif K. Body fatness and cancer—viewpoint of the IARC Working Group. *N Engl J Med.* 2016;375(8):794-798. See reference 1.
- World Cancer Research Fund/American Institute for Cancer Research. *Diet, Nutrition, Physical Activity and Cancer: A Global Perspective.* World Cancer Research Fund International; 2018. Accessed February 12, 2019. www.wcrf.org/dietandcancer. See reference 8.

among postmenopausal women. In a large prospective cohort within the Nurses' Health Study, women who had gained 25 kg or more since age 18 years were at an increased risk of breast cancer compared with those who had maintained their weight. Compared with women who had maintained their, women who had gained 10 kg or more since menopause were at an increased risk of breast cancer.[13] These data suggest that weight gain during adult life, and especially after menopause, increases breast cancer risk among postmenopausal women.

Intentional Weight Loss and Cancer Risk

Intentional weight loss may reduce cancer risk, particularly for breast and endometrial cancers.[1] The biological mechanisms proposed to link obesity and cancer—namely, increased insulin and insulin-like growth factors, increased estradiol, and inflammation—are potentially modifiable by weight loss.[14]

Two large studies show that weight loss may reduce cancer risk. In a large cohort of women from the Iowa Women's Health Study, when compared with women who had never had a weight loss episode of 20 lb (9.1 kg) or more, women who had experienced an intentional weight loss of 20 lb or more had an 11% lower incidence rate for any cancer and a 19% lower incidence rate for breast cancer. The women who had never experienced a weight loss of 20 lb or more or who had lost 20 lb or more unintentionally had a lower prevalence of overweight than the two groups reporting intentional weight loss episodes of 20 lb or greater. Although overweight women were at increased risk for several cancers, women who experienced intentional weight loss of 20 lb or more and were not currently overweight had an incidence of cancer similar to nonoverweight women who never lost weight.[15] Women in the Nurses' Health Study who had lost 22 lb (10 kg) or more following menopause and kept the weight off

were at a lower risk than those who maintained their weight (relative risk of 0.43 with a 95% confidence interval of 0.21 to 0.86),[13] showing that weight loss after menopause is associated with a decreased risk of breast cancer.

Of the three general modalities for intentional weight loss and maintenance, including lifestyle interventions, pharmacotherapy, and bariatric surgery, bariatric surgery leads to the largest and most sustained weight reduction.[16] Studies have shown bariatric surgery to reduce cancer risk.[14] In a systematic review and meta-analysis of bariatric surgery on oncologic outcomes, bariatric surgery reduced cancer risk and mortality in formerly obese patients, and the effect on oncological outcomes was protective in women but not in men.[17]

Energy Restriction and Cancer Risk

For centuries, fasting has been carried out for cultural, religious, and spiritual purposes. In 1914, Payton Rous first suggested limited food intake could decrease tumor growth.[18] In recent years, the interest in energy/calorie restriction (CR) and cancer growth has increased. CR, a chronic reduction of energy intake by approximately 30% without incurrence of malnutrition, results in decreased glucose levels and factors stimulating cell division and promotes autophagy-mediated recycling of cell components and clearance from damaging factors that influence tissue homeostasis and tumorigenesis.[19,20]

Most of the CR research regarding cancer has been done in prevention. A meta-analysis of animal studies on the impact of CR across multiple cancer types found a 75.5% reduction in tumor incidence.[21] Studies in humans are emerging and show that CR without malnutrition decreases adiposity and inflammation and results in maintenance of blood glucose levels in the low normal range, depletion of reduction of glycogen stores, mobilization of fatty acids and generation of ketones, a reduction of circulating leptin, and often elevation of adiponectin levels.[20,22] Interestingly, the results from the nonobese human trials regarding the metabolic and molecular changes are similar to those observed in rodent models.[20] Human studies have yet to reflect whether CR affects cancer rates. It is possible that CR may reduce cancer risk through its effects on cancer risk biomarkers, such as insulin, cytokines, and the adipokines leptin and adiponectin.[22]

Physical Activity and Cancer Risk

Data consistently show that a higher level of physical activity is associated with a lower risk of cancer, especially for colon,[23] breast,[24] and endometrial[25] cancers. In a pooled analysis of 12 prospective cohorts from the United States and Europe, Moore and colleagues[3] reported that physical activity is associated with a lower risk of 13 types of cancer. Interestingly, when the analysis was adjusted for BMI, the lowered risk from physical activity persisted except for liver, gastric, and endometrial cancer types, which suggests that physical activity can lower cancer risk regardless of weight status. When adjusted for smoking status, the lowered risk from physical activity remained for all cancer types except lung cancer.

For cancer prevention, the American Cancer Society (ACS) recommends that adults get at least 150 minutes of moderate-intensity activity or 75 minutes of vigorous activity (eg, running, walking briskly uphill or performing any activity that requires too much effort to talk while doing it) each week, and that children get at least 60 minutes of moderate or vigorous activity each day.[26] Similarly, the WCRF and AICR recommend being physically active every day. Furthermore, individuals are encouraged to aim for 150 minutes or more of moderate physical activity or at least 75 minutes of vigorous physical activity every week.[8] Physical activity guidelines are summarized in Box 3.1.[8,26-30]

Measures of Obesity and Energetics

Anthropometric Measures

BMI, which is a person's body weight (kg) divided by the person's height squared (m²), is a simple tool for categorizing patients as underweight (BMI <18.5), normal weight (BMI 18.5 to 24.99), overweight (BMI 25 to 29.99), and obese (BMI ≥30). Although BMI is the most common anthropometric tool for determining obesity, it is a poor reflection of body composition. And although BMI is the measurement tool most frequently used to correlate obesity to cancer risk, its major flaw lies in its inability to differentiate fat from muscle mass.[31] The assumption that the impact of weight is the same regardless of the degree of adiposity or skeletal muscle ignores the evidence that, in oncology, body composition has been shown to have a substantial impact on outcomes.[31,32]

Waist circumference, hip circumference, and waist to hip ratio are measurement tools that can detect central obesity and that have been used in association studies looking at the incidence or mortality from cancer.[33]

Direct Measures

Diagnostic tools that directly evaluate fat and muscle mass composition include bioimpedance analysis (BIA), dual-energy x-ray absorptiometry (DXA), magnetic resonance imaging (MRI), and computed tomography (CT). BIA measures tissue conductivity; however, it is a less reliable measurement tool than the others.[34] DXA scans accurately and reliably distinguish fat, bone mineral, and lean body mass and are accurate within 5% for assessing body fat percentage and changes in body fat over time.[34,35] MRI is ideal for quantifying skeletal muscle and fat, although this technique is generally reserved for the research setting.[35]

CT images are a standard of care in oncology, are routinely available, and offer a method for noninvasively and precisely quantifying skeletal muscle.[36] CT scans provide accurate and reliable information on muscle and different adipose tissue depots at the third lumbar vertebra cross-sectional area, an area chosen as the best correlate to whole body composition.[37] In a systematic review of the literature reporting quantitative evaluation of the cross-sectional area of the main tissues implicated in cancer cachexia, including muscle along with visceral, subcutaneous, and inter-muscular fat, in CT scans at the third lumbar vertebra, the reviewers found a consistent association between skeletal

Box 3.1
Physical Activity Guidelines for Cancer Prevention and Cancer Survivorship[8,26-30]

American Cancer Society

Cancer prevention recommendations	Adults should get 150 to 300 minutes of moderate intensity exercise or 75 to 150 minutes of vigorous intensity activity each week (or a combination of these).
Cancer survivorship recommendations	**During treatment:** When to initiate and how to maintain physical activity (PA) should be individualized to the patient's condition and personal preferences. Patient should return to baseline PA as soon as possible after diagnosis and avoid being sedentary. Be mindful of the special precautions for cancer survivors:

- Survivors with severe anemia should delay exercise, other than activities of daily living, until anemia improves.
- Survivors with compromised immune function should avoid public gyms and public pools until their white blood cell counts return to safe levels; after a bone marrow transplant, patients should avoid these exposures for 1 year.
- Survivors experiencing severe fatigue from therapy are encouraged to do 10 minutes of light exercise daily.
- Survivors undergoing radiation should avoid exposing irradiated skin to chlorine (eg, from swimming pools).
- Survivors with indwelling catheters or feeding tubes should be cautious or avoid pool, lake, or ocean water or other microbial exposures that may result in infections, as well as resistance training of muscles in the area of the catheter (to avoid dislodgement).
- Survivors with multiple comorbidities should consider program modification in consultation with their physician.
- Survivors with significant peripheral neuropathies or ataxia may do better with stationary reclining bicycles than with treadmills.

Over the long term:
At least 150 min/wk

Strength training exercises at least 2 d/wk

(continued)

Chapter 3 *Energy Balance, Body Composition, and Physical Activity for Cancer Prevention, Treatment, and Survivorship*

41

American College of Sports Medicine

Cancer prevention recommendations	At least 30 minutes of moderate to vigorous aerobic PA five times per week (2.5 h/wk)
	Muscle strengthening at least 2 d/wk; 8 to 12 repetitions suggested, one to three sets
Cancer survivorship recommendations	**During treatment:**
	Patient should avoid inactivity and return to normal PA as soon as possible after treatment.
	Conduct pre-exercise assessment and tumor site–specific assessments as needed.
	Over the long term:
	Adults aged 18 to 64 years: overall, 150 min/wk of moderate-intensity PA or 75 min/wk of vigorous-intensity PA, or equivalent combination (sessions of at least 10 minutes each and spread throughout the week)
	Muscle-strengthening PA of at least moderate intensity at least 2 d/wk for each major muscle group
	Stretching of major muscle groups and tendons on days other exercises are performed

World Cancer Research Fund/American Institute for Cancer Research

Cancer prevention recommendations	Daily PA
	At least 150 min/wk of moderate-intensity PA or 75 min/wk of vigorous-intensity PA
Cancer survivorship recommendations	**During Treatment:**
	Daily PA
	Over the Long Term:
	After treatment, follow recommendations for cancer prevention.

(continued)

muscle depletion and cancer outcomes, including chemotherapy response and toxicity, increased postsurgical complications, length of hospital stay, and mortality.[32] Other studies have corroborated these results. In a large-scale retrospective cohort study of patients with different stages of hepatocellular carcinoma who underwent CT imaging, researchers found that sarcopenia (severe muscle depletion), intramuscular fat deposition, and visceral adiposity independently predicted mortality.[38] Emerging studies examining body composition using CT imaging in cancer patients are finding that sarcopenia is underrecognized and occurs in 34% of patients with nonmetastatic breast cancer and 42% of patients with nonmetastatic colorectal cancer.[39,40]

CT is readily available for cancer patients, for both staging and surveillance, and commercial

National Comprehensive Cancer Network

Cancer prevention recommendations	N/A
Cancer survivorship recommendations	**During treatment:** Follow American Cancer Society and American College of Sports Medicine guidelines for cancer survivors.
	Over the long term: Overall, at least 150 min/wk of moderate-intensity PA or 75 min/wk of vigorous-intensity PA, or equivalent combination
	Two to three sessions per week of strength training that includes all major muscle groups
	Stretching of major muscle groups at least 2 d/wk
	Avoidance of prolonged sedentary behavior
	Resistance training as prescribed. Example resistance-training prescription:
	■ *Frequency:* Two to three times/wk; wait at least 48 hours between training sessions.
	■ *Intensity:* Two to three sets of 10 to 15 repetitions per set; consider increasing weight amount as tolerated when three sets of 10 to 15 repetitions becomes easy.
	■ *Time:* 20 minutes per session.
	■ *Rest:* 2- to 3-minute rest period between sets and exercises.

software programs are available to assess body composition.[39] The routine use of CT scans in nutritional assessments provides a more precise technique for assessing body composition and is recommended.

Biological Mechanisms Relating to Energetics and Cancer

Obesity-Related Mechanisms

Many of the pathologic features of obesity promote tumor growth, including metabolic imbalances, hormonal and growth factor imbalances, and chronic inflammation.[41] Visceral adiposity is strongly associated with the metabolic syndrome; visceral adipose tissue is biologically active and secretes adipokines, such as leptin and adiponectin, and other cytokines, such as tumor necrosis factor α (TNF-α) and interleukin-6 (IL-6), that contribute to insulin resistance and an inflammatory state that has been associated with cancer.[42]

People with obesity often have insulin resistance and increased insulin-like growth factor 1 (IGF-1), both of which may explain the link between obesity and cancer, at least in part. Insulin and IGF-1 can interact with the insulin receptor or the IGF-1 receptor, both of which have been associated with tumor development. IGF-1 drives insulin's anabolic and antiapoptotic effects.

Furthermore, IGF-1 is proangiogenic and induces tumor-related lymphangiogenesis.[43]

Insulin resistance and inflammation also occur in individuals with normal BMI. On the other hand, there are individuals with elevated BMI who are metabolically healthy. Again, determining obesity based solely on BMI is cautioned against, and BMI may be inadequate for identifying individuals with adipose inflammation.[44] Identifying the underlying perturbations may be more useful in determining the relationship between obesity and cancer. This approach was demonstrated in a systematic review that examined the effect of lifestyle interventions on adipose tissue gene expression. A change in subcutaneous adipose tissue gene expression was most commonly observed with dietary weight loss, with a pattern of decrease in leptin, TNF-α, and IL-6, as well as an increase in adiponectin. There was limited change with exercise-only interventions or study arms.[45]

Leptin, an adipokine produced by adipose tissue, is found at increased levels in people with obesity. It is thought to promote cancer development and progression. Leptin causes mitogenic, proinflammatory, antiapoptotic, and proangiogenic effects and may contribute to the regulation of estrogen signaling. Unlike leptin, the adipokine adiponectin is found at decreased levels in individuals with obesity. Adiponectin enhances insulin sensitivity, and its levels are inversely related to cancer occurrence and stage; adiponectin plays a protective role in cancer by indirectly acting against the development of insulin resistance.[43]

Estrogen may promote tumor development and progression through various complex mechanisms, including directly through stimulation of cellular proliferation and inhibition of apoptosis.[46] Before menopause, estrogen is predominantly produced in the ovaries, whereas after menopause, estrogen is produced to a much lesser degree mostly through adipose tissue. Hence, the increase in breast cancer risk with increasing BMI among postmenopausal women has been found to be largely the result of the associated increase in estrogen in obese women.[47]

Physical Activity–Related Mechanisms

The exact mechanisms by which physical activity inhibits carcinogenesis are not fully understood. Potential mechanisms include an indirect effect by preventing obesity and thereby modulating cytokines, glucose regulation, and hormones (estradiol,[48,49] estrogen,[50,51] sex hormone–binding globulin,[49] and insulin[52]).[53] Physical activity may directly decrease cancer risk by lowering chronic inflammation[52] and improving immune function.[53] Moderate and vigorous exercise may reduce colon cancer risk by activating peristalsis, which decreases transit time and the subsequent contact time between intestinal mucosa and carcinogens in the gut.

Energetics, Cancer Treatment, and Survivorship
Cachexia, Sarcopenia, and Sarcopenic Obesity

Cachexia is a metabolic syndrome driven by inflammation and characterized by loss of muscle with or without the loss of fat mass. It is a multifactorial syndrome that cannot be fully reversed by conventional nutritional support and that leads to progressive functional impairment.[54] In cancer cachexia, the tumor burden and host response induce increased inflammation, decreased anabolic tone, and suppressed appetite, which promote lipid mobilization and protein degradation, decreased protein synthesis, increased resting energy expenditure, and, ultimately, reduced body weight and quality of life. Cancer cachexia is most prevalent in gastric, pancreatic, esophageal, head and neck, lung, colorectal, and prostate cancers.[55]

A diagnosis of cancer cachexia is based on:

- weight loss of more than 5% over the past 6 months, in the absence of simple starvation; or
- BMI of less than 20 and any degree of weight loss greater than 2%; or
- appendicular skeletal muscle index consistent with sarcopenia (men, <7.26; women, <5.45) and any degree of weight loss greater than 2%.[54]

Criteria for defining cachexia, in addition to weight loss, include variable combinations of low BMI, low skeletal muscle mass, reduced dietary intake, and biological indicators of inflammation as markers of metabolic change. See Figure 3.2 for descriptions of the three stages of cancer cachexia, including precachexia, cachexia, and refractory cachexia.[54]

Sarcopenia is severe muscle depletion. First described as part of the frailty syndrome found in older persons, sarcopenia is now known to be prevalent in other conditions, including cancer. The prevalence of sarcopenia is about 15% in healthy individuals, compared to 40% to 50% in people of similar age with newly diagnosed cancer.[37] In cancer patients, sarcopenia has emerged to be an important prognostic factor for those with advanced cancer; it is associated with poor performance status, toxicity from chemotherapy, and shorter time of tumor control. Sarcopenia in patients with cancer could be attributed to age, comorbidities, malnutrition, physical inactivity, tumor-derived factors, cancer therapy, and supportive-care medications.[34]

Both sarcopenia and cachexia can be present in patients with any BMI, including in patients with obesity. The combination of low muscle mass and high adipose tissue, or sarcopenic obesity, is an emerging abnormal body composition phenotype. Obesity does not preclude the presence of cancer cachexia or sarcopenia and can mask its

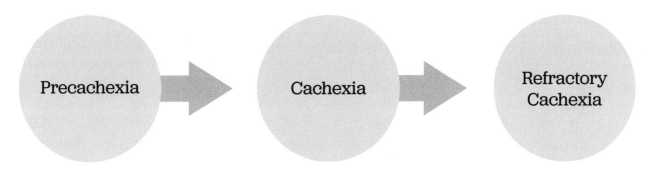

Precachexia → Cachexia → Refractory Cachexia

- Weight loss
- Anorexia
- Progression depends on cancer type and stage and on factors such as systemic inflammation, low food intake, and lack of response to anticancer therapy

- Weight loss of ≥5% over 6 months
- BMI <20 with >2% weight loss
- Sarcopenia and >2% weight loss
- Reduced food intake
- Presence of systemic inflammation

- Active catabolism
- Management of weight loss not possible
- Very advanced or rapidly progressive cancer unresponsive to anticancer therapy

Figure 3.2
Stages of cancer cachexia

Adapted from Fearon K, Strasser F, Anker SD, et al. Definition and classification of cancer cachexia: an international consensus. *Lancet Oncol.* 2011;12(5):489-495. See reference 54.

Box 3.2
Types of Energy Restriction Dietary Patterns[22]

Type	Description	Examples
Intermittent fasting	16 to 48 hours with little or no energy intake and with intervening periods of normal food intake, on a recurring basis	Complete fasting every other day 70% energy restriction every other day 500 to 700 kilocalorie intake on 2 consecutive d/wk
Periodic fasting	Fasting or a fasting-mimicking diet from 2 days to 21 days	4 to 5 days of a fasting-mimicking diet 2 to 5 days of water-only fasting 7 days of a fasting-mimicking diet
Time-restricted feeding	Food intake restricted to 8 h/d or less	

appearance.[37] Hence, cancer patients who have cachexia or sarcopenic obesity are often overlooked as having malnutrition or being at risk of malnutrition.

Energy Restriction

Although most of the research into cancer and CR has focused on prevention, the role of CR as an adjunct to chemotherapy and radiation therapy for a variety of cancers is evolving. Because CR may exacerbate weight loss, sarcopenia, and cachexia, the preferred modality in patients with cancer is intermittent fasting (IF), which results in similar metabolic and anti-inflammatory changes but without the potential negative effects.

IF involves having the patient go extended periods of time, such as 16 to 48 hours, with little or no energy intake and with intervening periods of normal food intake on a recurring basis. Periodic fasting is IF with periods of fasting or "fasting-mimicking diets" lasting from 2 to 21 or more days. The various types of CR and IF are described in Box 3.2.

In various animal models of cancer, short-term fasting has been shown to improve chemotherapeutic treatment with etoposide, mitoxantrone, oxaliplatin, cisplatin, cyclophosphamide, and doxorubicin. Alternate-day fasting has been shown to improve the radiosensitivity of mammary tumors in mice. Furthermore, fasting may improve the efficacy of anticancer therapies in part by controlling circadian rhythm.[20]

In a study of 10 patients with a variety of malignancies who fasted for 48 to 140 hours before chemotherapy, 5 to 56 hours after chemotherapy, or both, fasting was feasible, safe, and caused a reduction in a range of side effects.[56] Although results from trials in humans are limited, several trials using various forms of IF in different cancer types during treatment are underway or results are pending.[57] These trials and others may clarify whether fasting as an adjuvant cancer treatment reduces the cancer burden, which type of fasting that is most effective, and which cancer types and stages may be most responsive.

Excess Adiposity During Treatment and Survivorship

Excess adiposity, commonly approximated by BMI, is associated with poorer prognosis after cancer diagnosis. However, emerging studies have observed that among patients with cancer, elevated BMI is associated with improved survival compared with normal-weight patients, suggesting the existence of an obesity paradox. Specifically, the obesity paradox occurs when the risk of outcome, typically mortality, is significantly reduced for people with BMI values above 22.5, which is the widely accepted mid-reference point for normal weight.[58]

Evidence from clinical trials, pooling projects, and meta-analyses have shown that class 2 or 3 obesity (BMI >35) was associated with worse survival; however, studies have shown mixed associations with overweight or lower levels of obesity.[40,59,60] In patients with colorectal cancer, a BMI in the overweight range of 25 to less than 30 was associated with the lowest mortality risk.[61] Furthermore, 72% of patients in that BMI category had adequate muscle reserves, possibly providing the capacity to counter the catabolic consequences of tumor growth and cancer treatments. Only 19% had adiposity levels sufficiently high to influence the risk of survival.[39,61] Hence, it seems that overweight and mild obesity may have a protective effect on some types of patients with cancer.

Weight Management for Cancer Survivors

Cancer survivors have poorer health outcomes than the general population and are more likely to have multiple comorbid conditions, such as cardiovascular disease, than do individuals without cancer.[62] Obesity can exacerbate these conditions by further increasing the risk of developing cardiovascular disease, diabetes, osteoarthritis, and overall functional decline; postdiagnosis weight gain is linked to increased all-cause mortality in many cancer types.[63]

Evidence-based guidelines for the management of overweight and obesity in adults from the American Heart Association, the American College of Cardiology, and The Obesity Society recommend that patients who need to lose weight should receive a comprehensive intervention lasting at least 6 months that encompasses diet, physical activity, and behavior modification. Ideally, the intervention consists of on-site, high-intensity sessions (at least 14 in 6 months) provided in a group or individually by a trained interventionist for a period of 1 year or more.[64] Whether cancer survivors who are seeking weight loss should use programs available for the general population depends on the health of the survivor, the risk level associated with activity, and the comfort level of the survivor.[65]

Cancer survivors need a range of weight-management programs. Medically based programs, such as oncology registered dietitian nutritionist (RDN) services, are highly personalized yet have limited accessibility. Insurance coverage for oncology nutrition services varies among institutions and cancer centers. Insurance payers do not routinely cover ambulatory oncology nutrition services provided during treatment. Some institutions offer nutritional services to patients at no charge, and they are part of the center's overhead or part of a bundled payment. Other centers may bill patients directly or may contract with a third-party organization that provides funding for oncology nutrition services. Other patients do not have access to nutrition services unless they pay out of pocket, which may limit a patient's ability to seek nutritional care.[65] Theoretically, weight-loss programs in nononcology settings would be more accessible to patients, but many primary care providers are not adequately trained to discuss weight management and potential treatments.[65,66] Hence, weight-loss counseling or referral generally is not implemented. Box 3.3 on pages 48 and 49 identifies the types and characteristics of weight-management programs available to cancer survivors.

Chapter 3 *Energy Balance, Body Composition, and Physical Activity for Cancer Prevention, Treatment, and Survivorship*

47

Box 3.3
Types and Characteristics of Weight-Management Programs Available to Cancer Survivors[65]

Medically based programs

Program type	Description and comments	
Oncology Registered Dietitian Nutritionist services	<ul><li>Highly personalized</li><li>May be offered at no charge to the patient in some cancer treatment settings</li></ul>	<ul><li>Not routinely covered by insurance</li><li>Accessibility may be limited</li></ul>
Weight management in non-oncology settings	<ul><li>Convenient and generally accessible to patients</li><li>May provide obesity screening, weight-loss counseling, reduction of behavioral cardiovascular risk factors, medical weight-loss programs, and potentially bariatric surgery</li></ul>	<ul><li>May be covered by insurance and by Medicare for patients with a body mass index (BMI) of 30 or less and those with risk factors for cardiovascular disease</li><li>Services are not cancer-specific</li><li>Low rates of being implemented</li></ul>

Community-based programs

Program type	Description and comments	
Not-for-profit programs	<ul><li>Cancer-specific focus with a group or individual using an RDN, exercise specialist, or health educator</li><li>Community-based locations may be more convenient and provide in-person assistance (eg, LIVESTRONG at the YMCA)</li></ul>	<ul><li>Generally offered free of charge or at low cost</li><li>Not available in all communities</li></ul>
Work-site programs	<ul><li>Employers may include programs for cancer survivors as part of their health and wellness programs, which are convenient for participants and may provide built-in social support networks</li></ul>	<ul><li>May be offered at no cost or with cost sharing</li><li>Not widely available and may be less available or accessible to low-income workers and small businesses</li></ul>
Commercial programs	<ul><li>Convenient</li><li>Participant generally pays for the program or membership (eg, WW, formerly Weight Watchers)</li></ul>	<ul><li>Effectiveness unknown without cancer-specific content</li><li>May be costly and may not be evidence-based</li></ul>

(continued)

Physical Activity and Cancer Survivorship

A person diagnosed with cancer is a cancer survivor until the end of his or her life. Over one-third of adult cancer survivors report that they do not engage in any physical activity outside of work, although this trend is declining.[67]

Physical Activity During Cancer Treatment

The ACS guidelines recommend that after diagnosis, cancer survivors return to normal activity as soon as possible and avoid being sedentary.[27] Any risks associated with incorporating physical activity during treatment are low when contraindications to activity are screened for.[68] Survivors with peripheral neuropathy, lymphedema, or serious comorbidities may need to participate in a structured, medically based program before proceeding with physical activity on their own or in a community program or facility.[65] Physical limitations due to indwelling catheters, ostomies, and surgical wounds that could be disrupted by twisting or heavy lifting are also important to keep in mind. A framework for referral to services has been proposed that uses the least amount of medical screening and supervision necessary to keep patients safe based on their individual risk factors for physical activity and any existing comorbidities or impairments.[65,69] Future directions may include clinical algorithms to tailor exercise specific to underlying comorbidities and cancer-related adverse events.[70]

Resistance training increases muscular strength, improves muscle tone, and retains muscle mass. Data suggest that resistance training improves muscular strength and endurance with few reported adverse effects in patients undergoing treatment for breast cancer[71-73] and prostate cancer.[74-78] Presurgical physical activity also helped retain lean mass in patients undergoing chemotherapy for colon cancer in a small feasibility study.[79] Trials are currently underway for other cancer types.

Physical activity interventions may reduce chemotherapy-induced peripheral neuropathy (CIPN) and improve balance, yet most data are from small trials across a variety of different interventions.[80] However, exercise improved CIPN symptoms in a secondary analysis from a phase 3 randomized controlled trial of exercise primarily designed for fatigue reduction.[81]

An eight-week training program with endurance, resistance, and specific balance exercises also improved balance in patients undergoing chemotherapy for colorectal cancer compared to a control.[82] Balance also improved in patients on chemotherapy across four different studies that included specific balance-training exercises.[80]

Physical-activity interventions show a reduction in cancer-related fatigue and improved physical function. A recent meta-analysis showed that physical activity was more effective than using drugs to overcome fatigue across several studies including a total of 11,000 cancer survivors across all studies.[83] However, a systematic review of previous meta-analyses evaluating cancer and fatigue showed only a small effect on fatigue from the pooled results; importantly, these data also showed that fatigue did not worsen with exercise.[84] Resistance training with high-intensity interval training reduced cancer-related fatigue and reduced symptom burden compared to usual care in women during chemotherapy for breast cancer.[85] However, the most appropriate type and intensity of exercise to address fatigue would depend on an individual's baseline fitness, comorbidities, and clinical factors.

Physical activity improves quality of life.[86] Supervised physical activity has a larger effect on quality of life than unsupervised physical activity.[86,87] Small studies also show that cognitive function, especially processing speed, also improves with physical activity.[88,89]

Low lean mass and high total body fat have been associated with mortality in patients with nonmetastatic breast cancer.[40] Physical activity may counteract changes in body composition from hormone therapy. Data show that following the ACS guidelines of 150 minutes of physical activity per week with twice-weekly resistance training increased lean mass and decreased body fat in breast cancer survivors taking aromatase inhibitors.[90] Supervised resistance training three times per week increased lean mass and reduced body fat in patients with prostate cancer on androgen deprivation therapy.[78] Several trials are underway testing body composition in physical activity interventions of patients with cancer.

Weight-bearing exercise, especially resistance training, improves bone health and reduces fracture risk in general populations. In cancer populations, studies assessing change in bone mineral density with exercise interventions have shown mixed results, with some trials showing an improvement in bone mineral density with exercise,[91,92] and others showing maintained bone mineral density[93] or no significant difference.[90,94]

It is unclear whether physical activity during cancer treatment can overcome the decline of cardiorespiratory fitness induced by therapy.[95] The role of physical activity in preventing cardiotoxicity from cancer treatment is under investigation.[95-97]

Long-Term Survivorship

Regular physical activity after a cancer diagnosis reduces the risk of cancer recurrence and improves overall survival.[4] Delayed side effects from cancer and its treatment are common for many cancer types, while physical activity is associated with lower risk of chronic diseases and improved quality of life. Physical activity also helps manage weight and reduce fatigue.

Physical activity guidelines for cancer survivorship are summarized in Box 3.1 on pages 41 to 43. The guidelines generally recommend that cancer survivors get at least 150 minutes of physical activity each week and include at least 2 days of strength training each week. Adherence to physical activity guidelines is associated with 23% fewer cardiovascular disease events in women with breast cancer.[98]

Physical Activity Prescriptions and Referrals

Exercise prescription typically follows the FITT principle, incorporating frequency, intensity, time (duration), and type of exercise. In addition, the prescription includes a plan for advancing patients as their fitness improves. More sophisticated, long-term exercise prescriptions use periodization to optimize adaptation with planned changes in exercise volume, intensity, and rest.

Adhering to the exercise guidelines leads to many health benefits for cancer survivors. However, addressing specific side effects or desired health outcomes will require more specificity in the training program prescribed.[99]

Various programs are available to support exercise and rehabilitation during cancer therapy or during long-term survivorship.[65] Survivors should be evaluated and prescribed exercise programs based on their current health and activity goals.[65] Cancer survivors may seek trainers that understand their unique needs after cancer therapy. Exercise professionals with the Cancer Exercise Trainer certification from the American College of Sports Medicine may be found through the college's online database (www.acsm.org/get-stay-certified/find-a-pro). Survivors with physical limitations may need medically supervised rehabilitation programs with a physical therapist or a physiatrist.

Summary

Obesity and insufficient physical activity are associated with cancer recurrence risk, death from cancer, overall mortality, and risk of subsequent malignancies. Cancer survivors often develop cardiovascular disease and other comorbidities, for which obesity and physical inactivity are risk factors. As the prevalence of cancer risk factors, including obesity and physical inactivity, increases among the general US population, clinical and public health efforts should focus on identifying optimal preventive and screening measures. Increasing the availability and accessibility of lifestyle and behavior-change programs for cancer survivors and improving adherence to guidelines on nutrition and physical activity for cancer survivors have been proposed.[65] Specific action items include:

- expanding the availability of a range of evidence-based programs for weight management, nutrition counseling, and physical activity for cancer survivors;

- improving screening and referral of survivors to exercise, nutrition, and weight-management services;

- improving health care providers' capability and capacity to screen, assess, and refer survivors to weight-management, diet and exercise programs, information, and services;

- increasing and supporting the oncology-specific training and certification of RDNs, exercise professionals, physical therapists, and physiatrists to increase the competency of the workforce needed to appropriately deliver services to cancer survivors;

- expanding research on dissemination and implementation to test models for service delivery of evidence-based interventions; and

- advocating for and leveraging health care policy changes that support availability, access, affordability, and uptake of services.[65]

Chapter 3 *Energy Balance, Body Composition, and Physical Activity for Cancer Prevention, Treatment, and Survivorship*

51

References

1. Lauby-Secretan B, Scoccianti C, Loomis D, Grosse Y, Bianchini F, Straif K. Body fatness and cancer—viewpoint of the IARC Working Group. *N Engl J Med.* 2016;375(8):794-798.

2. Ogden CL, Carroll MD, Fryar CD, Flegal KM. Prevalence of obesity among adults and youth: United States, 2011–2014. *NCHS Data Brief.* 2015;(219):1-8.

3. Moore SC, Lee IM, Weiderpass E, et al. Association of leisure-time physical activity with risk of 26 types of cancer in 1.44 million adults. *JAMA Intern Med.* 2016;176(6):816-825.

4. Arem H, Moore SC, Park Y, et al. Physical activity and cancer-specific mortality in the NIH-AARP Diet and Health Study cohort. *Int J Cancer.* 2014;135(2):423-431.

5. Mishra SI, Scherer RW, Snyder C, Geigle PM, Berlanstein DR, Topaloglu O. Exercise interventions on health-related quality of life for people with cancer during active treatment. *Cochrane Database Syst Rev.* 2012;(8):CD008465.

6. Fong DY, Ho JW, Hui BP, et al. Physical activity for cancer survivors: meta-analysis of randomised controlled trials. *BMJ.* 2012;344:e70.

7. Schmid D, Leitzmann MF. Association between physical activity and mortality among breast cancer and colorectal cancer survivors: a systematic review and meta-analysis. *Ann Oncol.* 2014;25(7):1293-1311.

8. World Cancer Research Fund/ American Institute for Cancer Research. *Diet, Nutrition, Physical Activity and Cancer: A Global Perspective.* World Cancer Research Fund International; 2018. Accessed February 12, 2019. www.wcrf.org /dietandcancer

9. Massetti GM, Dietz WH, Richardson LC. Excessive weight gain, obesity, and cancer: opportunities for clinical intervention. *JAMA.* 2017;318(20):1975-1976.

10. Steele CB, Thomas CC, Henley SJ, et al. *Vital Signs*: Trends in incidence of cancers associated with overweight and obesity— United States, 2005–2014. *MMWR Morb Mortal Wkly Rep.* 2017;66(39):1052-1058.

11. American Institute for Cancer Research. The *AICR 2017 Cancer Risk Awareness Survey Report.* American Institute for Cancer Research; 2017. Accessed February 12, 2019. www.aicr .org/assets/docs/pdf/reports /AICR%20Cancer%20Awareness %20Report%202017_jan17 %202017.pdf

12. Keum N, Greenwood DC, Lee DH, et al. Adult weight gain and adiposity-related cancers: a dose-response meta-analysis of prospective observational studies. *J Natl Cancer Inst.* 2015;107(2).

13. Eliassen AH, Colditz GA, Rosner B, Willett WC, Hankinson SE. Adult weight change and risk of postmenopausal breast cancer. *JAMA.* 2006;296(2):193-201.

14. Schauer DP, Feigelson HS, Koebnick C, et al. Association between weight loss and the risk of cancer after bariatric surgery. *Obesity (Silver Spring).* 2017;25(suppl 2):S52-S57.

15. Parker ED, Folsom AR. Intentional weight loss and incidence of obesity-related cancers: the Iowa Women's Health Study. *Int J Obes Relat Metab Disord.* 2003;27(12):1447-1452.

16. National Academies of Sciences, Engineering, and Medicine. *The Challenge of Treating Obesity and Overweight: Proceedings of a Workshop.* National Academies Press; 2017.

17. Tee MC, Cao Y, Warnock GL, Hu FB, Chavarro JE. Effect of bariatric surgery on oncologic outcomes: a systematic review and meta-analysis. *Surg Endosc.* 2013;27(12):4449-4456.

18. Rous P. The influence of diet on transplanted and spontaneous mouse tumors. *J Exp Med.* 1914;20(5):433-451.

19. Kopeina GS, Senichkin VV, Zhivotovsky B. Caloric restriction—a promising anti-cancer approach: from molecular mechanisms to clinical trials. *Biochim Biophys Acta*. 2017;1867(1):29-41.

20. O'Flanagan CH, Smith LA, McDonell SB, Hursting SD. When less may be more: calorie restriction and response to cancer therapy. *BMC Med*. 2017;15(1):106.

21. Lv M, Zhu X, Wang H, Wang F, Guan W. Roles of caloric restriction, ketogenic diet and intermittent fasting during initiation, progression and metastasis of cancer in animal models: a systematic review and meta-analysis. *PLoS One*. 2014;9:e115147.

22. Mattson MP, Longo VD, Harvie M. Impact of intermittent fasting on health and disease processes. *Ageing Res Rev*. 2017;39:46-58.

23. Robsahm TE, Aagnes B, Hjartaker A, Langseth H, Bray FI, Larsen IK. Body mass index, physical activity, and colorectal cancer by anatomical subsites: a systematic review and meta-analysis of cohort studies. *Eur J Cancer Prev*. 2013;22(6):492-505.

24. Wu Y, Zhang D, Kang S. Physical activity and risk of breast cancer: a meta-analysis of prospective studies. *Breast Cancer Res Treat*. 2013;137(3):869-882.

25. Schmid D, Behrens G, Keimling M, Jochem C, Ricci C, Leitzmann M. A systematic review and meta-analysis of physical activity and endometrial cancer risk. *Eur J Epidemiol*. 2015;30(5):397-412.

26. Rock CL, Thomson C, Gansler T, et al. American Cancer Society guideline for diet and physical activity for cancer prevention. *CA A Cancer J Clin*. 2020;70: 245-271.

27. Rock CL, Doyle C, Demark-Wahnefried W, et al. Nutrition and physical activity guidelines for cancer survivors. *CA Cancer J Clin*. 2012;62(4):243-274.

28. Denlinger CS, Sanft T, Baker KS, et al. Survivorship, version 2.2017, National Comprehensive Cancer Network Clinical Practice Guidelines. *J Natl Compr Canc Netw*. 2017;15(9):1140-1163. doi:10.6004/jnccn.2017.0146

29. US Department of Health and Human Services. *Physical Activity Guidelines for Americans*. 2nd ed. US Department of Health and Human Services; 2018. Accessed January 10, 2020. https://health.gov/sites/default/files/2019-09/Physical_Activity_Guidelines_2nd_edition.pdf

30. Wolin KY, Schwartz AL, Matthews CE, Courneya KS, Schmitz KH. Implementing the exercise guidelines for cancer survivors. *J Support Oncol*. 2012;10(5): 171-177.

31. Strulov Shachar S, Williams GR. The obesity paradox in cancer—moving beyond BMI. *Cancer Epidemiol Biomarkers Prev*. 2017;26(1):13-16.

32. Kazemi-Bajestani SM, Mazurak VC, Baracos V. Computed tomography-defined muscle and fat wasting are associated with cancer clinical outcomes. *Semin Cell Dev Biol*. 2016;54:2-10.

33. Kyrgiou M, Kalliala I, Markozannes G, et al. Adiposity and cancer at major anatomical sites: umbrella review of the literature. *BMJ*. 2017;356:j477.

34. Chindapasirt J. Sarcopenia in cancer patients. *Asian Pac J Cancer Prev*. 2015;16(18): 8075-8077.

35. Seabolt LA, Welch EB, Silver HJ. Imaging methods for analyzing body composition in human obesity and cardiometabolic disease. *Ann N Y Acad Sci*. 2015;1353:41-59.

36. Martin L. Diagnostic criteria for cancer cachexia: data versus dogma. *Curr Opin Clin Nutr Metab Care*. 2016;19(3):188-198.

37. Prado CM, Cushen SJ, Orsso CE, Ryan AM. Sarcopenia and cachexia in the era of obesity: clinical and nutritional impact. *Proc Nutr Soc*. 2016;75(2):188-198.

Chapter 3 *Energy Balance, Body Composition, and Physical Activity for Cancer Prevention, Treatment, and Survivorship*

53

38. Fujiwara N, Nakagawa H, Kudo Y, et al. Sarcopenia, intramuscular fat deposition, and visceral adiposity independently predict the outcomes of hepatocellular carcinoma. *J Hepatol.* 2015;63(1):131-140.

39. Caan BJ, Meyerhardt JA, Kroenke CH, et al. Explaining the obesity paradox: the association between body composition and colorectal cancer survival (C-SCANS Study). *Cancer Epidemiol Biomarkers Prev.* 2017;26(7):1008-1015.

40. Caan BJ, Cespedes Feliciano EM, Prado CM, et al. Association of muscle and adiposity measured by computed tomography with survival in patients with nonmetastatic breast cancer. *JAMA Oncol.* 2018;4(6):798-804.

41. O'Flanagan CH, Bowers LW, Hursting SD. A weighty problem: metabolic perturbations and the obesity-cancer link. *Horm Mol Biol Clin Investig.* 2015;23(2):47-57.

42. Goodwin PJ, Stambolic V. Impact of the obesity epidemic on cancer. *Annu Rev Med.* 2015;66:281-296.

43. De Pergola G, Silvestris F. Obesity as a major risk factor for cancer. *J Obes.* 2013;2013: doi:10.1155/2013/291546

44. Iyengar NM, Gucalp A, Dannenberg AJ, Hudis CA. Obesity and cancer mechanisms: tumor microenvironment and inflammation. *J Clin Oncol.* 2016;34(35):4270-4276.

45. Campbell KL, Landells CE, Fan J, Brenner DR. A systematic review of the effect of lifestyle interventions on adipose tissue gene expression: implications for carcinogenesis. *Obesity (Silver Spring).* 2017;25(suppl 2):S40-S51.

46. Iyengar NM, Hudis CA, Dannenberg AJ. Obesity and cancer: local and systemic mechanisms. *Annu Rev Med.* 2015;66:297-309.

47. Key TJ, Appleby PN, Reeves GK, et al. Body mass index, serum sex hormones, and breast cancer risk in postmenopausal women. *J Natl Cancer Inst.* 2003;95(16):1218-1226.

48. Friedenreich CM, Woolcott CG, McTiernan A, et al. Alberta physical activity and breast cancer prevention trial: sex hormone changes in a year-long exercise intervention among postmenopausal women. *J Clin Oncol.* 2010;28(9):1458-1466.

49. Campbell KL, Foster-Schubert KE, Alfano CM, et al. Reduced-calorie dietary weight loss, exercise, and sex hormones in postmenopausal women: randomized controlled trial. *J Clin Oncol.* 2012;30(19):2314-2326.

50. Ziegler RG, Fuhrman BJ, Moore SC, Matthews CE. Epidemiologic studies of estrogen metabolism and breast cancer. *Steroids.* 2015;99(pt A):67-75.

51. Smith AJ, Phipps WR, Thomas W, Schmitz KH, Kurzer MS. The effects of aerobic exercise on estrogen metabolism in healthy premenopausal women. *Cancer Epidemiol Biomarkers Prev.* 2013;22(5):756-764.

52. Winters-Stone KM, Wood LJ, Stoyles S, Dieckmann NF. The effects of resistance exercise on biomarkers of breast cancer prognosis: a pooled analysis of three randomized trials. *Cancer Epidemiol Biomarkers Prev.* 2018;27(2):146-153.

53. McTiernan A. Mechanisms linking physical activity with cancer. *Nat Rev Cancer.* 2008;8(3):205-211.

54. Fearon K, Strasser F, Anker SD, et al. Definition and classification of cancer cachexia: an international consensus. *Lancet Oncol.* 2011;12(5):489-495.

55. Anderson LJ, Albrecht ED, Garcia JM. Update on management of cancer-related cachexia. *Curr Oncol Rep.* 2017;19:3.

56. Safdie FM, Dorff T, Quinn D, et al. Fasting and cancer treatment in humans: a case series report. *Aging (Albany NY).* 2009;1(12):988-1007.

57. US National Library of Medicine, National Institutes of Health. ClinicalTrials.gov. Accessed February 12, 2019. https://clinicaltrials.gov

58. Lennon H, Sperrin M, Badrick E, Renehan AG. The obesity paradox in cancer: a review. *Curr Oncol Rep.* 2016;18(9):56.

59. Kwan ML, Chen WY, Kroenke CH, et al. Pre-diagnosis body mass index and survival after breast cancer in the After Breast Cancer Pooling Project. *Breast Cancer Res Treat.* 2012;132(2):729-739.

60. Greenlee H, Unger JM, LeBlanc M, Ramsey S, Hershman DL. Association between body mass index and cancer survival in a pooled analysis of 22 clinical trials. *Cancer Epidemiol Biomarkers Prev.* 2017;26(1): 21-29.

61. Kroenke CH, Neugebauer R, Meyerhardt J, et al. Analysis of body mass index and mortality in patients with colorectal cancer using causal diagrams. *JAMA Oncol.* 2016;2(9):1137-1145.

62. Yabroff KR, Lawrence WF, Clauser S, Davis WW, Brown ML. Burden of illness in cancer survivors: findings from a population-based national sample. *J Natl Cancer Inst.* 2004;96(17):1322-1330.

63. Jain R, Denlinger CS. Incorporating weight management into clinical care for cancer survivors: challenges, opportunities, and future directions. *Obesity (Silver Spring).* 2017;25(suppl 2):S27-S29.

64. Jensen MD, Ryan DH, Apovian CM, et al. 2013 AHA/ACC/TOS guideline for the management of overweight and obesity in adults: a report of the American College of Cardiology/American Heart Association Task Force on Practice Guidelines and The Obesity Society. *J Am Coll Cardiol.* 2014;63:2985-3023.

65. Basen-Engquist K, Alfano CM, Maitin-Shepard M, et al. Agenda for translating physical activity, nutrition, and weight management interventions for cancer survivors into clinical and community practice. *Obesity (Silver Spring).* 2017;25(suppl 2):S9-S22.

66. Antognoli EL, Smith KJ, Mason MJ, et al. Direct observation of weight counselling in primary care: alignment with clinical guidelines. *Clin Obes.* 2014;4(2):69-76.

67. *Cancer Trends Progress Report.* National Cancer Institute, National Institutes of Health, Department of Health and Human Services; 2018.

68. Speck RM, Courneya KS, Masse LC, Duval S, Schmitz KH. An update of controlled physical activity trials in cancer survivors: a systematic review and meta-analysis. *J Cancer Surviv.* 2010;4(2):87-100.

69. Alfano CM, Cheville AL, Mustian K. Developing high-quality cancer rehabilitation programs: a timely need. *Am Soc Clin Oncol Educ Book.* 2016;35:241-249.

70. van der Leeden M, Huijsmans RJ, Geleijn E, et al. Tailoring exercise interventions to comorbidities and treatment-induced adverse effects in patients with early stage breast cancer undergoing chemotherapy: a framework to support clinical decisions. *Disabil Rehabil.* 2018;40(4):486-496.

71. Mijwel S, Backman M, Bolam KA, et al. Highly favorable physiological responses to concurrent resistance and high-intensity interval training during chemotherapy: the OptiTrain breast cancer trial. *Breast Cancer Res Treat.* 2018;169(1):93-103.

72. Wiskemann J, Schmidt ME, Klassen O, et al. Effects of 12-week resistance training during radiotherapy in breast cancer patients. *Scand J Med Sci Sports.* 2017;27(11):1500-1510.

73. Madzima TA, Ormsbee MJ, Schleicher EA, Moffatt RJ, Panton LB. Effects of resistance training and protein supplementation in breast cancer survivors. *Med Sci Sports Exerc.* 2017; 49(7):1283-1292.

74. Singh F, Newton RU, Baker MK, et al. Feasibility of presurgical exercise in men with prostate cancer undergoing prostatectomy. *Integr Cancer Ther.* 2017;16(3):290-299.

Chapter 3 *Energy Balance, Body Composition, and Physical Activity for Cancer Prevention, Treatment, and Survivorship*

55

75. Bourke L, Doll H, Crank H, Daley A, Rosario D, Saxton JM. Lifestyle intervention in men with advanced prostate cancer receiving androgen suppression therapy: a feasibility study. *Cancer Epidemiol Biomarkers Prev.* 2011;20(4):647-657.

76. Santa Mina D, Alibhai SM, Matthew AG, et al. A randomized trial of aerobic versus resistance exercise in prostate cancer survivors. *J Aging Phys Act.* 2013;21(4):455-478.

77. Keilani M, Hasenoehrl T, Baumann L, et al. Effects of resistance exercise in prostate cancer patients: a meta-analysis. *Support Care Cancer.* 2017;25(9):2953-2968.

78. Dawson JK, Dorff TB, Todd Schroeder E, Lane CJ, Gross ME, Dieli-Conwright CM. Impact of resistance training on body composition and metabolic syndrome variables during androgen deprivation therapy for prostate cancer: a pilot randomized controlled trial. *BMC Cancer.* 2018;18(1):368.

79. Singh F, Newton RU, Baker MK, Spry NA, Taaffe DR, Galvao DA. Feasibility and efficacy of presurgical exercise in survivors of rectal cancer scheduled to receive curative resection. *Clin Colorectal Cancer.* 2017;16: 358-365.

80. Duregon F, Vendramin B, Bullo V, et al. Effects of exercise on cancer patients suffering chemotherapy-induced peripheral neuropathy undergoing treatment: a systematic review. *Crit Rev Oncol Hematol.* 2018;121:90-100.

81. Kleckner IR, Kamen C, Gewandter JS, et al. Effects of exercise during chemotherapy on chemotherapy-induced peripheral neuropathy: a multicenter, randomized controlled trial. *Support Care Cancer.* 2018;26(4):1019-1028.

82. Zimmer P, Trebing S, Timmers-Trebing U, et al. Eight-week, multimodal exercise counteracts a progress of chemotherapy-induced peripheral neuropathy and improves balance and strength in metastasized colorectal cancer patients: a randomized controlled trial. *Support Care Cancer.* 2018;26(2):615-624.

83. Mustian KM, Alfano CM, Heckler C, et al. Comparison of pharmaceutical, psychological, and exercise treatments for cancer-related fatigue: a meta-analysis. *JAMA Oncol.* 2017;3(7):961-968.

84. Kelley GA, Kelley KS. Exercise and cancer-related fatigue in adults: a systematic review of previous systematic reviews with meta-analyses. *BMC Cancer.* 2017;17(1):693.

85. Mijwel S, Backman M, Bolam KA, et al. Adding high-intensity interval training to conventional training modalities: optimizing health-related outcomes during chemotherapy for breast cancer: the OptiTrain randomized controlled trial. *Breast Cancer Res Treat.* 2018;168(1):79-93.

86. Buffart LM, Kalter J, Sweegers MG, et al. Effects and moderators of exercise on quality of life and physical function in patients with cancer: an individual patient data meta-analysis of 34 RCTs. *Cancer Treat Rev.* 2017;52:91-104.

87. Baumann FT, Zopf EM, Bloch W. Clinical exercise interventions in prostate cancer patients—a systematic review of randomized controlled trials. *Support Care Cancer.* 2012;20(2):221-233.

88. Campbell KL, Kam JWY, Neil-Sztramko SE, et al. Effect of aerobic exercise on cancer-associated cognitive impairment: a proof-of-concept RCT. *Psychooncology.* 2018;27(1): 53-60.

89. Hartman SJ, Nelson SH, Myers E, et al. Randomized controlled trial of increasing physical activity on objectively measured and self-reported cognitive functioning among breast cancer survivors: The memory and motion study. *Cancer.* 2018;124(1):192-202.

90. Thomas GA, Cartmel B, Harrigan M, et al. The effect of exercise on body composition and bone mineral density in breast cancer survivors taking aromatase inhibitors. *Obesity (Silver Spring)*. 2017;25(2):346-351.

91. Almstedt HC, Grote S, Korte JR, et al. Combined aerobic and resistance training improves bone health of female cancer survivors. *Bone Rep*. 2016;5:274-279.

92. Winters-Stone KM, Dobek J, Nail LM, et al. Impact + resistance training improves bone health and body composition in prematurely menopausal breast cancer survivors: a randomized controlled trial. *Osteoporos Int*. 2013;24(5):1637-1646.

93. Dobek J, Winters-Stone KM, Bennett JA, Nail L. Musculoskeletal changes after 1 year of exercise in older breast cancer survivors. *J Cancer Surviv*. 2014;8:304-311.

94. Kim SH, Seong DH, Yoon SM, et al. The effect on bone outcomes of home-based exercise intervention for prostate cancer survivors receiving androgen deprivation therapy: a pilot randomized controlled trial. *Cancer Nurs*. 2018;41(5):379-388.

95. Scott JM, Nilsen TS, Gupta D, Jones LW. Exercise therapy and cardiovascular toxicity in cancer. *Circulation*. 2018;137(11):1176-1191.

96. Keats MR, Grandy SA, Giacomantonio N, MacDonald D, Rajda M, Younis T. EXercise to prevent AnthrCycline-based Cardio-Toxicity (EXACT) in individuals with breast or hematological cancers: a feasibility study protocol. *Pilot Feasibility Stud*. 2016;2:44.

97. Jacquinot Q, Meneveau N, Chatot M, et al. A phase 2 randomized trial to evaluate the impact of a supervised exercise program on cardiotoxicity at 3 months in patients with HER2 overexpressing breast cancer undergoing adjuvant treatment by trastuzumab: design of the CARDAPAC study. *BMC Cancer*. 2017(1);17:425.

98. Jones LW, Habel LA, Weltzien E, et al. Exercise and risk of cardiovascular events in women with nonmetastatic breast cancer. *J Clin Oncol*. 2016;34(23):2743-2749.

99. Jones LW, Eves ND, Scott JM. Bench-to-bedside approaches for personalized exercise therapy in cancer. *Am Soc Clin Oncol Educ Book*. 2017;37:684-694.

Chapter 3 *Energy Balance, Body Composition, and Physical Activity for Cancer Prevention, Treatment, and Survivorship*

57

Chapter 4
Nutrition Risk Screening and Assessment of the Oncology Patient

Rhone M. Levin, MEd, RDN, CSO, LD. FAND

Oncology treatment can create a physiologic burden that can overwhelm even a healthy person's nutritional reserve. Cancer treatment occurs over a lengthy period, even in early-stage, curative therapy. Treatment is cumulative, with total doses achieved over weeks and months. At the time of diagnosis, a treatment regimen is determined by the oncologist to provide the best outcome for cancer control or cure.

Good nutrition during oncology treatment is fundamental to meeting the nutritional demands that support the recovery process. Even those identified as being at low risk for malnutrition by diagnosis may experience unpredictable barriers to nutrition, lack basic nutrition knowledge, or practice nutrition behaviors that are inappropriate or nonconducive to healing.

Due to the complexity of cancer treatment, all oncology patients should be screened and rescreened throughout treatment for nutrition impact symptoms, clinical characteristics of malnutrition, and symptoms of cachexia and sarcopenia.[1] Nutrition assessment and early intervention that provide an individualized nutrition management plan are most effective in preserving the well-being of the patient with cancer.[2-4] Early intervention is essential, as attempts to reverse severe nutrition depletion or severe malnutrition in the patient with cancer are more challenging and less likely to succeed. The later oncology nutrition care is implemented, the more difficult it is to modify a patient's nutritional status.[5-9]

Effects of Malnutrition on the Patient With Cancer

Both cancer itself and its treatment can lead to malnutrition. Malnutrition has been defined as "a state of nutrition in which a deficiency or excess (or imbalance) of energy, protein, and other nutrients causes measurable adverse effects on tissue/body form (body shape, size, and composition) and function and clinical outcome."[10] The consequences of malnutrition include an impaired immune response, reduced muscle strength, increased fatigue, impaired wound healing, reduced quality of life, reduced response to prescribed oncology treatment, and, lastly, a potential increase in the cost of health care and length of hospital stay.[11] Malnutrition is frequently underreported in the oncology setting, and its presence is often ignored, despite evidence that nutrition intervention that prevents or limits malnutrition can significantly influence treatment schedules, therapeutic efficacy, and even treatment outcomes.[7,12]

Many patients experience anorexia and weight loss prior to cancer diagnosis and are at risk for malnutrition even at their first oncology visit. At the time of diagnosis, 40% to 80% of patients with gastrointestinal (GI), pancreatic, head and neck, and colorectal cancers have already experienced signs of nutritional impairment, even in the early stages of their disease.[13] Weight loss correlates with decreased performance status in a majority of tumor categories, and a weight loss of as little as 6% predicts a reduced response to oncology treatment, reduced survival, and reduced quality of life.[14]

Screening for Malnutrition

Screening for malnutrition leads to early identification of patients who are experiencing malnutrition or who are at risk for malnutrition. Implementation of a screening process is imperative to ensuring proactive nutrition care. The Academy of Nutrition and Dietetics defines nutrition screening as "the process of identifying patients who may have a nutrition diagnosis and benefit from nutrition assessment and intervention by a Registered Dietitian Nutritionist (RDN)."[15]

Malnutrition screening should be conducted on admission to oncology services and then repeated throughout treatment. Commonly, ambulatory cancer centers will use a malnutrition screening tool prior to physician visits: weekly during radiation therapy, every 2 to 3 weeks during chemotherapy, and at each follow-up visit. Facilities should incorporate the malnutrition screening process into their policies and procedures, and results should be documented in the electronic medical record (EMR).

Patients with all cancer types benefit from malnutrition screening and nutrition intervention. Several studies evaluating chemotherapy tolerance in patients with breast,[16] metastatic breast,[17] renal cell,[18] gastric,[19] hepatocellular,[20] and GI and colorectal cancers[21,22] demonstrate that patients with sarcopenia, weight loss, or low body mass are at risk for increased toxicity during cancer treatment and ultimately may receive less treatment than patients with adequate nutrition status. In the case of renal cell carcinoma, dose reductions were observed in 13% of patients, and treatment termination occurred in 21% of patients. In the treatment of nonmetastatic colon cancer, when comparing the sex-specific tertile having the highest muscle mass with the tertile having the lowest muscle mass, patients in the lowest tertile were more likely to experience toxicity and had twice the risk of adverse outcomes and early discontinuation of therapy. Toxicity from radiation treatment can lead to unplanned treatment breaks that result in lower locoregional control and survival rates in patients with head and neck cancer. In these patients, tumor control rate is reduced 1% for every day that the radiation therapy plan is interrupted.[23] It is vital to maintain weight and performance status,

as performance status scores are used in making decisions about treatment modality, amount of treatment, and timing of treatment. Treatment dosage reduction, the holding of treatment, and treatment termination have a negative impact on cancer outcomes.[24-28]

Nutrition Screening Tools

Several associations, including the Academy of Nutrition and Dietetics, the American Society for Parenteral and Enteral Nutrition (ASPEN), and the European Society for Clinical Nutrition and Metabolism (ESPEN), recommend nutrition screening of hospitalized and ambulatory cancer center patients.[11,29-31]

According to the Oncology Nutrition Evidence Analysis Work Group of the Academy of Nutrition and Dietetics, "The screening tool should be a valid identifier of malnutrition risk in adult oncology patients who would benefit from nutrition assessment and intervention by a Registered Dietitian Nutritionist. This tool should be able to detect a measurable adverse effect on body composition, function or clinical outcome."[11]

Tools used to screen patients with cancer should be valid identifiers of patients who are experiencing nutrition impact symptoms and the clinical characteristics of malnutrition. The tool itself should be easy to use, standardized, rapid, noninvasive, valid for the intended population, reliable, sensitive, and cost-effective.[31]

When choosing a malnutrition screening tool, several questions should be considered:

1. Which malnutrition screening tool is valid and reliable for the setting in which it will be used?

2. Which staff will perform the malnutrition screening? Can the screen be performed by health care paraprofessionals, such as a certified nursing assistant?

3. How long does the malnutrition screening process take?

4. When will the malnutrition screening be performed and how frequently?

5. How will the screening results be documented in the EMR?

6. How will referrals generated be sent to the oncology RDN? Is the EMR system capable of sending this referral automatically?

7. Is there adequate staff time for triaging, scheduling, and providing oncology nutrition interventions?

8. Can the results of the valid and reliable malnutrition screening tool be mined and used to document the need for adequate oncology RDN hours (full-time equivalents)?

Many nutrition screening tools are available, and several have been validated for use in hospitalized and ambulatory oncology patients. Screening tools include some or all of these data points: height and weight (or body mass index), weight change over time, presence of nutrition impact symptoms, disease severity, and presence of comorbidities.

Evidence-Based Nutrition Assessment

In the oncology setting, malnutrition is generally considered the presence of undernutrition and changes in body composition that are due to the cancer itself or the impact of the oncology treatment. Patients who are identified during screening as being at risk for malnutrition are referred to an RDN for a nutrition assessment. A nutrition assessment is the collection and analysis of in-depth information about the patient that allows the clinician to formulate a nutrition diagnosis and then develop the most appropriate intervention and follow-up plan.[32] See Chapter 5 for detailed information about assessing the nutritional needs of oncology patients.

In 2013, nutrition assessment interpretations were analyzed by the Evidence Analysis Library Oncology work group in its effort to develop a definition of nutrition assessment that was specific to adult oncology patients. According to the group's findings, an adult oncology nutrition assessment should "characterize and document the presence of, or expected potential for altered nutrition status and nutrition impact symptoms" that may result in a measurable adverse effect on body composition, function, quality of life, or clinical outcome, and may also include indicators of malnutrition.[11]

Identifying Cancer Cachexia

A key feature of malnutrition in the oncology patient is that it may or may not be associated with cancer cachexia syndrome. Up to 80% of patients with advanced cancer may be diagnosed with cancer cachexia.[33] Cancer cachexia has been defined as "a multifactorial syndrome characterized by an ongoing loss of skeletal muscle mass (with or without loss of fat mass) that cannot be fully reversed by conventional nutritional support and leads to progressive functional impairment."[2]

Cancer cachexia is indicated as a factor in the cause of death in 30% to 50% of all cancer patients.[8] The pathophysiology of cachexia is characterized by a negative protein and energy balance driven by reduced food intake or abnormal metabolism, or both. Regardless of the presence of cachexia, it is important to address the direct and indirect causes of decreased intake and intervene to address the factors and behaviors that can be manipulated. Key features to be assessed and any changes measured over time include anorexia, reduced food intake, catabolic drivers, and muscle mass and strength. There are three stages of cancer cachexia: precachexia, cachexia, and refractory cachexia (which may occur in the last 3 months of life).[2] See Chapter 3 for additional detail on diagnosis and criteria for defining cachexia, and the three stages of cancer cachexia (Figure 3.2).

Malnutrition and the Nutrition Care Process

The landmark consensus statement by the Academy of Nutrition and Dietetics and ASPEN, released simultaneously in May 2012 in both the *Journal of the Academy of Nutrition and Dietetics* and the *Journal of Parenteral and Enteral Nutrition*, proffers the clinical characteristics on which to base a nutrition assessment and diagnose malnutrition in adults.[34,35] The recommendations provided in this statement apply to all adult patients, including oncology patients. Interpretation specific to the oncology patient may be useful in guiding nutrition assessments and oncology nutrition interventions. The diagnostic nomenclature of the etiologically based inflammatory response in the definition of malnutrition incorporates the current understanding of the role of the inflammatory response on the incidence, progression, and resolution of disease. A patient's chief complaint and past medical history are evaluated by an RDN to identify the presence or absence of inflammation.

Box 4.1 provides oncology-specific guidance through the five domains of the Nutrition Assessment portion (step 1) of the Academy of Nutrition and Dietetics Nutrition Care Process and identification of malnutrition characteristics.

Box 4.1
Oncology-Related Nutrition Assessment (Based on the Five Domains of Nutrition Assessment as Part of the Nutrition Care Process)[a,2,7,14,36-46]

1. Food- and nutrition-related history

Diet history   Ask about:

- food records in the setting of the cancer treatment cycle (how it changes across the cycle)
- current portion size compared to usual intake
- patterns of meals and snacks
- use of medical nutrition foods (eg, shakes, smoothies, bars)
- use of alcohol
- food allergies, intolerances, or aversions
- foods that are currently tolerated

- use of a restricted diet, which may be liberalized in the context of overall decreased intake (eg, medical nutrition therapy for hypercholesterolemia, obesity, irritable bowel, diabetes)
- use of cancer prevention strategies potentially not appropriate in treatment (eg, the Gonzalez Regimen or a raw food diet, which may result in unintentional reduction in energy intake)

(continued)

---

[a] The Nutrition Care Process is a systematic approach to providing high-quality nutrition care. It consists of four distinct, interrelated steps: (1) Nutrition Assessment, (2) Nutrition Diagnosis, (3) Nutrition Intervention, and (4) Nutrition Monitoring/Evaluation (www.ncpro.org/nutition-care-process). Step 1, Nutrition Assessment, is organized into five domains: Food- and Nutrition-Related History; Anthropometric Measurements; Biochemical Data, Medical Tests, and Procedures; Nutrition-Focused Physical Findings; and Client History.

Box 4.1

Oncology-Related Nutrition Assessment (Based on the Five Domains of Nutrition Assessment as Part of the Nutrition Care Process)[a] *(continued)*

1. Food- and nutrition-related history *(continued)*

Medication history	Ask about: ■ the amount and frequency of prescribed medications and over-the-counter medications, including:

	■ narcotics		■ digestive enzymes
	■ antiemetics		■ vitamin, herbal, alternative, or natural botanical products
	■ steroids		■ probiotics and fiber supplements
	■ stool softeners and laxatives		

Ask about the use of medical marijuana or appetite stimulants.

Patient efforts	Ask about current strategies used by the patient to overcome difficulty with nourishment. Assess "what is working" and patient willingness to modify behaviors.

2. Anthropometric measurements[2,7,14,36,37]

Measurements	Measure, categorize, and assess the following:

	■ height, current weight, body mass index (BMI)		■ grip strength values compared to norms (also plot individual trend over time)
	■ usual weight and weight changes		■ triceps skinfold and mid-upper-arm circumference measured over time
	■ adjusted weight, if obese		

Unintended weight loss	Obtain baseline weight (defined as usual body weight taken from medical records). If not available, use the weight taken when admitted to oncology service, or if that is not available, use the patient's self-report of most recent usual weight. Assess for any recent weight loss, including before diagnosis and since diagnosis. Any weight loss has potential significance and may be associated with poor outcomes. Evaluate rate of weight loss over specified time frames. ■ For elderly patients, there is an association between increased mortality and BMI less than 20 or a weight loss of 5% in 30 days or any further weight loss after meeting these criteria. ■ For obese patients, sarcopenic obesity (decreased muscle mass masked by a mantle of fat) has a negative prognostic value. The shortest survival times are found among obese patients with sarcopenic weight loss. Identify the presence of precachexia, cachexia, and sarcopenia.

(continued)

Box 4.1

Oncology-Related Nutrition Assessment (Based on the Five Domains of Nutrition Assessment as Part of the Nutrition Care Process)[a] *(continued)*

3. Biochemical data, medical tests, and procedures [2,38-41]

Biochemical data	Assess for the following in the setting of chemotherapy, radiation, and biotherapy:

- hydration status
- electrolytes
- white blood cell count, red blood cell count, absolute neutrophil count
- anemias (ie, folate and vitamin B12)

- calcium
- liver function
- renal function
- blood glucose ranges

Assess inflammatory status with C-reactive protein (CRP); CRP ≥10 mg/L can be used as an indicator of inflammation, which determines the severity of each malnutrition characteristic.

Monitor trends across time and be aware that biochemical values may be altered due to oncology treatment (eg, glucose may be elevated due to steroid use; white blood cell count may be elevated or reduced due to treatment and medications; and liver function tests may be elevated due to chemotherapy).

Tests and procedures	Obtain bioimpedence results to evaluate lean body mass and changes over time.

Obtain computed tomography scans at the level of the third lumbar vertebra to evaluate the volume of muscle mass and changes in muscle volume over time.

Obtain gastrointestinal (GI) function tests (eg, gastric emptying, swallowing evaluations, stool elastase test).

Note: Evidence demonstrates that inflammatory status affects hepatic proteins (eg, albumin) and renders them inaccurate for nutrition-related decision-making. Currently, neither the Academy of Nutrition and Dietetics nor the American Society for Parenteral and Enteral Nutrition proposes any specific protein or hepatic protein markers for nutrition diagnostic purposes. However, the combination of CRP and albumin can be used to measure systemic inflammatory response and provide prognostic value, as in the Glasgow Prognostic Score and Modified Glasgow Prognostic Score.

(continued)

Box 4.1
Oncology-Related Nutrition Assessment (Based on the Five Domains of Nutrition Assessment as Part of the Nutrition Care Process)[a] *(continued)*

4. Nutrition-focused physical findings [7,42,43,46]

Nutrition impact symptoms	Identify nutrition impact symptoms that impede nutrition intake, digestion, absorption, or utilization, including, but not limited to: ■ anorexia ■ cachexia ■ muscle wasting ■ dysphagia ■ xerostomia ■ taste and smell changes ■ mucositis and stomatitis ■ nausea and vomiting ■ esophagitis ■ diarrhea ■ early satiety ■ gastroparesis ■ malabsorption ■ constipation ■ shortness of breath ■ dehydration
Vital signs	Check oxygenation, pulse, blood pressure, and temperature.
Nutrient deficiencies	Inspect for nutrient deficiencies by checking pallor, stomatitis, glossitis, anemia, quality of hair (if present), and appearance of nails (may be altered by chemotherapy).
Appearance	Check for observed cachectic muscle loss, observed loss of fat stores, sunken eyes, and presence of generalized edema (anasarca). ■ Reduced muscle mass, or sarcopenia, whether age-related, from oncology treatment, or from undernutrition, is an independent predictor of loss of independence, immobility, and mortality. It is associated with greater toxicity during cancer therapy. Assess grip strength and changes in grip strength over time in the individual patient. Ask about changes in functional status that may be described as reduced strength. ■ Loss of subcutaneous fat may occur with or without the presence of cachexia. If cachexia is present, lipolysis may occur even in the setting of adequate energy intake. ■ Localized or generalized fluid accumulation (edema) may mask weight loss. Track changes in the presence and severity of edema over time. Monitor intravenous fluid provision, as volume and frequency may alter weight status. Monitor for medications that promote fluid retention (eg, steroids). Monitor frequency of interventions used to reduce fluid accumulation (eg, tapping of fluid, drains, medications such as diuretics).

(continued)

Box 4.1
Oncology-Related Nutrition Assessment (Based on the Five Domains of Nutrition Assessment as Part of the Nutrition Care Process)[a] (continued)

4. Nutrition-Focused Physical Findings (continued)

Dermatologic	Assess for: - stomatitis - angular cheilitis - erythema from chemotherapy - presence and healing status of surgical wounds, radiation burns, and other wounds - skin turgor
Head and neck	Assess for: - pain - movement of head, neck, and face - presence of dysphagia for solids, dry foods, pills, and liquids of varying consistency - "lump" sensation after swallowing - obstruction or compression of esophagus - swallowing adequacy
Intraoral cavity	Assess for: - pain - motor strength for jaw movement and chewing, trismus - oral manipulation of a food bolus and tongue range of motion - oral ulcers, mucositis, infection or thrush, stomatitis - dental repair or recent edentulous status, fit of dentures, saliva quality and quantity - perceived tolerance of temperature, acidity, and texture - quality of taste that is present, absent, or altered
Abdomen	Assess for: - pain - bowel function and presence or absence of bowel sounds - frequency, quantity, and characteristic of stool, including steatorrhea - presence and health of a feeding tube site - frequency and quantity of urination - symptoms of dehydration - digestion (eg, of fat, fiber, lactose, and other food components) - digestion of pills or medication - GI symptoms stimulated by food intake and timing of the intake, including bloating gassiness, gastroparesis; reflux - presence of ascites (consider using girth measurements to monitor changes in abdominal ascites)

(continued)

5. Client history: personal, medical/health/family, and social[44,45]

Personal	Review cancer diagnosis and treatment regimen, anticipated side effects, timing of the treatment cycle, and timing of the side effects.
Medical/ health/ family	Assess for age over 65 years, other medical history, and comorbidities. Note that elderly patients with cancer are being assessed with geriatric assessment tools for frailty and anticipated ability to tolerate the rigors of chemotherapy and survival. Nutritional competency is included in these assessments.
Social	Take a social history, including family setting, caregiver support system, food security, ability to obtain and prepare food, religious and cultural factors, financial concerns, and level of literacy.
Comparative standards	Functional and quality-of-life assessments may be useful for assessing a patient's status and comparing function and quality of life over time. Examples include the Karnofsky Performance Status, the Eastern Cooperative Oncology Group Status, and the Functional Assessment of Cancer Therapy scales.

Clinical Characteristics of Malnutrition in the Oncology Patient

The Academy of Nutrition and Dietetics and ASPEN consensus statement provides guidelines and clinical characteristics to support a diagnosis of malnutrition in the context of acute illness or injury, chronic disease, and social or environmental circumstances.[34,35] It also distinguishes between severe malnutrition (inflammation is present) and nonsevere malnutrition (inflammation is absent). Regarding the guidelines' distinction between acute illness or injury and chronic disease, it is important to note that patients with cancer may experience "acute illness" at certain points of time, such as during rigorous treatment weeks, following oncologic surgery, following biotherapy treatment, and during the last weeks of head and neck or GI radiation therapy (and for weeks after radiation is completed). Patients who are in long-term and maintenance therapy may be described as experiencing "chronic disease" (a disease or condition that lasts 3 months or longer).

For a diagnosis of malnutrition, two or more of the six clinical characteristics described in Table 4.1 on pages 68 and 69 must be present, and documentation regarding all six characteristics represents a complete nutrition assessment. Upon review by the Oncology Nutrition Evidence Analysis Work Group, the characteristics listed in the consensus statement were accepted as appropriate for use in oncology patients and may form the outline of a nutrition assessment.[11,34,35]

Table 4.1
Clinical Characteristics That Support a Diagnosis of Malnutrition[a,34,35,47-56]

Clinical Characteristic[47,48,51]	Malnutrition in Acute Illness or Injury				
	Nonsevere (moderate) malnutrition		Severe malnutrition		
Energy intake Malnutrition is the result of inadequate food and nutrient intake or assimilation; thus, recent intake compared to estimated requirements is a primary criterion defining malnutrition. The clinician may obtain or review the food and nutrition history, estimate optimum energy needs, compare them with estimates of energy consumed, and report inadequate intake as a percentage of estimated energy requirements over time.	<75% of estimated energy requirement for >7 days		≤50% of estimated energy requirement for ≥5 days		
Interpretation of weight loss The clinician may evaluate weight in light of other clinical findings, including the presence of underhydration or overhydration. The clinician may assess weight change over time reported as a percentage of weight lost from baseline.	%	Time	%	Time	
	1-2	1 wk	>2	1 wk	
	5	1 mo	>5	1 mo	
	7.5	3 mo	>7.5	3 mo	
Physical findings[51-53] Malnutrition typically results in changes to the physical exam. The clinician may perform a physical exam and document any one of the physical exam findings below as an indicator of malnutrition.					
Body fat Loss of subcutaneous fat (eg, orbital, triceps, fat overlying the ribs).	Mild		Moderate		
Muscle mass Muscle loss (eg, wasting of the temples [temporalis muscle]; clavicles [pectoralis and deltoids]; shoulders [deltoids]; interosseous muscles; scapula [latissimus dorsi, trapezious, deltoids]; thigh [quadriceps], and calf [gastrocnemius]).	Mild		Moderate		
Fluid accumulation The clinician may evaluate generalized or localized fluid accumulation evident on exam (extremities; vulvar/scrotal edema or ascites). Weight loss is often masked by generalized fluid retention (edema) and weight gain may be observed.	Mild		Moderate to severe		
Reduced grip strength Consult normative standards supplied by the manufacturer of the measurement device.	N/A[b]		Measurably reduced		

[a] A minimum of two of the six characteristics above is recommended for diagnosis of either severe or non-severe malnutrition. Height and weight should be measured rather than estimated to determine body mass index. Usual weight should be obtained in order to determine the percentage and to interpret the significance of weight loss. Basic indicators of nutritional status such as body weight, weight change, and appetite may substantively improve with refeeding in the absence of inflammation. Refeeding and/or nutrition support may stabilize but not significantly improve nutrition parameters in the presence of inflammation. The National Center for Health Statistics defines *chronic* as a disease/condition lasting 3 months or longer.[12] Serum proteins such as albumin and prealbumin are not included as defining characteristics of malnutrition because recent evidence analysis shows that serum levels of these proteins do not change in response to changes in nutrient intake.[22,23,53-56]

Malnutrition in Chronic Illness				Malnutrition in Social or Environmental Circumstances			
Nonsevere (moderate) malnutrition		**Severe malnutrition**		**Nonsevere (moderate) malnutrition**		**Severe malnutrition**	
<75% of estimated energy requirement for ≥ 1 month		≤75% of estimated energy requirement for ≥ 1 month		<75% of estimated energy requirement for ≥ 3 months		≤50% of estimated energy requirement for ≥ 1 month	
%	**Time**	**%**	**Time**	**%**	**Time**	**%**	**Time**
5	1 mo	>5	1 mo	5	1 mo	>5	1 mo
7.5	3 mo	>7.5	3 mo	7.5	3 mo	>7.5	3 mo
10	6 mo	>10	6 mo	10	6 mo	>10	6 mo
20	1 y	>20	1 y	20	1 y	>20	1 y
Mild		Severe		Mild		Severe	
Mild		Severe		Mild		Severe	
Mild		Severe		Mild		Severe	
N/A[b]		Measurably reduced		N/A[b]		Measurably reduced	

[b] N/A=not applicable.

Reproduced with permission from White JV, Guenter P, Jensen G, Malone A, Schofield M; Academy Malnutrition Work Group; A.S.P.E.N. Malnutrition Task Force; A.S.P.E.N. Board of Directors. Consensus statement of the Academy of Nutriton and Dietetics/ American Society for Parenteral and Enteral Nutrition characteristics recommended for the identification and documentation of adult malnutrition (undernutrition). *J Acad Nutr Diet.* 112(5):730-738. doi:10.1016/j.jand.2012.03.012. See reference 34.

Weight Management in Early Oncology Treatment

The management of overweight and obesity during cancer treatment is an emerging area of importance. Patients with early-stage breast and prostate cancers, which are usually not associated with involuntary weight loss, may benefit from healthy weight control even during cancer treatment. The 2012 American Cancer Society Nutrition and Physical Activity Guidelines for Cancer Survivors introduced a new component of nutrition assessment and intervention for cancer survivors. These guidelines state, "For cancer survivors who are overweight or obese and who choose to pursue weight loss, there appears to be no contraindication to modest weight loss (ie, a maximum of 2 pounds per week) during treatment, as long as the treating oncologist approves, weight loss is monitored closely, and it does not interfere with treatment."[46] The evidence suggests that overweight and obesity are detrimental to long-term survival of some cancer patients; therefore, the oncology RDN should consider this concern and, when appropriate, transition patients to weight-management nutrition interventions. The oncology RDN should be involved in the patient's decision-making process regarding appropriateness of weight control in relation to the cancer diagnosis, oncology treatment type, type of weight-control regimen, and timing of weight-control intervention. The oncology RDN should supervise the adequacy of nutritional status during the intervention. All cancer survivors should have access to information about healthy weight management and intervention after cancer therapy has concluded as part of their survivorship plan.

References

1. Bozzetti F, SCRINIO Working Group. Screening the nutritional status in oncology: a preliminary report on 1,000 outpatients. *Support Care Cancer*. 2009;17(3):279-284. doi:10.1007/s00520-008-0476-3

2. Fearon K, Strasser F, Anker SD, et al. Definition and classification of cancer cachexia: an international consensus. *Lancet Oncol*. 2011;12(5):489-495. doi:10.1016/S1470-2045(10)70218-7

3. Ravasco P. Nutritional approaches in cancer: relevance of individualized counseling and supplementation. *Nutrition*. 2015;31(4):603-604. doi:10.1016/j.nut.2014.12.001

4. Ravasco P, Moteiro-Grillo I, Camilo M. Individualized nutrition intervention is of major benefit to colorectal cancer patients: long-term follow-up of a randomized controlled trial of nutritional therapy. *Clin Nutr*. 2012;96(6):1346-1353. doi:10.3945/ajcn.111.018838

5. Tong H, Isenring E, Yates P. The prevalence of nutrition impact symptoms and their relationship to quality of life and clinical outcomes in medical oncology patients. *Support Care Cancer*. 2009;17(1):83-90. doi:10.1007/s00520-008-0472-7

6. Isenring EA, Teleni L. Nutritional counseling and nutritional supplements: a cornerstone of multidisciplinary cancer care for cachectic patients. *Curr Opin Support Palliat Care*. 2013;7(4):390-395. doi:10.1097/SPC.0000000000000016

7. Fearon KCH. The 2011 ESPEN Arvid Wretlind lecture: cancer cachexia: the potential impact of translational research on patient-focused outcomes. *Clin Nutr*. 2012;31(5):577-582. doi:10.1016/j.clnu.2012.06.012

8. Aapro M, Arends J, Bozzetti F, et al. Early recognition of malnutrition and cachexia in the cancer patient: a position paper of a European School of Oncology Task Force. *Ann Oncol*. 2014;25(8). doi:10.1093/annonc/mdu085

9. Fearon K, Arends J, Baracos V. Understanding the mechanisms and treatment options in cancer cachexia. *Nat Rev Clin Oncol*. 2012;10(2):90-99. doi:10.1038/nrclinonc.2012.209

10. Stratton RJ, Hackston A, Longmore D, et al. Malnutrition in hospital outpatients and inpatients: prevalence, concurrent validity and ease of use of the "malnutrition universal screening tool" ("MUST") for adults. *Br J Nutr*. 2004;92(5):799-808. doi:10.1079/BJN20041258

11. Thompson KL, Elliott L, Fuchs-Tarlovsky V, Levin RM, Voss AC, Piemonte T. Oncology evidence-based nutrition practice guideline for adults. *J Acad Nutr Diet*. 2017;117(2):297-310. doi:10.1016/j.jand.2016.05.010

12. Santarpia L, Contaldo F, Pasanisi F. Nutritional screening and early treatment of malnutrition in cancer patients. *J Cachexia Sarcopenia Muscle*. 2011;2(1):27-35. doi:10.1007/s13539-011-0022-x

13. Muscaritoli M, Lucia S, Farcomeni A, et al. Prevalence of malnutrition in patients at first medical oncology visit: the PreMiO study. *Oncotarget*. 2017;8(45):79884-79896. doi:10.18632/oncotarget.20168

14. Dewys WD, Begg C, Lavin PT, et al. Prognostic effect of weight loss prior to chemotherapy in cancer patients. *Am J Med*. 1980;69(4):491-497. doi:10.1016/S0149-2918(05)80001-3

15. Field LB, Hand RK. Differentiating malnutrition screening and assessment: a nutrition care process perspective. *J Acad Nutr Diet*. 2015;115(5):824-828. doi:10.1016/j.jand.2014.11.010

16. Shachar SS, Deal AM, Weinberg M, et al. Body composition as a predictor of toxicity in patients receiving anthracycline and taxane-based chemotherapy for early-stage breast cancer. *Clin Cancer Res*. 2017;23(14):3537-3543. doi:10.1158/1078-0432.CCR-16-2266

17. Prado CMM, Baracos VE, McCargar LJ, et al. Sarcopenia as a determinant of chemotherapy toxicity and time to tumor progression in metastatic breast cancer patients receiving capecitabine treatment. *Clin Cancer Res*. 2009;15(8):2920-2926. doi:10.1158/1078-0432.CCR-08-2242

18. Antoun S, Baracos V, Birdsell L, et al. Low body mass index and sarcopenia associated with dose-limiting toxicity of sorafenib in patients with renal cell carcinoma. *Ann Oncol*. 2010;21(8):1594-1598. doi:10.1093/annonc/mdp605

19. Aoyama T, Yoshikawa T, Shirai J, et al. Body weight loss after surgery is an independent risk factor for continuation of S-1 adjuvant chemotherapy for gastric cancer. *Ann Surg Oncol*. 2013;20(6):2000-2006. doi:10.1245/s10434-012-2776-6

20. Mir O, Coriat R, Blanchet B, et al. Sarcopenia predicts early dose-limiting toxicities and pharmacokinetics of sorafenib in patients with hepatocellular carcinoma. *PLoS One.* 2012;7(5). doi:10.1371/journal.pone.0037563

21. Prado CMM, Baracos VE, McCargar LJ, et al. Body composition as an independent determinant of 5-fluorouracil-based chemotherapy toxicity. *Clin Cancer Res.* 2007;13(11):3264-3268. doi:10.1158/1078-0432.CCR-06-3067

22. Cespedes Feliciano EM, Lee VS, Prado CM, et al. Muscle mass at the time of diagnosis of nonmetastatic colon cancer and early discontinuation of chemotherapy, delays, and dose reductions on adjuvant FOLFOX: The C-SCANS study. *Cancer.* 2017;123(24):4868-4877. doi:10.1002/cncr.30950

23. Russo G, Haddad R, Posner M, Machtay M. Radiation treatment breaks and ulcerative mucositis in head and neck cancer. *Oncologist.* 2008;13(8):886-898. doi:10.1634/theoncologist.2008-0024

24. Ryan AM, Power DG, Daly L, Cushen SJ, Ní Bhuachalla E, Prado CM. Cancer-associated malnutrition, cachexia and sarcopenia: the skeleton in the hospital closet 40 years later. *Proc Nutr Soc.* 2016;75(2):199-211. doi:10.1017/S002966511500419X

25. Muscaritoli M, Molfino A, Lucia S, Rossi Fanelli F. Cachexia: a preventable comorbidity of cancer. A T.A.R.G.E.T. approach. *Crit Rev Oncol Hematol.* 2015;94(2):251-259. doi:10.1016/j.critrevonc.2014.10.014

26. Fukuda Y, Yamamoto K, Hirao M, et al. Prevalence of malnutrition among gastric cancer patients undergoing gastrectomy and optimal preoperative nutritional support for preventing surgical site infections. *Ann Surg Oncol.* 2015;22(suppl 3):S778-S785. doi:10.1245/s10434-015-4820-9

27. Kabata P, Jastrzębski T, Kąkol M, et al. Preoperative nutritional support in cancer patients with no clinical signs of malnutrition—prospective randomized controlled trial. *Support Care Cancer.* 2015;23(2):365-370. doi:10.1007/s00520-014-2363-4

28. Gangadharan A, Choi SE, Hassan A, et al. Protein calorie malnutrition, nutritional intervention and personalized cancer care. *Oncotarget.* 2017;8(14):24009-24030. doi:10.18632/oncotarget.15103

29. Cederholm T, Jensen GL, Correia MITD, et al. GLIM criteria for the diagnosis of malnutrition—a consensus report from the global clinical nutrition community. *Clin Nutr.* 2019;38(1):1-9. doi:10.1016/j.clnu.2018.08.002

30. Arends J, Baracos V, Bertz H, et al. ESPEN expert group recommendations for action against cancer-related malnutrition. *Clin Nutr.* 2017;36(5):1187-1196. doi:10.1016/j.clnu.2017.06.017

31. Skipper A, Ferguson M, Thompson K, Castellanos VH, Porcari J. Nutrition screening tools. *J Parenter Enter Nutr.* 2012;36(3):292-298. doi:10.1177/0148607111414023

32. Correia MITD. Nutrition screening vs nutrition assessment: what's the difference? *Nutr Clin Pract.* 2018;33(1):62-72. doi:10.1177/0884533617719669

33. Fox KM, Brooks JM, Gandra SR, Markus R, Chiou CF. Estimation of cachexia among cancer patients based on four definitions. *J Oncol.* 2009;2009:article ID 693458. doi:10.1155/2009/693458

34. White JV, Guenter P, Jensen G, et al. Consensus statement of the Academy of Nutrition and Dietetics/American Society for Parenteral and Enteral Nutrition: characteristics recommended for the identification and documentation of adult malnutrition (undernutrition). *J Acad Nutr Diet.* 2012;112(5)730-738. doi:10.1016/j.jand.2012.03.012

35. White JV, Guenter P, Jensen G, et al. Consensus statement: Academy of Nutrition and Dietetics and American Society for Parenteral and Enteral Nutrition: characteristics recommended for the identification and documentation of adult malnutrition (undernutrition). *JPEN J Parenter Enter Nutr.* 2012;36(3):275-283. doi:10.1177/0148607112440285

36. Grabowski DC, Ellis JE. High body mass index does not predict mortality in older people: analysis of the Longitudinal Study of Aging. *J Am Geriatr Soc.* 2001;49(7):968-979. doi:10.1046/j.1532-5415.2001.49189.x

37. Prado CM, Cushen SJ, Orsso CE, Ryan AM. Sarcopenia and cachexia in the era of obesity: clinical and nutritional impact. *Proc Nutr Soc.* 2016;75(2):188-198. doi:10.1017/S0029665115004279

38. Thibault R, Pichard C. The evaluation of body composition: a useful tool for clinical practice. *Ann Nutr Metab*. 2012;60(1):6-16. doi:10.1159/000334879

39. Kazemi-Bajestani SMR, Mazurak VC, Baracos V. Computed tomography-defined muscle and fat wasting are associated with cancer clinical outcomes. *Semin Cell Dev Biol*. 2016;54:2-10. doi:10.1016/j.semcdb.2015.09.001

40. Laird BJ, Kaasa S, McMillan DC, et al. Prognostic factors in patients with advanced cancer: a comparison of clinicopathological factors and the development of an inflammation-based prognostic system. *Clin Cancer Res*. 2013;19(19):5456-5464. doi:10.1158/1078-0432.CCR-13-1066

41. Proctor MJ, Morrison DS, Talwar D, et al. An inflammation-based prognostic score (mGPS) predicts cancer survival independent of tumour site: a Glasgow Inflammation Outcome Study. *Br J Cancer*. 2011;104(4):726-734. doi:10.1038/sj.bjc.6606087

42. Kubrak C, Olson K, Baracos VE. The Head and Neck Symptom Checklist©: an instrument to evaluate nutrition impact symptoms effect on energy intake and weight loss. *Support Care Cancer*. 2013;21(11):3127-3136. doi:10.1007/s00520-013-1870-z

43. Bozzetti F. Forcing the vicious circle: sarcopenia increases toxicity, decreases response to chemotherapy and worsens with chemotherapy. *Ann Oncol*. 2017;28(9):2107-2118. doi:10.1093/annonc/mdx271

44. O'Donovan A, Mohile SG, Leech M. Expert consensus panel guidelines on geriatric assessment in oncology. *Eur J Cancer Care (Engl)*. 2015;24(4):574-589. doi:10.1111/ecc.12302

45. Wilkinson R, Arensberg ME, Hickson M, Dwyer JT. Frailty prevention and treatment: why registered dietitian nutritionists need to take charge. *J Acad Nutr Diet*. 2017;117(7):1001-1009. doi:10.1016/j.jand.2016.06.367

46. Rock CL, Doyle C, Demark-Wahnefried W, et al. Nutrition and physical activity guidelines for cancer survivors. *CA Cancer J Clin*. 2012;62(4):242-274. doi:10.3322/caac.2114246

47. Kondrup J. Can food intake in hosptials be improved? *Clin Nutr*. 2001;20(suppl 1):153-160.

48. Blackburn GL, Bistrian BR, Maini BS, Schlamm HT, Smith MF. Nutritonal and metabolic assessment of the hospitalized patient. *JPEN J Parenter Enteral Nutr*. 1977;1(1):11-22.

49. Klein S, Kinney J, Jeejeebohy K, et al. Nutrition suport in cllinical practice: review of published data and recommendations for ruture research directions. National Institutes of Health, American Society for Parenteral and Enteral Nutrtiion and American Society for Clinical Nutrition. *JPEN J Parenter Enteral Nutr*. 1977;21:133-136.

50. Rosenbaum K, Wang J, Pierson RN, Kotler DP. Time-dependent variation in weight and body composition in health adults. *JPEN J Parenter Enteral Nutr*. 2000;24(2):52-55.

51. Keys A. Chronic undernutrition and starvation with notes on protein deficiency. *JAMA*. 1948;138(7):500-511.

52. Sacks GS, Dearman K, Replogle WH, Cora VL, Meeks M, Canada T. Use of subjective global assessment to identify nutrition-associated complications and death in long-term care facility residents. *J Am Coll Nutr*. 2000;19(5):570-577.

53. Norman K, Stobaus N, Gonzalez MC, Schulzke J-D, Pirlich M. Hand grip strength: outcome predictor and marker of nutritional status. *Clin Nutr*. 2011;30(2):135-142.

54. Hagan JC. Acute and chronic diseases. In: Mulner RM, ed. *Encyclopedia of Health Services Research*. Vol 1: Sage; 2009:25.

55. Academy of Nutrition and Dietetics Evidence Analysis Library. Does serum prealbumin correlate with weight loss in four models of prolonged protein-energy restriction: anorexia nervosa, non-malabsorptive gastric partitioning bariatric surgery, calorie-restricted diets or starvation. Accessed April 30, 2020. www.adaevidencelibrary.com/conclusion.cfm?conclusion_statement_id=251313.&highlight=prealbumin&home=1

56. Academy of Nutrition and Dietetics Evidence Analysis Library. Does serum prealbumin correlate with nitrogen balance? Accessed April 30, 2020. www.adaevidencelibrary.com/conclusion.cfm?conclusion_statement_id=251313&highlight=prealbumin&home=1

Chapter 5
Nutritional Needs of the Adult Oncology Patient

Kathryn K. Hamilton, MA, RDN, CSO, CDN, FAND

The nutritional status of individuals diagnosed with cancer influences their disease prognosis, treatment tolerance, and quality of life. Medical nutrition therapy provided by a registered dietitian nutritionist (RDN) uses various strategies to improve or maintain nutritional status, manage side effects of cancer treatments, and improve functional status, including determining the most appropriate nutrition prescription for meeting the patient's needs.

These interventions, which are documented as part of the Nutrition Care Process, are evidence-based or evidence-informed and identify nutritional needs of non–critically ill and critically ill adults. This chapter reviews current recommendations to measure and estimate the nutritional needs of adult patients with cancer.

Metabolic Changes Associated With Cancer

Evidence for observed variation in metabolic states for different cancer diagnoses is limited, with several of the largest studies demonstrating slight increases in energy expenditures in select oncology patient populations but other individuals with cancer measuring similarly to the healthy control population.[1,2] ESPEN guidelines on nutrition in cancer patients published in 2016 describe the difficulty in predicting the metabolic rate for this patient population due to differences in individual metabolism, cancer diagnoses, anticancer treatment effects, and the extent of inflammation present.[1,3] Cancer both causes and is affected by inflammation. The effects of inflammation contribute to the development and progression of cancer and can alter nutritional requirements resulting in "metabolic derangements."[4] This phenomenon is largely driven by the presence of cytokines and will continue as long as the inflammation is present. Systemic inflammation also impacts macronutrient metabolism as outlined in Box 5.1. For some individuals with cancer, when the severity or persistence of inflammation results in a decrease in lean body mass causing functional impairment, it is considered disease-related malnutrition with inflammation or cachexia.[1,5] The inflammatory process may limit the effectiveness of nutrition interventions and the resulting malnutrition may further compromise the clinical response to anticancer treatment.

For this reason, in chronic disease-related malnutrition with inflammation (cachexia) successful nutrition intervention must involve addressing both the underlying cancer and the individual's nutritional needs.[6,7]

Box 5.1
Effects of Systemic Inflammation on Macronutrient Metabolism[1]

Protein metabolism: changes in protein synthesis and degradation, a loss of fat and muscle mass, and an increase in the production of acute-phase proteins, such as C-reactive protein

Carbohydrate metabolism: increased insulin resistance and impaired glucose tolerance

Lipid metabolism: maintained or increased lipid oxidation, particularly in the presence of weight loss

Body Composition Changes Associated With Cancer

Individuals with cancer are at increased risk for loss of muscle mass resulting from two conditions: sarcopenia (an age-related muscle breakdown) and cachexia.[1,8] This muscle depletion has been shown to decrease quality of life and negatively affect morbidity from cancer treatments through postoperative complications, cancer treatment toxicities, and mortality. Additional information on sarcopenia and cachexia-related muscle loss can be found in Chapter 4.

Several studies have attempted to differentiate and describe energy expenditures among the cancer types. In a large study looking at resting energy expenditure (REE)—particularly measured REE (mREE) and predicted REE (pREE)—in people with newly diagnosed cancer, approximately 40% were found to be hypermetabolic, 50% were found to be normometabolic, and 10% were found to be hypometabolic; however, it is important to recognize that the control group had individuals in the hypermetabolic (25%), normometabolic (50%), and hypometabolic (25%) groups too, thereby underscoring the controversy and difficulty predicting energy requirements in this population.[2,9]

While recognizing that individual energy needs fall along a spectrum, these studies and others have identified people with pancreatic, gastric, bile duct, kidney, adrenal, non–small cell lung, and head and neck cancers as being hypermetabolic, and those with breast, colorectal, and bladder cancers as normometabolic or not statistically significantly different from the control group.[1,2,9-13]

Estimation of each cancer patient's nutritional needs is based on anthropometric data as well as physical assessment and observation, and the clinician should assess a patient's needs and then reassess them at regular intervals, based on achievement of predetermined goals. The ESPEN Guidelines on Nutrition in Cancer patients rate the level of evidence for energy expenditure recommendations in cancer survivors as "low," not because the evidence is perceived as inaccurate but because it is lacking.[1] More research is needed to identify energy expenditures related to individual types of cancer and factors that affect those expenditures.

Research results have been mixed when evaluating the energy expenditure in individuals with advanced cancer. Some studies find energy needs to be higher, and some have reported lower energy needs estimations. Metastatic cancer to the liver is estimated to cause an increase in energy requirements due to higher than normal energetic demands of the liver.[14] Explanations offered for findings of reduced energy expenditures in the presence of stage IV disease involved a difference in physical activity, cancer treatment, and the fact that those with earlier-stage disease likely have more metabolically active tissue.[2,9] These conflicting results indicate the need for more study.

In light of continued controversy regarding unique energy expenditures and research evidence demonstrating many cancer survivors expend similar levels of energy as individuals without cancer, the following information is available for use when assessing the energy needs of cancer patients.

Dietary Reference Intakes

The Dietary Reference Intakes (DRIs) were published between 1997 and 2010 by the Food and Nutrition Board of the Institute of Medicine (now the Health and Medicine Division of the National Academies of Sciences, Engineering, and Medicine). These nutrient reference values for Americans and Canadians are based on average estimated amounts of energy and nutrients needed for defined life stages and sexes. They include Recommended Dietary Allowances (RDAs) and Adequate Intakes (AIs), which estimate intakes needed for good health, and Tolerable Upper

Intake Levels (ULs), which identify intakes that pose a risk of adverse effects. Estimates of nutrient needs for various health conditions are based on these data.[15]

The DRIs provide reliable information for groups of people but cannot be used to ensure adequate or safe levels of intake for individuals. They can be used as reference points or approximations, as an individual's actual requirements might be more or less than the DRI value.[16]

Macronutrient Needs

Protein
Protein is essential for a range of life-sustaining functions, such as building and repairing cells and maintaining muscle mass. The DRI for protein for healthy individuals is 0.8 grams per kilogram of body weight per day (g/kg/d).[15,16] The ESPEN Guidelines on Nutrition for Cancer Patients recommend a protein intake of more than 1 g/kg/d, and, if possible, 1.5 g/kg/d.[1] The adequacy of recommended protein levels can be assessed using nitrogen balance.

Normoweight (body mass index [BMI] 18.5–24.9) or obese (BMI >30) individuals experiencing hepatic dysfunction, renal dysfunction, or both should not automatically be placed on standard protein restriction but instead should be individually assessed for needs.[16] Table 5.1 lists protein requirements in health and various disease states.

Carbohydrates and Fats
Carbohydrates and fats are the primary energy sources. Adequate kilocalories from carbohydrates and fats are needed each day to spare protein intake for its essential function and to preserve lean muscle. Regarding the feeding of patients with cancer, the optimal ratio of carbohydrates and fats has not been determined.[1] Due to lack of evidence, the RDA is used to guide carbohydrate intake. The RDA for carbohydrates is 130 g/d for healthy adults.[15,16] No estimated average requirement (EAR), AI, or RDA has been determined for fats, though there is a need for essential fatty acids that can usually be met when linoleic acid and linolenic acid provide approximately 2% to 4% of total energy intake.[15]

Table 5.1
Protein Requirements in Health and Disease[1,6,17]

Condition	Protein requirement (g/kg/d)[a]
Dietary Reference Intake	0.8
Adult maintenance	0.8-1.0
Healthy older adult	At least 1.0-1.2
Acutely or chronically ill older adult	1.2-1.5
Adult with cancer	1.0-1.5
Adult with cancer cachexia	1.5-2.5
Adult undergoing hematopoietic stem cell transplant	1.5

[a] kg of actual body weight, unless specified otherwise

Table 5.2
Acceptable Macronutrient Distribution Ranges for Adults[15]

Macronutrient	Recommendations
Fat	20%-35% total energy intake
Carbohydrate	45%-65% total energy intake
Protein	10%-35% total energy intake
Dietary cholesterol	As low as possible while consuming a nutritionally adequate diet
Trans fatty acids	As low as possible while consuming a nutritionally adequate diet
Saturated fatty acids	As low as possible while consuming a nutritionally adequate diet

The DRIs suggest a distribution range for macronutrients and other dietary components, which is provided in Table 5.2.

Fluid Requirements

Adequate hydration is important to sustain life and is particularly important during nephrotoxic chemotherapy, such as cisplatin, or in the presence of anticancer-treatment nutrition impact symptoms, such as constipation, diarrhea, and vomiting. Thirst is the main determinant but is not always a reliable gauge for fluid needs. Underhydration is often a problem for individuals with cancer due to decreased fluid intake (difficulty obtaining and consuming fluids) and excessive fluid losses (volume depletion due to vomiting and diarrhea). Adequate hydration is especially a problem in the older oncology population due to impaired thirst mechanisms and access issues stemming from decreased mobility. Table 5.3 lists factors that influence fluid needs and the corresponding increase in fluids required to maintain adequate hydration.[18]

Intravenous (IV) hydration may be recommended for people with cancer who are at high risk for dehydration and unable to achieve adequate hydration orally. Repletion must be determined on an individual basis, taking fluid intake and output into consideration. Overhydration can occur with excessive IV hydration and can complicate underlying conditions of congestive heart failure, pulmonary edema, and renal dysfunction.[19]

Several methods are used to calculate fluid requirements.[15,16,20] These three methods—weight, body surface area, and RDA—have not been validated but have been widely referenced in peer-reviewed journals. More research is needed to provide evidence regarding the estimation of fluid needs.

Weight (or Holliday-Segar) method[21]
- Body weight of 0 to 10 kg: 100 mL of fluid per kg
- Body weight of 10 to 20 kg: 1,000 mL of fluid + 50 mL of fluid for each kg over 10 kg
- Body weight of 20 kg and higher:
    - Age 50 years and younger: 1,500 mL of fluid + 20 mL of fluid for each kg over 20 kg
    - Age greater than 50 years: 1,500 mL of fluid + 15 mL of fluid for each kg over 20 kg

Body surface area (BSA) method[16]
1,500 mL of fluid per m² (or BSA × 1,500 mL)

RDA (or energy) method[15]
1 mL of fluid per kcal of estimated needs

Table 5.3
Factors That Affect Fluid Requirements

Factors	Increase in fluid requirement
Fever	12.5% for every 1° C above normal
Sweating	10%-25%
Hyperventilation	10%-60%
Hyperthyroidism	25%-50%
Extraordinary gastric and/or renal losses	Varies based on output

Reprinted with permission from Laura Matarese. From Whitmere SJ. Fluid, electrolytes, and acid-base balance. In: Matarese L, Gottschlich M, eds. *Contemporary Nutrition Support Practice*. WB Saunders; 1998: 131. See reference 18.

Micronutrient Needs

Micronutrients are required in small amounts but are essential for triggering a range of biochemical reactions essential for life. Micronutrient deficiencies in an already ill person can affect various biochemical processes and enzyme functions that can lead to organ dysfunction, muscle weakness, poor wound healing, and altered immunity; correction should be considered a priority.[22] In the presence of normal values, supplementation in excess of the DRIs may not result in elevated serum levels and may, in fact, be detrimental.[1,22] Cancer patients should aim for an intake of 100% of the RDAs and AIs for micronutrients unless otherwise advised by a physician or indicated by the results of an abnormal laboratory test, nutrition-focused physical exam for micronutrient deficiencies, or nutrition assessment.

Effect of Inflammation on Micronutrient Status

Vitamins, minerals, and trace elements are needed in adequate amounts for a functioning immune system.[23] Serum levels of some micronutrients decrease with inflammation, but the significance of these fluctuations is unclear. During the inflammatory process, selenium, copper, iron, and zinc levels decrease due to sequestration, possibly in the liver and reticuloendothelial system, though increased urinary losses and protein catabolism also contribute to overall decreased levels. Thiamine, riboflavin, vitamin B12, and folate levels are usually not affected by inflammation; consequently, low levels may be related to actual deficiencies.[22]

Box 5.2 on page 80 summarizes the medical conditions and cancer-related treatments that influence micronutrient levels and how they may affect those levels.

Estimating Energy Needs

Energy drives biological reactions and essential processes in the body, such as respiration and circulation. Consequences of underfeeding and overfeeding can be obvious, as evidenced by the presence of malnutrition and obesity. However, body composition can mask underlying significant changes in fat-free mass and fat mass that also may influence organ function and outcomes of cancer treatment. See Box 5.3 on page 81 for terminology

Box 5.2
General Medical Conditions and Cancer-Related Treatments Affecting Micronutrient Levels[22,24,25]

Medical condition	Possible resulting change in micronutrient levels
Alcoholic liver	Decrease in folate, thiamine, pyridoxine, and vitamin A
Renal failure	Decrease in pyridoxine, folate, and vitamin C
Gastrointestinal (GI) fistulas and diarrhea	Decrease in all vitamins and multiple trace minerals, especially zinc and selenium
Loss of bile	Decrease in fat-soluble vitamins
Pancreatitis	Decrease in absorption of vitamin B12
Chyle leaks and fistulas (with large protein-rich fluid losses)	Decrease in micronutrients
Gastrectomy or terminal ileum resection	Decrease in iron and vitamin B12
Bariatric surgery (Roux-en-Y gastric bypass and gastric banding procedures)	Decrease in fat-soluble vitamins, water-soluble vitamins, and minerals, such as iron and zinc
Critical illness	Decrease in vitamin C despite supplementation
Syndrome of inappropriate antidiuretic hormone (SIADH)	Decrease in sodium
Cisplatin (chemotherapy)	Decrease in magnesium

associated with energy expenditure. There are two primary methods for assessing energy requirements:

- **Indirect calorimetry (IC)**, the "gold standard," uses oxygen consumption and carbon dioxide production, but the equipment is not always available or possible to use.[16,18] IC is used to measure REE—that is, to determine mREE.

- **Predictive equations**, some validated, some not, are developed for select patient populations and are used to assess energy needs. The appropriate method or equation depends on an individual's clinical status and the results of available clinical data.[16,18] These equations are used to predict REE—that is, to determine pREE.

Indirect Calorimetry

While impractical to use to assess the needs of all patients with cancer, IC is used frequently in oncology nutrition research to measure the resting metabolic rate (RMR) and is thought to be a more accurate way to estimate energy requirements as

Box 5.3
Energy Expenditure Terminology[16,19,26]

Basal energy expenditure (BEE): minimum amount of energy expended to be compatible with life

Basal metabolic rate (BMR): measurement made early in the morning before activity and 10 to 12 hours after ingestion of food, beverage, or nicotine

Resting metabolic rate (RMR): measurement taken when any requirement for BMR is not met, also in the fasted state (at least 5 hours); generally 10% to 20% higher than BMR

Resting energy expenditure (REE): energy needed to maintain normal body functions measured after 30 minutes of recombinant rest

Estimated energy expenditure (EEE): energy needed per day to maintain normal body functions

Estimated energy requirement (EER): average predicted nutrition intake for maintenance of energy balance and good health based on age, sex, weight, height, and activity level

Physical activity level (PAL): four activity levels—*sedentary, low active, active, very active*—as are defined by the National Academy of Medicine

Respiratory quotient (RQ): calculation derived from indirect calorimetry using carbon dioxide expended and oxygen consumed

Body mass index (BMI): calculation of the degree of adiposity

---

compared with predictive equations. Considered "the standard for determination of RMR in critically ill patients," IC has been shown to both closely predict actual expenditures and account for changes in metabolic state.[16,20,27]

IC is often conducted in a clinical setting using a metabolic cart. RDNs are trained to conduct the test. IC measures carbon dioxide production (VCO_2) and oxygen consumption (VO_2) and provides a respiratory quotient (RQ). The RQ can then be inserted into a modified Weir formula to determine REE in kcal/d.

Weir formula:

$$REE = (3.9\ VO_2 + 1.1\ VCO_2) \times 1.44$$

RQ readings below 0.7 and above 1.0 warrant a repeat test because, according to the Academy of Nutrition and Dietetics Evidence Analysis Library (EAL), an RQ below 0.7 suggests hypoventilation or prolonged fasting and an RQ above 1.0 in the absence of overfeeding represents hyperventilation or inaccurate gas collection.[27]

Predictive Equations

When assessment with IC is not possible, predictive equations can be used to determine energy needs in the oncology population. There are more than 200 published predictive equations, and because of their inherent limitations, use of these equations in nutrition assessment requires supplemental clinical judgment. Energy equations have been developed

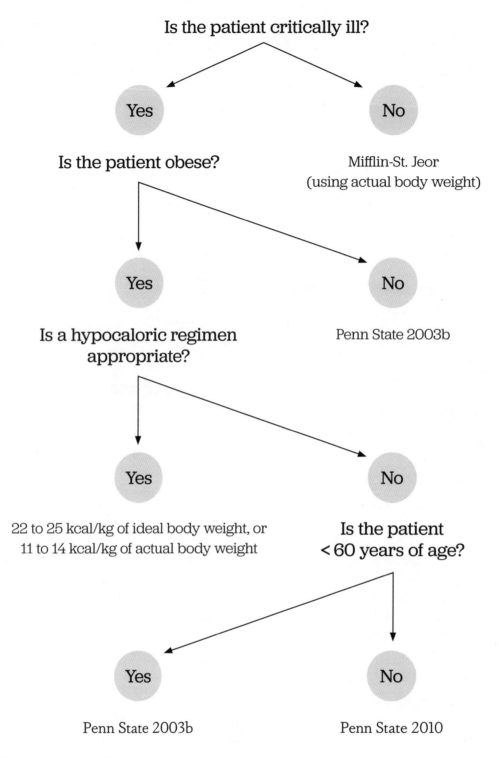

Figure 5.1
Decision tree for identifying appropriate predictive equation for energy needs

Reprinted with permission from Malone A, Russell MK. Nutrient requirements. From Charney P, Malone A, eds. *Academy of Nutrition and Dietetics Pocket Guide to Nutrition Assessment.* 3rd ed: Academy of Nutrition and Dietetics Publications; 2016. See reference 16.

for specific medical conditions and for populations of individuals; consequently, it is important to apply the most appropriate calculations to the individual or population being assessed and to have the information available to use in calculation, such as age, weight, height, and sex. In most cases, researchers compared predictive equations to IC to assess the accuracy of their equations.[28] Formulas have been developed for use in healthy, non–critically ill, critically ill, and obese populations.[28,29] Predictions for the latter three groups are most applicable to patients undergoing cancer treatment and in active recovery (see Figure 5.1).

Alternative equations or adjustments to equations may need to be considered, as in the case of patients with ascites, edema, and other conditions affecting body weight. Although limited research exists, actual body weight (ABW) and ideal body weight (IBW) have both been used when assessing energy and protein needs in critically ill, obese patients when a hypocaloric, high-protein feeding has been prescribed. IBW has also been used for people with amputations. In most other circumstances, ABW is recommended when assessing energy, protein, and fluid needs.[29]

In addition to accurately assessing a person's degree of health or illness, the following factors should be considered when estimating energy requirements in patients with cancer[30]:

- medical (cancer) diagnosis
- presence and extent of comorbid conditions
- intent of treatment (cure, control, palliation)
- anticancer treatment modalities
- presence and extent of malnutrition
- stress factors (such as fever and infection)
- presence of advanced directives, if appropriate

Equations for the Noncritically Ill Population

Because research has shown that many patients with cancer are normometabolic, the Mifflin-St. Jeor equation, the Harris-Benedict equation, and the DRIs for energy, which were initially developed to assess energy needs of healthy, non–critically ill people, may be considered for use in patients with cancer.[31] The Mifflin-St. Jeor equation has been judged to have the best predictive value in this population. In addition, it is a component of several equations used to assess energy needs in critically ill patients.

Mifflin-St. Jeor Equation This equation was created by studying healthy men and women, then comparing the predictive results to the IC readings. The Mifflin-St. Jeor equation, using ABW, is useful when predicting RMR in healthy nonobese and obese populations, aged 20 to 82 years.[16,18,31]

Men:
RMR (kcal/d)=(9.99×weight in kg)+ (6.25×height in cm)–(4.92×age in years)+5

Women:
RMR (kcal/d)=(9.99×weight in kg)+ (6.25×height in cm)–(4.92×age in years)–161

Equations for the Critically Ill Population

According to the Academy of Nutrition and Dietetics 2012 Critical Illness Evidence-Based Nutrition Practice Guideline, the Penn State equation (2003b) is a good predictor of energy needs in critically ill mechanically ventilated adults with obesity who are under 60 years of age, and the Penn State equation (2010) is a good predictor of energy needs in critically ill mechanically ventilated adults with obesity who are over 60 years of age.[20]

Penn State Equations The Penn State equations were developed by David Frankenfield and colleagues at Pennsylvania State University.[32]

The 2003b Penn State equation was validated in 2009 and is called the Penn State equation. This was the second of three equations titled Penn State.[33] It requires the use of the Mifflin-St. Jeor equation.

RMR=(Mifflin-St. Jeor×0.96)
+(minute ventilation in L/min×31)
+(maximum daily body temperature in ° C×167)
−6,212

The third Penn State equation was validated in 2010 and is referred to as the modified Penn State equation. It, too, requires the use of the Mifflin-St. Jeor equation.

RMR=(Mifflin-St. Jeor×0.71)
+(minute ventilation in L/min×64)
+(maximum daily body temperature in ° C×85)
−3,085

Weight-Based Equation

Guidelines published by the Society of Critical Care Medicine (SCCM) and the American Society of Parenteral and Enteral Nutrition (ASPEN) recommend using a weight-based equation (kilocalories per kilogram of ABW) to estimate energy needs and suggest an initial assessment starting range of 25 to 35 kcal/kg/d for normoweight (BMI 18.5 to 24.9) adults, with ongoing adjustments made based on the patient's clinical response.[34] This equation lacks evidence-based validation, though it is frequently used as a baseline estimate and then adjusted after comparison to outcome goals (see Table 5.4).

Special Considerations for the Obese Population

With rising rates of obesity, there is a likelihood that clinicians will be required to assess energy needs in non–critically ill or critically ill patients with cancer who are obese (BMI ≥30). Standard

Table 5.4

Estimated Energy Needs Based on Body Weight[16,34]

Medical condition	Estimated energy needs (kcal/kg/d)
Cancer, repletion, weight gain	30-35
Cancer, inactive, nonstressed	25-30
Cancer, hypermetabolic, stressed	35
Sepsis	25-30
Hematopoietic cell transplant	30-35
Non–critically ill and critically ill, obese	11-14 (actual body weight) 22-25 (ideal body weight)

predictive equations for energy needs may overestimate the nutritional needs of patients who are overweight or obese, or possibly underestimate the needs of cancer patients who are obese.[35,36] To help clinicians avoid making this mistake, much attention has been paid to accurately assessing the needs for this population.

The best way to assess energy needs for a patient with obesity is to use IC, but if it is not available, predictive equations for hypocaloric high-protein feedings are suggested in patients who do not have advanced cancer, severe renal disease, or hepatic disease.[16] While clinical discretion should be used in the nutrition management of a patient with a cancer known to be hypermetabolic, the use of hypocaloric, high-protein formulas in critically ill overweight or obese patients has been shown to positively affect protein anabolism and minimize complications from overfeeding, such as hyperglycemia and hyperlipidemia.[34] Hypocaloric, high-protein feeding should not be confused with permissive underfeeding.[16,34,37]

Hypocaloric, high-protein feedings should not exceed 65% to 70% of estimated energy needs and should provide less than 14 kcal/kg and at least 1.2 g of protein per kg of ABW or 2 to 2.5 g of protein per kg of IBW.[16,34]

Special Considerations for the Older Adult Population

The findings of the Academy of Nutrition and Dietetics Unintended Weight Loss in Older Adults guideline (2009) suggest use of the weight-based formulas of 25 to 35 kcal/kg/d in healthy women and 30 to 40 kcal/kg/d in healthy men. They also suggest using the weight-based formula of 25 to 30 kcal/kg/d, or higher energy levels, for weight gain in underweight or ill older adults (aged 64 to 84 years and older). It is estimated that energy requirements in the older adult population are decreased due to changes in body composition and decreased physical activity.[38]

Actual, Ideal, or Adjusted Body Weight

Some predictive equations use ABW, some IBW, and some adjusted body weight. Unless specified, it is suggested to use ABW. In the presence of edema or ascites, the SCCM and ASPEN guidelines for nutrition support in critically ill adults advise the use of dry or usual weight.[34]

Refeeding Syndrome

Refeeding syndrome is a potential result of aggressive and rapid refeeding (restoration of normal nutrition) in a person who has had inadequate nutritional intake resulting in starvation-related malnutrition or significant weight loss for an extended period of time. The syndrome is characterized by electrolyte disturbances and a significant, possibly life-threatening metabolic shift. Phosphorus, magnesium, and potassium levels are depleted from cells, but serum levels remain normal due to regulation by the kidneys. The restart of feeding introduces carbohydrates into the system and triggers the release of insulin, which drives phosphorus, magnesium, and potassium back into the cells. Hypophosphatemia, one hallmark sign of refeeding syndrome, usually occurs within 3 days of starting nutrition intervention.[16,39,40]

Conditions seen in the cancer patient population, such as long-standing alcohol abuse with or without cirrhosis, prolonged undernutrition, and morbid obesity with substantial weight loss, are risk factors for refeeding syndrome.[16]

For patients at risk for refeeding syndrome, energy repletion should start at low levels, estimated at 25% of estimated needs, and advance to the target goal slowly over 3 to 5 days while monitoring electrolyte levels and watching for signs of the syndrome.[16,39] Thiamine supplementation may be added for patients at risk for refeeding syndrome, especially for critically ill patients with reported alcohol abuse, but it is thought to be beneficial to all others to help stabilize blood glucose levels and address potential thiamine deficiencies.[39-41]

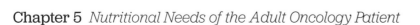

References

1. Arends J, Bachman P, Baracos V, et al. ESPEN guidelines on nutrition in cancer patients. *Clin Nutr.* 2017;36(1):11-48.

2. Cao D, Wu G, Zhang B, et al. Resting energy expenditures and body composition in patients with newly detected cancer. *Clin Nutr.* 2010;29(1):72-77.

3. Kumar, NB. Assessment of malnutrition and nutrition therapy approaches in cancer patients. In: *Nutritional Management of Cancer Treatment Effects.* Springer-Verlag; 2012:7-41.

4. Diakos CI, Charles KA, McMillan DC, Clarke SJ. Cancer-related inflammation and treatment effectiveness. *Lancet Oncol.* 2014;15(11):e493-503.

5. Cederholm T, Barazzoni R, Austin P, et al. ESPEN guidelines on definitions and terminology of clinical nutrition. *Clin Nutr.* 2017;36(1):49-64.

6. Ryan AM, Power DG, Daly L, et al. Cancer associated malnutrition, cachexia and sarcopenia: the skeleton in the hospital closet 40 years later. *Proc Nutr Soc.* 2016;75(2):199-211.

7. Guenter P, Jennes G, Patel V, et al. Addressing disease-related malnutrition in hospitalized patients: a call for a national goal. *Jt Comm J Qual Saf.* 2015;41(10):469-473.

8. Peterson SJ, Mozer M. Differentiating sarcopenia and cachexia among patients with cancer. *Nutr Clin Pract.* 2017;32(1):30-39.

9. Alves ALC, Zuconi CP, Correia MI. Energy expenditure in patients with esophageal, gastric and colorectal cancer. *JPEN J Parenter Enteral Nutr.* 2016;40(4):499-506.

10. Head and Neck Guideline Steering Committee. Evidence-based practice guidelines for the nutritional management of adult patients with head and neck cancer. Cancer Council Australia. Accessed July 30, 2020. https://wiki.cancer.org.au/australia/COSA:Head_and_neck_cancer_nutrition_guidelines

11. Langius JAE, Kruizenga HM, Uitdehaah BMJ, et al. Resting energy expenditure in head and neck cancer patients before and during radiotherapy. *Clin Nutr.* 2012;31(4):549-554.

12. Zuconi CP, Ceolin Alves AL, Toulson Davisson Correia MI. Energy expenditure in women with breast cancer. *Nutrition.* 2015;31(4):556-559.

13. Xu WP, Cao DX, Lin ZM, et al. Analysis of energy utilization and body composition in kidney, bladder and adrenal cancer. *Urol Oncol.* 2012;30(5):711-718.

14. Purcell SA, Elliott SA, Baracos VE, et al. Key determinants of energy expenditure in cancer and implications for clinical practice. *Eur J Clin Nutr.* 2016;70(11): 1230-1238.

15. Institute of Medicine. DRI tables and application reports. US Department of Agriculture National Agricultural Library website. Accessed July 30, 2020. https://www.nal.usda.gov/fnic/dri-application-reports.

16. Malone A, Russell MK. Nutrient requirements. In: Charney P, Malone A, eds. *Academy of Nutrition and Dietetics Pocket Guide to Nutrition Assessment.* 3rd ed. Academy of Nutrition and Dietetics; 2016:181-182, 213-236.

17. Deutz NEP, Baur JM, Barazzoni R, et al. Protein intake and exercise for optimal muscle function with aging: recommendations from the ESPEN Expert Group. *Clin Nutr.* 2014;33(6):929-936.

18. Whitmere SJ. Fluid, electrolytes, and acid-base balance. In: Matarese L, Gottschlich M, eds. *Contemporary Nutrition Support Practice.* WB Saunders; 1998: 131.

19. Claure-Del Granado R, Mehta R. Fluid overload in the ICU: evaluation and management. *BMC Nephrol.* 2016;17(1):109.

20. Academy of Nutrition and Dietetics Evidence Analysis Library website. Critical Illness (CI) Guideline (2012). Accessed July 30, 2020. https://www.andeal.org/topic.cfm?menu=4800

21. Holliday MA, Segar WE. The maintenance need for water in parenteral fluid therapy. *Pediatrics.* 1957;19:823-832.

22. Sriram K, Lonchyna VA. Micronutrient supplementation in adult nutrition therapy practical considerations. *JPEN J Parenter Enteral Nutr.* 2009;33(5):548-562.

23. Zitvogel L, Pietrocola F, Krowmer G. Nutrition, inflammation and cancer. *Nat Immunol.* 2017;18(8):843-850.

24. Vermeulen EA, Vervloet MG, Lubach CH, Nurmohamed SA, Penne EL. Feasibility of long-term continuous subcutaneous magnesium supplementation in a patient with irreversible magnesium wasting due to cisplatin. *Neth J Med.* 2017;75(1):35-38.

25. Iyer P, Ibrhim M, Siddiqui W, Dirweesh A. Syndrome of inappropriate secretion of anti-diuretic hormone (SIADH) as an initial presenting sign of non small cell lung cancer-case report and literature review. *Respir Med Case Rep.* 2017;22:164-167.

26. Academy of Nutrition and Dietetics Evidence Analysis Library. Energy expenditure glossary (2005). Accessed July 30, 2020. https://www.andeal.org/topic.cfm?menu=5299&cat=1520

27. Academy of Nutrition and Dietetics Evidence Analysis Library. Measuring resting metabolic rate (RMR) in the critically ill guideline (2013). Accessed July 30, 2020. https://www.andeal.org/topic.cfm?menu=5299&cat=5017

28. Fraipout V, Preiser JC. Energy estimation and measurement in critically ill patients. JPEN *J Parenter Enteral Nutr.* 2013;17(6):705-713.

29. Ireton-Jones C. Adjusted body weight, con: why adjust body weight in energy expenditure calculations? *Nutr Clin Pract.* 2005; 20(4):474-479.

30. Grant BL. Nutrition assessment of energy and nutrient requirements in cancer. In: *Pocket Guide to Nutrition Care Process and Cancer.* Academy of Nutrition and Dietetics; 2015: 59-73.

31. Mifflin MD, St. Jeor ST, Hill LA, Scott BJ, Daugherty SA, Koh YO. A new predictive equation for resting energy expenditure in healthy individuals. *Am J Clin Nutr.* 1990;51(2):241-247.

32. Frankenfield D. Validation of an equation for resting metabolic rate in older obese critically ill patients. *JPEN J Parenter Enteral Nutr.* 2011;35(2):264-269.

33. Academy of Nutrition and Dietetics Evidence Analysis Library. In adult critically ill patients, what is the relationship between resting metabolic rate (RMR) and RMR predicted by the Penn State equations?. Accessed July 30, 2020. https://www.andeal.org/topic.cfm?cat=4311&evidence_summary_id=251026&highlight=Penn%20state&home=1

34. McClave SA, Taylor BE, Martindale RG, et al. Guidelines for the provision and assessment of nutrition support therapy in the adult critically ill patient: Society of Critical Care Medicine (SCCM) and the American Society of Parenteral and Enteral Nutrition (A.S.P.E.N.). *JPEN J Parenter Enteral Nutr.* 2016;40(2):159-211.

35. Tajchman SK, Tucker AM, Cardenas-Turanzas M, Nates JL. Validation study of energy requirements in critically ill obese cancer patients. *JPEN J Parenter Enteral Nutr.* 2016;40(6):806-813.

36. Choban P, Dickerson R, Malone A, Worthington P, Compher C; American Society for Parenteral and Enteral Nutrition. A.S.P.E.N. clinical guidelines: nutrition support of hospitalized adult patients with obesity. *JPEN J Parenter Enteral Nutr.* 2013;37(6):714-744.

37. Dickerson RN, Medling TL, Smith AC, et al. Hypocaloric, high-protein nutrition therapy in older vs younger critically ill patients with obesity. *JPEN J Parenter Enteral Nutr.* 2013;37(3):342-351.

38. Academy of Nutrition and Dietetics Evidence Analysis Library. Unintended weight loss in older adults guideline (2009). Accessed July 30, 2020. https://www.andeal.org/topic.cfm?menu=5294

39. Friedli N, Staga Z, Sobotka L, et al. Revisiting the refeeding syndrome: results of systematic review. *Nutrition.* 2017;35:151-160.

40. McCray S, Parrish CR. Refeeding the malnourished patient: lessons learned. *Pract Gastroenterol.* 2016;155:56-66.

41. Manzanares W, Hardy G. Thiamine supplementation in the critically ill. *Curr Opin Clin Nutr Metab Care.* 2011;14(6):610-617.

Chapter 6
Integrative Oncology: The Role of Mind-Body Interventions and Practices in Cancer

Sandeep (Anu) Kaur, MS, RDN, RYT-500
Cheryl D. Toner, MS, RDN

Acknowledgment: The authors would like to thank Alicia A. Livinski, MPH, MA, of the NIH Library, National Institutes of Health, for conducting the literature review and assisting with the bibliography.

Over the last two decades, it has become increasingly common and more widely accepted to use health care modalities that are not typical of mainstream Western health care systems.[1] In particular, there has been an increased demand for such approaches among people with cancer, as evidenced by expanded offerings at the National Institutes of Health (NIH) National Cancer Institute (NCI)–Designated Cancer Centers.[2]

Such modalities include energy-based therapies (eg, Reiki), manipulative and body-based methods (eg, chiropractic care, massage, acupuncture, yoga), alternative medical systems (eg, Ayurveda, traditional Chinese medicine), and natural products and supplements (eg, herbs).[1,3]

Because the mind-body modalities covered in this chapter are not typical of Western medicine, they are still variably referred to as alternative medicine (if used instead of mainstream medicine) or complementary medicine (if used along with mainstream medicine). The term *complementary and alternative medicine* (CAM) is common in the published literature, and *complementary* is still used by the NIH in reference to modalities not traditionally used in allopathic (conventional) medicine. *Integrative medicine* (IM) is a more recent term that emphasizes the integration of conventional practices with those that have been considered complementary or alternative and are supported by evidence of safety and effectiveness. At the heart of IM is a focus on the whole person and their environment, patient involvement in the treatment process, and incorporation of experience-based therapeutic knowledge.[4] IM is used in this chapter to refer to the integration of these modalities into overall medical care. CAM is also used where appropriate, based on the context of how the modality is being discussed and how it was studied in specific referenced papers.

The NIH National Center for Complementary and Integrative Health classifies complementary health approaches into two broad categories: biological products and mind-body practices.[1] Biological products, including dietary supplements and special diets, are the most commonly used complementary approaches among patients with cancer and survivors of cancer in the United States, according to the National Health Interview Survey.[5] For additional information on supplements, diets, and metabolic therapies, see Chapter 7. Modalities such as deep breathing, qigong meditation, tai chi, and yoga are examples of mind-body interventions (MBIs)[6] and are the focus of this chapter (see Box 6.1 on page 90).

This chapter provides an overview of the research on MBIs in patients with cancer and survivors of cancer. This research has focused primarily on quality of life (QOL), fatigue, anxiety, depression, pain, nausea, vomiting, intestinal function after surgery, appetite, and dry mouth. It is well known that these outcomes have both direct and indirect effects on nutrition status, as do cancer and cancer treatments.[7]

Some MBI modalities are related to whole medical systems—complete systems that encompass mind-body, biologically based, manipulative- and body-based, and energy-medicine approaches to treatment.[8] Though allopathic medicine can be practiced in this manner, whole medical systems are typically characteristic of traditional, ancient cultures. Traditional Chinese medicine (TCM) includes a range of mind-body modalities, such as acupuncture, qigong, tai chi, and Chinese therapeutic massage, as well as biological products, musical intervention, and other approaches.

Box 6.1
Selected Popular Mind-Body Interventions[6,9]

Mind-body intervention	Description or premise
Acupuncture	Acupuncture originated as a traditional Chinese medicine (TCM) modality at least 2,000 years ago. Needles are inserted into the skin at specific "acupoints," then the acupoints are stimulated either manually or with electricity. According to TCM, acupuncture is used to stimulate the flow of "qi" (pronounced *chee*), or energy, throughout the body. Research suggests it may work through specific neuronal and cortical pathways to cause release of endorphins at the spinal and supraspinal levels.
Acupressure	Acupressure uses fingers or other dull objects to apply pressure to the acupoints and move qi throughout the body.
Meditation	Meditation is a set of practices that train attention and awareness to control mental processes. Most types of meditation require four components: a quiet, relatively distraction-free location; a comfortable posture; focus of attention on something specific; and an open, judgment-free attitude toward thoughts that arise during the process. Meditation may or may not include a spiritual or belief component. Mantra meditation involves focused attention on repetition of a sound or word, while in mindfulness meditation thoughts and distractions are allowed to come and go from attention without judgment.
Mindfulness-based stress reduction (MBSR)	Based on the work of Jon Kabat-Zinn, MBSR is a structured 6-to-8-week mindfulness-meditation group program. It incorporates a body scan, sitting meditation, walking meditation, loving-kindness practice, and gentle hatha yoga postures. Throughout the program, participants practice both with a group and individually at home. It is designed to cultivate increasing levels of mindfulness in day-to-day life.
Qigong	Qigong, a TCM modality, incorporates movement, meditation, controlled breathing, self-massage, and sound to move and use energy for therapeutic purposes. The physical postures may be gentle or vigorous. Qigong is used to move qi throughout, into, or out of the body, which is accomplished with "gong" (pronounced *gung*), or skill cultivated through steady practice.
Tai chi	Tai chi originated in ancient China as a combination of martial art and qigong. Forms, or sets of movements, are executed and may be followed by breath work. Tai chi principles are based on Taoism and the need for balance between the opposites of yin and yang. The practice is used to unblock and improve the flow of qi throughout the body. It is thought to integrate mind and body, control movements and breathing, and generate internal energy, mindfulness, loosening, and serenity.
Yoga	Yoga dates back 4,000 years to its roots in Indian philosophy. The name captures the traditional intent of yoga to unite (or yoke) the individual with the totality of the universe. The techniques of yoga include ethical daily living (yamas and niyamas), physical postures (asanas), breathing techniques (pranayamas), and meditation training (dhyana) to elicit the relaxation response, a physiological condition characterized by reduced activity in the sympathetic nervous system.

Meditation and yoga are MBIs that are closely related to Ayurveda, a whole medical system that offers guidelines on herbs, diet, exercise, and lifestyle regimens.[10] Homeopathy is an example of a whole medical system that is biologically based, using highly diluted natural substances thought to restore the body's innate ability to heal.[11]

It is important for practitioners to understand the relationships between MBIs and whole medical systems and to be aware that research does not yet consistently recognize these relationships or describe such details of practice. Yet these details (eg, what form of meditation is practiced) may provide important context in assessing the effectiveness of an MBI across multiple studies.

Use of Complementary and Alternative Medicine in Cancer Treatment and Survivorship

Prevalence

In 2012, the National Health Interview Survey found that one-third (33.2%) of US adults use some form of CAM, primarily for wellness rather than for treating a condition.[5] Of the MBIs named, deep-breathing was the most common (11.6%), followed by yoga (9.5%), meditation (7.6%), and massage therapy (6.9%). Among US adults with a cancer diagnosis, 35.3% had used CAM in the past year, and 43.6% with breast cancer had done so. Among those with a recent cancer diagnosis, 3.7% used whole medical systems (eg, Ayurveda, TCM) and 14.9% used MBIs; and of those with a recent breast cancer diagnosis, 6.1% used whole medical systems and 26.2% used MBIs.[12] A systematic review of 45 NCI-Designated Cancer Center websites found that IM information was included on the websites for a range of MBIs, but few centers offered actual on-site services.[2] The most commonly offered MBI information and services at NCI-Designated Cancer Centers in 2016 were acupuncture (73%), meditation (69%), yoga (69%), tai chi (42 %), and qigong (36%).[2]

The use of CAM is known to be high (40% to 66%) in young adult women[13-15]; however, only a limited number of studies have been conducted in women with cancers other than breast, such as gynecologic cancers.[16,17] Abdallah and colleagues[18] evaluated CAM practices among women with a gynecologic malignancy who were treated at an NCI-Designated Cancer Center and found that 30.6% stated they used an MBI. The most commonly used CAM therapies were vitamin and mineral supplements (78%) and herbal supplements (27.9%) in addition to mind-body practices; spiritual healing and prayer (15.1%); and deep-breathing relaxation exercises (13.1%), with nominal use of energy therapies and alternative medical systems. Abdallah and colleagues also found that CAM use was greatest in women aged 20 to 30 years and older than 60 years, and more prevalent among widowed, retired, and highly educated women. These findings are mostly consistent with previous studies.[13-15,19,20]

Motivators

Why do patients with cancer and cancer survivors use CAM? CAM decision-making is complex, influenced not only by social relationships but also by cultural, spiritual, and religious beliefs that consequently affect people's beliefs about the risks and benefits of conventional treatment and CAM modalities.[21,22] Individuals may be influenced to use CAM by practitioners, family, friends, and even casual acquaintances met in waiting rooms and support groups. CAM provides patients with a way to be more involved in their cancer care and manage their feelings of vulnerability, loss, and uncertainty.[21,23,24] While many use these modalities complementary to chemotherapy or radiation to decrease side effects of treatment, a smaller number use them as an alternative to conventional treatment.[3] For cancer survivors, the goal of CAM is often to improve QOL and decrease recurrence. Certain psychological and physical symptoms that are common in cancer make patients and survivors more likely to use CAM; these include depression and anxiety,[25] peripheral neuropathy, chemotherapy-induced nausea and vomiting, cancer-related fatigue and pain, cognitive dysfunction, sleep disturbances, and overall detriments to QOL.[7,26]

Though there is little research on the use of CAM by men with cancer, one secondary analysis of participants in an Australian survey provides interesting insights into potential motivators for these men and their caregivers. The study found that high CAM use in men with cancer was associated with routines and rituals (eg, functional, meaningful, and mental or spiritual). CAM routines provided men with certainty and control, and CAM rituals functioned for them and their significant others as a way to create meaning in the face of the uncertainty of a cancer diagnosis. In fact, significant others were often influential in initiating and maintaining CAM use, leading to enhanced closeness and interpersonal bonding.[27]

Ojukwu and colleagues[28] looked at the prevalence of CAM use among US cancer survivors and examined whether weight and body mass index (BMI) status played a role in CAM use. Of 1,785 cancer survivors from the 2007 National Health Interview Survey, nearly 90% had used at least one type of CAM in the past year, and use was higher among those who were overweight versus normal-to-underweight or obese.[28]

Proposed Mechanisms of Action for Mind-Body Interventions and Stress

Common among patients with cancer is the stress response associated with the initial diagnosis and treatment, evolving into chronic stress with survival.[29-31] MBIs work in the cancer population by addressing the negative mental and biological impacts of stress.[32,33] Stress affects people emotionally and spiritually[7,34] and has a physiological impact via neuroendocrine pathways.[31,35-37] Stress is also associated with poor outcomes for those with cancer.[26,29,30,38,39]

There are multidirectional relationships between stress, cancer etiology, and cancer treatments[40-42] that can inhibit immune response and increase inflammation.[29,30] Stress has been shown to indirectly increase inflammatory cytokines, promote angiogenesis, reduce anoikis and apoptosis, decrease cell-mediated immunity, shorten telomeres, cause neuroendocrine changes, and even decrease the efficiency of chemotherapy.[26,39,43-45] Stress among caregivers of those with chronic illness has been correlated with genome-wide changes in transcription,[46,47] and psychosocial stress has been shown to physiologically promote depressive symptoms.[48] Perhaps related to these effects is the observation that higher depressive-symptom scores among patients with renal cell cancer were correlated with decreased survival rates as well as increased expression of genes in circulating leukocytes that are proinflammatory and prometastatic.[29,30]

The stress response involves the autonomic nervous system (ANS), which is an important regulator of allostasis (the process of maintaining homeostasis or managing stress),[49] immune function, and the inflammatory cytokine network.[50,51] Chronic activation of the sympathetic nervous system (SNS), a branch of the ANS (see Figure 6.1), can lead to increased inflammation along with the dysregulation of the hypothalamic-pituitary-adrenal (HPA) axis.[43,52,53] Conversely, increased activation of the parasympathetic nervous system leads to decreased inflammation.[52,54] Both the SNS and the HPA axis are stress response systems that, when activated, elicit release of stress hormones and promote tumor growth.[31,36,39,55,56]

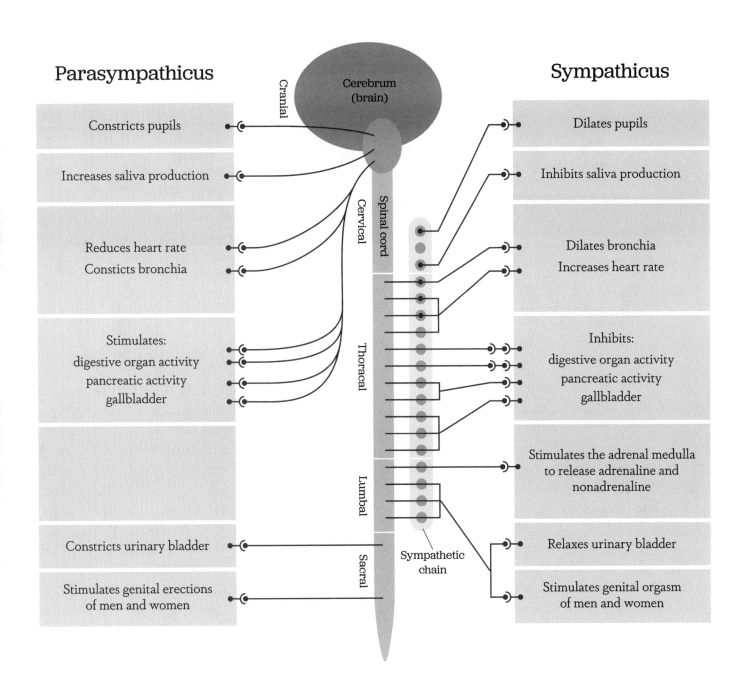

Parasympathicus

Constricts pupils

Increases saliva production

Reduces heart rate
Consticts bronchia

Stimulates:
digestive organ activity
pancreatic activity
gallbladder

Constricts urinary bladder

Stimulates genital erections
of men and women

Sympathicus

Dilates pupils

Inhibits saliva production

Dilates bronchia
Increases heart rate

Inhibits:
digestive organ activity
pancreatic activity
gallbladder

Stimulates the adrenal medulla
to release adrenaline and
nonadrenaline

Relaxes urinary bladder

Stimulates genital orgasm
of men and women

Cranial

Cerebrum
(brain)

Cervical

Spinal cord

Thoracal

Lumbal

Sacral

Sympathetic
chain

Figure 6.1
The autonomic nervous system

Adapted under CCO 1.0 from Geo-Science-International, Wikimedia Commons.

Box 6.2
Evidence Grades Used by the Society for Integrative Oncology in Its Clinical Guidelines for the Use of Integrative Therapies With Breast Cancer[9]

The only clinical guidelines for integrative therapies and breast cancer based on comprehensive systematic reviews of randomized controlled trials are those published by the Society for Integrative Oncology (SIO). The authors of the guidelines note, "It is important to define the use of the term 'recommendation' in these clinical practice guidelines.... Here, in the setting of integrative oncology, we use the term 'recommendation' to infer that the therapy should be considered as a viable but not singular option for the management of a specific symptom or side effect." The authors use the following grades to describe the quality and strength of the evidence for their recommendations (Grades D and H are also used but are not listed here, as they do not apply to any of the mind-body interventions to be discussed in this chapter):

Grade A: The SIO recommends the modality. There is high certainty that the net benefit is substantial. Offering and providing this modality is recommended.

Grade B: The SIO recommends the modality. There is high certainty that the net benefit is moderate, or there is moderate certainty that the net benefit is moderate to substantial. Offering and providing this modality is recommended.

Grade C: The SIO recommends selectively offering or providing this service to individual patients based on professional judgment and patient preferences. There is at least moderate certainty that the net benefit is small. Offering and providing this modality is recommended for selected patients depending on individual circumstances.

Over the last few decades there has been a growing body of basic science and clinical research indicating that MBIs may play a role in improving health outcomes and overall well-being.[57-59] Muehsam and colleagues[57] hypothesized that MBIs have both top-down and bottom-up effects on stress. The contemplative components of MBIs, (eg, deep-breathing and meditation) are said to be top-down, influencing stress through stimulation of the vagus nerve.[35,60] Musculoskeletal exertion and cardiovascular output resulting from the physical components of MBIs elicit bottom-up effects on stress and immune function via the HPA axis, SNS, and parasympathetic nervous system.[57]

Evidence for Specific Mind-Body Interventions for Cancer

The following section takes a closer look at some of the current evidence related to MBIs as complementary approaches to addressing cancer symptoms and cancer-treatment side effects, focusing specifically on acupuncture, qigong, and tai chi (all TCM interventions),[61] as well as meditation and yoga.[62] Research on these MBIs focuses on their role as biobehavioral interventions (incorporating psychological, social, and behavioral processes) to manage the stress response and influence cancer biology.[26,33,43,63,64] The conclusions of systematic reviews of the evidence for each modality are presented, one of which formed the basis of clinical practice guidelines (see Box 6.2).[9,61,65-69] Based on trends in MBI practices and the volume of research available in the peer-reviewed literature, there is a greater focus on yoga in this chapter.[5,13,70]

Acupuncture

Acupuncture was one of the most popular services provided at NCI-Designated Cancer Centers in 2016 (provided by 73% of centers).[2] There is emerging research on acupuncture as an adjunct therapy in various types of cancer and for various symptoms and side effects of treatment. Acupuncture has been examined for lung cancer and immunomodulatory effects (eg, natural killer cells, T-cell subtypes),[71] managing chemotherapy-induced nausea and vomiting,[72] and management of postoperative symptoms after cancer surgery.[61,73]

Acupuncture and acupressure were evaluated in a systematic review of 13 randomized controlled trials (RCTs) with 969 cancer patients; the reviewers found that acupuncture had a quicker and longer-lasting analgesic effect than conventional pain treatments.[66] Another systematic review and meta-analysis of research on acupuncture and pain with cancer sought to distinguish the effects on pain from different sources by analyzing studies on acupuncture for pain from cancer (17 papers), chemotherapy or radiotherapy (11), surgery (5), and hormone therapy (1).[68] Acupuncture was found to reduce cancer pain overall as well as malignancy- and surgery-related pain. There was no significant effect of acupuncture on pain related to chemotherapy, radiotherapy, or hormonal therapy. Notably, heterogeneity among trials was noted for the subgroups in which no significant effect was detected.

Acupuncture has also been found to significantly improve QOL, fatigue, diarrhea, and time to flatulence following surgery, but not depression, in a meta-analysis of 11 trials in 968 Chinese patients with cancer.[61] Findings from a systematic review of CAM and cancer-fatigue management indicated that acupuncture may also relieve cancer-related fatigue, particularly after chemotherapy and radiation treatment, but that larger studies are needed to justify clinical recommendations.[67,74]

The Society for Integrative Oncology (SIO) guidelines qualify the evidence for acupuncture in people with breast cancer as Grade B for use with antiemetic drugs to help control chemotherapy-induced nausea and vomiting. They rate the evidence for acupuncture for reducing anxiety and stress, hot flashes, cancer-related pain, and cancer fatigue, and improving mood disturbances, depressive symptoms, and QOL as Grade C.[9]

To view the literature through a whole medical system lens, one can group studies of individual modalities that stem from one type of whole medical system together for analysis. For example, research papers examining the use of psychobehavioral interventions in Chinese patients with cancer following treatment were identified through systematic review, including 16 papers on interventions rooted in TCM (11 on acupuncture, 4 on therapeutic Chinese massage, and 1 on qigong) and 51 papers on non-TCM psychobehavioral interventions.[61] Collectively, the TCM modalities were found to have a significant positive impact on QOL, pain, depression, sleep quality, fatigue, diarrhea, and intestinal function following surgery. Non-TCM modalities were also effective in improving QOL, depression, sleep quality, pain, and intestinal function following surgery, as well as anxiety and mood, but not fatigue or gastrointestinal symptoms.[75]

One of the limitations in acupuncture studies is inadequate description of the acupuncture intervention—that is, prescribed acupuncture points or specific use of TCM theory. Dose or frequency of acupuncture treatments were described in the literature as either twice a week or once a week, which may be suboptimal to effect change in cancer-related fatigue.[76]

Chiu and colleagues[68] noted that, of the 29 trials assessed in their acupuncture meta-analysis, only 4 claimed that the acupuncture intervention was carried out according to TCM theory. Likewise, much of the meditation literature does not distinguish whether the meditation is practiced in isolation or in conjunction with yoga, mindfulness-based stress reduction, or other modalities. These inconsistencies in research design and reporting, as well as differences in intervention frequency, are sources of heterogeneity in the literature.

Qigong and Tai Chi

Less research has been published on qigong and tai chi (compared with acupuncture) as interventions for patients with cancer or cancer survivors. The SIO qualifies the evidence for qigong as an intervention to improve QOL for people with breast cancer as Grade C (see Box 6.2 on page 94).[9] However, the research that continues to emerge indicates further investigation is worthwhile.

Combining the tai chi and qigong research published through January 30, 2017, Wayne and colleagues[69] conducted a qualitative review of 22 papers that met inclusion criteria and a meta-analysis of data from 15 studies that were RCTs. Notably, 12 of the 15 RCTs were found to have low risk of bias according to assessment with the Cochrane Collaboration's risk-of-bias tool. Significant beneficial effects were documented for tai chi and qigong with respect to fatigue, sleep difficulty, depression, and QOL, as well as a non-significant reduction in pain.

Tao and colleagues[61] found that five studies examining tai chi effects on QOL in cancer patients were of high quality but could not be evaluated via meta-analysis due to heterogeneity of assessment methods. These RCTs were noted to have documented improvements in postoperative upper-limb lymphedema, lung function, sleep quality, limb muscle strength, fatigue, and distress in patients using tai chi versus control patients.

Risks associated with tai chi and qigong are quite limited but do exist. Robins and colleagues[77] found an initial increase in perceived stress among patients with breast cancer with the initiation of chemotherapy for those in the tai chi intervention group, but not for those in the control or comparative treatment groups. Stress decreased for all groups after 6 weeks and was not different between groups. The authors speculate that the initial increase in stress perception could be an early effect of increasing mindfulness.

Meditation

Meditation is a contemplative and self-regulating practice[78] that may be practiced alone or as a component of other MBIs, with the ultimate goal of meditation being two-fold: to cultivate self-awareness with either a *focused attention* or *single point* and also to monitor one's thoughts with openness.[60] Mediation is being studied in cancer patients for its ability to enhance QOL and foster resilience throughout the spectrum of cancer care.

Studies on meditation have exponentially increased in the last two decades, particularly on mindfulness-based stress reduction (MBSR). In the cancer population, particularly in patients with breast cancer,[79-81] MBSR has been shown to have positive psychological outcomes, including fewer symptoms of stress, anxiety, and depressed mood.[9,82] The formal practices in MBSR are intended to enhance mindfulness, which is characterized by being present in the moment with an openness and curiosity that allows for acceptance (compassionate self-observation) of an experience and can be a useful biobehavioral approach for people living with cancer.[83] MBSR is a program that encourages cultivating this practice in one's day-to-day life habits and encourages a daily home practice.

In a meta-analysis of MBSR's impact on psychological distress, survivors of breast cancer had a significant improvement in depression, anxiety, stress, and overall improvement of QOL.[84] Consistently, the SIO clinical practice guidelines for breast cancer describe the quality of evidence for meditation and reduced anxiety, treatment of mood disturbance and depressive symptoms (especially MBSR), and improved QOL as Grade A. The effect of MBIs, such as MBSR and various types of mediation, on biomarkers are few in number and are in the preliminary stages of investigation. One systematic review of six studies looked at the relationship of MBSR and other mindful meditation modalities to biomarkers (cytokines, neuropeptides, and C-reactive protein) in 360 study participants with cancer and concluded that MBIs may have an impact on cytokine levels (increasing interleukin-4 and decreasing interferon-γ) and aid the immune system.[85]

Overall, meditation does not seem to pose much risk; however, intense meditation practices may not be suitable for all people. Due to the limitations imposed by cancer symptoms and treatment side effects, it may be difficult for some patients to attend meditation sessions in person; this is being addressed with online options and the provision of instructions for a home-based practice.[86] To assist cancer patients who may have limited energy, MBSR programs can be adapted, as seen in mindfulness-based cancer recovery (MBCR), a program similar to MBSR but with shorter sessions and specific educational material dealing with cancer.[83,87] More studies are needed to compare meditation directly to other MBIs and other active interventions or therapies, such as cognitive behavioral therapy or individual counseling, to tease out confounding factors such as "participant's engagement and commitment to the practice."[9] Overall, a more rigorous RCT design is needed to evaluate the impact of different types of MBI programs on biomarkers and other aspects of cancer.

Yoga

Yoga comes from the Sanskrit word *yug*, which means "union," "yoke," or "to join,"[78] and is a multicomponent MBI modality that has been practiced for thousands of years as a method of maintaining mental, physical, and spiritual wellness.[88] The 2016 Yoga in America study reported a significant increase in the number of yoga practitioners to 36.7 million, up from 20.4 million in 2012.[89] The last five decades[88] have shown a renewed interest in yoga for health benefits and an exponential increase in yoga therapy research.[90]

Yoga services were provided at 68.9% of NCI-Designated Comprehensive Cancer Centers surveyed in 2016.[2] Yoga has been used for managing mood-related matters (eg, anxiety, stress, depression, and fatigue) and is considered a gentle option, depending on the lineage of yoga, for increasing physical activity (see Box 6.3 on pages 98 and 99).[6,7,91,92] For the oncology dietitian, it is important to seek training to understand which yoga lineage may be best suited for a particular patient based on that patient's symptoms and cultural beliefs; in the absence of such training, the oncology dietitian should be prepared to refer the patient to a practitioner with the appropriate expertise.

Although there is a wide variety of forms and styles of yoga, hatha yoga is one of the most common in the United States and Canada, and it forms the basis for all classic approaches to yoga. Hatha yoga emphasizes postures (asanas) and often breathing exercises (pranayama).[9] Many forms or lineages of yoga emphasize yogic philosophy, which includes intention, relaxation, and static and dynamic movement that incorporates breath and hand gestures that stimulate the body and are based on an Ayurvedic framework meant to stimulate the nadis (energy lines).[9,91] A broader approach to multicomponent yoga practice may deepen the benefits to patients with cancer and survivors of cancer by influencing the patient's worldview and stress response.

Culos-Reed and colleagues[93] reviewed and analyzed 15 studies (7 of which were RCTs and 8 with other study designs) with survivors (98% women) with varying cancer diagnoses (eg, breast, prostate, colorectal, lung, lymphoma, and others). Yoga styles included Viniyoga (2 studies), Iyengar yoga (6 studies), hatha-based yoga (7 studies), and specially designed yoga protocols for cancer such as Yoga of Awareness,[94] Yoga Thrive,[95] and Yoga for Cancer Survivors[96] that use specific, documented combinations of postures, breathing, and meditation. According to the authors, these preliminary

Box 6.3
Selected Yoga Lineages[6,9,91,92,97-101]

Yoga lineage	Online resource	Description of style of yoga
Anusara	www.anusarayoga.com	Holistic approach that integrates traditional yogic philosophy (the Vedic roots of yoga) with hatha yoga and an emphasis on spiritual growth through the practice of combining intent with movement
Ashtanga	www.ashtanga.com	Continuous movement or "flow" from one posture to the next coupled with breath work as taught by Sri K. Pattabhi Jois
Bikram	www.bikramyoga.com	Twenty-six hatha poses practiced in a heated room, developed by Bikram Choudhury, founder of Bikram's Yoga College of India
Iyengar	www.bksiyengar.com	Developed by B. K. S. Iyengar, a hatha-style yoga distinguished by an emphasis on precise structural alignment with postures, use of props, and sequencing of poses; also emphasizes postures and breathing techniques for therapeutic purposes and targeting specific cancer symptoms (eg, the "legs up the wall" posture to help move lymph)
Kripalu	www.kripalu.org	Inquiry-based learning and practice, characterized by highlighting awareness and acceptance of sensations, emotions, and thoughts that occur during yoga practice; developed by Yogi Amrit Desai and the Kripalu Center for Yoga and Health in Massachusetts
Kundalini	www.3ho.org/kundalini-yoga	Uses a variety of mediation techniques with an emphasis on movement with the breath and a mantra for a focus on spiritual awakening, as taught by Yogi Bhajan
Restorative	www.restorativeyogateachers.com www.judithhansonlasater.com	Derived from Iyengar yoga, uses props to adapt poses for individuals healing from cancer or other medical conditions so they can practice yoga with less strain or pain; popularized in the 1970s by B. K. S. Iyengar's student Judith Lasater, founder of Yoga Journal
Viniyoga	www.viniyoga.com	A therapeutic approach tailored to the individual with an emphasis on breath; developed by T. Krishnamacharya, "father of modern yoga," and his son, T. K. V. Desikachar
Vinyasa	www.yogajournal.com	Adaptable yoga practice that uses breath and movement; developed by T. Krishnamacharya; caution advised for patients with cancer when considering heated and more vigorous adaptations

(continued)

Box 6.3
Selected Yoga Lineages[6,7,91-97] *(continued)*

Yoga lineage	Online resource	Description of style of yoga
Yin Yoga	www.yinyoga.com	Involves holding postures for 3 to 5 minutes to work with deep connective tissues and fascia; should be done with care; introduced by Paulie Zink
Yoga nidra	www.irest.us	Soothing guided imagery based on yogic teaching for deep rest; IRest yoga nidra is a modern-day practice developed by Richard Miller, PhD
Yoga therapy	www.iayt.org	Therapeutic approach that works specifically with imbalances; ideally suited for people with cancer Emerging profession of yoga in health care; certified yoga therapist (C-IAYT) must complete 800 hours of yoga training from approved schools accredited by the International Association of Yoga Therapists

studies indicate that yoga as an MBI may be effective both physiologically and psychosocially for cancer survivors.

Although certain yoga lineages may be better suited for cancer patients, more research is needed for clarity on this point. Limited adverse events have been reported in the yoga research.[92] However, the gap in adverse-event reporting, variations in yoga protocols and interventions, variations in frequency and duration of practice, and different outcome measurements complicate comparisons and limit conclusions.[88,93]

Yoga elicits physiological changes relevant to cancer. For example, yoga has been shown to increase heart rate variability, a measure of ANS activity that can be low with stress-related imbalances between the sympathetic and parasympathetic nervous systems.[102] Lower heart rate variability is associated with higher fatigue in survivors of breast cancer, including younger survivors.[50,103] Yoga has also been shown to increase the release of dopamine[104] and the neurotransmitter γ-aminobutyric acid, and lower salivary cortisol levels.[105,106] In a targeted, 12-week, restorative Iyengar yoga intervention, cancer survivors with persistent fatigue were observed to have reduced inflammation-related gene expression. These findings suggest that a targeted yoga program may have beneficial effects on inflammatory activity in this patient population, with potential relevance for mental and physical well-being.[107] Specifically, improvements with yoga have been documented for fatigue, sleep quality, depression, anxiety, and QOL.[62] Conversely, yoga does not appear to have a significant effect on physical functioning and vasomotor outcomes (eg, hot flashes).[9]

Yoga has been investigated most often in patients with breast cancer for symptoms and side effects widespread among most cancer patients. In a 2017 Cochrane review,[65] 24 studies on yoga and breast cancer were evaluated. The studies included 2,166 women who were receiving active treatment or had completed cancer treatment. Compared to no intervention, yoga was found to be more effective in improving QOL and sleep and reducing fatigue. Improvements in measures of depression and anxiety were also found to be greater with yoga than with psychosocial or educational interventions, such as counseling. The Cochrane review authors recommended that future studies assess the impact of specific yoga lineages.

The SIO concluded that the evidence for yoga on reduced anxiety and improved mood, depressive symptoms, QOL, and sleep were Grade B. For reduced fatigue, the evidence was a Grade C.

Long-term increases in body fat are increasingly common in survivorship, and higher body-fat proportion is associated with increased risk for certain cancers.[108] The adoption of a physically active lifestyle is considered integral to long-term improvements in body composition and is increasingly recommended for patients with cancer and survivors of cancer (for more information, refer to the discussion of energetics in Chapter 3). The positive effects of yoga practice on reduced stress, improved body satisfaction, and improved mood suggest it could play a positive role in regulating body weight, as these factors are also associated with improved eating and exercise behaviors and body composition. Experts hypothesize that yoga's usefulness in stress and binge eating involves the downregulation of the SNS and HPA axis.[109]

Epidemiological studies have documented positive associations between yoga practice and reduced weight, healthier diet patterns, and more physical activity for those who practice yoga regularly compared to those who do not.[110] Female yoga practitioners tend to weigh less with increasing years of experience.[111] And frequency of yoga practice has been found to be associated with lower BMI, higher fruit and vegetable consumption, fewer sleep disturbances, and improved mindfulness and subjective well-being.[109] Causation cannot be inferred from these retrospective, cross-sectional studies.

Preliminary evidence from yoga weight-loss trials in overweight and obese persons, along with epidemiological findings and biological plausibility, indicates that such research in patients with cancer and survivors of cancer is warranted. Following a 3-month, uncontrolled pilot weight-loss intervention based on Ayurvedic and yoga therapy practices, participants lost weight and reported high levels of self-efficacy for exercise and diet changes, as well as improved stress perception, energy, well-being, QOL, and self-awareness at the 9-month follow-up.[112] A group-based Ayurvedic program using yoga for weight loss was tested for feasibility in yoga-naïve and yoga-experienced women who were overweight or obese.[113] Findings indicated improved self-reported psychosocial factors, such as mindful eating and body image, and feasibility of the intervention in both groups. And participants in a 5-day residential Kripalu yoga program reported improved eating behaviors and psychosocial factors, as well as self-reported weight loss at 1-year follow-up.[114]

Controlled studies with larger sample sizes are needed to evaluate the effectiveness of yoga to reduce excess body-fat mass and improve sustainability of diet and physical-activity behavior changes, particularly in cancer survivors, and to prevent cancer in the general public. Research to date supports the feasibility and safety of conducting larger yoga studies and more RCTs in both the adult and pediatric cancer populations.[62]

Practical Applications

Whether newly diagnosed, in treatment, or a survivor, people with cancer will at some point experience symptoms or side effects that may be helped by MBIs. Clinicians working with cancer patients and survivors may have a positive impact on their patients' QOL by better understanding the potential role of MBIs in managing not only nutrition-impact symptoms but also overall symptom burden.[115] A cancer diagnosis often leads to social changes, such as relationship strain, social isolation, stress, and spiritual challenges related to concerns about the uncertainty of disease progression or fear of death.[83] These troubling matters are not always directly addressed by health professionals.[42,116-118] At the same time, patients with cancer indicate that they have stress and anxiety over using MBI approaches due to a lack of information or support from health professionals, as well as the individual responsibility of choosing CAM.[22]

With the interdisciplinary team, the registered dietitian nutritionist (RDN) can play an important role in assessing many of these symptoms and side effects; assessing past, current, and intended physical activities and use of mind-body modalities; making appropriate referrals; recommending safe practice of MBIs; and monitoring progress. Because MBIs may be either helpful or contraindicated, it is important for the RDN to initiate conversations with their patients about whether mind-body approaches are being used. The Standards of Practice and Standards of Professional Performance for Registered Dietitian Nutritionists (Competent, Proficient, and Expert) in Oncology Nutrition states that the RDN evaluates "physical activity habits and restrictions" as a standard in the nutrition assessment process.[119] During the assessment process, expressing support for those IM approaches that are backed by high-quality research may open the door to more complete information sharing by the patient and also strengthen the patient-provider relationship.

In order to guide patients to explore those MBIs that may be best suited for their individual situations, it is important for practitioners to seek the necessary training and knowledge. This chapter is only an introduction. Resources like Cochrane reviews and clinical practice guidelines are useful in understanding the strength of the evidence overall.[9,65] It is important to be clear about the search inclusion and exclusion criteria used in any systematic review, how the research reviewed is graded for quality, and the intentions of the grading. As noted by the SIO, for example, the clinical guidelines developed for integrative therapies in breast cancer specifically evaluated the strength of the evidence with respect to the use of modalities as complements to conventional care. The grading, therefore, should inform recommendations for adjuvant therapy based on clinical judgment and with close monitoring by the health care team, rather than standalone treatment.

Practitioners should also keep in mind the limitations of their own knowledge base. Develop a strong network of both conventional and credentialed integrative practitioners to whom referrals can be made (see Box 6.4 on page 102). For example, the yoga therapist credential requires more extensive training than the yoga teacher credential, and these professionals are specifically dedicated to yoga as a healing art. It is also advisable to investigate IM offerings at local cancer-care facilities in order to understand local offerings and also make connections and foster dialogue with IM practitioners.

Summary

As evidence continues to emerge regarding the usefulness of MBIs for patients with cancer and survivors of cancer to help counter stress and the many related nutrition-impact symptoms, and as these patients and survivors increasingly adopt MBIs with or without supporting evidence, it will be increasingly important for the oncology RDN to assess and monitor mind-body practices and even recommend them as appropriate. It is important to read the literature and to engage in dialogue about the literature and practice implications with both conventional and integrative oncology practitioners. The RDN has an opportunity to emerge as a leader by advancing such dialogue, seeking opportunities to share knowledge and practice experience with other practitioners (eg, organizing journal clubs, delivering professional presentations, developing continuing education programs), encouraging and participating in the development of protocols for MBI recommendations with respect to nutrition-related outcomes, and collaborating on research.

Box 6.4

Mind-Body Intervention Resources

Complementary alternative medicine modality	Resource
Acupuncture, acupressure, traditional Chinese medicine	Accreditation Commission for Acupuncture and Oriental Medicine: www.acaom.org
	American Association of Acupuncture and Oriental Medicine: www.aaaomonline.org
	National Certification Commission for Acupuncture and Oriental Medicine: www.nccaom.org
Ayurveda	National Ayurvedic Medical Association: www.ayurvedanama.org
	Kripalu School of Ayurveda: www.kripalu.org/schools/kripalu-school-ayurveda
Qigong, tai chi	Center for Taiji Studies: www.centerfortaiji.com
	American Tai Chi and Qigong Association: www.americantaichi.org
	National Qigong Association: www.nqa.org
Meditation, mindfulness	Center for Mindful Eating: www.tcme.org
	Center for Mindfulness in Medicine, Health Care, and Society at the University of Massachusetts Medical School: www.umassmed.edu/cfm/mindfulness-based-programs/mbsr-courses
Yoga	International Association of Yoga Therapists: www.iayt.org
	Yoga Alliance: www.yogaalliance.org
	Yoga International: www.yogainternational.com

References

1. Complementary, alternative, or integrative health: what's in a name? National Center for Complementary and Integrative Health website. July 2018. Accessed April 29, 2019. https://nccih.nih.gov/health /integrative-health

2. Yun H, Sun L, Mao JJ. Growth of integrative medicine at leading cancer centers between 2009 and 2016: a systematic analysis of NCI-Designated Comprehensive Cancer Center websites. *J Natl Cancer Inst Monogr.* 2017;2017(52).

3. Smith PJ, Clavarino A, Long J, Steadman KJ. Why do some cancer patients receiving chemotherapy choose to take complementary and alternative medicines and what are the risks? *Asia Pac J Clin Oncol.* 2014;10(1):1-10.

4. Salamonsen A. Use of complementary and alternative medicine in patients with cancer or multiple sclerosis: possible public health implications. *Eur J Public Health.* 2016;26(2): 225-229.

5. Clarke TC, Black LI, Stussman BJ, Barnes PM, Nahin RL. Trends in the use of complementary health approaches among adults: United States, 2002-2012. *Natl Health Stat Report.* 2015;(79):1-16.

6. Ospina MB, Bond K, Karkhaneh M, et al. Meditation practices for health: state of the research. *Evid Rep Technol Assess (Full Rep).* 2007:(155):1-263.

7. National Cancer Institute. Nutrition in cancer care (PDQ)– health professional version. Published May 2020. Accessed July 31, 2020. www.cancer.gov /about-cancer/treatment/side -effects/appetite-loss/nutrition -hp-pdq

8. National Center for Complementary and Alternative Medicine. *Expanding Horizons of Health Care: Strategic Plan 2005–2009.* National Institutes of Health; 2004. Accessed July 31, 2020. https://nccih.nih.gov/sites /nccam.nih.gov/files/about/plans /2005/strategicplan.pdf

9. Greenlee H, DuPont-Reyes MJ, Balneaves LG, et al. Clinical practice guidelines on the evidence-based use of integrative therapies during and after breast cancer treatment. *CA Cancer J Clin.* 2017;67(3):194-232.

10. Frawley D. *Yoga and Ayurveda Self-Healing and Self-Realization.* Lotus Press; 1999.

11. Frenkel M. Is there a role for homeopathy in cancer care? Questions and challenges. *Curr Oncol Rep.* 2015;17(9):43.

12. Clarke TC. The use of complementary health approaches among U.S. adults with a recent cancer diagnosis. *J Altern Complement Med.* 2018;24(2):139-145.

13. Barnes PM, Bloom B, Nahin RL. Complementary and alternative medicine use among adults and children: United States, 2007. *Natl Health Stat Report.* 2008;(12):1-23.

14. Richardson MA, Sanders T, Palmer JL, Greisinger A, Singletary SE. Complementary/ alternative medicine use in a comprehensive cancer center and the implications for oncology. *J Clin Oncol.* 2000;18(13):2505-2514.

15. Helyer LK, Chin S, Chui BK, et al. The use of complementary and alternative medicines among patients with locally advanced breast cancer—a descriptive study. *BMC Cancer.* 2006;6:39.

16. Molassiotis A, Browall M, Milovics L, Panteli V, Patiraki E, Fernandez-Ortega P. Complementary and alternative medicine use in patients with gynecological cancers in Europe. *Int J Gynecol Cancer.* 2006;16(suppl 1):219-224.

17. Navo MA, Phan J, Vaughan C, et al. An assessment of the utilization of complementary and alternative medication in women with gynecologic or breast malignancies. *J Clin Oncol.* 2004;22(4):671-677.

18. Abdallah R, Xiong Y, Lancaster JM, Judson PL. Complementary and alternative medicine use in women with gynecologic malignancy presenting for care at a comprehensive cancer center. *Int J Gynecol Cancer.* 2015;25(9):1724-1730.

19. Fouladbakhsh JM, Balneaves L, Jenuwine E. Understanding CAM natural health products: implications of use among cancer patients and survivors. *J Adv Pract Oncol.* 2013;4(5):289-306.

20. Gross AM, Liu Q, Bauer-Wu S. Prevalence and predictors of complementary therapy use in advanced-stage breast cancer patients. *J Oncol Pract.* 2007;3(6):292-295.

21. Mulkins AL, McKenzie E, Balneaves LG, Salamonsen A, Verhoef MJ. From the conventional to the alternative: exploring patients' pathways of cancer treatment and care. *J Complement Integr Med.* 2016;13(1):51-64.

22. Weeks L, Balneaves LG, Paterson C, Verhoef M. Decision-making about complementary and alternative medicine by cancer patients: integrative literature review. *Open Med.* 2014;8(2): e54-66.

23. Verhoef MJ, Balneaves LG, Boon HS, Vroegindewey A. Reasons for and characteristics associated with complementary and alternative medicine use among adult cancer patients: a systematic review. *Integr Cancer Ther.* 2005;4(4):274-286.

24. Singh H, Maskarinec G, Shumay DM. Understanding the motivation for conventional and complementary/alternative medicine use among men with prostate cancer. *Integr Cancer Ther.* 2005;4(2):187-194.

25. Cramer H, Lange S, Klose P, Paul A, Dobos G. Yoga for breast cancer patients and survivors: a systematic review and meta-analysis. *BMC Cancer.* 2012;12:412.

26. Bower JE, Lamkin DM. Inflammation and cancer-related fatigue: mechanisms, contributing factors, and treatment implications. *Brain Behav Immun.* 2013;30(suppl):S48-57.

27. Klafke N, Eliott JA, Olver IN, Wittert GA. The role of complementary and alternative medicine (CAM) routines and rituals in men with cancer and their significant others (SOs): a qualitative investigation. *Support Care Cancer.* 2014;22(5):1319-1331.

28. Ojukwu M, Mbizo J, Leyva B, Olaku O, Zia F. Complementary and alternative medicine use among overweight and obese cancer survivors in the United States. *Integr Cancer Ther.* 2015;14(6):503-514.

29. Cohen S, Janicki-Deverts D, Doyle WJ, et al. Chronic stress, glucocorticoid receptor resistance, inflammation, and disease risk. *Proc Natl Acad Sci U S A.* 2012;109(16):5995-5999.

30. Cohen L, Cole SW, Sood AK, et al. Depressive symptoms and cortisol rhythmicity predict survival in patients with renal cell carcinoma: role of inflammatory signaling. *PLoS One.* 2012;7(8):e42324.

31. Antoni MH. Psychosocial intervention effects on adaptation, disease course and biobehavioral processes in cancer. *Brain Behav Immun.* 2013;30(suppl):S88-98.

32. Andersen BL, Kiecolt-Glaser JK, Glaser R. A biobehavioral model of cancer stress and disease course. *Am Psychol.* 1994;49(5):389-404.

33. Subnis UB, Starkweather AR, McCain NL, Brown RF. Psychosocial therapies for patients with cancer: a current review of interventions using psychoneuroimmunology-based outcome measures. *Integr Cancer Ther.* 2014;13(2):85-104.

34. Stress. National Center for Complementary and Integrative Health website. Accessed July 30, 2020. https://nccih.nih.gov/health /stress

35. Porges SW. The polyvagal perspective. *Biol Psychol.* 2007;74(2):116-143.

36. Glaser R, Kiecolt-Glaser JK. Stress-induced immune dysfunction: implications for health. *Nat Rev Immunol.* 2005;5(3):243-251.

37. Cohen S, Janicki-Deverts D, Miller GE. Psychological stress and disease. *JAMA.* 2007;298(14):1685-1687.

38. Satin JR, Linden W, Phillips MJ. Depression as a predictor of disease progression and mortality in cancer patients: a meta-analysis. *Cancer.* 2009;115(22):5349-5361.

39. Armaiz-Pena GN, Cole SW, Lutgendorf SK, Sood AK. Neuroendocrine influences on cancer progression. *Brain Behav Immun.* 2013;30(suppl):S19-25.

40. Powell ND, Tarr AJ, Sheridan JF. Psychosocial stress and inflammation in cancer. *Brain Behav Immun.* 2013;30(suppl):S41-47.

41. Antoni MH, Lutgendorf SK, Cole SW, et al. The influence of bio-behavioural factors on tumour biology: pathways and mechanisms. *Nat Rev Cancer.* 2006;6(3):240-248.

42. Chandwani KD, Ryan JL, Peppone LJ, et al. Cancer-related stress and complementary and alternative medicine: a review. *Evid Based Complement Alternat Med.* 2012;2012:79213. doi:10.155.2012.979213

43. Lutgendorf SK, Sood AK. Biobehavioral factors and cancer progression: physiological pathways and mechanisms. *Psychosom Med.* 2011;73 (9):724-730.

44. Wu Y, Antony S, Meitzler JL, Doroshow JH. Molecular mechanisms underlying chronic inflammation-associated cancers. *Cancer Lett.* 2014;345(2):164-173.

45. Epel ES, Blackburn EH, Lin J, et al. Accelerated telomere shortening in response to life stress. *Proc Natl Acad Sci U S A.* 2004;101(49):17312-17315.

46. Miller GE, Chen E, Sze J, et al. A functional genomic fingerprint of chronic stress in humans: blunted glucocorticoid and increased NF-kappaB signaling. *Biol Psychiatry.* 2008;64(4):266-272.

47. Miller GE, Murphy ML, Cashman R, et al. Greater inflammatory activity and blunted glucocorticoid signaling in monocytes of chronically stressed caregivers. *Brain Behav Immun.* 2014;41:191-199.

48. Slavich GM, Irwin MR. From stress to inflammation and major depressive disorder: a social signal transduction theory of depression. *Psychol Bull.* 2014;140(3):774-815.

49. Juster RP, McEwen BS, Lupien SJ. Allostatic load biomarkers of chronic stress and impact on health and cognition. *Neurosci Biobehav Rev.* 2010;35(1):2-16.

50. Crosswell AD, Lockwood KG, Ganz PA, Bower JE. Low heart rate variability and cancer-related fatigue in breast cancer survivors. *Psychoneuroendocrinology.* 2014;45:58-66.

51. McEwen BS, Wingfield JC. The concept of allostasis in biology and biomedicine. *Horm Behav.* 2003;43(1):2-15.

52. Thayer JF, Sternberg E. Beyond heart rate variability: vagal regulation of allostatic systems. *Ann N Y Acad Sci.* 2006; 1088:361-372.

53. Irwin MR, Cole SW. Reciprocal regulation of the neural and innate immune systems. *Nat Rev Immunol.* 2011;11(9):625-632.

54. Uebelacker L, Lavrertsky H, Tremont G. Yoga therapy for depression. In: Khalsa SBS, Cohen L, McCall T, Telles S, eds. *The Principles and Practice of Yoga in Health Care.* Handspring Publishing; 2016:73-93.

55. Cole SW, Mendoza SP, Capitanio JP. Social stress desensitizes lymphocytes to regulation by endogenous glucocorticoids: insights from in vivo cell trafficking dynamics in rhesus macaques. *Psychosom Med.* 2009;71(6):591-597.

56. Kiecolt-Glaser JK, Preacher KJ, MacCallum RC, Atkinson C, Malarkey WB, Glaser R. Chronic stress and age-related increases in the proinflammatory cytokine IL-6. *Proc Natl Acad Sci U S A.* 2003;100(15):9090-9095.

57. Muehsam D, Lutgendorf S, Mills PJ, et al. The embodied mind: a review on functional genomic and neurological correlates of mind-body therapies. *Neurosci Biobehav Rev.* 2017;73:165-181.

58. Ernst E, Pittler MH, Wider B, Boddy K. Mind-body therapies: are the trial data getting stronger? *Altern Ther Health Med.* 2007;13(5):62-64.

59. Jonas WB, Eisenberg D, Hufford D, Crawford C. The evolution of complementary and alternative medicine (CAM) in the USA over the last 20 years. *Forsch Komplementmed*. 2013;20 (1):65-72.

60. Schmalzl L, Streeter C, Khalsa SBS. Research on the psychophysiology of yoga. In: Khalsa SBS, Cohen L, McCall T, Telles S, eds. *The Principles and Practice of Yoga in Health Care*. Handspring Publishing; 2016: 49-68.

61. Tao W, Luo X, Cui B, et al. Practice of traditional Chinese medicine for psycho-behavioral intervention improves quality of life in cancer patients: a systematic review and meta-analysis. *Oncotarget*. 2015;6(37):39725-39739.

62. Danhauer SC, Addington EL, Sohl SJ, Chaoul A, Cohen L. Review of yoga therapy during cancer treatment. *Support Care Cancer*. 2017;25(4):1357-1372.

63. Kiecolt-Glaser JK, Bennett JM, Andridge R, et al. Yoga's impact on inflammation, mood, and fatigue in breast cancer survivors: a randomized controlled trial. *J Clin Oncol*. 2014;32(10):1040-1049.

64. Payne JK. State of the science: stress, inflammation, and cancer. *Oncol Nurs Forum*. 2014;41(5):533-540.

65. Cramer H, Lauche R, Klose P, Lange S, Langhorst J, Dobos GJ. Yoga for improving health-related quality of life, mental health and cancer-related symptoms in women diagnosed with breast cancer. *Cochrane Database Syst Rev*. 2017(1):CD010802. doi:10 .1002/14651858.CD010802.pub2

66. Lau CH, Wu X, Chung VC, et al. Acupuncture and related therapies for symptom management in palliative cancer care: systematic review and meta-analysis. *Medicine*. 2016;95(9):e2901.

67. Finnegan-John J, Molassiotis A, Richardson A, Ream E. A systematic review of complementary and alternative medicine interventions for the management of cancer-related fatigue. *Integr Cancer Ther*. 2013;12(4):276-290.

68. Chiu HY, Hsieh YJ, Tsai PS. Systematic review and meta-analysis of acupuncture to reduce cancer-related pain. *Eur J Cancer Care (Engl)*. 2017;26(2).

69. Wayne PM, Lee MS, Novakowski J, et al. Tai Chi and Qigong for cancer-related symptoms and quality of life: a systematic review and meta-analysis. *J Cancer Surviv*. 2018;12(2):256-267.

70. Clarke T.C, Barnes PM, Black LI, Stussman BJ, Nahin RL. Use of yoga, meditation, and chiropractors among U.S. adults aged 18 and over. *NCHS Data Brief* 2018;(325):1-8.

71. Chen HY, Li SG, Cho WC, Zhang ZJ. The role of acupoint stimulation as an adjunct therapy for lung cancer: a systematic review and meta-analysis. *BMC Complement Altern Med*. 2013;13:362.

72. Li QW, Yu MW, Yang GW, et al. Effect of acupuncture in prevention and treatment of chemotherapy-induced nausea and vomiting in patients with advanced cancer: study protocol for a randomized controlled trial. *Trials*. 2017;18(1):185.

73. Kim KH, Kim DH, Kim HY, Son GM. Acupuncture for recovery after surgery in patients undergoing colorectal cancer resection: a systematic review and meta-analysis. *Acupunct Med*. 2016;34(4):248-256.

74. Balk J, Day R, Rosenzweig M, Beriwal S. Pilot, randomized, modified, double-blind, placebo-controlled trial of acupuncture for cancer-related fatigue. *J Soc Integr Oncol*. 2009;7(1):4-11.

75. Shen J, Wenger N, Glaspy J, et al. Electroacupuncture for control of myeloablative chemotherapy-induced emesis: A randomized controlled trial. *JAMA*. 2000;284(21):2755-2761.

76. Grant SJ, Smith CA, de Silva N, Su C. Defining the quality of acupuncture: the case of acupuncture for cancer-related fatigue. *Integr Cancer Ther*. 2015;14(3):258-270.

77. Robins JL, Elswick RK, Jr., Sturgill J, McCain NL. The effects of tai chi on cardiovascular risk in women. *Am J Health Promot.* 2016;30(8):613-622.

78. Carlson LE, Zelinski E, Toivonen K, et al. Mind-body therapies in cancer: what is the latest evidence? *Curr Oncol Rep.* 2017;19(10):67.

79. Zainal NZ, Booth S, Huppert FA. The efficacy of mindfulness-based stress reduction on mental health of breast cancer patients: a meta-analysis. *Psychooncology.* 2013;22(7):1457-1465.

80. Shennan C, Payne S, Fenlon D. What is the evidence for the use of mindfulness-based interventions in cancer care? A review. *Psychooncology.* 2011;20(7):681-697.

81. Matchim Y, Armer JM, Stewart BR. Mindfulness-based stress reduction among breast cancer survivors: a literature review and discussion. *Oncol Nurs Forum.* 2011;38(2):E61-71.

82. Santorelli S. Mindfulness-based stress reduction (MBSR): standards of practice. Center for Mindfulness in Medicine, Health Care, and Society, University of Massachusetts Medical School; 2014. Accessed May 31, 2019. www.umassmed.edu /contentassets/24cd221488 584125835e2eddce7dbb89/mbsr _standards_of_practice_2014.pdf

83. Carlson LE. Mindfulness-based interventions for coping with cancer. *Ann N Y Acad Sci.* 2016;1373(1):5-12.

84. Huang HP, He M, Wang HY, Zhou M. A meta-analysis of the benefits of mindfulness-based stress reduction (MBSR) on psychological function among breast cancer (BC) survivors. *Breast Cancer.* 2015;23(4): 568-576.

85. Sanada K, Alda Diez M, Salas Valero M, et al. Effects of mindfulness-based interventions on biomarkers in healthy and cancer populations: a systematic review. *BMC Complement Altern Med.* 2017;17(1):125.

86. Zernicke KA, Campbell TS, Speca M, McCabe-Ruff K, Flowers S, Carlson LE. A randomized wait-list controlled trial of feasibility and efficacy of an online mindfulness-based cancer recovery program: the eTherapy for cancer applying mindfulness trial. *Psychosom Med.* 2014;76(4):257-267.

87. Carlson LE, Tamagawa R, Stephen J, Drysdale E, Zhong L, Speca M. Randomized-controlled trial of mindfulness-based cancer recovery versus supportive expressive group therapy among distressed breast cancer survivors (MINDSET): long-term follow-up results. *Psychooncology.* 2016;25 (7):750-759.

88. Agarwal RP, Maroko-Afek A. Yoga into cancer care: a review of the evidence-based research. *Int J Yoga.* 2018;11(1):3-29.

89. The 2016 Yoga in America Study Conducted by Yoga Journal and Yoga Alliance [press release]. January 13, 2016. Accessed August 1, 2020. www .yogaalliance.org/Portals/0/YIAS %20Press%20Release%20with %20YA%20contact%20info.pdf

90. Jeter PE, Slutsky J, Singh N, Khalsa SB. Yoga as a therapeutic intervention: a bibliometric analysis of published research studies from 1967 to 2013. *J Altern Complement Med.* 2015;21(10):586-592.

91. Schmalzl L, Powers C, Henje Blom E. Neurophysiological and neurocognitive mechanisms underlying the effects of yoga-based practices: towards a comprehensive theoretical framework. *Front Hum Neurosci.* 2015;9:235:1-19.

92. Sovik R, Bhavanani AB. History, philosophy, and practice of yoga. In: Khalsa SBS, Cohen L, McCall T, Telles S, eds. *The Principles and Practice of Yoga in Health Care.* Handspring Publishing; 2016:17-29.

93. Culos-Reed SN, Long R, Walter A, Van Puymbroeck M. Yoga Therapy for cancer survivors. In: Khalsa SBS, Cohen L, McCall T, Telles S, eds. *The Principles and Practice of Yoga in Health Care.* Handspring Publishing; 2016:375–398.

94. Carson JW, Carson KM, Porter LS, Keefe FJ, Seewaldt VL. Yoga of Awareness program for menopausal symptoms in breast cancer survivors: results from a randomized trial. *Support Care Cancer*. 2009;17(10):1301-1309.

95. Mackenzie MJ, Carlson LE, Ekkekakis P, Paskevich DM, Culos-Reed SN. Affect and mindfulness as predictors of change in mood disturbance, stress symptoms, and quality of life in a community-based yoga program for cancer survivors. *Evid Based Complement Alternat Med*. 2013;2013:419496. doi:10.1155/2013/419496

96. Mustian KM, Sprod LK, Janelsins M, et al. Multicenter, randomized controlled trial of yoga for sleep quality among cancer survivors. *J Clin Oncol*. 2013;31(26):3233-3241.

97. McCall T, Satish L, Tiwari, S. History, philosophy, and practice of yoga therapy. In: Khalsa SBS, Cohen L, McCall T, Telles S, eds. *The Principles and Practice of Yoga in Health Care*. Handspring Publishing; 2016:31-46.

98. Shannahoff-Khalsa DS. Patient perspectives: kundalini yoga meditation techniques for psycho-oncology and as potential therapies for cancer. *Integr Cancer Ther*. 2005;4(1):87-100.

99. McCall T. During cancer treatment: clinical insights. In: Khalsa SBS, Cohen L, McCall T, Telles S, eds. *The Principles and Practice of Yoga in Health Care*. Handspring Publishing; 2016:370-372.

100. Seitz D. An overview of regulatory issues for yoga, yoga therapy, and ayurveda. *Int J Yoga Therap*. 2010;20:34-40.

101. Yin yoga. Yoga Journal website. Accessed July 31, 2020. www.yogajournal.com/yoga-101/types-of-yoga/yin

102. Schubert C, Lambertz M, Nelesen RA, Bardwell W, Choi JB, Dimsdale JE. Effects of stress on heart rate complexity—a comparison between short-term and chronic stress. *Biol Psychol*. 2009;80(3):325-332.

103. Fagundes CP, Murray DM, Hwang BS, et al. Sympathetic and parasympathetic activity in cancer-related fatigue: more evidence for a physiological substrate in cancer survivors. *Psychoneuroendocrinology*. 2011;36(8):1137-1147.

104. Kjaer TW, Bertelsen C, Piccini P, Brooks D, Alving J, Lou HC. Increased dopamine tone during meditation-induced change of consciousness. *Brain Res Cogn Brain Res*. 2002;13(2):255-259.

105. Streeter CC, Gerbarg PL, Saper RB, Ciraulo DA, Brown RP. Effects of yoga on the autonomic nervous system, gamma-aminobutyric-acid, and allostasis in epilepsy, depression, and post-traumatic stress disorder. *Med Hypotheses*. 2012;78(5):571-579.

106. Streeter CC, Whitfield TH, Owen L, et al. Effects of yoga versus walking on mood, anxiety, and brain GABA levels: a randomized controlled MRS study. *J Altern Complement Med*. 2010;16(11):1145-1152.

107. Bower JE, Greendale G, Crosswell AD, et al. Yoga reduces inflammatory signaling in fatigued breast cancer survivors: a randomized controlled trial. *Psychoneuroendocrinology*. 2014;4:20-29.

108. World Cancer Research Fund/American Institute for Cancer Research. *Diet, Nutrition, Physical Activity and Cancer: A Global Perspective*. Continuous Update Project Expert Report 2018. Accessed July 31, 2020. www.wcrf.org/dietandcancer

109. Ross A, Friedmann E, Bevans M, Thomas S. Frequency of yoga practice predicts health: results of a national survey of yoga practitioners. *Evid Based Complement Alternat Med*. 2012;2012:983258. doi:10.1155/2012/983258

110. Kristal AR, Littman AJ, Benitez D, White E. Yoga practice is associated with attenuated weight gain in healthy, middle-aged men and women. *Altern Ther Health Med.* 2005;11(4):28-33.

111. Moliver N, Mika E, Chartrand M, Burrus S, Haussmann R, Khalsa S. Increased Hatha yoga experience predicts lower body mass index and reduced medication use in women over 45 years. *Int J Yoga.* 2011;4(2):77-86.

112. Rioux J, Thomson C, Howerter A. A pilot feasibility study of whole-systems Ayurvedic medicine and yoga therapy for weight loss. *Glob Adv Health Med.* 2014;3(1):28-35.

113. Braun TD, Park CL, Gorin AA, Garivaltis H, Noggle JJ, Conboy LA. Group-based yogic weight loss with ayurveda-inspired components: a pilot investigation of female yoga practitioners and novices. *Int J Yoga Therap.* 2016;26(1):55-72.

114. Braun TD, Park CL, Conboy LA. Psychological well-being, health behaviors, and weight loss among participants in a residential, Kripalu yoga-based weight loss program. *Int J Yoga Therap.* 2012(22):9-22.

115. Viscuse PV, Price K, Millstine D, Bhagra A, Bauer B, Ruddy KJ. Integrative medicine in cancer survivors. *Curr Opin Oncol.* 2017;29(4):235-242.

116. Bailey DE Jr, Wallace M, Mishel MH. Watching, waiting and uncertainty in prostate cancer. *J Clin Nurs.* 2007;16(4):734-741.

117. Mishel MH, Germino BB, Lin L, et al. Managing uncertainty about treatment decision making in early stage prostate cancer: a randomized clinical trial. *Patient Educ Couns.* 2009;77(3):349-359.

118. Spiegel D. Psychosocial aspects of breast cancer treatment. *Semin Oncol.* 1997;24(1 suppl 1):S1-36-S1-47.

119. Charuhas Macris P, Schilling K, Palko R. Academy of Nutrition and Dietetics: revised 2017 standards of practice and standards of professional performance for registered dietitian nutritionists (competent, proficient, and expert) in oncology nutrition. *J Acad Nutr Diet.* 2018;118(4):736-748.e742.

Chapter 7
Diets, Functional Foods, and Dietary Supplements for Cancer Prevention and Survival

Maureen S. Leser, MS, RDN, LD
Natalie Ledesma, MS, RD, CSO

Rigorous research suggests a plant-based diet is protective against the development of cancer and other chronic diseases.[1-3] This finding is reflected in the population-focused *2020–2025 Dietary Guidelines for Americans*,[3] which include recommended daily intake amounts for a healthy US-style eating pattern[4] as recommended by the US Department of Agriculture (USDA), and it is the basis for diet and nutrition recommendations published by the American Cancer Society[5] and jointly by the World Cancer Research Fund and the American Institute for Cancer Research.[1]

A healthy vegetarian eating pattern[6] and a healthy Mediterranean-style eating pattern,[7] as outlined in the Dietary Guidelines, are also consistent with this research. A comprehensive review of diet and cancer prevention is provided in Chapter 2. Appendix A outlines evidence-based diets with cancer-prevention benefits, and Appendix B summarizes some alternative and unfounded dietary patterns, which may not meet evidence-based recommendations but are nevertheless proposed for cancer prevention and treatment by some centers and practitioners. Appendix C summarizes select dietary supplements and functional foods that may be used by patients for cancer prevention or treatment.

The remainder of this chapter focuses on the emerging relationship between functional foods, dietary supplements, and cancer.

Functional Foods and Cancer

Through the mid-20th century, foods were primarily valued for their ability to satisfy hunger, provide energy, help children grow into strong and healthy adults, and provide vitamins and minerals indispensable for life. These goals are achieved by consuming appropriate amounts of energy, macronutrients, and micronutrients naturally present in a varied diet. The realization that food provides an additional layer of bioactive compounds, primarily phytochemicals that modulate metabolism and health, surfaced in the second half of the 20th century.[8] Thousands of phytochemicals present in small amounts in foods act as antioxidants and anti-inflammatory agents, facilitate normal cell division, help establish a healthy gut microbiota, protect the cellular integrity of normal cells, and promote the destruction of abnormal cells that contribute to cancer formation, among other functions. Whole foods that are natural sources of these phytochemicals are considered functional foods, but research has also fostered interest in creating functional foods during food processing by adding bioactive functional ingredients that modulate metabolism over and above basic nutrition needs.[8-11] Food manufacturers already replace nutrients lost in food processing via food fortification and add nutrients not normally found in some foods via food enrichment. While whole fruits, whole vegetables, and whole grains are natural cancer-fighting functional foods, creating functional foods by adding physiologically active compounds that potentially prevent or treat a health condition or disease is a continuation of the goal of maximizing health benefits via food.[10-12]

Definition of Functional Foods

The term *functional food* was first defined in the 1980s in Japan, when that nation's government sought a food-based system for improving health and decreasing the rising incidence of chronic disease. Rather than adopting a "dietary guidelines" approach (first developed in the United States in 1980), the Japanese government encouraged its population to consume more functional foods, hoping this would lead to a natural improvement in overall diet and, in turn, better health. Japan defined a food as "functional" if it provided "basic nutrition, a positive sensory or satisfaction experience, and physiological benefits," and the government used a food labeling system to identify such foods.[13] The US government—via the Food and Drug Administration (FDA) or the USDA—has never proposed such a definition, but many definitions can be found in the literature. A 2017 article described functional foods as doing more than simply providing nutrients because they "help to maintain health and thereby reduce the risk of disease."[10] The Academy of Nutrition and Dietetics has published the most comprehensive definition, stating that functional foods are "whole foods along with fortified, enriched, or enhanced foods that have a potentially beneficial effect on health when consumed as part of a varied diet on a regular basis at effective levels based on significant standards of evidence."[14]

Effects of Functional Foods on Carcinogenesis

Bioactive compounds within plants influence every stage of carcinogenesis and have the potential to prevent and slow its initiation and progression. These compounds are sometimes referred to as nutraceuticals—foods or parts of foods with health benefits and the ability to treat disease—and also as phytochemicals—chemicals within plants with medicinal properties.[15-16] The terms *nutraceutical* and *phytochemical* are sometimes used interchangeably, and functional foods can be categorized under either term because they are used in an overall plan to improve health and treat disease. In the case of cancer, functional

foods are those that have potential to prevent, slow, or reverse tumorigenesis.[10] Appendix C addresses the cancer-fighting functions of selected functional foods and ingredients. Functional foods may become increasingly important, as only a small percentage of cancers (less than 10%) are believed to originate predominantly from inborn genetic errors, such as *BRCA1* and *BRCA2* gene mutations.[17] In contrast, the majority of cancers are influenced mainly by modifiable risk factors, including diet.

The *2020–2025 US Dietary Guidelines for Americans* report that "about eighty percent of the American population has an eating pattern that is low in vegetables, fruits, and dairy," and more than half of the population is meeting or exceeding total grain food and total protein food recommendations.[3] Americans who consume inadequate portions of these important foods are missing out on many cancer-fighting nutrients, phytochemicals, and other bioactive compounds.

Ongoing strategies to improve American diets through education and government-based nutrition programs are continuing, and functional foods have the potential to assist these efforts.

Examples of and Evidence for Functional Foods

Food manufacturers are adding fermented brown rice flour to their products to increase whole-grain content of otherwise refined breads and other refined-flour products.[18] Green-banana flour, a source of resistant starch, can be added to flours and other food products. It helps prevent DNA damage in cells while also moving digestive contents through the gastrointestinal (GI) tract faster and preventing changes to the intestinal mucosa that are favorable to the development of colon cancer.[19] Natural sources of resistant starch, which is a prebiotic, include bananas (resistant starch content drops as bananas ripen), legumes, beans, brown rice, quinoa, lentils, raw oat products, and raw potato starch. It is challenging for anyone following a traditional Western diet to consume amounts of resistant starch associated with physiologic benefits (estimated at 6 g per meal), as the usual US daily intake is estimated at 5 g/d.[20] Functional-food sources of resistant starch could help close that gap.

Flaxseed is a prime choice for a functional food ingredient, owing to its abundant nutritive and bioactive compound content. The brown-seeded flaxseed grown in Canada and the yellow-seeded flaxseed grown in the United States are the best nonfish sources of omega-3 fatty acids, in the form of α-linolenic acid. Flaxseed also has an amino acid profile similar to soy, is gluten free, and provides both soluble and insoluble fibers including lignan, which has phytoestrogen properties.[21] Flaxseed is versatile enough to be incorporated in muffins and other baked products, meat patties, pasta, dairy products, protein and snack bars, beverages, and spreads.[22] It must be ground to be digested, but that is easily done during the manufacturing process.

Chicory root is one of the best sources of inulin-type fructans, which are prebiotics not digested in the upper GI tract.[23] Like other prebiotics, rather than being digested or absorbed in the small intestine, inulin-type fructans pass through to the large intestine where, via fermentation, they form short-chain fatty acids (SCFAs). SCFAs are the major energy source for cells within the colon. Inulin, one of several bioactive compounds in chicory, also has potential as a functional food ingredient. It improves glucose tolerance, promotes bowel regularity, improves absorption of magnesium and calcium, and increases amounts of healthy bacteria while reducing levels of pathogenic bacteria in the colon.[24,25] Butyrate, an SCFA formed from inulin, inhibits the growth of colon tumor cells and promotes apoptosis. Mice studies suggest prebiotic fructans reduce the incidence of colon cancer.[26]

Oat by-products are well-known functional ingredients and are added to a wide range of foods, including breads, pastas, biscuits, cookies, snack bars, probiotic drinks, and breakfast cereals. Oats are a natural source of many micronutrients and potentially cancer-fighting phytochemicals, including resistant starch, vitamin E, zinc, phytic acid, lignans, flavonoids, and β-glucan.[27] Approximately 25% of the total starch in oats is resistant starch, and oats are also a source of avenanthramides—phenolic compounds with antioxidant, anti-inflammatory, and antiproliferative activity.[28] Data on the effect of whole-grain intake (most studies reflect intake of multiple whole-grain products rather than individual grains such as oats) on cancer risk are inconsistent. Researchers found lower all-cause mortality with higher intake of total whole-grain products in a large Scandinavian cohort.[29] For all-cause mortality, researchers found lower mortality in the highest intake quartile compared with the lowest quartile for breakfast cereals, nonwhite bread, total whole-grain products, oat, rye (only in men), wheat, and total whole-grain types. Data from the Iowa Women's Health Study and Norwegian County Study showed a nonsignificant reduced cancer mortality risk among eaters of whole grains.[30-32]

For years, algae have been used by food manufacturers as a source of thickening agents, but they are increasingly being considered as functional food ingredients. Nutritional values of algae vary by species, but the protein quality of some forms of algae is as good as that of eggs. Manufacturers are working to identify the best strategies for storing and handling algae as well as trying to understand the ways in which processing affects the nutritional composition of final products. Nevertheless, algae are already being added to foods, such as salad dressings, liquid condiments, beverages, and baked goods. Planktonic algae are a predominant source of omega-3 fatty acids in fish and provide both eicosapentaenoic acid (EPA) and docosahexaenoic acid (DHA).[33] DHA may influence carcinogenesis by enhancing anti-inflammatory actions and inducing apoptosis. Ongoing research is also exploring the ability of DHA to promote cell cycle arrests that provide time for a cell to repair any abnormalities.[34] Understanding that consumers are looking to food for health as well as taste, food manufacturers continue to explore functional ingredients in order to expand their market line.

Regulation of Functional Foods

FDA regulations for functional foods fall under those for conventional foods. Health claims must meet the requirements of the Nutrition Labeling and Education Act of 1990, which characterize relationships between bioactive substances and disease risk reduction based on a "standard of significant scientific agreement." Qualified health claims also describe diet-disease relationships; they are used when research results do not reach the highest level of evidence. Claims are allowed between foods (including functional foods) and six disease categories, cancer being one.[35]

Incorporating Functional Foods in the Cancer Nutrition Care Process

Registered dietitian nutritionists (RDNs) who specialize in oncology develop nutrition care plans best suited to the unique nutritional needs, diagnoses, and treatment statuses of their individual cancer patients. For prevention and survivorship, this requires inclusion of recommended amounts of whole foods, such as fruits, vegetables, and whole grains, and their component functional ingredients, such as fibers, carotenoids, polyphenols, and others, as tolerated and appropriate. RDNs also advise cancer patients on potential functional foods that may not be appropriate for their unique nutritional needs because they are also high in sugar, saturated fat, or both. The *2020–2025 Dietary Guidelines for Americans*[3] present three options for healthy eating patterns, Healthy US-Style Eating Pattern,[4] Healthy Vegetarian Eating Pattern,[6] and Healthy Mediterranean-Style Eating Pattern,[7] which advise consumers on the amounts of fruits, vegetables, whole grains, protein foods, and dairy foods recommended for good health (at 12 calorie levels) and, if adopted, would increase functional-food intake. These recommended eating patterns may be appropriate for nutrition intervention for some cancer patients, or they may be the starting point, with recommendations for additional and specific functional foods and ingredients being included in the nutrition care plan as needed. RDNs will consider the medical diagnoses, cancer stage, medical treatment plan, GI integrity, and baseline nutritional status before determining whether, and which, functional foods should play a role in nutrition intervention.

Dietary improvement, dietary fortification and enrichment, and the inclusion of appropriate, cancer-fighting functional foods in a diet can prevent nutrient insufficiencies and deficiencies, promote cancer prevention and survivorship, and improve overall health.

Dietary improvement, as the first goal, requires the inclusion of functional foods as a valid and versatile source of nutrients and other bioactive compounds. To fully apply current literature to the Nutrition Care Process for cancer patients, RDNs should be knowledgeable about the wide range of functional foods in the marketplace and their applicability to cancer prevention, treatment, and survivorship. Additional resources for functional foods are provided in Box 7.1.

Dietary Supplements and Cancer

The use of dietary supplements is widespread, particularly among those with cancer. Many studies

Box 7.1
Resources on Functional Foods

Source	Document or article
Micronutrient Information Center, Linus Pauling Institute, Oregon State University	Phytochemicals. Micronutrient Information Center website. https://lpi.oregonstate.edu/mic/dietary-factors/phytochemicals
Journal of Developments in Sustainable Agriculture	Figures supporting the discussion of cancer and functional foods in Benninghoff AD, Lefevre M, Hintze KJ, Ward RE, Broadbent JR. Fighting cancer with functional foods: new approaches to investigate the interactions of dietary bioactive chemicals and the gut microbiome. *Journal of Developments in Sustainable Agriculture*. 2015;10:34-54. www.jstage.jst.go.jp/article/jdsa/10/1/10_34/_pdf
American Journal of Cancer Research	Table 1: Sources, function, and effects of different functional foods in cancer prevention in Aghajanpour M, Nazer MR, Obeidavi Z, Akbari M, Ezati P, Kor NM. Functional foods and their role in cancer prevention and health promotion: a comprehensive review. *Am J Cancer Res*. 2017;7(4):740-769. www.ncbi.nlm.nih.gov/pmc/articles/PMC5411786
Canadian Foundation for Dietetic Research	Duncan AM, Hilary A. Dunn HA, Vella MN, Stratton LM. *Functional Foods for Healthy Aging: A Toolkit for Registered Dietitians*. Department of Human Health and Nutritional Sciences, University of Guelph; 2012. www.cfdr.ca/Downloads/Presentations/Functional-Foods-For-Healthy-Aging-TOOLKIT-January.aspx
The World Bank	Williams M, Pehu E, Ragasa C. Functional foods: opportunities and challenges for developing countries. *Agricultural and Rural Development Notes*. 2016;(19):1-4. http://siteresources.worldbank.org/INTARD/Resources/Note19_FunctionalFoods_web.pdf

report that use of dietary supplements by cancer patients is much greater than by cancer-free individuals.[36-40] Interest in herbal or other botanical supplements and vitamin and mineral supplements surged in the latter half of the 20th century, as many Americans came to consider these products natural and, therefore, safer than prescription medicines. By the 1980s, with sales skyrocketing, it was clear that new legislation was needed to define dietary supplements. When debating the proposed Dietary Supplement Health and Education Act of 1994, the US Senate Committee on Labor and Human Resources summarized a widely held consumer view of herbal products, stating, "Unlike many drugs, the role of herbal dietary supplements is to enhance the diet by adding safe and natural plants and their constituents to support and protect bodily functions and processes."[41]

While most consumers of supplements use these products to maintain or improve health, health care provider recommendations account for less than 25% of use.[42] As health care providers, RDNs need to understand the safety, uses, and efficacy of dietary supplements. Nutrition assessments should document dietary supplement use, including ingredients and dosage. It is paramount that health care providers openly discuss the use of dietary supplements with patients and present safe, evidence-based recommendations.

Prevalence

The use of dietary supplements remained relatively stable between 1999 and 2012, with 52% of US adults reporting use of any supplements in 2011 through 2012.[43] While vitamin and mineral products are the most popular supplements used in the United States, approximately 20% of Americans and 23% of people with cancer take herbal or other botanical supplements.[44,45]

Dietary supplements fuel a multibillion-dollar industry. Sales of dietary supplements amounted to approximately $18.8 billion in 2003 and surpassed $30 billion in 2011, with an expected growth in sales of 7% annually.[46,47]

Safety

Dietary supplements and their manufacture, sale, and use are overseen in the United States by several federal agencies with overlapping jurisdiction—they are regulated by the FDA and the Federal Trade Commission; enforcement of the regulations falls to the State Attorneys General Offices and the Department of Justice; and the Centers for Disease Control and Prevention monitors (but does not regulate) their use.[48] In 1994, the US Congress, when passing the Dietary Supplement Health and Education Act, defined and established a regulatory framework for dietary supplements. Dietary supplements were defined as products taken by mouth that provide ingredients intended to supplement the diet; they may include vitamins and minerals, herbal and other botanical products, amino acids, and other nutritive and dietary substances.[49] The regulatory framework assigned responsibilities for ensuring that products are safe before being marketed by the manufacturer. The burden of taking action against any unsafe dietary supplement was assigned to the FDA.[49]

By law, dietary supplement packaging must provide contact information for reporting adverse events; in turn, manufacturers and distributors of dietary supplements are required to forward reports of serious adverse effects to the FDA.[50] Consumers can report adverse effects associated with dietary supplements to the FDA's MedWatch program.[51] In 2011, the FDA reported receiving 1,777 adverse event reports from the dietary supplement industry,[52] though US poison control centers reported receiving 29,000 calls regarding adverse effects experienced after taking a dietary supplement.[53] The supplements *Larrea tridentate* (chaparral), *Ephedra sinica*, and symphytum (comfrey) are inherently unsafe and have been banned in the United States. *Mentha pulegium* (pennyroyal) is also unsafe but is still available in the marketplace. These products have been linked with serious liver toxicity and should never be consumed. The National Library of Medicine, under the auspices of the National Institute of Diabetes and Digestive and Kidney Diseases of the National Institutes of Health, has established the website LiverTox (https://livertox.nih.gov) to help people identify herbal and dietary supplements, as well as conventional medications, that have been linked with liver toxicity.[54] LiverTox also includes a case submission registry that allows users to submit case reports.

Though dietary supplement use has been associated with a healthier lifestyle (normal weight, never smoking, and better diet), a French cohort study reported that 18% of dietary supplement users engaged in potentially harmful supplement practices; these included the simultaneous use of vitamin E and anticoagulant or antiplatelet agents, the use of β-carotene and smoking, and the use of phytoestrogens by hormone-dependent cancer patients.[39] This evidence points to the importance

Plants and Pharmaceuticals

Approximately 40% of pharmaceutical products are derived from plants. Various plant-derived compounds are currently being investigated for use in cancer therapy, and many other active but perhaps untested plant compounds are widely available in dietary supplements.[55]

Plants and dietary supplements made from their parts (eg, leaves and stems) possess a variety of active compounds that influence carcinogenesis. Some help regulate cell cycles; others modulate inflammation, promote DNA repair, and reduce oxidative stress. They may influence drug metabolism, and by increasing or decreasing a drug's blood level can influence its therapeutic effect. Interactions can result from alterations in absorption, bioavailability, and drug clearance.[56] Phytochemicals, secondary plant metabolites, are thought to play a role in cancer chemoprevention due to their ability to suppress oxidative stress-induced DNA damage.[57] Because dietary supplements are not required to undergo premarket evaluation, adverse side effects may not be recognized until reported by consumers.

The cytochrome P-450 (CYP) enzyme system is important to drug metabolism, particularly given its key role in detoxification.[58] Genetics, prescription drugs, food, and dietary supplements may influence the activity of these enzymes, potentially decreasing drug efficacy or resulting in adverse effects. *Hypericum perforatum* (St. John's wort) may influence the CYP system and can potentially reduce concentrations of some drugs, including imatinib and irinotecan, which are commonly used in cancer treatments; *Allium sativum* (garlic), *Panax ginseng*, and *Gingko biloba* also may interact with CYP substrates.[59]

Some data suggest that *Silybum marianum* (milk thistle) may reduce the clearance of various drugs via inhibition of CYP enzymes.[58] In vitro studies have reported that milk thistle can significantly inhibit CYP3A4 induction by rifampicin, erlotinib, and paclitaxel,[60] but this interaction has not been replicated in human studies. Lack of absorption might explain why many clinical trials of natural products, including milk thistle, have shown no drug interactions even though interactions were predicted during preclinical studies.[61]

Research trials in humans have found only four botanical dietary supplements that cause supplement-drug interactions, including *Hypericum perforatum* (St. John's wort), *Hydrastis canadensis* (goldenseal), *Echinacea purpurea* (echinacea), and Allium (garlic) oil.[58] Many popular botanical dietary supplements, such as *Aloe vera*, kelp, chia seeds and oil, maca, ginger, cinnamon, and elderberry, have not been reported to pose risks of interaction with drugs.[61]

Vitamin-Mineral Supplements

Research examining the role of vitamin and mineral supplementation in cancer prevention has failed to consistently demonstrate a benefit. However, patients with cancer who have difficulty eating because of nutrition impact symptoms may be at risk of malnutrition or nutrient deficiency and thus may benefit from a multivitamin and mineral (MVM) supplement. An intake analysis of 19 micronutrients from natural foods, fortified and enriched food, and nutrient-based dietary supplements found that vitamin and mineral supplements made important contributions to total micronutrient intake, thus demonstrating their benefit.[62]

Several trials have assessed the relationship between MVM supplements and cancer risk and mortality. Findings are somewhat mixed. Results from the Women's Health Initiative, the largest cohort of women with postmenopausal breast cancer, suggest that MVM use may reduce breast cancer mortality in postmenopausal women with invasive breast cancer.[63] In the Life After Cancer

Epidemiology Study, persistent MVM supplement use (both prediagnosis and postdiagnosis, three or more times a week), compared to never use, was associated with a nonsignificant reduction in the risk of cancer recurrence, breast cancer mortality, and total mortality.[64] Interestingly, women who used MVM supplements and were in the top quartile for fruit and vegetable intake (at least 5.5 servings per day) had a significantly reduced risk of total mortality compared to women who were in the bottom quartile (at most 2.4 servings per day). Similarly, persistent multivitamin use among women who were physically active 16 h/wk was associated with a reduced risk of total mortality compared to women who were physically active less than 8 h/wk. Findings from the Physicians' Health Study II stated that men who used MVM supplements had a statistically significant 8% reduced risk of cancer.[65] This benefit was even greater in men with a history of cancer: Cancer incidence was 27% lower in MVM users versus nonusers. Results from the Multiethnic Cohort Study, however, found no association between MVM use and cancer risk or cancer mortality.[66]

MVM supplements providing 100% of the Daily Value for each nutrient can be considered safe and likely adequate for healthy persons, but in patients with cancer, it is important to evaluate the needs of each patient individually according to his or her specific cancer diagnosis, symptoms, and treatments. When a diet includes many fortified, enriched, and functional foods, it may already be providing the recommended nutrient needs.

Antioxidant Supplements

Despite many years of research into the use of antioxidant supplementation in cancer, controversy remains regarding the safety and efficacy of these complementary treatments. Antioxidant intake does indeed seem to influence the effectiveness of antitumor therapy and its adverse effects.

There is a long-standing belief that antioxidant supplementation may protect against oxidative stress associated with the development of certain diseases, such as cancer.[67] Hence, it has become commonplace for many to consume antioxidant supplements for health purposes. Research suggests that antioxidants may slow or possibly prevent the development of cancer due to their effects on cell cycle regulation, inflammation, the inhibition of tumor cell proliferation and invasiveness, the induction of apoptosis, and the stimulation of the detoxifying enzyme activity.[68,69]

Cancer cells appear to have a higher level of oxidative stress compared to normal cells. This greater amount of stress is associated with an increased production of reactive oxygen species (ROS).[69] Tumor cells become highly dependent on antioxidant agents during cancer development because of higher levels of ROS; a balance of ROS and antioxidants is needed to promote growth of cancer cells. Hence, a high antioxidant load that reduces levels of free radicals has the potential to promote cancer cell development and proliferation.[68] The considerable formation of ROS in tumor cells could damage DNA and promote genetic instability and chemoresistance.[69,70] There is hope that new therapeutic strategies will be developed to counteract damage caused by ROS.

Concurrent Use of Antioxidant Supplements and Chemotherapy or Radiotherapy

Research regarding antioxidant supplementation concurrent with chemotherapy or radiotherapy, or both, is mixed and results are somewhat contradictory. Studies in animals have found the coadministration of antioxidants and chemotherapeutic agents to be effective and promising.[71-75] Reproducing those results in humans, however, has proven to be challenging. Though it has been proposed that antioxidant supplements during cancer treatment may protect healthy cells and mitigate side effects from treatment while simultaneously augmenting the cancer treatment, they may reduce the effectiveness of the therapy. Currently, no general recommendation on the use of supplemental antioxidants during treatment can be made for humans. The interaction of supplements and chemotherapy or radiotherapy will likely vary based on the type of cancer, the mechanism of action of the drug or drugs used in the treatment, and the type of antioxidant(s). The literature has yielded mixed results. A review of 52 clinical trials examining the effects of combining antioxidant supplementation (eg, glutathione compounds, vitamin E, selenium, coenzyme Q10, and zinc) with conventional treatment found that a number of antioxidants studied conferred a benefit (eg, reduced side effects), but no conclusion could be reached because of the wide variability in the type of compound tested, dosage, and method of administration (eg, at least five different types of vitamin E have been tested, in doses ranging from 100 mg to 3,200 IU).[76]

Supplemental antioxidants should be used carefully in patients undergoing cancer therapy; those patients seeking a curative regimen should use them with great caution. Khurana and colleagues[71] reported that antioxidant supplementation concurrent with treatment should be discouraged because of the potential for tumor protection and reduced survival. Greater leeway should be granted for those undergoing palliative regimens. Well-designed studies that consider the "complexity and diversity"[77] of antioxidants are needed before clinicians can confidently provide cancer patients undergoing active treatment with much needed evidence-based advice.

Navigating Dietary Supplements

Most cancer patients use dietary supplements. Some supplements may be safe, but others may be unsafe and have the potential to interfere with cancer treatments. RDNs should integrate questions regarding supplement use into the nutrition assessment process and incorporate their findings into the nutrition care plan. RDNs can also recommend conventional and functional foods that may meet the patient's desired health goals.

RDNs already educate and counsel cancer patients on diets that meet their unique needs. It is equally important for RDNs to become leaders in advising the medical team on potential effects of dietary supplements on cancer treatment and in educating patients with cancer on evidence-based and appropriate use of dietary supplements. Box 7.2 on page 120 provides resources on dietary supplements. Appendix C summarizes the evidence on select supplements commonly used by the cancer population.

Summary

The use of diet, functional foods, and supplements for cancer prevention and survival is common among the population in the United States and across the world. RDNs serve in the vital role of assisting the public in understanding the scientific evidence regarding diets, functional foods, and supplements and providing individualized, safe, and effective nutrition interventions for cancer prevention and survivorship.

Box 7.2
Resources on Dietary Supplements

Source	Document or article
Memorial Sloan Kettering Cancer Center	About herbs, botanicals, and other products. Memorial Sloan Kettering Cancer Center website. www.mskcc.org/cancer-care/diagnosis-treatment/symptom-management/integrative-medicine/herbs
Office of Dietary Supplements, National Institutes of Health	Dietary supplement fact sheets. Office of Dietary Supplements website. http://ods.od.nih.gov/factsheets/list-all
Academy of Nutrition and Dietetics	Position of the Academy of Nutrition and Dietetics: Micronutrient supplementation (2018). Academy of Nutrition and Dietetics website. www.eatrightpro.org/-/media/eatrightpro-files/practice/position-and-practice-papers/position-papers/micronutrientsupplementation.pdf
Therapeutic Research Center	Natural Medicines database. Natural Medicines website. naturalmedicines.therapeuticresearch.com An evidence-based database with product monographs including safety, efficacy, and interaction information (requires subscription).
Linus Pauling Institute, Oregon State University	Micronutrient Information Center website. http://lpi.oregonstate.edu/mic
US Food and Drug Administration	Dietary Supplements. US Food and Drug Administration website. www.fda.gov/food/dietary-supplements Includes alerts, safety information, and adverse event reporting.

References

1. World Cancer Research Fund/ American Institute for Cancer Research. *Diet, Nutrition, Physical Activity and Cancer: A Global Perspective*. Continuous Update Project Expert Report 2018. Accessed April 23, 2019. www.wcrf.org/dietandcancer

2. Lohse T, Faeh D, Bopp M, Rohrmann S. Adherence to the cancer prevention recommendations of the World Cancer Research Fund/American Institute for Cancer Research and mortality: a census-linked cohort. *Am J Clin Nutr*. 2016;104(3): 678-685.

3. US Department of Health and Human Services, US Department of Agriculture. *2020–2025 Dietary Guidelines for Americans*. 9th ed. US Department of Agriculture; 2020. Accessed January 6, 2021. https://dietaryguidelines.gov

4. US Department of Health and Human Services, US Department of Agriculture. Appendix 3. USDA dietary patterns: Healthy US-style dietary pattern. In: *2020–2025 Dietary Guidelines for Americans*. 9th ed. US Department of Agriculture; 2020. Accessed January 6, 2021. https://dietaryguidelines.gov

5. Rock CL, Thomson C, Gansler T, et al. American Cancer Society guideline for diet and physical activity for cancer prevention. *CA A Cancer J Clin*. 2020;70: 245-271.

6. US Department of Health and Human Services, US Department of Agriculture. Appendix 3. USDA dietary patterns: healthy vegetarian dietary pattern. In: *2020–2025 Dietary Guidelines for Americans*. 9th ed. US Department of Agriculture; 2020. Accessed January 6, 2021. https://dietaryguidelines.gov

7. US Department of Health and Human Services and US Department of Agriculture. Appendix 3. USDA dietary patterns: Healthy Mediterranean-Style dietary pattern. In: *2020–2025 Dietary Guidelines for Americans*. 9th ed. US Department of Agriculture; 2020. Accessed January 6, 2021. https://dietaryguidelines.gov

8. Messina M, Messina V. The second golden age of nutrition. In Huang M-T, Osawa T, Ho C-T, Rosen RT, eds. *Food Phytochemicals for Cancer Prevention I*. American Chemical Society; 1993:382-387. doi:10.1021/bk-1994-0546.ch032

9. Zubair H, Azim S, Ahmad A. Cancer chemoprevention by phytochemicals: nature's healing touch. *Molecules*. 2017;22(3):395. doi:10.3390/molecules22030395

10. Aghajanpour M, Nazer MR, Obeidai Z, et al. Functional foods and their role in cancer prevention and health promotion: a comprehensive review. *Am J Cancer Res*. 2017;7(4):740-769.

11. Lobo V, Patil A, Phatak A, Chandra N. Free radicals, antioxidants and functional foods: impact on human health. *Pharmacogn Rev*. 2010;4(8):118-126.

12. Backstrand JR. The history and future of food fortification in the United States: a public health perspective. *Nutr Rev*. 2002;60(1):15-26.

13. Shimizu T. Health claims on functional foods: the Japanese regulations and an international comparison. *Nutr Res Rev*. 2004;16(2):241-252.

14. Crowe K, Francis C. Position of the Academy of Nutrition and Dietetics: functional foods. *J Acad Nutr Diet*. 2013;113(8):1096-1103. doi:10.1016/j.jand.2013.06.002

15. Dillard CJ, German BJ. Review: phytochemicals: nutraceuticals and human health. *J Sci Food Agric*. 2000;80:1744-1756.

16. Salami A, Seydi E, Pourahmad. Use of nutraceuticals for prevention and treatment of cancer. *Iran J Pharm Res*. 2013;12(3):219-220.

17. Kapinova A, Kubatka P, Golubnitschaja O, et al. Dietary phytochemicals in breast cancer research: anticancer effects and potential utility for effective chemoprevention. *Environ Health Prev Med*. 2018;23(1):36. doi:10.1186/s12199-018-0724-1

18. Ilowefah M, Chinma C, Bakar J, et al. Fermented brown rice as functional food ingredient. *Foods*. 2013;3(1):149-159.

19. Haugabrooks E. *Evaluating the Use of Resistant Starch as a Beneficial Dietary Fiber and Its Effect on Physiological Response of Glucose, Insulin, and Fermentation* (Dissertation). Iowa State University; 2013. Accessed February 1, 2019. https://lib.dr.iastate.edu/cgi/viewcontent.cgi?article=4632&context=etd

20. Birt D, Boylston T, Hendrich S, et al. Resistant starch: promise for improving human health. *Adv Nutr*. 2013;4(6):587-601.

21. Morris DH. Description and composition of flax. In: *Flax—a Health and Nutrition Primer*. Flax Council of Canada; 2007. Accessed April 23, 2019. https://flaxcouncil.ca/wp-content/uploads/2015/03/FlxPrmr_4ed_Chpt1.pdf

22. Kajla P, Sharma A, Sood DR. Flaxseed—a potential functional food source. *J Food Sci Technnol*. 2015;52(4):1857-1871.

23. Roberfroid MG. Inulin-type fructans: functional food ingredients. *J Nutr*. 2007;137(11 suppl); 2493S-2502S. doi:10.1093/jn/137.11.2493S

24. Rivera-Huerta M, Lizarraga-Grimes VL, Castro-Torres IG, et al. Functional effects of prebiotic fructans in colon cancer and calcium metabolism in animal models. *Biomed Res Int*. 2017;2017: 9758982. doi:10.1155/2017/9758982

25. Franco-Robles E, Lopez MG. Implication of fructans in health: immunomodulatory and antioxidant mechanisms. *ScientificWorldJournal*. 2015;2015:289267. doi:10.1155/2015/289267

26. Hu S, Dong TS, Dalad SR, et al. The microbe-derived short chain fatty acid butyrate targets miRNA-dependent 21 gene expression in human colon cancer. *PLoS One*. 2011;6(1):e16221. doi:10.1371/journal.pone.0016221.e16221

27. Rasane P, Jha A, Sabikhi L, Kumar A, Unnikrishnan VS. Nutritional advantages of oats and opportunities for its processing as value added foods   a review. *J Food Sci Technol*. 2015;52(2):662-675.

28. Sibakov J. *Processing of Oat Dietary Fibre for Improved Functionality as a Food Ingredient* (Thesis). VTT Technical Research Centre; 2014.

29. Johnsen NF, Frederiksen K, Christensen J, et al. Whole-grain products and whole-grain types are associated with lower all-cause and cause-specific mortality in the Scandinavian HELGA cohort. *Br J Nutr*. 2015.114(4):608-623.

30. Jacobs DR Jr, Andersen LF, Blomhoff R. Whole-grain consumption is associated with a reduced risk of noncardiovascular, noncancer death attributed to inflammatory diseases in the Iowa Women's Health Study. *Am J Clin Nutr*. 2007;85(6):1606-1614.

31. Jacobs DR Jr, Meyer KA, Kushi LH, Folsom AR. Is whole grain intake associated with reduced total and cause-specific death rates in older women? The Iowa Women's Health Study. *Am J Public Health*. 1999;89(3):322-329.

32. Jacobs DR Jr, Meyer HE, Solvoll K. Reduced mortality among whole grain bread eaters in men and women in the Norwegian County Study. *Eur J Clin Nutr*. 2001;55(2):137-143.

33. Wells M, Potin P, Craigie JS. Algae as nutritional and functional food sources: revisiting our understanding. *J Appl Phycol*. 2017;29(2):949-982.

34. Newell M, Baker K, Postovit LM, Field CJ. A critical review on the effect of docosahexaenoic acid (DHA) on cancer cell cycle progression. *Int J Mol Sci*. 2017;18(8):1784. doi:10.3390/ijms18081784

35. Office of Nutrition and Food Labeling. *Guidance for Industry: A Food Labeling Guide*. US Food and Drug Administration; January 2013. Accessed September 17, 2019. www.fda.gov/regulatory-information/search-fda-guidance-documents/guidance-industry-food-labeling-guide

36. Song S, Youn J, Lee YJ, et al. Dietary supplement use among cancer survivors and the general population: a nation-wide cross-sectional study. *BMC Cancer*. 2017;17(1): 891.

37. Lee V, Goyal A, Hsu CC, Jacobson JS, Rodriguez RD, Siegel AB. Dietary supplement use among patients with hepatocellular carcinoma. *Integr Cancer Ther*. 2015;14(1):35-41.

38. Frenkel M, Sierpina V. The use of dietary supplements in oncology. *Curr Oncol Rep*. 2014;16(11):411.

39. Pouchieu C, Fassier P, Druesne-Pecollo N, et al. Dietary supplement use among cancer survivors of the NutriNet-Santé cohort study. *Br J Nutr*. 2015;113(8):1319-1329.

40. Bardia A, Greeno E, Bauer BA. Dietary supplement usage by patients with cancer undergoing chemotherapy: does prognosis or cancer symptoms predict usage? *J Support Oncol*. 2007;5(4):195-198.

41. Committee on Labor and Human Resources. S Rep No. 410, 103rd Cong, 2d Sess, at 16 (1994). Dietary Supplement Health and Education Act of 1994, Pub L No. 103–417, 103rd Cong (October 25, 1994).

42. Bailey RL, Gahche JJ, Miller PE, Thomas PR, Dwyer JT. Why US adults use dietary supplements. *JAMA Intern Med*. 2013;173(5):355-361.

43. Kantor ED, Rehm CD, Du M, White E, Giovannucci EL. Trends in dietary supplement use among US adults from 1999–2012. *JAMA*. 2016;316(14):1464-1474.

44. Bailey RL, Gahche JJ, Lentino CV, et al. Dietary supplement use in the United States, 2003–2006. *J Nutr*. 2011;141(2):261-266.

45. Ferrucci LM, McCorkle R, Smith T, Stein KD, Cartmel B. Factors related to the use of dietary supplements by cancer survivors. *J Alt Complem Med*. 2009;15(6):673.

46. Nutrition Business Journal. Executive summary. In: *NBJ's Supplement Business Report 2012*. Penton Media; 2012. Accessed February 8, 2020. www.newhope.com/sites/newhope360.com/files/uploads/2012/10/TOC_SUMM120928.supp%20report%20FINAL%20standard.pdf

47. Cassileth BR, Heitzer M, Wesa K. The public health impact of herbs and nutritional supplements. *Pharm Biol*. 2009;47(8):761-767.

48. Brown AC. An overview of herb and dietary supplement efficacy, safety and government regulations in the United States with suggested improvements. Part 1 of 5 series. *Food Chem Toxicol*. 2017;107(pt A):449-471.

49. Gauche J, Bailey R, Burt V, et al. *Dietary Supplement Use Among U.S. Adults Has Increased Since NHANES III (1988–1994)*. NCHS Data Brief, No. 61. National Center for Health Statistics; 2011.

50. For industry: dietary supplements. Reporting an adverse event, at a glance. US Food and Drug Administration website. Accessed February 8, 2020. www.fda.gov/food/dietary-supplements/information-industry-dietary-supplements

51. MedWatch online voluntary reporting form. US Food and Drug Administration website. Accessed February 8, 2020. www.accessdata.fda.gov/scripts/medwatch

52. Adverse Event Reporting and Recordkeeping for Dietary Supplements as Required by the Dietary Supplement and Nonprescription Drug Consumer Protection Act. Fed Regist. 2012;77(57):17076-17077. Accessed February 8, 2020. www.govinfo.gov/content/pkg/FR-2012-03-23/pdf/FR-2012-03-23.pdf

53. Bronstein AC, Spyker DA, Cantilena LR Jr, et al. 2009 annual report of the American Association of Poison Control Centers' National Poison Data System (NPDS): 27th annual report. *Clin Toxicol (Phila)*. 2010;48(10):979–1178.

54. US National Library of Medicine. LiverTox: Clinical and Research Information on Drug-Induced Liver Injury website. Accessed February 8, 2020. www.ncbi.nlm.nih.gov/books/NBK547852

55. Nirmala MJ Samundeeswari A, Sankar PD. Natural plant resources in anti-cancer therapy—a review. *Res Plant Biol*. 2011;1(3):1-14.

56. Boullata JI, Hudson LM. Drug-nutrient interactions: a broad view with implications for practice. *J Acad Nutr Diet*. 2012;112(4):506-517.

57. Chikara S, Nagaprashantha LD, Singhal J, et al. Oxidative stress and dietary phytochemicals: role in cancer chemoprevention and treatment. *Cancer Lett*. 2018;413:122-134.

58. Wanwimolruk S, Prachayasittikul V. Cytochrome P450 enzyme mediated herbal drug interactions (Part 1). *EXCLI J*. 2014;13:347-391.

59. Mathijssen RHJ, Verweij J, de Bruijn P, Loos WJ. Effects of St. John's wort on irinotecan metabolism. *J Natl Cancer Inst*. 2002;94(16):1247-1249.

60. Mooiman KD, Maas-Bakker RF, Moret EE, et al. Milk thistle's active components silybin and isosilybin: novel inhibitors of PXR-mediated CYP3A4 induction. *Drug Metab Dispos*. 2013;41(8):1494–1504.

61. Sprouse A, van Breemen RB. Pharmacokinetic interactions between drugs and botanical dietary supplements. *Drug Metab Dispos*. 2016;44(2):162–171.

62. Fulgoni VL, Keast DR, Bailey RL, Dwyer J. Foods, fortificants, and supplements: where do Americans get their nutrients? *J Nutr*. 2011;141(10):1847-1854.

63. Wassertheil-Smoller S, McGinn AP, Budrys N, et al. Multivitamin and mineral use and breast cancer mortality in older women with invasive breast cancer in the women's health initiative. *Breast Cancer Res Treat*. 2013;141(3):495-505.

64. Kwan ML, Greenlee H, Lee VS, et al. Multivitamin use and breast cancer outcomes in women with early-stage breast cancer: the Life After Cancer Epidemiology study. *Breast Cancer Res Treat*. 2011;130(1):195-205.

65. Hardy ML, Duvall K. Multivitamin/multimineral supplements for cancer prevention: implications for primary care practice. *Postgrad Med*. 2015;127(1):107-116.

66. Park S-Y, Murphy SP, Wilkens LR, Henderson BE, Kolonel LN. Multivitamin use and the risk of mortality and cancer incidence: the Multiethnic Cohort Study. *Am J Epidemiol*. 2011;173(8):906-914.

67. Mut-Salud N, Álvarez PJ, Garrido JM, et al. Antioxidant intake and antitumor therapy: toward nutritional recommendations for optimal results. *Oxid Med Cell Longev*. 2016;2016:6719534. doi:10.1155/2016/6719534

68. Valko M, Leibfritz D, Moncol J, et al. Free radicals and antioxidants in normal physiological functions and human disease. *Intl J Biochem Cell Biol*. 2007;39(1):44-84.

69. Bennett L, Rojas S, Seefeldt T. Role of antioxidants in the prevention of cancer. *J Exper Clin Med.* 2012;4(4):215-222.

70. Matés JM, Segura JA, Alonso FJ, Márquez J. Oxidative stress in apoptosis and cancer: an update. *Arch Toxicol.* 2012;86(11):1649-1665.

71. Khurana RK, Jain A, Jain A, et al. Administration of antioxidants in cancer: debate of the decade. *Drug Discov Today.* 2018;23(4):763-770.

72. Yang Q, Wang B, Zang W, et al. Resveratrol inhibits the growth of gastric cancer by inducing G1 phase arrest and senescence in a Sirt1-dependent manner. *PLoS One.* 2013;8(11):e70627.

73. Mansour HH, Hafez HF, Fahmy NM. Silymarin modulates cisplatin-induced oxidative stress and hepatotoxicity in rats. *J Biochem Mol Biol.* 2006;39(6):656-661.

74. Malekinejad H, Janbaz-Acyabar H, Razi M, Varasteh S. Preventive and protective effects of silymarin on doxorubicin-induced testicular damages correlate with changes in c-myc gene expression. *Phytomedicine.* 2012;19(12):1077-1084.

75. Palipoch S, Punsawad C, Koomhin P, Suwannalert P. Hepatoprotective effect of curcumin and alpha-tocopherol against cisplatin-induced oxidative stress. *BMC Complem Altern Med.* 2014;14:111.

76. Olayinka ET, Ore A, Adeyemo OA, et al. Quercetin, a flavonoid antioxidant, ameliorated procarbazine-induced oxidative damage to murine tissues. *Antioxidants (Basel).* 2015;4(2):304-321.

77. Nakayama A, Alladin K, Igbokwe O, White J. Systematic review: generating evidence-based guidelines on the concurrent use of dietary antioxidants and chemotherapy or radiotherapy. *Cancer Invest.* 2011;29(10):655-667.

Chapter 8
Nutrition and Cancer Survivorship

Cynthia A. Thomson, PhD, RDN, FAND, FTOS
Tracy E. Crane, PhD, MS, RDN

Cancer survivorship is an expanding area of clinical dietetics practice. More than 22 million Americans will be living with a history of a cancer by 2030, primarily because survival rates have steadily improved for many cancers over the past several decades. Close to 70% of patients in whom cancer is diagnosed survive beyond the 5-year monitoring period, which is considered a benchmark for cancer treatment.[1]

The designation "cancer survivor" encompasses individuals in active treatment and recovery as well as those with advanced disease commonly receiving palliative care; however, for the purpose of this chapter, the focus is on those living after initial cancer therapy, and primarily those who are disease-free or who have stable disease.

While cancer survivors may have undergone treatment for a wide variety of neoplasms, survivors of breast, prostate, and colon cancers represent the majority of this population. These cancers are more commonly diagnosed through early-detection screening plans, resulting in relatively high survival rates. For example, more than 98% of women with an early-stage breast cancer diagnosis will be living 10 years after diagnosis; they account for approximately 40% of female cancer survivors.[2]

Notably for nutrition professionals, cancer survivors represent a motivated segment of the patient population for medical nutrition therapy (MNT), as they actively seek information and counseling to improve their overall health through reduced treatment-related symptoms and enhanced quality of life.[3,4] More importantly, survivors report personal attempts to improve dietary selections at the time of or shortly after diagnosis, which indicates that they are highly motivated candidates for dietary change.[5] In fact, people who survive cancer seem to be more likely to adopt dietary behaviors over other cancer-preventive lifestyle behaviors (eg, physical activity, smoking cessation, alcohol restriction), a trend that holds true even among racially and ethnically diverse survivors.[6]

The usual dietary behaviors of patients at the time of cancer diagnosis are increasingly identified as indicators of survival after cancer.[7-9] This suggests that those at risk for cancer, including family members of cancer survivors, would benefit from adopting healthy eating habits to reduce risk, independent of the influence on health if cancer is diagnosed.[10-12]

Early Posttreatment: Symptom Management

The weeks and months following therapy leave many oncology patients at nutritional risk. The early survival period following therapy is generally up to 12 months[1]; during that time, eating may be difficult due to persistent issues, such as nausea, xerostomia, loss of dentition, and radiation enteritis. During this period, efforts to reduce persistent therapy-related side effects within the gastrointestinal tract should be a primary focus of nutritional care. Box 8.1 on pages 128 to 131 summarizes many of the common symptoms and health issues survivors contend with during this period and the appropriate nutritional approaches that can be used to effectively intervene. See Chapter 11 and cancer-specific chapters for additional details on addressing side effects of treatment.

Of note, a significant number of patients lose lean mass (due to the cancer itself as well as subsequent treatment, including surgery and chemotherapy), suffer fatigue related to radiation therapy

Box 8.1

Long-Term Nutrition-Related Side Effects and Interventions for Common Cancers

Cancer site	Common nutrition complications	Common nutritional interventions[a]
All sites	Fatigue	Develop an individualized eating plan and encourage caretakers to get involved in the plan.
		Use foods that are easy to prepare and easy to eat.
		Use medical nutrition beverages as needed.
		Monitor weight and nutrition status.
		Promote physical activity as tolerated.
	Weight change, change in body composition	Monitor weight.
		Ensure nutrient intake is balanced to maintain or achieve a healthy weight.
		Promote physical activity and include weight bearing exercise and resistance training as needed.
Breast	Impaired bone health	Ensure adequate intake of calcium and vitamin D.
		Promote weight-bearing exercises, if appropriate.
	Weight gain, metabolic syndrome	Adjust energy, carbohydrate, fat, and fiber intakes to promote a healthy weight and achieve recommended levels of blood glucose, circulating insulin, and circulating lipids.
		Promote physical activity to meet current guidelines for survivors.
	Cardiovascular complications	Recommend a plant-based diet.
		Promote weight control.
Prostate	Impaired bone health	Ensure adequate intake of calcium and vitamin D.
		Promote weight-bearing exercises, if appropriate.
	Enteritis, chronic diarrhea	Increase fluid intake and balance electrolytes.
		Decrease fat intake, alter fiber intake, and limit dairy intake as needed.
Lung and bronchus	Esophageal pain, dysphagia	Alter food and beverage consistency, and use medical nutrition beverages as needed.
		Alter food temperature and avoid alcohol, spicy foods, and other irritant-containing foods (eg, acidic foods).
		Monitor nutrition status and weight.
	Respiratory failure	Monitor and correct fluid balance.
		Decrease carbohydrate intake, if indicated.

(continued)

[a] Modify approaches according to results of nutrition assessment.

Box 8.1
Long-Term Nutrition-Related Side Effects and Interventions for Common Cancers *(continued)*

Cancer site	Common nutrition complications	Common nutritional interventions[a]
Colon and rectum	Malabsorption	Increase intake or modify sources of nutrients that are malabsorbed. Monitor nutrition status and weight.
	Altered liver function, cirrhosis	Increase intake of nutrients that are malabsorbed. Monitor liver enzymes. If cirrhotic, follow evidence-based medical nutrition therapy for liver cirrhosis.
	Weight change	Monitor weight. Ensure balanced nutrient intake for maintaining or achieving a healthy weight. Balance energy intake with physical activity.
	Irregular bowel movements	Alter fiber intake as needed. Consume adequate fluids; monitor fluid intake. Use probiotics or prebiotics, if appropriate.
	Enteritis, chronic diarrhea	Increase fluid intake and balance electrolytes. Decrease fat intake, alter fiber intake, and limit dairy as needed.
	Bowel strictures or obstructions	Depending on the location of the stricture or obstruction and presence of bowel sounds, provide enteral or parenteral nutrition support as appropriate.
Urinary bladder	Irregular bowel movements	Alter fiber intake as needed. Consume adequate fluids, monitor fluid intake, and balance electrolytes.
Uterine corpus	Impaired bone health	Ensure adequate intake of calcium and vitamin D. Promote weight-bearing exercises, if appropriate.
Thyroid	Hypothyroidism	Adjust energy intake to maintain a healthy weight. Promote physical activity to meet current guidelines for survivors.

(continued)

Box 8.1

Long-Term Nutrition-Related Side Effects and Interventions for Common Cancers *(continued)*

Cancer site	Common nutrition complications	Common nutritional interventions[a]
Non-Hodgkin lymphoma	Metabolic syndrome	Adjust energy, carbohydrate, fat, and fiber intakes to promote a healthy weight and achieve recommended levels of blood glucose, circulating insulin, and circulating lipids.
		Promote physical activity to meet current guidelines for survivors.
	Hypothyroidism	Adjust energy intake to maintain a healthy weight.
		Promote physical activity to meet current guidelines for survivors.
Kidney	Decreased creatinine clearance	Monitor renal laboratory test results, and adjust nutrient intake as needed following evidence-based medical nutrition therapy for renal disease.
	Hypertension	Monitor sodium intake, and adjust (most commonly reduce) sodium intake as needed.
		Promote weight control and physical activity as appropriate.
		Promote adequate intake of potassium and calcium.
	Renal failure	Monitor renal laboratory test results, and adjust nutrient intake as needed following evidence-based medical nutrition therapy for renal disease.
Oral cavity and pharynx	Xerostomia	Ensure nutrient requirements are met via oral intake, if possible.
		Promote consumption of "wet" foods.
		Promote good oral care.
		Alter food and beverage consistency as needed.
		Use medical nutrition beverages and supplemental energy, protein, and nutrient products as indicated.
		Consider nutrition support, if needed.
	Dysphagia	Alter food and beverage consistency as needed.
		Use medical nutrition beverages and supplemental energy, protein, and nutrient products as needed.
		Monitor nutrition status and weight.
		Consult with a speech-language pathologist.

(continued)

[a] Modify approaches according to results of nutrition assessment.

Box 8.1
Long-Term Nutrition-Related Side Effects and Interventions for Common Cancers (continued)

Cancer site	Common nutrition complications	Common nutritional interventions[a]
Oral cavity and pharynx (continued)	Tooth decay, periodontal disease	Alter food and beverage consistency as needed. Use medical nutrition beverages and supplemental energy, protein, and nutrient products as needed. Alter food temperature if tooth sensitivity is an issue. Alter types of food consumed if dysgeusia is an issue. Consult a dental professional.
Leukemia	Kidney stones	Increase fluid intake to recommended levels.
	Impaired bone health	Ensure adequate intake of calcium and vitamin D. Promote weight-bearing exercises, if appropriate.
	Metabolic syndrome	Adjust energy, sugar, and fat intakes to promote a healthy weight and achieve recommended levels of blood glucose, circulating insulin, and circulating lipids. Promote physical activity to meet current guidelines for survivors.
	Hypothyroidism	Adjust energy intake to maintain a healthy weight. Promote physical activity to meet current guidelines for survivors.
Ovary	Impaired bone health	Ensure adequate intake of calcium and vitamin D. Promote weight-bearing exercises, if appropriate.
	Bowel strictures or obstructions	Depending on the location of the stricture or obstruction and presence of bowel sounds, provide enteral or parenteral nutrition support as appropriate.
	Irregular bowel movements	Alter fiber intake as needed. Consume adequate fluids, monitor fluid intake, and balance electrolytes.
Pancreas	Malabsorption	Modify intake of nutrients that are unabsorbed, if indicated. Consider use of pancreatic enzymes replacement therapy. Monitor weight, nutrition, and fluid status.
	Irregular bowel movements	Alter fiber intake. Use probiotics or prebiotics, if appropriate.

and chemotherapy, and experience anxiety or become depressed as a result of having a life-threatening illness.[13,14] Treatment-associated symptoms that continue after treatment can compromise a person's nutritional status, but these concerns are, fortunately, responsive to dietary counseling.[10-12,15-18] Further, weight gain is common during this period, with many patients demonstrating a rise in their fat mass without a concomitant increase in lean mass, placing many of them at risk for sarcopenic obesity.[19,20] See Chapter 3 for additional information on cancer survivorship.

Identifying Inadequacies Through Nutritional Assessment

Chapter 4 reviews nutrition screening and assessment in cancer care. Over the longer term, dietetics professionals need to evaluate clients in terms of their unique nutritional inadequacies that can result from either treatment sequelae or adoption of highly restrictive diets (fasting, vegan, ketogenic), or both. See Appendix B for more details on these diets. Assessments should include anthropometric evaluation to identify changes in central adiposity by measuring waist circumference and assessing lean- and fat-mass status by using computed tomography (CT), bioelectrical impedance, or dual-energy x-ray absorptiometry (DXA). Serial assessments are an important aspect for the provision of care to ensure that lean mass is maintained and to implement a nutrition and activity plan to promote lean mass. Many patients who have undergone extensive surgery or long-term therapies require ample protein intake and regular physical activity, particularly resistance training, in order to increase lean mass (see Chapter 3).[21] Partnering registered dietitian nutritionists with exercise physiologists and physical therapists is advised for optimal progress in these patients.

Body-composition assessment data acquired from DXA or CT scan can be used to assess bone health and provide MNT to optimize skeletal health; this may include a calcium- and magnesium-rich eating plan, vitamin D supplementation, and regular impact and strength-training exercise.[22,23] Beyond body composition, the physical examination should include a comprehensive, systems-level review to identify potential nutrient deficiencies.

Additionally, the nutrition assessment should review prior medical and oncology-related history to identify comorbidities that guide MNT (eg, diabetes, hypertension, heart disease, osteoporosis) as well as possible drug-nutrient interactions. To best understand and intervene on potential nutrition-related medical and pharmacological interactions, dietetic professionals should routinely evaluate biochemical measures. Early in survivorship the focus tends to be on biochemical indexes associated with nutritional deficiencies, including anemia, hypoalbumenia, and specific diet-related undernutrition associated with restricted eating (eg, deficiencies in vitamin D, vitamin E, calcium, and other nutrients). However, it is also imperative that the patient's laboratory values for hyperglycemia, hyperlipidemia, and inflammation (high-sensitivity C-reactive protein) be evaluated to determine the need for additional dietary interventions.

Perhaps the most significant component of nutritional status assessment is dietary intake. Dietetics professionals should evaluate usual dietary intake early in the survivorship period and at regular intervals across the survivorship continuum to identify altered eating as a result of changes in taste, nausea, irregular bowel or gastrointestinal function, and dysgeusia or dysphagia. These symptoms will guide the appropriate nutritional therapy over the survivorship continuum, with the understanding that most of these symptoms will improve or resolve with time. Furthermore, evidence suggests that patients with more toxic therapies have difficulty meeting micronutrient needs without oral nutritional supplementation.[24]

Recovering Nutritional Status: Postsymptom Diet Therapy

After the initial 12 months following treatment, most survivors' cancer treatment–related symptoms have improved, and they are able to tolerate all food groups and textures. Nutrition therapy shifts toward health promotion and cancer prevention. In this longer-term period, many cancer survivors gain weight and put themselves at risk for chronic disease and cancer recurrence.[20] Figure 8.1 on page 134 summarizes the metabolic and physical concerns that can result in increased risk for chronic disease and decreased quality of life in individuals treated for cancer.

During the 12-month period following treatment, many survivors express interest in improving lifestyle choices to enhance health. Convincing evidence suggests that obesity is associated with risk for 13 different cancers.[25] Obesity may predict a poorer prognosis and decreased survival for patients with several cancer types,[26-29] including breast and gynecological,[30,31] colorectal,[32] and prostate.[33] This association is particularly concerning in patients who demonstrate lower lean mass[34-36] and correlates with the presence of comorbid obesity-related disease, such as diabetes.[37]

Medical Nutrition Therapy for Posttreatment Weight Management

Coping with a cancer diagnosis and with the side effects of therapy as well may contribute to obesity risk after treatment. The most common symptoms after a cancer diagnosis are fatigue, depression, and anxiety. These symptoms may lead survivors to alter their eating habits in an effort to increase energy levels and reduce anxiety. For example,

data from the SUCCEED trial of obese survivors of endometrial cancer suggest that women seek high-energy foods as a reward.[38] Other research has shown that fatigue may be a significant driver of high-energy-food–seeking behavior in cancer survivors.[39] Understanding these relationships between food intake and emotions can promote healthier choices. Limited but intriguing data suggest mindfulness approaches can have therapeutic benefit for diet.[40-42] Lifestyle coaching for survivors who are eating to reward themselves has also demonstrated efficacy.[38] For survivors who are experiencing fatigue, weight-loss success may require an integrated approach, with strategies to manage fatigue in addition to diet intervention.

To decrease cancer recurrence and other disease risk, survivors with excess body weight or body fat should be counseled to achieve a healthy body weight and composition. Several studies, primarily in breast cancer survivors,[43-47] demonstrated efficacy of weight loss in relation to improvements in metabolic and cardiovascular biomarkers and quality of life, all factors that have been associated with overall cancer mortality.[48] The ideal weight-loss approach should promote healthy food choices, meal patterns, and portion control; incorporate physical activity; and provide behavior modification support tailored to the individual survivor. Most cancer survivors should be encouraged to undertake a regular activity regime that includes a variety of aerobic, weight-bearing, and resistance-training activities to promote a healthy body composition following treatment.[49] This is an important aspect of weight management during cancer survivorship and a factor that may be insufficiently addressed in the practice setting. Even in normal-weight individuals with cancer, higher rates of metabolic abnormalities, such as hyperglycemia, hypertension, and hyperlipidemia, will respond to healthier food choices when combined with regular physical activity that includes resistance training. Recent studies suggest that

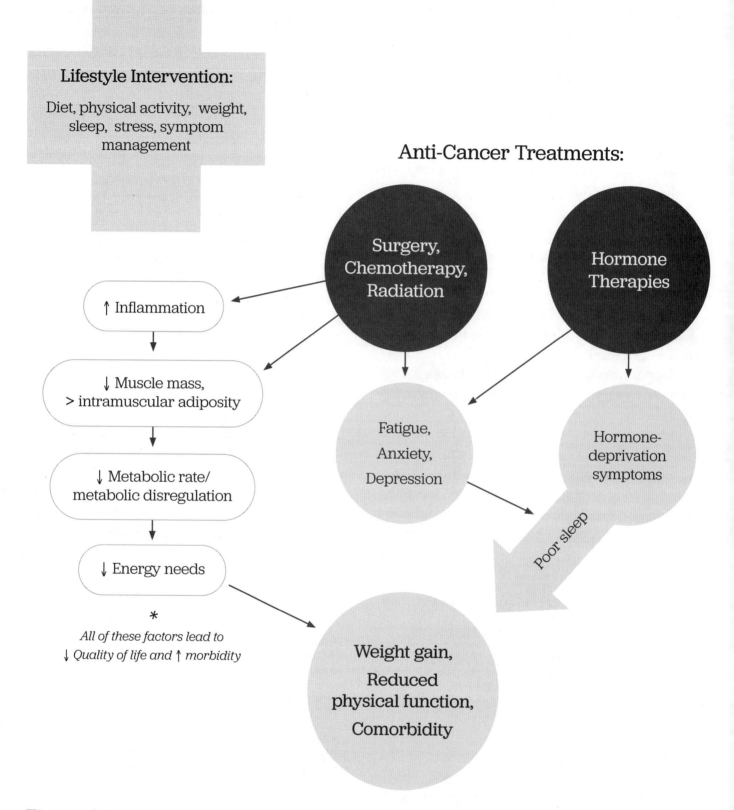

Figure 8.1
Lifestyle interventions for symptoms experienced by cancer survivors

oncology providers do not feel equipped to discuss body weight and weight management, making the role of the nutrition professional particularly important.[4]

Although the majority of the studies listed in Table 8.1 on pages 136 to 143 were conducted in survivors of breast and endometrial cancer, efficacy in promoting weight loss is demonstrated. Of note, these interventions are most effective when provided on-site as well as through a variety of distributed coaching and support interventions.[50]

Evidence Supporting Lifestyle Guidelines in Cancer Survivors

Several studies have been conducted in the past two decades to determine the effects of posttherapy lifestyle interventions on cancer survival. The majority have been conducted in breast cancer survivors, as this is the most commonly diagnosed cancer in women, and survival rates provide for a large study. While findings may not be generalized to all cancer survivors, the results do provide early evidence that (1) cancer survivors can make substantial changes in eating behavior, and (2) healthy eating and lifestyle choices may promote overall health in survivors, including improvements in functional health, weight control, and quality of life. Evidence relating diet and lifestyle changes to increased progression-free survival has not generally been demonstrated.

Table 8.2 on pages 144 to 145 describes select published and ongoing intervention trials in cancer survivors.

Most of the intervention trials were developed with a strong theoretical underpinning to promote behavioral change. Successful behavioral strategies for improving diet and physical activity in survivors include self-efficacy, motivational interviewing, and self-determination theory.[51-53]

Cancer Survivorship Guidelines and Adherence

Appendix A summarizes the current organizational guidelines for healthy diet after cancer. Across organizations, such as the American Cancer Society, American Institute for Cancer Research, the National Comprehensive Cancer Network, and the World Cancer Research Fund International, there is generally consistency in recommendations. These include maintaining a healthy body weight, restricting alcohol, and adopting plant-based eating patterns with higher vegetable and fiber intake and lower intake of red or processed meats.

Dietary Patterns and Diet Quality

Much of the guidance for a healthy diet after a cancer diagnosis focuses on specific food groups that have been associated with cancer survival. Briefly, the evidence suggests that alcohol may be problematic, particularly in relation to breast cancer outcomes.[54] Alcohol may alter folate status, influence aromatase activity, contribute low-nutrient energy, or promote intake of energy-dense snacks as a combined intake pattern. Limiting or avoiding alcohol is recommended for all cancer survivors. Alcohol avoidance is particularly relevant for patients diagnosed with head and neck, esophageal, hepatobiliary, and breast cancers, in which alcohol intake after diagnosis is predictive of poorer overall survival.[54-56] Thus, alcohol avoidance should be addressed routinely in the MNT for cancer survivorship, as recommended in a statement from the American Society for Clinical Oncology.[57]

In contrast, selected individual dietary components have been associated with improved outcomes (including mortality) after cancer, albeit less consistently. These include diets higher in vegetables and fruit,[58] higher in fiber,[59] and lower in fat.

Table 8.1
Summary of Dietary Intervention and Physical Activity Studies[9,44-47,60-80]

Lead author and study name (year)	Cancer type	Number of participants, mean age or age range, and other characteristics
Clinically based, supervised programs		
Thompson[60] The CHOICE Study (2015)	Breast, postmenopausal	n = 249 54.9 years
Swisher[61] GetFit for Fight (2015)	Breast, triple-negative	n = 28 53.7 years
Thomson[62] Modified-Atkins (2010)	Breast, stage I and II	n = 40 56 years
McCarroll[47] Survivors of Uterine Cancer Empowered by Exercise and Healthy Diet (SUCCEED) (2014)	Endometrial, stage I and II	n = 75 Age not reported
Saxton[63] (2014)	Breast	n = 85 56 years

Adapted with permission from Thomson CA, Bea JW. The role of diet, physical activity and body composition in cancer prevention. In: Alberts DS, Hess LM, eds. *Fundamentals of Cancer Prevention*. 4th ed. Springer-Verlag; 2017:53-110. See reference 50.

Intervention	Duration	Weight change (kg)
Registered dietitian nutritionist (RDN) counseling; 42-day cycle menu, low-fat or low-carbohydrate diet; deficit of 3,500 kcal/wk; physical activity (PA) of 10,000 steps daily	6 months	Low fat, –8.9 Low carbohydrate, –10.5 Control, –0.3
RDN counseling to decrease fat intake by 200 kcal/wk; exercise physiologist–supervised moderate aerobic PA three times weekly and twice weekly unsupervised plus stretching and resistance training	12 weeks	Intervention, –3.0 Control, –0.4
RDN counseling; low-fat or low-carbohydrate diet; deficit of 500 kcal/d	6 months	Low fat, –6.3 Low carbohydrate, –5.9
Physician-led group and individual counseling; 16 sessions: diet, PA, and behavior modification	6 months	Intervention, –1.5 kg/m^2 (change in BMI) Usual care, +0.1 kg/m^2
Three small-group, supervised exercise sessions weekly; aerobic exercise and strength training; individualized dietary advice and written information; with 600 kcal/d deficit; weekly small-group nutrition seminars	6 months	Intervention, –1.1 Usual care, –0.4

(continued)

Table 8.1
Summary of Dietary Intervention and Physical Activity Studies[9,44-47,60-80] *(continued)*

Lead author and study name (year)	Cancer type	Number of participants, mean age or age range, and other characteristics
Mixed-modality programs (clinically based plus telephone counseling)		
Rock[64] Exercise and Nutrition to Enhance Recovery and Good Health for You (ENERGY) (2015)	Breast, stage I through III	n = 692 56 years
Von Gruenigan[65] (2008)	Endometrial, stage I and II	n = 45 54.5 years
Sheppard[66] Stepping Stone (2016)	Breast	n = 22 (analytic cases) Black
Telephone counseling		
Harrigan[67] Lifestyle, Exercise, and Nutrition (LEAN) (2016)	Breast	n = 100 59 years
Harris[68] Cancer Survival Through Lifestyle Change (CASTLE) (2013)	Breast, stage I through IIIa	n = 52 52.8 years

Intervention	Duration	Weight change (kg)
RDN-led, 4 months of weekly group sessions, tapering to biweekly, then monthly; reinforced by one-on-one telephone or email; deficit of 500-1,000 kcal/d; 60 min/d of PA; tailored print materials	2 years	Group plus telephone, –3.6 Control, –0.9
RDN- and physician-led group sessions weekly, then biweekly, then monthly; telephone or newsletter every week the group does not meet; walk 5 d/wk for >45 min	6 months	Group plus telephone, –3.3 Usual care, +2.1
Individually tailored, group sessions led by nutritionist and exercise physiologist twice monthly with alternate-week telephone counseling by a trained survivor coach; survivor and interventionist tool kit; American Cancer Society (ACS) guidelines for diet (lower fat plus fruits and vegetables); PA of 10,000 steps daily	12 weeks	Intervention, –0.8 Control, +0.2
RDN- and exercise physiologist–delivered; one-on-one weekly for 4 weeks, then biweekly for 8 weeks, then monthly for 3 months; Diabetes Prevention Program adaptation with –500 kcal /25% fat kcal from fat, and 150 min/wk of PA (walking, lower sedentary time), plus mindfulness; self-monitoring	6 months	Three-arm randomized control trial (in-person, telephone, control): In-person, –5.6 Telephone, –4.8 Control (usual care), –1.7
Health professionals employed by TrestleTree provided 15-60 minutes of telephone coaching weekly for 25 weeks, then monthly for 6 months; behavioral targets: diet and PA	12 months	Telephone, –4.0 In-person, –3.3

(continued)

Table 8.1
Summary of Dietary Intervention and Physical Activity Studies[9,44-47,60-80] *(continued)*

Lead author and study name (year)	Cancer type	Number of participants, mean age or age range, and other characteristics
Telephone counseling (continued)		
Goodwin[45] The LISA Trial (2014)	Breast, T1-3N01-3 M0, on letrozole	n = 338 61 years
Befort[69] (2016)	Breast, stage I through III	n = 210 (n = 172 in phase 2) 58 years Rural
Community-based programs		
Greenlee[70] Cocinar Para Su Salud (2015)	Breast, stage 0 through III, Hispanic	n = 70 56.6 years
Commercial programs		
Djuric[71] Weight Watchers (WW) (2002)	Breast, stage I and II	n = 48 36-70 years
Greenlee[72] Curves (2013)	Breast, stage 0 through IIIa	n = 42 50.6 years Hispanic, Black

Intervention	Duration	Weight change (kg)
Trained lifestyle coaches; 19 calls plus workbook-directed call content adapted from Diabetes Prevention Program; deficit of 500-1,000 kcal/d; 150-200 min/wk of PA; behavior modification	24 months	Telephone, −3.1 Print material alone, −0.3 (All received general health educational print material)
As above (phase 1) Maintenance: new kilocalorie goal; two meal replacements daily; 225 min/wk of PA; continued biweekly group conference calls or mailed newsletter	6 months and 12 months	Group telephone, −12.2 kg Newsletter, − 13.2 kg Regain: Group telephone, +3.3 Newsletter, +4.9
RDN, physician, health educators, and trialists delivered four 2-hour nutrition-education roundtables, three 3.5-hour cooking sessions, and two food-shopping field trips over 12 weeks (24 h); culturally tailored Cook for Your Life curriculum	12 weeks	Intervention, −2.5 Control, +3.8
Weekly Weight Watchers (WW) meetings vs one-on-one meetings with RDN weekly for 3 months, then biweekly for 3 months, then monthly for 6 months; both promoted low fat intake, 500-1,000 kcal/d deficit, and self-monitoring	12 months	Control, −2.6 WW alone, −8.0 Individual (RDN counseling), −9.4 WW plus individual, −0.85
Curves weight management program curriculum led by Curves staff; exercise at Curves for 30 minutes three times weekly plus 2 days at home; bidirectional strength training plus low-impact aerobic PA; 60% increasing to 75% maximal heart rate; six 1-hour weekly nutrition classes; 1,200 kcal/d increasing to 1,600 kcal/d plus weekly motivational-interviewing telephone calls	6 months	Curves program, −2.87 Waitlist control, −1.42

(continued)

Table 8.1

Summary of Dietary Intervention and Physical Activity Studies[9,44-47,60-80] *(continued)*

Lead author and study name (year)	Cancer type	Number of participants, mean age or age range, and other characteristics
Telephone counseling (continued)		
Morey[73] Reach out to Enhance Wellness (RENEW) (2009)	Breast Prostate Colorectal	n = 641 73 years
Demark-Wahnefried[44] Daughters And MothErS Against Breast Cancer (DAMES) (2014)	Breast, stage 0 through III	n = 136 (68 mothers, 68 daughters)
Technology-based programs		
Huang[74] Fit4Life (2014)	Acute lymphoblastic leukemia	n = 38 13 years
Haggerty[46] Text4Diet (2016)	Endometrial, pre and stage I	n = 20 60.5 years

Intervention	Duration	Weight change (kg)
Intervention delivered by health counselor; personally tailored workbook, quarterly newsletters, 15 telephone counseling sessions, and 8 prompts; 15 minutes of strength training twice weekly and 30 minutes of aerobic PA daily; diet high in fruits and vegetables and low in saturated and total fat; kcal restriction to promote up to 0.45 kg/wk weight loss	12 months	Intervention, –2.06 Control, –0.92
Tailored print materials; ACS and *2020–2025 Dietary Guidelines for Americans*; deficit of 500-1,000 kcal/d; removal or substitute of three identified highly caloric food sources; 150 min/wk of PA; self-monitoring	12 months	In mothers: Individual, –3.77 Control, –0.87
Professional, caregiver and parent plus survivor input to material development; 4-month web-based, text (short messaging service, or SMS), and telephone counseling; ACS and Children's Oncology Group guidelines for healthy weight; kilocalorie deficit, 60 min/d moderate-vigorous PA; 15,000 steps daily; self-monitoring	4 months	Web, SMS, and telephone, –0.1 Control, +1.4
Telemedicine-adapted Diabetes Prevention Program delivered by physician and master's level clinician; weekly telephone and Wi-Fi weigh-ins daily for 6 month; Text4Diet received via SMS text message with three to five personalized SMS texts daily with monthly themes; two-way communication, weekly Wi-Fi weigh-ins; all participants educated to consume 1,200-1,500 kcal/d; self-monitoring	6 months	Telemedicine group –9.7 kg SMS group –3.9 kg

Table 8.2
Dietary Intervention Trials in Cancer Survivors[63,73,75-80]

Lead author and study name (year)	Cancer type	Number of participants, mean age or age range, and other characteristics
Pierce[75] Women's Healthy Eating and Living (WHEL) (2007)	Breast cancer survivors	n = 3,088
Chlebowski[76] Women's Intervention Nutrition Study (WINS) (2006)	Breast cancer survivors	n = 2,437
Morey[73] Reach Out to Enhance Wellness in Older Survivors (RENEW) (2009)	Overweight, older breast and prostate cancer survivors	n = 641
Demark-Wahnefried[77] FRESH START (2007)	Breast and prostate cancer survivors	n = 543
Hawkes[78] CanChange (2013)	Colorectal cancer survivors	n = 410
Thomson[79] Lifestyle Intervention for Ovarian Cancer Enhanced Survival (LIVES) (2016)	Ovarian cancer survivors	n = 1,200
Ligibel[80] Breast Cancer Weight Loss (BWEL) (2017)	Breast cancer survivors	n = 3,136

Intervention	Duration	Outcome
Randomized controlled trial (RCT) of a telephone-based intervention of five servings of vegetables daily, 16 oz of vegetable juice daily, three servings of fruit daily, and 30 g of fiber daily, vs usual care (five servings of fruits and vegetables a day)	7.3 year follow-up	No difference in breast cancer recurrence between groups; however, secondary analyses revealed women in the highest quartile of plasma carotenoids experienced a reduced risk of recurrence.
RCT of an in-person intervention of low-fat diet with <15% of energy coming from fat, vs usual care	60 month follow-up	No difference was observed between groups for overall disease progression; however, survival differences were observed by hormone status for women most adherent to the diet.
RCT of a home-based, tailored, print- and telephone-based intervention aimed at increasing healthy lifestyle behaviors, vs waitlist control	12 months	Significant increases were seen in physical activity, diet quality, and quality of life, and there was a 2-kg weight-loss difference in intervention vs control participants.
RCT of nontailored print vs tailored print materials for promotion of healthy lifestyle behaviors	10 month intervention; 1 year follow-up	Both groups improved, but the tailored-print group experienced greater gains in exercise (+59 min/wk vs +39 min/wk), servings of fruits and vegetables per day (+1.1 serving vs +0.6 servings), and change in body mass index (BMI) (–0.3 vs +0.1).
RCT of telephone-based health-coaching intervention vs usual care	6 months	Participants in the intervention increased their moderate to vigorous physical activity by 28.5 min/wk and their intake of fruits and vegetables by 0.4 servings per day compared to control participants, and they decreased their energy from fat by 7% and their BMI by 0.9.
RCT of low-fat diet higher in vegetables, fruits, and fiber, vs usual care	24 months	Ongoing
RCT of telephone-based weight-loss intervention vs health education	2 year intervention 2 year follow-up	Ongoing

The role of vegetables and fruit in cancer survivorship is not clearly established. Intervention trials such as the Women's Healthy Eating and Living, (WHEL) study, wherein survivors consumed increased amounts of plant foods on a regular basis, showed no survival advantage versus the control condition, which included five servings of fruits and vegetables daily.[75] However, vegetables and fruit may improve the health of cancer survivors for noncancer outcomes and overall mortality. In a subgroup analysis, eating five vegetables and fruits daily along with 30 minutes of moderate activity reduced overall mortality in breast cancer survivors by 44% during the study observation period.[81] Vegetables and, to a slightly lesser extent, fruit are nutrient-dense, high-fiber, lower-energy options that may promote increased satiety. These foods also support increased exposure to numerous bioactive food components with chemopreventive activity, such as carotenoids, allyl sulfides, isothiocyanates, and anthocyanins.[82]

No specific daily fiber recommendation exists explicitly for cancer survivors. Survivors should strive to meet the dietary guidelines for the US population of 25 to 30 g of fiber daily. Fiber intake has been associated with favorable shifts in hormone concentrations, reduced bowel transit time, improved glucose and lipid control, and improved satiety. Each of these mechanisms of action holds promise for improving outcomes in a variety of cancers. However, no fiber-specific interventions to evaluate cancer outcomes have been conducted. A systematic review of flaxseed (a source of fiber and omega-3 fatty acids) and its association with breast cancer demonstrated a 31% lower mortality after breast cancer among those with greater intake.[83] Fiber also holds potential to reduce gastroenteritis resulting from cancer therapies[84] and has demonstrated efficacy in promoting healthy gut microbiota.[85]

The role of dietary fat in cancer survivorship also is not well established. Intriguing evidence from the Women's Intervention Nutrition Study (WINS) did suggest that very low-fat diets were associated with lower breast cancer recurrence in women with estrogen-receptor-negative disease.[76] However, the low-fat diet consumed by women enrolled in the WHEL study was not associated with reduced recurrence of breast cancer.[75] Of note, the low-fat diet intervention of the Women's Health Initiative was shown to reduce mortality after breast cancer in a secondary analysis.[86]

In relation to diet and cancer survival, an increasing emphasis is being placed on dietary patterns of intake rather than nutrients, foods, or food groups. Biologically, this makes sense in that people consume whole diets, and it is the totality of diet exposure that is most likely to be associated with health outcomes after cancer. As an example, an analysis from Switzerland showed a 15% to 18% higher overall survival among men who followed a diet pattern that predominantly included fish and high-fiber foods compared to men who consumed a low-variety diet.[87] Similarly, a systematic review and meta-analysis of cohort studies suggested a prudent (ie, low-fat, high-quality) diet pattern was associated with lower cancer mortality, whereas Western diets are associated with greater mortality.[88] Importantly, healthy eating patterns, such as the Mediterranean diet pattern, have been associated with lower cardiovascular and all-cause mortality after a cancer diagnosis, including evidence of a 52% lower mortality after colorectal cancer[89] and a 10% reduction in any cancer mortality in an analysis of observational studies.[90] Similarly, a dietary pattern associated with the intake of foods that cause inflammation, as measured by the inflammatory index, such as processed and fried foods, showed an increase in cardiovascular-specific death but not overall or cancer-specific mortality in postmenopausal patients with breast cancer, suggesting that pattern of intake may have a differential impact on mortality across cancer diagnoses.[91] Overall, data are limited, and a recent systematic review suggested that, other than a protective association between the prudent diet and mortality in breast cancer survivors, the evidence to date does not support a protective effect of diet patterns on cancer mortality.[92]

Role of Lean Mass and Physical Activity in Long-Term Survivorship

Age is a leading risk factor for cancer, and it is also a primary risk factor for increased loss of bone mineral density, reduced physical function, and, in the advanced stages of cancer, sarcopenia. For individuals who survive beyond age 75 years, there is a common and steady reduction in skeletal muscle mass, an increase in fat-to-lean-mass ratio, and an increase in osteopenia and osteoporosis.[93] These clinical consequences of aging are more prominent in those who have experienced a cancer diagnosis,[94] suggesting that older cancer patients represent a high-risk group that could benefit from MNT.

While physical activity that includes weight-bearing, resistance, and balance exercises is central to improving musculoskeletal health, dietary selections also influence musculoskeletal health. Adequate protein to reduce frailty is an important first-line nutritional therapy. In a study of healthy postmenopausal women, protein intakes above 1.2 g/kg/d were associated with reduced frailty.[95] This same level of protein intake is recommended to meet the protein requirements of cancer survivors who are over age 50 years.

Dietary Supplementation

The literature shows that 64% to 81% of cancer survivors are known to consume dietary supplements, which is a higher frequency of use than in the overall population.[96] There is limited evidence that multivitamin and mineral supplementation or individual nutrient supplements are protective against recurrence or mortality after cancer. A meta-analysis and a subsequent cohort analysis found no protection from antioxidant supplementation, despite these nutrients' being a common choice among cancer survivors who take supplements.[97,98] Summary evidence suggests that, with a lack of evidence of efficacy and concerns for safety from prior studies, dietary supplementation should be directed toward correcting nutrient deficiencies rather than presuming survival benefit after cancer.[99] Dietetic professionals should guide patients to obtain nutrients through varied food choices to meet individual nutritional needs. See Chapter 7 and Appendix C for additional information on dietary supplements.

Resources for Supporting Dietary Health and Overall Well-Being After Cancer

Box 8.2 on pages 148 to 149 provides a list of online resources available to health care providers to support overall well-being and lifestyle behavior change in their patients.

Box 8.2
Nutrition Resources in Cancer Survivorship

Organization	Website or webpage	Synopsis
Academy of Nutrition and Dietetics	Academy of Nutrition and Dietetics (www.eatright.org)	Provides general information on healthy eating, including cancer prevention and nutrition during cancer treatment
	Oncology Nutrition (www.oncologynutrition.org)	Dietetic practice group of the Academy of Nutrition and Dietetics; provides nutrition information for clinicians, patients, and families
American Cancer Society	American Cancer Society (www.cancer.org)	Provides information for cancer patients at all stages
	Cancer Survivors Network (http://csn.cancer.org)	Connects survivors for support
American Institute for Cancer Research	Reduce Your Cancer Risk: Physical Activity (www.aicr.org/reduce-your-cancer-risk/physical-activity/reduce_physical_getting_started.html)	Provides information on increasing physical activity
American Society of Clinical Oncology	Cancer.Net: Survivorship (www.cancer.net/survivorship)	Provides information about health promotion and care management after cancer
CancerCare	CancerCare (www.cancercare.org)	Connects survivors with social workers, financial support, and support groups
Centers for Disease Control and Prevention	Cancer Survivors (www.cdc.gov/cancer/survivors)	Provides information on cancer survivorship–related prevalence, support for caregivers, and general information
National Cancer Institute	Office of Cancer Survivorship (https://cancercontrol.cancer.gov/ocs)	Provides information on science findings about cancer survivorship and current efforts
National Cancer Institute and the American Cancer Society	Springboard Beyond Cancer (https://survivorship.cancer.gov)	Provides self-management tools and related resources to promote health and well-being after a cancer diagnosis

(continued)

Box 8.2
Box 8.2
Nutrition Resources in Cancer Survivorship *(continued)*

Organization	Website or webpage	Synopsis
National Coalition for Cancer Survivorship	National Coalition for Cancer Survivorship (www.canceradvocacy.org)	Cancer-survivor advocacy organization; primarily focuses on policy that affects care and provides a toolbox and other information for survivors
Oncology Nursing Society	Putting Evidence into Practice (https://voice.ons.org/conferences /how-to-use-onss-putting-evidence -into-practice-resources)	Synthesizes the evidence to date for patient-centered outcomes, such as symptoms; provides information on what interventions are effective in preventing and treating specific patient-centered outcomes for cancer survivors
World Cancer Research Fund and American Institute for Cancer Research	Diet, Nutrition, Physical Activity and Cancer: A Global Perspective— Continuous Update Project (www.wcrf.org/dietandcancer)	Continuous update of the science on diet, physical activity, and body weight and cancer risk and survival by leading cancer epidemiologists

References

1. American Cancer Society. *Cancer Treatment & Survivorship Facts & Figures 2019-2021*. American Cancer Society; 2019. Accessed February 19, 2021. www.cancer .org/content/dam/cancer-org /research/cancer-facts-and -statistics/cancer-treatment -and-survivorship-facts-and -figures/cancer-treatment-and -survivorship-facts-and-figures -2019-2021.pdf

2. DeSantis CE, Fedewa SA, Goding Sauer A, Kramer JL, Smith RA, Jemal A. Breast cancer statistics, 2015: convergence of incidence rates between Black and White women. *CA Cancer J Clin*. 2016;66(1):31-42.

3. Jones LW, Demark-Wahnefried W. Diet, exercise, and complementary therapies after primary treatment for cancer. *Lancet Oncol*. 2006;7(12): 1017-1026.

4. Beeken R, Williams K, Wardle J, Croker H. "What about diet?" A qualitative study of cancer survivors' views on diet and cancer and their sources of information. *Eur J Cancer Care*. 2016;25(5):774-783.

5. Thomson CA, Flatt SW, Rock CL, Ritenbaugh C, Newman V, Pierce JP. Increased fruit, vegetable and fiber intake and lower fat intake reported among women previously treated for invasive breast cancer. *J Amer Diet Assoc*. 2002;102(6):801-808.

6. Nayak P, Paxton RJ, Holmes H, Thanh Nguyen H, Elting LS. Racial and ethnic differences in health behaviors among cancer survivors. *Amer J of Prev Med*. 2015;48(6):729-736.

7. Thomson CA, Crane TE, Wertheim BC, et al. Diet quality and survival after ovarian cancer: results from the Women's Health Initiative. *J Natl Cancer Inst*. 2014;106(11):dju314.

8. Thomson CA, McCullough ML, Wertheim BC, et al. Nutrition and physical activity cancer prevention guidelines, cancer risk, and mortality in the Women's Health Initiative. *Cancer Prev Res*. 2014;7(1):42-53.

9. Arthur AE, Peterson KE, Rozek LS, et al. Pretreatment dietary patterns, weight status, and head and neck squamous cell carcinoma prognosis. *Amer J Clin Nutr*. 2013;97(2):360-368.

10. Duffy SA, Ronis DL, McLean S, et al. Pretreatment health behaviors predict survival among patients with head and neck squamous cell carcinoma. *J Clin Onc*. 2009;27(12):1969-1975.

11. Shen G-P, Xu F-H, He F, et al. Pretreatment lifestyle behaviors as survival predictors for patients with nasopharyngeal carcinoma. *PLoS One*. 2012;7(5):e36515.

12. Dolecek TA, McCarthy BJ, Joslin CE, et al. Prediagnosis food patterns are associated with length of survival from epithelial ovarian cancer. *J Amer Diet Assoc*. 2010;110(3):369-382.

13. Cleeland CS. Symptom burden: multiple symptoms and their impact as patient-reported outcomes. *J Natl Cancer Inst Monogr*. 2007;(37):16-21.

14. Sunga A, Eberl MM, Oeffinger KC, Hudson MM, Mahoney MC. Care of cancer survivors. *Amer Fam Physician*. 2005;71(4):699-706.

15. Marin Caro MM, Laviano A, Pichard C. Nutritional intervention and quality of life in adult oncology patients. *Clin Nutr*. 2007;26(3):289-301.

16. Ravasco P, Monteiro Grillo I, Camilo M. Cancer wasting and quality of life react to early individualized nutritional counselling. *Clin Nutr*. 2007;26(1):7-15.

17. Ravasco P, Monteiro-Grillo I, Vidal PM, Camilo ME. Dietary counseling improves patient outcomes: a prospective, randomized, controlled trial in colorectal cancer patients undergoing radiotherapy. *J Clin Oncol*. 2005;23(7):1431-1438.

18. Rock CL. Dietary counseling is beneficial for the patient with cancer. *J Clin Oncol*. 2005;23(7):1348-1349.

19. Demark-Wahnefried W, Peterson BL, Winer EP, et al. Changes in weight, body composition, and factors influencing energy balance among premenopausal breast cancer patients receiving adjuvant chemotherapy. *J Clin Onc*. 2001;19(9):2381-2389.

20. Baracos VE, Arribas L. Sarcopenic obesity: hidden muscle wasting and its impact for survival and complications of cancer therapy. *Ann Onc*. 2018;29(suppl 2):ii1-ii9.

21. Winters-Stone KM, Dobek J, Nail L, et al. Strength training stops bone loss and builds muscle in postmenopausal breast cancer survivors: a randomized, controlled trial. *Breast Cancer Res Treat.* 2011;127(2):447-456.

22. Sanudo B, de Hoyo M, Del Pozo-Cruz J, et al. A systematic review of the exercise effect on bone health: the importance of assessing mechanical loading in perimenopausal and postmenopausal women. *Menopause.* 2017;24(10):1208-1216.

23. Tai V, Leung W, Grey A, Reid IR, Bolland MJ. Calcium intake and bone mineral density: systematic review and meta-analysis. *BMJ.* 2015;351:h4183. doi:10.1136/bmj.h4183

24. Nejatinamini S, Kubrak C, Alvarez-Camacho M, et al. Head and neck cancer patients do not meet recommended intakes of micronutrients without consuming fortified products. *Nutr Cancer.* 2018;70(3):474-482.

25. Steele CB, Thomas CC, Henley SJ, et al. Vital Signs: trends in incidence of cancers associated with overweight and obesity—United States, 2005–2014. *MMWR Morb Mort Wkly Rep.* 2017;66(39):1052-1058.

26. Arem H, Irwin ML. Obesity and endometrial cancer survival: a systematic review. *Inter J Obes.* 2013;37(5):634-639.

27. Freedland SJ. Obesity and prostate cancer: a growing problem. *Clin Cancer Res.* 2005;11(19 pt 1):6763-6766.

28. Patterson RE, Flatt SW, Saquib N, et al. Medical comorbidities predict mortality in women with a history of early stage breast cancer. *Breast Cancer Res Treat.* 2010;122(3):859-865.

29. Protani M, Coory M, Martin JH. Effect of obesity on survival of women with breast cancer: systematic review and meta-analysis. *Breast Cancer Res Treat.* 2010;123(3):627-635.

30. McTiernan A, Irwin M, Vongruenigen V. Weight, physical activity, diet, and prognosis in breast and gynecologic cancers. *J Clin Oncol.* 2010;28(26):4074-4080.

31. McTiernan A. Weight, physical activity and breast cancer survival. *Proc Nutr Soc.* 2018;77(4):403-411.

32. Siegel EM, Ulrich CM, Poole EM, Holmes RS, Jacobsen PB, Shibata D. The effects of obesity and obesity-related conditions on colorectal cancer prognosis. *Cancer Control.* 2010;17(1):52-57.

33. Efstathiou JA, Bae K, Shipley WU, et al. Obesity and mortality in men with locally advanced prostate cancer: analysis of RTOG 85-31. *Cancer.* 2007;110(12):2691-2699.

34. Caan BJ, Cespedes Feliciano EM, Prado CM, et al. Association of muscle and adiposity measured by computed tomography with survival in patients with nonmetastatic breast cancer. *JAMA Oncol.* 2018;4(6):798-804.

35. Caan BJ, Meyerhardt JA, Kroenke CH, et al. Explaining the obesity paradox: the association between body composition and colorectal cancer survival (C-SCANS Study). *Cancer Epidemiol Biomarkers Prev.* 2017;26(7):1008-1015.

36. Fujiwara N, Nakagawa H, Kudo Y, et al. Sarcopenia, intramuscular fat deposition, and visceral adiposity independently predict the outcomes of hepatocellular carcinoma. *J Hepat.* 2015;63(1):131-140.

37. Erickson K, Patterson RE, Flatt SW, et al. Clinically defined type 2 diabetes mellitus and prognosis in early-stage breast cancer. *J Clin Oncol.* 2011;29(1):54-60.

38. Nock NL, Dimitropolous A, Tkach J, Frasure H, von Gruenigen V. Reduction in neural activation to high-calorie food cues in obese endometrial cancer survivors after a behavioral lifestyle intervention: a pilot study. *BMC Neurosci.* 2012;13:74.

39. Guest DD, Evans EM, Rogers LQ. Diet components associated with perceived fatigue in breast cancer survivors. *Eur J Cancer Care (Engl).* 2013;22(1):51-59.

40. Carmody JF, Olendzki BC, Merriam PA, Liu Q, Qiao Y, Ma Y. A novel measure of dietary change in a prostate cancer dietary program incorporating mindfulness training. *J Acad Nutr Diet.* 2012;112(11):1822-1827.

41. Chung S, Zhu S, Friedmann E, et al. Weight loss with mindful eating in African American women following treatment for breast cancer: a longitudinal study. *Support Care Cancer.* 2016;24(4):1875-1881.

42. Lucas AR, Focht BC, Cohn DE, Buckworth J, Klatt MD. A mindfulness-based lifestyle intervention for obese, inactive endometrial cancer survivors: a feasibility study. *Integr Cancer Ther.* 2017;16(3):263-275.

43. Befort CA, Klemp JR, Austin HL, et al. Outcomes of a weight loss intervention among rural breast cancer survivors. *Breast Cancer Res Treat.* 2012;132(2):631-639.

44. Demark-Wahnefried W, Jones LW, Snyder DC, et al. Daughters and Mothers Against Breast Cancer (DAMES): main outcomes of a randomized controlled trial of weight loss in overweight mothers with breast cancer and their overweight daughters. *Cancer.* 2014;120(16):2522-2534.

45. Goodwin PJ, Segal RJ, Vallis M, et al. Randomized trial of a telephone-based weight loss intervention in postmenopausal women with breast cancer receiving letrozole: the LISA trial. *J Clin Oncol.* 2014;32(21):2231-2239.

46. Haggerty AF, Huepenbecker S, Sarwer DB, et al. The use of novel technology-based weight loss interventions for obese women with endometrial hyperplasia and cancer. *Gynecol Oncol.* 2016;140(2):239-244.

47. McCarroll ML, Armbruster S, Frasure HE, et al. Self-efficacy, quality of life, and weight loss in overweight/obese endometrial cancer survivors (SUCCEED): a randomized controlled trial. *Gynecol Oncol.* 2014;132(2):397-402.

48. Gathirua-Mwangi WG, Song Y, Monahan PO, Champion VL, Zollinger TW. Associations of metabolic syndrome and C-reactive protein with mortality from total cancer, obesity-linked cancers and breast cancer among women in NHANES III. *Int J Cancer.* 2018;143(3):535-542.

49. Vallance JK, Courneya KS, Taylor LM, Plotnikoff RC, Mackey JR. Development and evaluation of a theory-based physical activity guidebook for breast cancer survivors. *Health Educ Behav.* 2008;35(2):174-189.

50. Thomson CA, Bea JW. The role of diet, physical activity and body composition in cancer prevention. In: Alberts DS, Hess LM, eds. *Fundamentals of Cancer Prevention.* 4th ed. Springer-Verlag; 2017:53-110.

51. Bennett JA, Young HM, Nail LM, Winters-Stone K, Hanson G. A telephone-only motivational intervention to increase physical activity in rural adults: a randomized controlled trial. *Nurs Res.* 2008;57(1):24-32.

52. Spencer JC, Wheeler SB. A systematic review of motivational interviewing interventions in cancer patients and survivors. *Patient Educ Couns.* 2016;99(7):1099-1105.

53. Patrick H, Williams GC. Self-determination theory: its application to health behavior and complementarity with motivational interviewing. *Int J Behav Nutr Phys Act.* 2012;9:18.

54. Ekwueme DU, Allaire BT, Parish WJ, et al. Estimation of breast cancer incident cases and medical care costs attributable to alcohol consumption among insured women aged <45 years in the U.S. *Amer J Prev Med.* 2017;53(3s1):S47-S54.

55. Fortin A, Wang CS, Vigneault E. Influence of smoking and alcohol drinking behaviors on treatment outcomes of patients with squamous cell carcinomas of the head and neck. *Int J Radiat Oncol Biol Phys.* 2009;74(4):1062-1069.

56. Barrera S, Demark-Wahnefried W. Nutrition during and after cancer therapy. *Oncology (Williston Park).* 2009;23(2 suppl):15-21.

57. LoConte NK, Brewster AM, Kaur JS, Merrill JK, Alberg AJ. Alcohol and cancer: a statement of the American Society of Clinical Oncology. *J Clin Oncol.* 2018;36(1):83-93.

58. Aune D, Giovannucci E, Boffetta P, et al. Fruit and vegetable intake and the risk of cardiovascular disease, total cancer and all-cause mortality—a systematic review and dose-response meta-analysis of prospective studies. *Int Journal Epidemiol.* 2017;46(3):1029-1056.

59. Hajishafiee M, Saneei P, Benisi-Kohansal S, Esmaillzadeh A. Cereal fibre intake and risk of mortality from all causes, CVD, cancer and inflammatory diseases: a systematic review and meta-analysis of prospective cohort studies. *Br J Nutr.* 2016;116(2):343-352.

60. Thompson HJ, Sedlacek SM, Playdon MC, et al. Weight loss interventions for breast cancer survivors: impact of dietary pattern. *PLoS One.* 2015;10(5):e0127366.

61. Swisher AK, Abraham J, Bonner D, et al. Exercise and dietary advice intervention for survivors of triple-negative breast cancer: effects on body fat, physical function, quality of life, and adipokine profile. *Support Care Cancer.* 2015;23(10):2995-3003.

62. Thomson CA, Stopeck AT, Bea JW, et al. Changes in body weight and metabolic indexes in overweight breast cancer survivors enrolled in a randomized trial of low-fat vs. reduced carbohydrate diets. *Nutr Cancer.* 2010;62(8):1142-1152.

63. Saxton JM, Scott EJ, Daley AJ, et al. Effects of an exercise and hypocaloric healthy eating intervention on indices of psychological health status, hypothalamic-pituitary-adrenal axis regulation and immune function after early-stage breast cancer: a randomised controlled trial. *Breast Cancer Res.* 2014;16(2):R39. doi:10.1186/bcr3643

64. Rock CL, Flatt SW, Byers TE, et al. Results of the Exercise and Nutrition to Enhance Recovery and Good Health for You (ENERGY) Trial: a behavioral weight loss intervention in overweight or obese breast cancer survivors. *J Clin Oncol.* 2015;33(28):3169-3176.

65. von Gruenigen VE, Courneya KS, Gibbons HE, Kavanagh MB, Waggoner SE, Lerner E. Feasibility and effectiveness of a lifestyle intervention program in obese endometrial cancer patients: a randomized trial. *Gynecol Oncol.* 2008;109(1):19-26.

66. Sheppard VB, Hicks J, Makambi K, Hurtado-de-Mendoza A, Demark-Wahnefried W, Adams-Campbell L. The feasibility and acceptability of a diet and exercise trial in overweight and obese Black breast cancer survivors: the Stepping STONE study. *Contemp Clin Trials.* 2016;46:106-113.

67. Harrigan M, Cartmel B, Loftfield E, et al. Randomized trial comparing telephone versus in-person weight loss counseling on body composition and circulating biomarkers in women treated for breast cancer: the Lifestyle, Exercise, and Nutrition (LEAN) Study. *J Clin Oncol.* 2016;34(7):669-676.

68. Harris MN, Swift DL, Myers VH, et al. Cancer survival through lifestyle change (CASTLE): a pilot study of weight loss. *Int J Behav Med.* 2013;20(3):403-412.

69. Befort CA, Klemp JR, Sullivan DK, et al. Weight loss maintenance strategies among rural breast cancer survivors: the rural women connecting for better health trial. *Obesity.* 2016;24(10):2070-2077.

70. Greenlee H, Gaffney AO, Aycinena AC, et al. Randomized controlled trial of a culturally based dietary intervention among Hispanic breast cancer survivors. *J Acad Nutr Diet.* 2015;115(5 suppl):S42-S56.e3.

71. Djuric Z, DiLaura NM, Jenkins I, et al. Combining weight-loss counseling with the Weight Watchers plan for obese breast cancer survivors. *Obes Res.* Jul 2002;10(7):657-665.

72. Greenlee HA, Crew KD, Mata JM, et al. A pilot randomized controlled trial of a commercial diet and exercise weight loss program in minority breast cancer survivors. *Obesity (Silver Spring).* 2013;21(1):65-76.

73. Morey MC, Snyder DC, Sloane R, et al. Effects of home-based diet and exercise on functional outcomes among older, overweight long-term cancer survivors: RENEW: a randomized controlled trial. *JAMA.* 2009;301(18):1883-1891.

74. Huang JS, Dillon L, Terrones L, et al. Fit4Life: a weight loss intervention for children who have survived childhood leukemia. *Pediatr Blood Cancer.* 2014;61(5):894-900.

75. Pierce JP, Natarajan L, Caan BJ, et al. Influence of a diet very high in vegetables, fruit, and fiber and low in fat on prognosis following treatment for breast cancer: the Women's Healthy Eating and Living (WHEL) randomized trial. *JAMA*. 2007;298(3):289-298.

76. Chlebowski RT, Blackburn GL, Thomson CA, et al. Dietary fat reduction and breast cancer outcome: interim efficacy results from the Women's Intervention Nutrition Study. *J Natl Cancer Inst*. 2006;98(24):1767-1776.

77. Demark-Wahnefried W, Clipp EC, Lipkus IM, et al. Main outcomes of the FRESH START trial: a sequentially tailored, diet and exercise mailed print intervention among breast and prostate cancer survivors. *J Clin Oncol*. 2007;25(19):2709-2718.

78. Hawkes AL, Chambers SK, Pakenham KI, et al. Effects of a telephone-delivered multiple health behavior change intervention (CanChange) on health and behavioral outcomes in survivors of colorectal cancer: a randomized controlled trial. *J Clin Oncol*. 2013;31(18): 2313-2321.

79. Thomson CA, Crane TE, Miller A, Garcia DO, Basen-Engquist K, Alberts DS. A randomized trial of diet and physical activity in women treated for stage II–IV ovarian cancer: rationale and design of the Lifestyle Intervention for Ovarian Cancer Enhanced Survival (LIVES): an NRG Oncology/Gynecologic Oncology Group (GOG-225) Study. *Contemp Clin Trials*. 2016;49: 181-189.

80. Ligibel JA, Barry WT, Alfano C, et al. Randomized phase III trial evaluating the role of weight loss in adjuvant treatment of overweight and obese women with early breast cancer (Alliance A011401): study design. *NPJ Breast Cancer*. 2017;3:37.

81. Pierce JP, Stefanick ML, Flatt SW, et al. Greater survival after breast cancer in physically active women with high vegetable-fruit intake regardless of obesity. *J Clin Oncol*. 2007;25(17):2345-2351.

82. Mates JM, Segura JA, Alonso FJ, Marquez J. Anticancer antioxidant regulatory functions of phytochemicals. *Curr Med Chem*. 2011;18(15):2315-2338.

83. Flower G, Fritz H, Balneaves LG, et al. Flax and breast cancer: a systematic review. *Integr Cancer Ther*. 2014;13(3):181-192.

84. Wedlake L, Shaw C, McNair H, et al. Randomized controlled trial of dietary fiber for the prevention of radiation-induced gastrointestinal toxicity during pelvic radiotherapy. *Am J Clin Nutr*. 2017;106(3):849-857.

85. Han M, Wang C, Liu P, Li D, Li Y, Ma X. Dietary fiber gap and host gut microbiota. *Protein Pept Lett*. 2017;24(5):388-396.

86. Chlebowski RT, Aragaki AK, Anderson GL, et al. Low-fat dietary pattern and breast cancer mortality in the Women's Health Initiative randomized controlled trial. *J Clin Oncol*. 2017;35(25):2919-2926.

87. Krieger JP, Cabaset S, Pestoni G, Rohrmann S, Faeh D. Dietary patterns are associated with cardiovascular and cancer mortality among Swiss adults in a census-linked cohort. *Nutrients*. 2018;10(3):e313.

88. Schwedhelm C, Boeing H, Hoffmann G, Aleksandrova K, Schwingshackl L. Effect of diet on mortality and cancer recurrence among cancer survivors: a systematic review and meta-analysis of cohort studies. *Nutr Rev*. 2016;74(12):737-748.

89. Ratjen I, Schafmayer C, di Giuseppe R, et al. Postdiagnostic Mediterranean and healthy Nordic dietary patterns are inversely associated with all-cause mortality in long-term colorectal cancer survivors. *J Nutr*. 2017;147(4):636-644.

90. Schwingshackl L, Hoffmann G. Adherence to Mediterranean diet and risk of cancer: a systematic review and meta-analysis of observational studies. *Int J Cancer.* 2014;135(8):1884-1897.

91. Zheng J, Tabung FK, Zhang J, et al. Association between post-cancer diagnosis dietary inflammatory potential and mortality among invasive breast cancer survivors in the Women's Health Initiative. *Cancer Epidemiol Biomarkers Prev.* 2018;27(4):454-463.

92. Jochems SHJ, Van Osch FHM, Bryan RT, et al. Impact of dietary patterns and the main food groups on mortality and recurrence in cancer survivors: a systematic review of current epidemiological literature. *BMJ Open.* 2018;8(2):e014530.

93. Bijlsma AY, Meskers CG, Westendorp RG, Maier AB. Chronology of age-related disease definitions: osteoporosis and sarcopenia. *Ageing Res Rev.* 2012;11(2):320-324.

94. Wickham R. Osteoporosis related to disease or therapy in patients with cancer. *Clin J Oncol Nurs.* 2011;15(6):e90-e104.

95. Beasley JM, Newcomb PA, Trentham-Dietz A, et al. Post-diagnosis dietary factors and survival after invasive breast cancer. *Breast Cancer Res Treat.* 2011;128(1):229-236.

96. Velicer CM, Ulrich CM. Vitamin and mineral supplement use among US adults after cancer diagnosis: a systematic review. *J Clin Oncol.* 2008;26(4):665-673.

97. Davies AA, Davey Smith G, Harbord R, et al. Nutritional interventions and outcome in patients with cancer or preinvasive lesions: systematic review. *J Natl Cancer Inst.* 2006;98(14):961-973.

98. Pocobelli G, Peters U, Kristal AR, White E. Use of supplements of multivitamins, vitamin C, and vitamin E in relation to mortality. *Amer J Epidemiol.* 2009;170(4):472-483.

99. Vernieri C, Nichetti F, Raimondi A, et al. Diet and supplements in cancer prevention and treatment: Clinical evidences and future perspectives. *Crit Rev Oncol Hematol.* 2018;123:57-73.

Chapter 9
Nutritional Effects of Cancer Treatment: Medical Oncology

Barbara L. Grant, MS, RDN, CSO, FAND

Conventional modalities of cancer treatment include medical oncology, radiation oncology, and surgical oncology, used alone or in combination to prevent, cure, control, or palliate cancer. This chapter provides an overview of cancer treatment and a discussion of medical oncology therapies, as well as their mechanisms of action, routes of administration, and specific effects and impact on nutritional status for people with cancer undergoing treatment.

Chapter 10 provides a similar overview for radiation oncology therapies, and Chapters 13 through 25 address site-specific surgical oncology as it relates to the removal of involved or suspicious malignant tissue in different areas of the body, either as a sole modality or used in combination with medical and radiation oncology. Recommendations for managing cancer-related symptoms and treatment-related side effects are presented in Chapter 11.

More than 70% of all people who receive and are treated for a cancer diagnosis in the United States receive care in the more than 1,500 cancer centers accredited by the American College of Surgeons Commission on Cancer (CoC).[1] The CoC's standards specify that all accredited programs provide patients with access to a full scope of care to enhance patient outcomes. Their program standards include a provision of oncology nutrition services by a registered dietitian nutritionist (RDN), either on-site or by referral. Best practice for RDNs working in cancer centers should include ongoing professional education and competence in oncology nutrition. The CoC also recommends attendance at weekly tumor boards and representation at cancer committee meetings.[1]

Medical Oncology Overview

Medical oncology is the prevention, diagnosis, treatment, and palliation of cancer using antineoplastic therapies, which may include chemotherapy, targeted therapy, immunotherapy, and hormone therapy (see Figure 9.1 on page 158). An oncologist prescribes a patient's cancer treatment regimen according to established National Comprehensive Cancer Network (NCCN) guidelines or clinical trial protocol guidelines.[2] Other patient-related factors include the following[3-5]:

- type of cancer
- tumor size, location, and if it has metastasized
- age and general health
- medical and social history and comorbid conditions
- previous cancer treatments
- genetic testing
- cancer pharmacogenomics

Box 9.1 on page 158 summarizes the factors affecting a patient's response to cancer treatment. Box 9.2 on page 159 outlines goals for the types of cancer therapy used to prevent, cure, control, or palliate cancer.

Chemotherapy

Chemotherapy is the use of chemical agents or drugs to systemically kill cancer cells.[4] Chemotherapy has a cytotoxic effect on all cells (both healthy and malignant); therefore, some side effects and toxicities can result due to damage to rapidly dividing healthy cells, such as those lining the mouth (called mucositis). However, normal cells

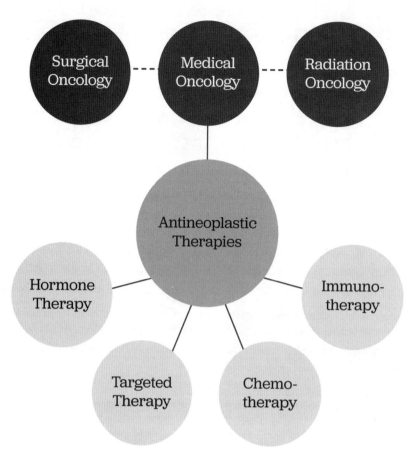

Figure 9.1
Conventional modalities of cancer treatment

Box 9.1
Cancer-Specific Factors Affecting Response to Cancer Treatment[6,7]

Factor	Definition	Effect on response
Tumor burden or tumor load	The size of the tumor or the amount of cancer in the body	As tumor mass increases in size, its growth rate can slow, thus reducing the effectiveness of cancer treatments.
Tumor growth rate	The proportion of cancer cells within the tumor that are growing and dividing to form new cancer cells	Rapidly growing tumors usually are more responsive to treatment.
Drug resistance	The failure of cancer cells to respond to a drug used to kill or weaken them	Cancer cells may be resistant at the beginning of treatment or may develop resistance after exposure to treatment.

Box 9.2
Goals of Cancer Therapy Approaches[3,7-9]

Approach	Goals	Examples
Prevention	Use of medicines or other agents to reduce the risk of cancer or delay its development	Hormone therapy (an antiestrogen agent) to reduce the risk of breast cancer in a woman who is at high risk for developing the disease Immunization of adolescents (male and female) to decrease the risk for human papillomavirus–related cervical, vaginal, anal, mouth or throat, and penis cancers
Preventative surgery	Use of surgery to reduce the risk of cancer or delay its development	Total colectomy in a person who has familial adenomatous polyposis and who carries the adenomatous polyposis coli (APC) gene Prophylactic bilateral mastectomy and salpingo-oophorectomy on a premenopausal woman with a strong family history of breast and ovarian cancer
Adjuvant therapy	Use of additional cancer treatment after the primary therapy to reduce the risk of cancer recurrence and to decrease the incidence of metastatic disease	Chemotherapy given after a lobectomy for treatment of lung cancer Chemotherapy, hormone therapy, and monoclonal antibody therapy given after a lumpectomy for treatment of breast cancer
Definitive therapy[a]	Use of radiation therapy as the primary treatment modality, with or without chemotherapy	Radiation therapy to treat prostate cancer
Neoadjuvant therapy[a]	Use of one or more treatment modalities before the primary therapy to reduce the size of the primary tumor, improve the effectiveness of surgery, and decrease the incidence of metastatic disease	Chemotherapy and external-beam radiation therapy given before an esophagogastrectomy to treat esophageal cancer Chemotherapy before surgery to treat resectable non–small cell lung cancer
Palliation[a]	Use of cancer treatment modalities, when disease cure and control cannot be achieved, to relieve side effects and symptoms caused by cancer and other serious illnesses, and to improve quality of life	External-beam radiation therapy to palliate painful bony lesions consequent to metastatic prostate cancer; systemic supportive therapy drug, such as a zolendronic acid can also be given to decrease complications (slows bone breakdown) created by bone metastasis
Prophylactic therapy[a]	Use of radiation therapy to relieve symptoms, such as pain, bleeding, neurological compromise, or airway obstruction to improve quality of life or treat life-threatening problems	Whole-brain irradiation in asymptomatic individuals diagnosed with cancers that have a high risk for metastases (eg, small cell lung cancer)

[a] Multimodal approaches to medical oncology treatment that includes radiation therapy

are better able to repair themselves than malignant cells, and most toxicities are reversible. Body cells with rapid turnovers that are especially susceptible to the effects of chemotherapy agents include the following:

- bone marrow (eg, blood cells)
- hair folliclos
- gonads (eg, testes and ovaries)
- gastrointestinal mucosa (eg, mouth, esophagus, stomach, intestines)

Mode of Action

Chemotherapeutic agents interfere with cell division and ultimately lead to cell death. These agents affect the cell during a specific phase of the cell cycle, defined as the period of time and activities that take place between cell divisions. The five phases of the cell cycle are as follows[8]:

- **G0** (resting phase), during which cells are temporarily out of the cycle and have stopped dividing;
- **G1** (postmitotic phase), during which cells begin the first phase of reproduction by synthesizing protein and RNA necessary for cell division;
- **S** (synthesis phase), during which DNA is synthesized;
- **G2** (premitotic phase), during which cells prepare to divide; and
- **M** (mitotic phase), during which cell growth and protein production stops, and cellular energy is focused on the orderly division into two daughter cells.

Agents Used

Chemotherapy agents are classified according to their mechanism of action and effect on cell reproduction. Cell cycle–nonspecific agents are drugs that damage cells in all phases of the cell cycle and include the following, among others[8]:

- alkylating agents
- antitumor antibiotics
- hormone therapies
- nitrosoureas

Cell cycle–specific agents, on the other hand, exert their effect within a specific phase of the cell cycle. They include the following[8]:

- antimetabolites (synthesis phase)
- camptothecins (synthesis phase)
- plant alkaloids and taxanes (mitosis phase)
- miscellaneous agents (various phases)

Administration

Chemotherapy and other antineoplastic agents are administered in a variety of ways. Routes of administration include oral, intraperitoneal, intravenous, intrathecal, intraventricular, intrapleural, intra-arterial, subcutaneous or intramuscular, and topical. Antineoplastic therapy is given in cycles. By giving agents (or a combination of agents) at specific times, cancer cells can be the most susceptible and normal cells can recover from the damage. There are three important factors in the delivery of these agents[8,10]:

- frequency of cycles—daily, weekly, every 14 or 21 days, monthly, or continuously;
- length of cycles—lasting minutes, hours, days, or years, whether by injection, bolus infusion, or continuous infusion; and
- number of cycles—as determined by research and clinical trials.

Side Effects and Nutritional Implications

Just as chemotherapy agents differ, short- and long-term side effects differ depending on the agent and the prescribed treatment regimen.[8] Whether an individual experiences a specific side effect and how long that side effect lasts depend on several factors, such as personal health history, the amount of the agent given, the way it is delivered, the length of time it is given, and other agents and drugs that may have been given previously. Most side effects are temporary and resolve quickly. However, in some cases it can take weeks, months, and even years for treatment-related side effects to resolve. In other instances, long-term side effects occur; permanent effects may include damage to the lungs, heart, liver, kidneys, reproductive organs, nerves, and bone marrow.[8] The effects of chemotherapy on patients' nutritional status are shown in Box 9.3 on pages 162 to 169. (See Chapter 11 for guidance regarding the management of the nutrition implications of these side effects.)

Personalized Medicine

Personalized medicine—also called precision medicine—uses a patient's genetic information to prevent, diagnose, or treat cancer.[11,12] Genetic testing is performed on a sample of a patient's tumor to detect mutations in the DNA of the cancer cells. Knowing if a patient has a genetic mutation helps guide oncologists in customizing and recommending certain treatments that may be more effective. The absence or presence of certain genetic mutations can predict if a patient may benefit from receiving an agent and whether the patient is more likely to respond to one specific treatment over another.[11] This is an evolving area of intense medical and research interest and is becoming a routine component of all oncologists' treatment planning and decision-making. Genetic tests for targeted cancer therapy for specific cancers include but are not limited to the following[12]:

- *ALK* mutation: non–small cell lung cancer
- *BCR-ABL* mutation: chronic myelogenous leukemia and acute lymphoblastic leukemia
- *BRCA* mutation: breast cancer and ovarian cancer
- *BRAF* mutation: melanoma, lung cancer, and breast cancer
- *EGFR* mutation: non–small cell lung cancer
- Estrogen and progesterone receptor status: breast cancer
- *ERBB2* (formerly HER2 or HER2/neu) status: breast cancer
- *JAK2* mutation: bone marrow disorders and myleoproliferative diseases
- *KRAS* mutation: colon cancer and non–small cell lung cancer

Pharmacogenomics is the study of how a patient's genes affect the way the body processes and responds to certain drugs. Genetic differences between patients can mean that while one patient may tolerate a certain cancer drug, another patient receiving the same drug may experience serious side effects. Pharmacogenomics looks at small variations within genes and determines whether the gene activates or deactivates certain drugs.[13] Genetic evaluation helps oncologists select the safest and most effective drugs, and appropriate dosages, for a patient. For example, testing for a genetic variation that can cause decreased levels of the enzyme dihydropyrimidine dehydrogenase (DPD) can help determine the appropriate dose of the chemotherapy agent fluorouracil (5-FU).[14] The body requires the DPD enzyme to metabolize 5-FU. Patients who have a DPD deficiency and are receiving 5-FU can experience significant and often life-threatening side effects (eg, neutropenia,

Box 9.3
Possible Side Effects and Nutritional Implications of Chemotherapy Agents[8,16-18]

Cell cycle–nonspecific drugs: active throughout the cell cycle

Classification and mechanism of action	Medication name,[a] route of administration, and indication	Possible side effects and nutritional implications
Alkylating agents *Mechanism of Action:* Interfere with DNA bases, causing breaks in DNA helix strands, thus preventing DNA replication and transcription of RNA	**Bendamustine (Treanda)** *Route:* intravenous (IV) *Indication:* B-cell non-Hodgkin lymphoma (NHL), chronic lymphocytic leukemia (CLL)	▪ Myelosuppression ▪ Mild nausea and vomiting, fatigue ▪ Other: hypersensitivity infusion reactions (fever, chills, pruritis, rash), tumor lysis syndrome
	Busulfan (Myleran) *Route:* oral **Busulfan (Busulfex)** *Route:* IV *Indication:* chronic myelogenous leukemia (CML), hematopoietic cell transplantation (HCT) preparation, polycythemia vera	▪ Myelosuppression ▪ Nausea, vomiting, diarrhea, mucositis ▪ Hepatic toxicity ▪ Adrenal insufficiency ▪ Other: pulmonary symptoms (eg, cough, dyspnea), insomnia, dizziness, anxiety, alopecia
	Carboplatin (Paraplatin) *Route:* IV *Indication:* cancers of the breast, bladder, cervix, endometrium, esophagus, germ cell, head and neck, lung, and ovaries; sarcomas	▪ Myelosuppression ▪ Hypomagnesemia ▪ Nausea, vomiting ▪ Renal toxicity ▪ Other: hypersensitivity reaction, mild alopecia, peripheral neuropathy, taste change
	Carmustine (BCNU) (may also be classified as a nitrosourea) *Route:* IV *Indication:* brain cancer, Hodgkin disease (HD), NHL, multiple myeloma (MM), cutaneous T-cell lymphoma	▪ Myelosuppression ▪ Nausea, vomiting ▪ Hepatic toxicity ▪ Renal toxicity ▪ Pulmonary toxicity

(continued)

[a] The medications listed in this box are examples; this is not intended to be a comprehensive list. Consult the National Comprehensive Cancer Network guidelines for current recommendations since publication. See reference 2.

Box 9.3
Possible Side Effects and Nutritional Implications of Chemotherapy Agents[8,16-18] *(continued)*

Cell cycle–nonspecific drugs: active throughout the cell cycle (continued)

Classification and mechanism of action	Medication name,[a] route of administration, and indication	Possible side effects and nutritional implications
Alkylating agents (continued) *Mechanism of Action:* Interfere with DNA bases, causing breaks in DNA helix strands, thus preventing DNA replication and transcription of RNA	**Chlorambucil (Leukeran)** *Route:* oral *Indication:* CLL, HD, NHL; cancers of the breast, ovaries, and testes	■ Nausea, vomiting ■ Hyperuricemia ■ Pulmonary toxicity ■ Other: skin rash, seizure risk in children
	Cisplatin (Platinol, CDDP) *Route:* IV *Indication:* cancers of the bladder, cervix, esophagus, head and neck, lung, prostate, ovaries, stomach, and testes; NHL *Note:* hydration given for urological protection	■ Myelosuppression ■ Nausea, vomiting (acute and delayed), metallic taste ■ Renal toxicity ■ Hypomagnesemia, low calcium, low potassium levels ■ Other: syndrome of inappropriate antidiuretic hormone (SIADH), ototoxicity, hypersensitivity infusion reaction, peripheral neuropathy
	Cyclophosphamide (Cytoxan, CTX) *Route:* IV, oral, intrapleural (IP) *Indication:* cancers of the breast, endometrium, lung, ovaries, and testes; CLL; NHL; HD; MM; mycosis fungoides; neuroblastoma; Wilms' tumors; sarcomas	■ Myelosuppression ■ Nausea, vomiting ■ Bladder toxicity ■ Cardiac toxicity ■ Other: SIADH, alopecia
	Dacarbazine (DTIC) *Route:* IV *Indication:* HD, malignant melanoma, neuroblastoma, sarcomas, medullary thyroid cancer	■ Myelosuppression ■ Nausea, vomiting ■ Other: flu-like symptoms (eg, fever, chills), central nervous system toxicity, photosensitivity
	Ifosfamide (Ifex) *Route:* IV *Indication:* cancers of the bladder, cervix, germ cell, head and neck, and lung; HD; NHL; sarcomas *Note:* mesna and hydration given for urological protection	■ Myelosuppression ■ Nausea, vomiting, anorexia ■ Bladder toxicity (eg, hemorrhagic cystitis, dysuria) ■ Other: SIADH, neurotoxicity (eg, seizure, lethargy), alopecia

(continued)

Box 9.3
Possible Side Effects and Nutritional Implications of Chemotherapy Agents[8,16-18] (continued)

Cell cycle–nonspecific drugs: active throughout the cell cycle (continued)

Classification and mechanism of action	Medication name,[a] route of administration, and indication	Possible side effects and nutritional implications
Alkylating agents (continued) *Mechanism of Action:* Interfere with DNA bases, causing breaks in DNA helix strands, thus preventing DNA replication and transcription of RNA	**Mechlorethamine; also known as nitrogen mustard** *Route:* IV *Indication:* CLL, CML, HD, NHL, mycosis fungoides, breast and lung cancers	▪ Myelosuppression ▪ Nausea, vomiting ▪ Hyperuricemia ▪ Other: pain or inflammation at injection site, alopecia
	Melphalan (Alkeran) *Route:* IV, oral *Indication:* breast and ovarian cancers, MM, HCT, polycythemia vera, neuroblastoma	▪ Myelosuppression ▪ Nausea, vomiting, mucositis, diarrhea ▪ Other: hypersensitivity infusion reaction
	Oxaliplatin (Eloxatin) *Route:* IV *Indication:* colorectal cancer, pancreatic cancer	▪ Myelosuppression ▪ Nausea, vomiting, diarrhea ▪ Neurotoxicity (eg, peripheral neuropathy, sensitivity to cold, laryngopharyngeal dysesthesia) ▪ Hepatic toxicity ▪ Other: allergic reaction
	Temozolomide (Temodar) *Route:* oral *Indication:* astrocytoma, glioblastoma	▪ Myelosuppression ▪ Nausea, vomiting, fatigue ▪ Headache ▪ Hepatic toxicity ▪ Constipation ▪ Other: photosensitivity, rash
	Thiotepa (Thioplex) *Route:* IV, intramuscular (IM), intrathecal (IT), subcutaneous (SC) *Indication:* bladder, breast, and ovarian cancers; HD; NHL	▪ Myelosuppression ▪ Nausea, vomiting, mucositis ▪ Renal toxicity (eg, hemorrhagic cystitis) ▪ Other: skin changes (eg, rash, bronzing of skin)

(continued)

[a] The medications listed in this box are examples; this is not intended to be a comprehensive list. Consult the National Comprehensive Cancer Network guidelines for current recommendations since publication. See reference 2.

Box 9.3
Possible Side Effects and Nutritional Implications of Chemotherapy Agents[8,16-18] (continued)

Cell cycle–specific drugs

Classification and mechanism of action	Medication name[a], route of administration, and indication	Possible side effects and nutritional implications
Antimetabolites *Mechanism of Action:* Interfere with DNA synthesis by acting as false metabolites; incorporated into the DNA strand or block essential enzymes	**Azacitidine (Vidaza)** *Route:* SC, IV *Indication:* CML, myelodysplastic syndrome (MDS)	▪ Myelosuppression ▪ Nausea, vomiting, diarrhea, fatigue ▪ Constipation ▪ Hypokalemia ▪ Renal toxicity
	Capecitabine (Xeloda) *Route:* oral *Indication:* cancers of the colon, esophagus, pancreas, rectum, and (metastatic) breast	▪ Myelosuppression ▪ Nausea, vomiting, diarrhea, fatigue ▪ Increased bilirubin ▪ Other: hand-foot syndrome
	Cytarabine (ARA-C) *Route:* IV, SC, IT, IM *Indication:* acute lymphoblastic leukemia (ALL), acute promyelocytic leukemia (APL), acute myelogenous leukemia (AML), CML, NHL	▪ Myelosuppression ▪ Nausea, vomiting, mucositis, anorexia, acute pancreatitis ▪ Neurotoxicity (eg, lethargy, confusion) ▪ Hepatic toxicity ▪ Pulmonary toxicity ▪ Other: conjunctivitis, keratitis
	Fludarabine (Fludara) *Route:* IV *Indication:* CLL, NHL, acute leukemias	▪ Myelosuppression ▪ Nausea, vomiting, diarrhea ▪ Neurotoxicity ▪ Other: rash
	Fluorouracil (5-FU) *Route:* IV, topical *Indication:* cancers of the breast, colon and rectum, cervix, gastrointestinal (GI) tract, head and neck, pancreas, ovaries, and stomach; unknown primary cancer; hepatobiliary cancer; neuroendocrine cancer; thymic cancer	▪ Myelosuppression ▪ Nausea, vomiting, diarrhea, mucositis ▪ Other: hand-foot syndrome, cardiac toxicity, photosensitivity, taste changes
	Gemcitabine (Gemzar) *Route:* IV *Indication:* cancers of the bladder, breast, lung, ovaries, and pancreas; NHL; sarcoma	▪ Myelosuppression ▪ Nausea, vomiting ▪ Pulmonary toxicity ▪ Other: rash, flu-like symptoms (eg, fever, chills)

(continued)

Box 9.3

Possible Side Effects and Nutritional Implications of Chemotherapy Agents[8,16-18] *(continued)*

Cell cycle–specific drugs (continued)

Classification and mechanism of action	Medication name,[a] route of administration, and indication	Possible side effects and nutritional implications
Antimetabolites (continued) *Mechanism of Action:* Interfere with DNA synthesis by acting as false metabolites; incorporated into the DNA strand or block essential enzymes	**Hydroxyurea (Hydrea)** *Route:* oral *Indication:* CML; blood disorders; cancers of the head and neck, and ovaries	▪ Myelosuppression ▪ Nausea, vomiting, diarrhea, mucositis ▪ Other: darkening and/or thickening of the nails
	Mercaptopurine (6-MP) *Route:* oral *Indication:* ALL; APL; lymphoma; ulcerative colitis; Crohn disease	▪ Myelosuppression ▪ Nausea, vomiting, mucositis, diarrhea ▪ Hepatic toxicity ▪ Hyperuricemia
	Methotrexate (MTX) *Route:* IM, IV, IT, oral *Indication:* cancers of the bladder, breast, and head and neck; NHL; ALL; osteosarcoma; rheumatoid arthritis	▪ Myelosuppression ▪ Nausea, mucositis, oral and GI ulcerations ▪ Renal toxicity ▪ Hepatic toxicity ▪ Other: photosensitivity
	Pemetrexed (Alimta) *Route:* IV *Indication:* mesothelioma, lung cancer	▪ Myelosuppression ▪ Nausea, vomiting, diarrhea, fatigue ▪ Patients treated with pemetrexed usually require folic acid and vitamin B12 supplementation to reduce side effects ▪ Other: rash
	Thioguanine (6-TG) *Route:* oral *Indication:* AML, CML	▪ Myelosuppression ▪ Nausea, vomiting, mucositis, diarrhea ▪ Hepatic toxicity ▪ Renal toxicity ▪ Other: rash

(continued)

[a] The medications listed in this box are examples; this is not intended to be a comprehensive list. Consult the National Comprehensive Cancer Network guidelines for current recommendations since publication. See reference 2.

Box 9.3
Possible Side Effects and Nutritional Implications of Chemotherapy Agents[8,16-18] *(continued)*

Cell cycle–specific drugs (continued)

Classification and mechanism of action	Medication name,[a] route of administration, and indication	Possible side effects and nutritional implications
Antitumor antibiotics *Mechanism of Action:* Inhibit cell division by binding to DNA and interfering with RNA synthesis	**Bleomycin (Blenoxane)** *Route:* IV, SC, IM *Indication:* HD; NHL; head and neck cancer; squamous cell cancers of the skin, cervix, vulva, and testes; melanoma; malignant pleural effusions	■ Pulmonary toxicity ■ Renal toxicity ■ Other: hyperpigmentation, skin and nail changes, hypersensitivity infusion reaction
	Dactinomycin (Actinomycin D) *Route:* IV *Indication:* Ewing sarcoma, rhabdomyosarcoma, Wilms tumor, testicular cancer	■ Myleosuppression ■ Nausea, vomiting, mucositis, diarrhea, anorexia ■ Other: alopecia
	Mitomycin-C (Mutamycin) *Route:* IV *Indication:* cancers of the anus, bladder, breast, esophagus, head and neck, lung, pancreas, and stomach	■ Myelosuppression ■ Nausea, vomiting, mucositis, diarrhea, anorexia ■ Pulmonary toxicity ■ Renal toxicity ■ Other: alopecia
Anthracycline antitumor antibiotics *Mechanism of Action:* Inhibit cell division by binding to DNA and interfering with RNA synthesis	**Daunorubicin (Daunomycin)** *Route:* IV *Indication:* ALL, AML, APL	■ Myelosuppression ■ Nausea, vomiting, diarrhea, mucositis, anorexia ■ Hyperuremia ■ Other: cardiotoxicity, alopecia, red urine, hyperpigmentation
	Doxorubicin (Adriamycin) *Route:* IV *Indication:* cancers of the breast, liver, lung, ovaries, prostate, and stomach; NHL; HD; MM; ALL; AML; squamous cell cancer of the head and neck; sarcomas	■ Myelosuppression ■ Nausea, vomiting, diarrhea, mucositis, anorexia ■ Other: cardiotoxicity, hand-foot syndrome, hyperpigmentation, alopecia, red-orange urine

(continued)

Box 9.3
Possible Side Effects and Nutritional Implications of Chemotherapy Agents[8,16-18] *(continued)*

Cell cycle–specific drugs (continued)

Classification and mechanism of action	Medication name,[a] route of administration, and indication	Possible side effects and nutritional implications
Anthracycline antitumor antibiotics (continued) *Mechanism of Action:* Inhibit cell division by binding to DNA and interfering with RNA synthesis	**Doxorubicin liposomal (Doxil)** *Route:* IV *Indication:* AIDS-related Kaposi sarcoma; cancers of the breast and ovaries and other solid tumors	▪ Myelosuppression ▪ Nausea, vomiting, diarrhea, mucositis ▪ Other: cardiotoxicity, hand-foot syndrome, hyperpigmentation, alopecia, red-orange urine, infusion reaction
	Epirubicin (Ellence) *Route:* IV *Indication:* breast cancer	▪ Myelosuppression ▪ Nausea, vomiting, diarrhea, mucositis ▪ Other: cardiotoxicity, skin rash, alopecia, red-orange urine
	Idarubicin (Idamycin) *Route:* IV *Indication:* AML, ALL, CML, MDS	▪ Myelosuppression ▪ Nausea, vomiting, diarrhea, mucositis ▪ Other: cardiotoxicity, alopecia, hand-foot syndrome, elevation of liver enzymes, red urine
Epipodophyllotoxins *Mechanism of Action:* Damage the cell prior to mitosis, late S and G2 phases; inhibits topoisomerase II	**Etoposide (Vepesid, VP-16)** *Route:* IV, oral *Indication:* cancers of the bladder, lung, prostate, stomach, and uterus; HD; NHL; germ cell cancer (testicular)	▪ Myelosuppression ▪ Nausea, vomiting, diarrhea, mucositis, anorexia ▪ Other: metallic taste during infusion, hypersensitivity reaction, alopecia, orthostatic hypertension, yellowing of the skin or eyes
	Teniposide (Vumon, VM-26) *Route:* IV *Indications:* childhood ALL	▪ Myelosuppression ▪ Nausea, vomiting ▪ Other: hypotension, pulmonary toxicity

(continued)

[a] The medications listed in this box are examples; this is not intended to be a comprehensive list. Consult the National Comprehensive Cancer Network guidelines for current recommendations since publication. See reference 2.

Cell cycle–specific drugs *(continued)*

Classification and mechanism of action	Medication name,[a] route of administration, and indication	Possible side effects and nutritional implications
Taxanes *Mechanism of Action:* Active in the mitosis phase of the cell cycle; antimicrotubule agents, which lead to inhibition of mitosis and cell division	**Paclitaxel (Taxol)** *Route:* IV *Indication:* cancers of the bladder, breast, esophagus, head and neck, lung, ovaries, pancreas, and prostate	▪ Myelosuppression ▪ Swelling of feet and ankles ▪ Nausea, vomiting, diarrhea, mucositis ▪ Peripheral neuropathy ▪ Other: hypersensitivity reaction, alopecia, arthralgia, myalgia
	Docetaxel (Taxotere) *Route:* IV *Indication:* cancers of the bladder, breast, head and neck, lung, ovaries, pancreas, prostate, and stomach; sarcomas	▪ Myelosuppression ▪ Mucositis, diarrhea, nausea, vomiting ▪ Peripheral neuropathy ▪ Other: fluid retention syndrome, skin and nail changes, hypersensitivity reaction, alopecia
	Paclitaxel protein bound (Abraxane) *Route:* IV *Indication:* cancers of the breast and pancreas; non–small cell lung cancer	▪ Myelosuppression ▪ Nausea, vomiting, diarrhea, mucositis ▪ Arthralgia, myalgia ▪ Peripheral neuropathy ▪ Other: alopecia, swelling of the feet and ankles, eye problems
Vinca alkaloids *Mechanism of Action:* Bind to protein tubulin, disrupt mitotic spindle formation, and prevent cell division in the mitosis phase	**Vincristine (Oncovin)** *Route:* IV *Indication:* ALL, AML, HD, NH, rhabdomyosarcoma, neuroblastoma, Ewing sarcoma, Wilms tumor, brain and thyroid cancers	▪ Myelosuppression ▪ Peripheral neuropathy ▪ Constipation, abdominal cramps, nausea, taste changes, mucositis ▪ Other: SIADH, hypersensitivity reactions, jaw pain, alopecia
	Vinblastine (Velban) *Route:* IV *Indication:* cancers of the bladder, breast, testes, head and neck, and lung; HD; NHL; sarcomas; blood disorders	▪ Myelosuppression ▪ Mucositis, stomatitis, constipation, taste changes ▪ Other: hypertension, alopecia, jaw pain
	Vinorelbine (Navelbine) *Route:* IV *Indication:* cancers of the breast and ovaries; non–small cell lung cancers; HD	▪ Myelosuppression ▪ Nausea, vomiting, constipation, stomatitis, anorexia ▪ Other: transient elevations in liver function tests, alopecia

diarrhea, mucositis), because the drug is not effectively metabolized.[15] Pharmacogenomics research is constantly evolving and changing, and cancer researchers are continually identifying new gene variations that can affect responses to cancer drugs and treatment.[13] This has precipitated "personalized" cancer medicine and targeted treatments based on how certain drugs target specific cancer genes and proteins.[4] These efforts are leading the way for the development of promising agents in ongoing clinical trials and their use in consensus protocol treatment guidelines.

Targeted Therapy

Targeted therapies use drugs or other substances that are specific to a certain tumor type or they concentrate on the genetic change instead of the type of cell. Targeted therapies fall into two types: one targets specific genes or proteins found in cancer cells, and the other acts on the tissue environment related to cancer cell growth and survival, such as blood vessel cells. Monoclonal antibodies act like the naturally occurring antibodies in the body to target a specific protein on the outside of the cancer cell or cell surface. Small-molecule drugs block the processes that allow cancer cells to grow and metastasize.

Side Effects of Targeted Therapy

Genes influence the molecular transformation of normal cells to malignant cells and then to metastatic disease. By "targeting," or focusing on, the molecular changes that are specific to cancer, molecularly targeted therapies show promise of being more effective than systemic treatments (chemotherapy) or localized treatments (radiation therapy) and less toxic to normal cells.[11,19] However, this observation has not proven to be entirely the case. As the use of targeted agents increases, their side effects are proving not to be less toxic to normal cells but just very different.[20] Whereas the common side effects of systemic chemotherapy agents include

myelosuppression, mucositis, nausea, vomiting, and alopecia, the common side effects of targeted agents include vascular, coagulatory, dermatologic, immunologic, ocular, and pulmonary toxicities.[20]

Monoclonal Antibodies

Monoclonal antibodies target specific receptors on the outside of tumor cells that then activate pathways inside the cell to disrupt cell function and cause cell apoptosis (cell death). These agents are used alone or in combination with other cancer therapies and can also serve as delivery vehicles for radioactive molecules (eg, tositumomab).[21] Monoclonal antibodies can also be used to block certain proteins made by some types of immune system cells by affecting critical cell pathways to control growth. New agents, known as immune checkpoint inhibitors (eg, ipilimumab [Yervoy], nivolumab [Opdivo], and pembrolizumab [Keytruda]), block specific pathways to stop or to slow cancer growth.[20]

Molecular targets with signaling effects on the outside of cancer cells include:

- *BRAF V600E*: cell growth signaling protein
- *CD20*: B-lymphocyte antigen CD20
- *EGFR*: epidermal growth factor receptor
- *ERBB2*: human epidermal growth factor receptor 2
- *PD-1/PD-L1*: programmed cell death ligand 1
- *RANKL*: receptor-activated nuclear factor κB ligand
- *VEGF*: vascular endothelial growth factor

Side effects of monoclonal antibodies can include infusion-related symptoms, such as fever, chills, urticaria, flushing, fatigue, headache, dyspnea, hypotension, or hypertension.[10,22] Muscular-skeletal side effects may involve muscle aches and pains, and skin-related changes may include skin rash, facial erythema, and hand-foot syndrome. Gastrointestinal (GI) side effects may include mouth sores, nausea, vomiting, diarrhea, and decreased appetite. Some monoclonal antibodies can result in cardiotoxicities, such as dyspnea, peripheral edema, and reduced left ventricular function, and there is increased risk if given in combination with an anthracycline-based regimen. There is greater risk of myelosuppression when monoclonal antibodies are administered with chemotherapeutic agents. Pulmonary toxicity symptoms of monoclonal antibodies may include increased cough, dyspnea, pulmonary infiltrates, and pleural effusions.[8,10,22]

Box 9.4 on pages 172 to 173 provides a comprehensive overview of the classification, mechanisms of action, route of administration, and possible side effects of monoclonal antibodies.

Small-Molecule Drugs

Small-molecule drugs can be protein-targeted agents or apoptosis inhibitors. Protein-targeted therapy uses small molecules that penetrate malignant cell membranes to interact with specific areas of the target proteins.[23] These agents disrupt cell function, which causes or induces cell apoptosis. Box 9.5 on page 174 provides examples of protein-targeted agents.

Possible skin-related side effects of small-molecule drugs may include skin rash, facial erythema, and hand-foot syndrome. Hair depigmentation may occur with sunitinib (Sutent), which causes hair to turn white while on therapy. Cardiotoxicities, such as QT prolongation and possible sudden death may also occur, so it is important to monitor patients with a previous history of cardiovascular disease, left ventricular dysfunction, hypertension, bleeding, and myocardial infarction. GI symptoms such as nausea, vomiting, diarrhea, decreased appetite, and taste changes, alter a patient's ability to maintain normal dietary intake.[8,18]

Another category of small-molecule drugs is angiogenesis inhibitors (known as antiangiogenesis therapy), which hinder the formation of new blood vessels in primary tumors and metastatic tumors, thus preventing their growth, invasion, and spread.[16]

Box 9.6 on page 175 provides examples of anti-angiogenetic agents.

Other possible side effects of angiogenesis inhibitors can include hypertension and arterial thromboembolic events, such as myocardial infarction, angina, and stroke. Patients may experience nosebleeds, hemoptysis, hematuria, GI bleeding, GI perforation, or vaginal bleeding. Factors linked to increased risk for GI perforation are a tumor at an anastomotic site, abdominal carcinomatosis, bowel obstruction, history of abdominal or pelvic radiation therapy, or recent colonoscopy.[8,17] Proteinuria may occur in nearly one-third of patients treated with bevacizumab. Hypothyroidism can occur in some patients, and they may experience related symptoms, including increased sensitivity to cold, dry skin, weight gain, fatigue, myalgias, arthralgias, and depression.

Immunotherapy

Immunotherapy, also known as biological therapy or biotherapy, is defined as treatment to boost or restore the ability of the immune system to fight cancer, infection, and other diseases by inducing, enhancing, or suppressing an individual's own immune response.[8,16] Immunotherapy has revolutionized cancer treatment by using the body's immune system to either directly or indirectly fight the disease.[16,23] Immunotherapy agents consist of substances made by the body or produced in a laboratory. They can be used alone or in combination with chemotherapeutic agents. The action of immunotherapy agents also may be short-term, as is the case with monoclonal antibodies and small-molecule drugs, or long-lasting, as with therapeutic cancer vaccines.

Box 9.4

Side Effects and Nutritional Implications of Monoclonal Antibodies[8,16-18,20,21]

Target	Medication name,[a] route of administration, and indication	Possible side effects and nutritional implications
CD20	**Ibritumomab tiuxetan (Zevalin)** *Route:* Intravenous (IV) *Indication:* non-Hodgkin lymphoma (NHL), follicular lymphoma	▪ Myelosuppression ▪ Asthenia ▪ Infections ▪ Nausea, vomiting—generally mild ▪ Other: possible infusion reaction, cough, dyspnea, sinusitis
	Rituximab (Rituxan) *Route:* IV *Indication:* NHL, chronic lymphocytic leukemia (CLL)	▪ Myelosuppression ▪ Nausea, vomiting—generally mild ▪ Tumor lysis syndrome ▪ Other: possible infusion reaction, skin reaction
CD52	**Alemtuzumab (Campath)** *Route:* IV *Indication:* CLL	▪ Myelosuppression ▪ Nausea, vomiting ▪ Other: possible infusion reaction
ERBB2	**Pertuzumab (Perjeta)** *Route:* IV *Indication:* ERBB2+ breast cancer	▪ Myelosuppression ▪ Diarrhea, nausea, vomiting ▪ Other: possible infusion reaction, rash
	Trastuzumab (Herceptin) *Route:* IV *Indication:* ERBB2+ breast cancer, gastric cancer	▪ Myleosuppression (rarely) ▪ Nausea, vomiting, diarrhea—generally mild ▪ Cardiotoxicity ▪ Other: possible infusion reaction, pulmonary toxicity
	Ado-trastuzumab emtansine (Kadcyla) *Route:* IV *Indication:* ERBB2+ metastatic breast cancer	▪ Myelosuppression ▪ Nausea ▪ Peripheral neuropathy ▪ Other: possible infusion reaction, increased liver enzymes, decreased serum potassium
EGFR	**Cetuximab (Erbitux)** *Route:* IV *Indication:* metastatic colorectal cancer, non–small cell lung cancer, squamous cell cancer of the head and neck; squamous cell skin cancer	▪ Nausea, vomiting, diarrhea, anorexia ▪ Pulmonary toxicity ▪ Hypomagnesemia ▪ Other: possible infusion reaction, skin rash, pruritus

(continued)

[a] The medications listed in this box are examples; this is not intended to be a comprehensive list. Consult the National Comprehensive Cancer Network guidelines for current recommendations since publication. See reference 2.

Box 9.4
Side Effects and Nutritional Implications of Monoclonal Antibodies[8,16-18,20,21] *(continued)*

Target	Medication name,[a] route of administration, and indication	Possible side effects and nutritional implications
EGFR (continued)	**Panitumumab (Vectibix)** *Route:* IV *Indication:* colorectal cancer	■ Possible infusion reaction ■ Acneiform skin rash, pruritis ■ Pulmonary toxicity ■ Hypomagnesemia ■ Diarrhea ■ Malaise
RANKL	**Denosumab (Xgeva)** *Route:* IV *Indication:* bone metastases, giant cell tumor of the bone	■ Nausea, vomiting, diarrhea ■ Hypocalcemia ■ Risk for osteonecrosis of the jaw
	Denosumab (Prolia) *Route:* IV *Indication:* osteoporosis with high risk of fracture	■ Nausea, vomiting, diarrhea ■ Hypocalcemia ■ Risk for osteonecrosis of the jaw
PD-1/ PD-L1	**Ipilimumab (Yervoy)** *Route:* IV *Indication:* melanoma	■ Anemia ■ Nausea, vomiting, diarrhea ■ Other: rash, pruritus, pulmonary symptoms
	Nivolumab (Opdivo) *Route:* IV *Indication:* melanoma, non–small cell lung cancer, renal cell cancer	■ Myelosuppression ■ Colitis, nausea, vomiting, constipation ■ Hyponatremia, hypokalemia, hypomagnesemia ■ Other: pruritus, pulmonary symptoms, pneumonia
PD-1	**Pembrolizumab (Keytruda)** *Route:* IV *Indication:* melanoma, non–small cell lung cancer, squamous cell cancer of the head and neck, endometrial cancer	■ Anemia ■ Nausea ■ Hyperglycemia ■ Hyponatremia, hypoalbuminemia ■ Other: pruritus, pulmonary symptoms, increased liver enzymes

Box 9.5
Small-Molecule Drugs: Protein-Targeted Agents[8,16-18,21]

Drug class and mechanism of action	Medication name[a]	Indication
Tyrosine kinase inhibitors: inhibit several receptor tyrosine kinases, which are involved in tumor growth, angiogenesis, and metastasis	Erlotinib (Tarceva)	Locally advanced or metastatic non–small cell lung cancer or pancreatic cancer
	Gefitinib (Iressa)	Refractory non–small cell lung cancer
	Imatinib (Gleevec)	Philadelphia chromosome positive (Ph+) chronic myelogenous leukemia (CML), gastrointestinal stromal tumor (GIST), myelodysplastic syndrome (MDS), refractory Ph+ acute lymphoblastic leukemia (ALL)
	Sorafenib (Nexavar)	Renal cell cancer, thyroid cancer, hepatocellular cancer
	Sunitinib (Sutent)	GIST, renal cell cancer, pancreatic neuroendocrine tumors
	Crizotinib (Xalkori)	anaplastic lymphoma kinase positive (ALK+) or *ROS1*+ non–small cell lung cancer
	Dasatinib (Syprcel)	Ph+ CML, Ph+ ALL
Mammalian target of rapamycin (*mTOR*) inhibitors: block angiogenesis by preventing the release of vascular endothelial growth factor (*VEGF*) and platelet-derived growth factor (*PDGF*), thus blocking tumor cell proliferation and causing cell death	Temsirolimus (Torisel)	Renal cell cancer
	Everolimus (Affinitor)	Renal cell cancer, pancreatic neuroendocrine tumors, estrogen receptor positive advanced breast cancer
Proteasome inhibitors: inhibit breakdown of intracellular proteins and disrupt the proteasome pathway	Bortezomib (Velcade)	Multiple myeloma, mantle cell lymphoma
BRAF inhibitors: target the mutant form of the *BRAF* protein	Vemurafenib (Zelboraf)	Melanoma

[a] The medications listed in this box are examples; this is not intended to be a comprehensive list. Consult the National Comprehensive Cancer Network guidelines for current recommendations since publication. See reference 2.

Box 9.6
Small-Molecule Drugs: Angiogenesis Inhibitors[16-18]

Target	Medication name[a] and mechanism of action	Indication	Side effects
Vascular endothelial growth factor (*VEGF*)	**Bevacizumab (Avastin)** Recognizes and binds to *VEGF*, thus stopping it from activating the *VEGF* receptor. This action helps to arrest endothelial cell proliferation and angiogenesis.	Metastatic colorectal cancer, non–small cell lung cancer, metastatic breast cancer, glioblastoma, metastatic renal cell cancer	Generalized weakness, pain, abdominal pain, nausea and vomiting, reduced appetite, upper respiratory infection, low white cell count
Ubiquitin E3 ligase cereblon	**Lenalidomide (Revlimide)** Interacts with the ubiquitin E3 ligase cereblon and targets this enzyme to degrade the Ikaros transcription factors *IKZF1* and *IKZF3*. Inhibits tumor angiogenesis, tumor secreted cytokines, and tumor proliferation.	Multiple myeloma, mantle cell lymphoma, myelodysplastic syndrome	Diarrhea, nausea, vomiting, constipation, rash, tiredness, fever, itching
	Thalidomide (Thalomid) Mechanism of action is not fully understood. Inhibits tumor angiogenesis and proinflammatory tumor secreted cytokines (eg, tumor necrosis factor α (*TNF*-α), interleukin-1 β (*IL-1*β), interleukin-6 (*IL-6*).	Multiple myeloma, renal cell cancer, glioblastoma multiforme	Headache, dizziness, drowsiness, weakness, tired feeling, anxiety, agitation, confusion, tremors, muscle weakness, nausea, reduced appetite, contipation, edema, dyspnea, weight gain or loss, rash, dry skin

[a] The medications listed in this box are examples; this is not intended to be a comprehensive list. Consult the National Comprehensive Cancer Network guidelines for current recommendations since publication. See reference 2.

Agents Used and Modes of Action

The following describes the categories of immunotherapy agents and their modes of action[11,23]:

- Nonspecific immunotherapies stimulate a broad-based immune response, as opposed to generating a targeted response to a specific tumor antigen.

- Oncolytic viral therapies use genetically modified viruses to kill cancer cells.

- T-cell therapies use T lymphocytes (T cells) removed from a patient's blood that are then changed in the laboratory in order to attach specific protein receptors. The altered cells are then returned to the body, where they seek out and destroy cancer cells.

- Cancer vaccines expose the immune system to an antigen, which triggers an immune response that recognizes and destroys that antigen or related materials. Cancer vaccine therapies are still under clinical investigation.

- Radiopharmaceuticals are a type of immunotherapy monoclonal antibody therapy that delivers radioactive molecules to specific cancer cells. These agents are discussed in Chapter 10.

Nonspecific Immunotherapy

Nonspecific immunotherapy stimulates a broad-based immune response. Box 9.7 provides examples of this treatment.

Possible side effects of nonspecific immunotherapies can include fatigue, anorexia, nausea, vomiting, diarrhea, and flu-like symptoms, such as fever, chills, headache, arthralgias, and myalgias. Myelosuppression may also occur, causing leukopenia, thrombocytopenia, and anemia. Other side effects, such as renal toxicity and cardiotoxicity, may trigger renal insufficiency and capillary leak syndrome.[8,17,18]

Oncolytic Viral Therapy

Oncolytic viral therapy uses a genetically modified virus to kill cancer cells.[24] The altered virus is injected into the tumor, and as the virus replicates, it releases antigens to trigger an immune response. The patient's immune system targets other cells in the body with those antigens, and the cancer cells are infected and destroyed. One

---

Box 9.7
Nonspecific Immunotherapies[8,17,18]

Medication name and mechanism of action[a]	Indication
Interleukin-2 (Aldesleukin) Stimulates the growth and activity of immune cells (lymphocytes) to kill cancer cells	Metastatic melanoma, renal cell cancer
Interferon-α 2b (Intron A) Interferes with cancer cells' ability to divide; indirectly modifies the body's immune response to the cancer cells	Hairy cell leukemia, malignant melanoma, follicular lymphoma, AIDS-related Kaposi sarcoma, and chronic hepatitis B and C

[a] The medications listed in this box are examples; this is not intended to be a comprehensive list. Consult the National Comprehensive Cancer Network guidelines for current recommendations since publication. See reference 2.

Oncology Nutrition *for* Clinical Practice

example is talimogene laherparepvec (Imlygic), or T-VEC for short, a genetically modified and weakened live herpes simplex virus used to treat melanoma.[12] Side effects can include fatigue, fever, chills, nausea, flu-like symptoms, and pain at the injection site.[17,24] Currently, T-VEC is the first and only oncolytic virus approved by the US Food and Drug Administration (FDA) for use in patients. Other viruses are currently under investigation for use in treating different cancers.

Chimeric Antigen Receptor T-Cell Therapy

T-cell therapy involves collecting and using a patient's own immune cells (T lymphocytes, or T cells) to treat cancer. The patient's T cells are obtained through apheresis. These cells are then sent to a laboratory where they are genetically modified by the addition of DNA to create cells that contain a chimeric antigen receptor (CAR) site on their surface.[24] Once the T cells are re-engineered in this manner, they can recognize antigens on targeted tumor cells. The FDA has approved two CAR T-cell therapies, one to treat acute lymphoblastic leukemia in children and the other to treat advanced large β-cell lymphoma in adults.[25] See Chapter 14 for more information. Research is currently underway to modify T cells for treating other types of cancer.

Acute side effects of CAR T-cell therapy include cytokine release syndrome (characterized by nausea, headache, chills, and fatigue) and neurological symptoms, such as confusion, weakness, coordination difficulty, aphasia, and seizures.[26] Late effects of therapy can include increased risk for cytopenia, infection, endocrine dysfunction, and possible infertility.[26]

Cancer Vaccines

Cancer vaccines can be either preventive or therapeutic. The FDA has approved two types of preventive vaccines for use in healthy people: one to protect against hepatitis B virus, which can lead to hepatocellular carcinoma (liver cancer), and the other a recombinant HPV quadrivalent vaccine (Gardasil) and recombinant HPV bivalent vaccine (Cervarix) to protect against human papillomavirus (HPV), which increases one's risk of cervical and oral cancers.[27,28]

Unlike targeted therapies, cancer treatment vaccines do not act on a certain pathway in tumor cells.[24] Rather, this type of therapy is designed to stimulate an individual's own immune system against abnormal and foreign cells, such as cancer cells. The FDA has approved only one cancer treatment vaccine: sipuleucel-T, for use in men with hormone-refractory metastatic prostate cancer.[17] The side effects most commonly experienced with sipuleucel-T include flu-like symptoms, nausea, vomiting, muscle aches, and difficulty breathing. Clinical trials are currently underway for developing treatment vaccines for other types of cancer.

Hormone Therapy

Hormone therapy, also called endocrine therapy, is used to treat hormone-sensitive cancers (eg, breast, ovarian, prostate) by these mechanisms of action:

- stopping or reducing the body's ability to produce hormones
- interfering with or blocking hormone receptors
- substituting chemically similar agents for active hormones but that cannot be used by the tumor[29]

Classification of Hormonal Agents, Side Effects, and Nutritional Implications

Hormone therapy is categorized by the type of hormone that is affected and its function (see Box 9.8 on pages 178 to 179). The agent's side effects and nutritional implications are also described.

Box 9.8
Hormonal Agents Used in Cancer Treatment[10,18,29]

Medication type and examples[a]	Mechanism of action
Selective estrogen receptor modulators, or antiestrogens *Examples*: tamoxifen citrate (Novaldex) toremifene citrate (Fareston) raloxifene (Evista)	These nonsteroidal antiestrogen agents compete with estrogen for binding to estrogen receptors.
Aromatase inhibitors *Examples*: anastrozole (Arimidex) letrozole (Femara) exemestane (Aromasin)	These nonsteroidal and/or steroidal inhibitors of aromatase block the production of estrogen by inhibiting the conversion of adrenal androgens to estrogens. They are primarily used in postmenopausal women because premenopausal women produce too much aromatase for the agents to effectively block.
Progesterones *Example*: megestrol acetate (Megace)	These agents possess antiestrogenic effects and inhibit the stability, availability, and turnover of estrogen receptors.
Antiandrogens *Examples*: bicalutamide (Casodex) flutamide (Eulexin)	These agents bind to androgen receptors and block the effects of testosterone in androgen-sensitive prostate cancer cells.
Luteinizing hormone-releasing hormone (LHRH) agonists *Examples:* leuprolide acetate (Lupron) goserelin (Zoladex)	These synthetic proteins, which are similar to naturally occurring LHRH, signal the pituitary gland to stop producing luteinizing hormone, which results in the suppression of testosterone to manage the growth and spread of prostate cancer. They can also be used to suppress ovarian function by interfering with signals from the pituitary gland that stimulate the ovaries to produce estrogen.

[a] The medications listed in this box are examples; this is not intended to be a comprehensive list. Consult the National Comprehensive Cancer Network guidelines for current recommendations since publication. See reference 2.

Indication	Side effects and nutritional implications	
Tamoxifen and toremifene citrate: breast cancer Raloxifene: osteoporosis or postmenopausal women at risk for breast cancer	■ Menstrual symptoms: hot flashes, sweating, nausea, menstrual irregularities, vaginal dryness, mood changes, decreased libido, fatigue ■ Fluid retention and peripheral edema	■ Increased risk of endometrial changes and cancer ■ Thromboembolic complications ■ Skin changes, rash ■ Joint aches and pains ■ Weight gain
Breast cancer	■ Hot flashes ■ Arthralgias ■ Nausea and vomiting—generally mild ■ Asthenia	■ Thromboembolic events ■ High cholesterol (letrozole) ■ Fever, malaise, myalgias ■ Joint aches and pains
Breast, endometrial, renal cell cancers Prescribed as an appetite stimulant in cancer and HIV/AIDS	■ Weight gain (fluid retention) ■ Thromboembolic events ■ Nausea and vomiting	■ Menstrual bleeding, hot flashes, sweating, and mood change ■ Hyperglycemia
Prostate cancer	■ Weight gain ■ Hot flashes, fatigue ■ Decreased libido, impotence ■ Bone pain	
Prostate and ovarian cancers	■ Hot flashes, fatigue ■ Decreased libido, impotence ■ Bone pain	■ Gynecomastia ■ Headache ■ Muscle weakness

References

1. American College of Surgeons Commission on Cancer. Standard 4.7: oncology nutrition services. Optimal Resources for Cancer Care (2020 Standards). Effective January 2020. Accessed January 27, 2020. www.facs.org/quality -programs/cancer/coc/2020 -standards

2. NCCN guidelines and clinical resources. National Comprehensive Cancer Network website. Accessed June 17, 2019. www.nccn.org/professionals /physician_gls

3. American Society of Clinical Oncology. Understanding chemotherapy. Cancer.Net website. Accessed June 17, 2019. www.cancer.net/navigating -cancer-care/how-cancer-treated /chemotherapy/understanding -chemotherapy

4. American Society of Clinical Oncology. What is personalized cancer medicine? Cancer.Net website. Accessed June 17, 2019. www.cancer.net/navigating -cancer-care/how-cancer-treated /personalized-and-targeted -therapies/what-personalized -cancer-medicine

5. Precision medicine in cancer treatment. National Cancer Institute website. Accessed June 17, 2019. www.cancer.gov /about-cancer/treatment/types /precision-medicine

6. NCI Dictionary of Cancer Terms. National Cancer Institute website. Accessed June 17, 2019. www.cancer.gov/publications /dictionaries/cancer-terms

7. American Society of Clinical Oncology website. Accessed June 17, 2019. www.cancer.net

8. Polovich M, Olsen M, Lefebvre K. *Chemotherapy and Biotherapy Guidelines and Recommendations for Practice*. 4th ed. Oncology Nursing Society; 2014.

9. Iwamoto RR, Haas ML, Gosselin TK. *Oncology Nursing Society's Manual for Radiation Oncology Nursing Practice and Education*. 4th ed. Oncology Nursing Society; 2012.

10. Wilkes GM, Barton-Burke, M. *Oncology Nursing Drug Handbook*. Jones and Bartlett Learning; 2018.

11. American Society of Clinical Oncology. Understanding targeted therapy. Cancer.Net website. Accessed June 17, 2019. www.cancer.net/navigating -cancer-care/how-cancer-treated /personalized-and-targeted -therapies/understanding -targeted-therapy

12. American Association for Clinical Chemistry. Genetic tests for targeted cancer therapy. Lab Tests Online website. Accessed June 17, 2019. https://labtestsonline.org/tests /genetic-tests-targeted-cancer -therapy

13. American Society of Clinical Oncology. Understanding pharmacogenomics. Cancer. Net website. Accessed June 17, 2019. www.cancer.net/navigating -cancer-care/how-cancer-treated /personalized-and-targeted -therapies/understanding -pharmacogenomics

14. Omura K. Clinical implications of dihydropyrimidine dehydrogenase (DPD) activity in 5-FU based chemotherapy: mutations in the DPD gene, and DPD inhibitory fluoropyrimidines. *Int J Clin Oncol*. 2003;8(3)132-138.

15. Vogel WH. Hypersensitivity reactions to antineoplastic drugs. In: Yarbo CH, Wujcik D, Holmes Gobel B, eds. *Cancer Symptom Management*. 4th ed. Jones and Bartlett Learning; 2014:115–117.

16. Biological therapies for cancer. National Cancer Institute website. Accessed June 17, 2019. www.cancer.gov/about-cancer /treatment/types/immunotherapy /bio-therapies-fact-sheet

17. Chemotherapy drugs and drugs often used during chemotherapy. Chemocare website. Accessed June 17, 2019. http://chemocare .com/chemotherapy/drug-info

18. Chu E, DeVita VT. Chemotherapeutic and biologic drugs. In: *Physicians' Cancer Chemotherapy Drug Manual: 2018*. Jones and Bartlett Learning; 2018:5-476.

19. Targeted cancer therapies. National Cancer Institute website. Accessed June 17, 2019. www.cancer.gov/cancertopics/factsheet/Therapy/targeted

20. Dy GK, Adjei AA. Understanding, recognizing, and managing toxicities of targeted anticancer therapies. *CA Cancer J Clin*. 2013(4);63:249-279.

21. Targeted therapy: monoclonal antibodies. Chemocare website. Accessed January 27, 2020. http://chemocare.com/chemotherapy/what-is-chemotherapy/targeted-therapy.aspx

22. American Society of Clinical Oncology. Side effects of immunotherapy. Cancer.Net website. Accessed June 17, 2019. www.cancer.net/navigating-cancer-care/how-cancer-treated/immunotherapy-and-vaccines/side-effects-immunotherapy

23. American Society of Clinical Oncology. Understanding immunotherapy. Cancer.Net website. Accessed June 17, 2019. www.cancer.net/navigating-cancer-care/how-cancer-treated/immunotherapy-and-vaccines/understanding-immunotherapy

24. Chimeric antigen receptor (CAR) T-cell therapy. Leukemia and Lymphoma Society website. Accessed June 4, 2019. https://lls.org/treatment/types-of-treatment/immunotherapy/chimeric-antigen-receptor-car-t-cell-therapy#FDA%20Approved%20Treatments

25. CAR T-cells: engineering patients' immune cells to treat their cancers. National Cancer Institute website. Accessed June 17, 2019. www.cancer.gov/about-cancer/treatment/research/car-t-cells

26. Becze E. Survivorship considerations after CAR T-cell therapy. *ONS Voice*. 2019;6(34):16-17.

27. National Cancer Institute. Liver (hepatocellular) cancer prevention (PDQ)—health professional version. Accessed June 17, 2019. www.cancer.gov/types/liver/hp/liver-prevention-pdq

28. Preventing cervical cancer: the development of HPV cancer vaccines. National Cancer Institute website. Accessed June 17, 2019. www.cancer.gov/research/progress/discovery/hpv-vaccines

29. Hormone therapy to treat cancer. National Cancer Institute website. Accessed June 17, 2019. www.cancer.gov/about-cancer/treatment/types/hormone-therapy

Chapter 10
Nutritional Effects of Cancer Treatment: Radiation Oncology

Barbara L. Grant, MS, RDN, CSO, FAND

Radiation oncology is the diagnosis, treatment, palliation, and prophylaxis of cancer using a spectrum of ionizing radiation to a localized area of the body. It is used alone or in combination with surgery, chemotherapy, immunotherapy, and hormonal therapy. In the United States, approximately two-thirds of all people diagnosed with cancer receive radiation therapy to cure or to palliate the disease.[1] Radiation oncology, also referred to as radiation therapy, uses high-energy x-rays (ionizing radiation) or other radioactive particles, such as electrons, neutrons, protons, β particles, or γ rays.

See Chapter 9 Box 9.2 Goals of Cancer Therapy Approaches (page 159), which describes several combination approaches to treatment.

Ionizing radiation can be used to treat local, regional, or systemic disease and benign conditions.[2] The goal of therapy is to eradicate tumor cells while minimizing injury to healthy, normal tissues in a specific area of treatment.[3] Ionizing radiation damages the DNA and other cellular components within the cells through direct and indirect interactions producing varying effects.[2-4]

- Direct effects include:

  - physical damage that is caused within the cells by the excitation and ionization of atoms or molecules

  - biological damage that is brought about by damage to critical cellular genetic material.

- Indirect effects include chemical damage that is caused by the formation of highly reactive free radicals within the cells.

Although these changes occur to cancer cells as well as normal cells, they prevent cancer cells from reproducing, resulting in cell death. Radiation oncologists determine which type of radiation therapy is selected and how it will be prescribed for treatment, based on the following factors[4]:

- type, size, and location of the cancer in the body

- proximity of the cancer to normal tissues, structures, and organs

- distance the radiation needs to travel

- the individual's general health, medical history, age, and performance status

- use of other cancer therapies, such as chemotherapy, immunotherapy, or surgery

Types of radiation therapy include external beam radiation therapy, brachytherapy, and radio-pharmaceutical therapy:

- External beam radiation therapy (EBRT), also called teletherapy, uses photons, electrons, and protons. Ionizing radiation is delivered from outside of the body to treat a specific treatment field (ie, area of the body).

- Brachytherapy, or internal radiation therapy, uses sealed sources of radiation, which are temporarily or permanently placed inside a body cavity, tissue, or surface.

- Radiopharmaceutical therapy uses unsealed sources of radiation to treat cancer systemically.

External Beam Radiation Therapy

In EBRT, megavoltage machines deliver ionizing radiation to a specific treatment field. Treatments with curative intent typically are given over the course of several weeks, depending on the type of cancer and the total dose of radiation to be delivered. Palliative radiation therapy can be delivered to improve quality of life and to manage cancer and cancer-related symptoms[2]; for example, it can be used to:

- shrink a metastatic brain or liver lesion that has spread from primary cancer to another area of the body;

- shrink an obstructing tumor near the esophagus to facilitate swallowing; or

- treat a metastatic bony lesion (eg, on the spine, pelvis, or rib) to alleviate pain.

EBRT directs a beam of radiation from outside the body to a tumor or cancerous tissues inside the body. Types of EBRT include the following:

- **Three-dimensional conformal radiation therapy (3D-CRT)** uses special computed tomography (CT) scanning and a sophisticated planning system to deliver a prescribed dose of radiation to a precise 3-D target area using multileaf beam-shaping devices (collimators) or customized blocks to minimize the dose of radiation to the surrounding normal tissue while maximizing the dose to cancer cells.

- **Intensity-modulated radiation therapy (IMRT)** is an advanced form of 3D-CRT that uses computer-controlled, movable "leaves" to customize the radiation beam by modulating or varying the amount delivered to different parts of the specific area being treated. The goal of therapy is to reduce radiation exposure to surrounding normal tissue while delivering more radiation to cancer cells.

- **Image-guided radiation therapy (IGRT)** guides treatment to improve the precision of the delivery of EBRT, 3D-CRT, or IMRT and is often used in tissues that move, such as the heart. It uses repeated imaging scans, which are taken during a prescribed treatment, to help increase the accuracy of therapy to specific targeted tissue. Images taken during treatment are compared to images that were taken during the planning process to take into account changes in the patient's position and tumor location.

- **Stereotactic radiosurgery (SRS)** and **stereotactic radiation therapy (SRT)** are noninvasive types of therapy that use image-guided and precise patient positioning and immobilization (eg, a head frame or other devices) to deliver tumor-targeted treatments. SRS is given in a single dose, and SRT is delivered in a fractionated manner over a specific time period. These therapies are commonly used to treat malignant, metastatic, and benign brain tumors, liver and prostate cancers, and other conditions, such as arteriovenous malformations.

- **Total body irradiation (TBI)** delivers a large dose of radiation to the entire body to treat cancer cells that may be present throughout the body. Treatment can range from a single dose to twice-daily fractions over a 3-day period, depending on the treatment protocol. TBI is often given in conjunction with high-dose chemotherapy as an immunosuppressive treatment during hematopoietic cell transplantation for hematological malignancies such as leukemias, myelomas, and lymphomas.

- **Intraoperative radiation therapy (IORT)** delivers radiation into a tumor during surgery by using either external or internal radiation therapy (brachytherapy). Healthy tissue is surgically moved away in advance of the procedure. IORT spares healthy tissue and vital organs that may be close to the target area.

Dosage

Total dose, the amount of an individual dose, number of fractions (treatment of a particular dose size), and the duration of treatment are determined by the type of cancer and the tolerance of normal tissues in the treatment field.[3] Dividing doses into multiple fractions helps limit damage to healthy tissue. The amount of ionizing radiation is measured in gray (Gy) units. Most types of EBRT are given once a day in a single dose (a daily fraction) up to 5 days a week. However, some treatments may be delivered in different ways, such as[4]:

- hyperfractionation—smaller doses given more than once per day;

- hypofractionation—larger doses given once per day or less often to reduce the number of fractions; or

- accelerated fractionation—doses given in larger daily or weekly doses to reduce the number of weeks in a prescribed treatment.

Side Effects

Side effects occur from radiation damage to the normal cells within the treatment field and depend on a number of factors, including the body area being treated, total amount of radiation given, dose per fraction, overall treatment course, and whether or not radiation therapy is combined with other treatment modalities, such as chemotherapy or surgery, and in what manner they are given (eg, concurrently or sequentially).[2] Early and acute side effects occur during or immediately after completing the course of radiation therapy (see Figure 10.1 on page 186). Late side effects (see Box 10.1 on page 187) can occur months to even

years after radiation therapy has been given and are usually a result of damage to microcirculation within the irradiated area. Effects are more severe when a higher dose per fraction is given.[2] Side effects related to TBI are listed in Box 10.2 on page 188. See Chapter 11 for strategies to address nutrition-related side effects.

A comprehensive review conducted by the American Cancer Society found that adult cancer survivors cope with the long-term physical effects of cancer treatment, as well as lasting physiological sequelae that affect their quality of life. Therefore, health care professionals are encouraged to provide ongoing assessment and management of lingering or late-occurring side effects.[6] The incidence of radiation therapy–related second cancers in adults is estimated to be 8%, on average.[7]

Brachytherapy

Brachytherapy involves temporary or permanent placement of radioactive material directly into tumors or next to tumors.[2] *Brachy* comes from the Greek word *brachys*, meaning short, as in a short distance. The types of brachytherapy placement are listed in Box 10.3 on page 188, and Box 10.4 on page 189 describes types of brachytherapy based on duration.

Radioactive isotopes are sealed inside tiny pellets or "seeds"[8] and placed in a person via a variety of specialized applicators, such as needles or catheters. The treatment is designed to precisely deliver radiation therapy in an individualized and targeted manner to spare normal tissue.[13] It can be used alone or in combination with EBRT. Brachytherapy is used to boost the delivery of radiation to a tumor and to spare surrounding healthy tissue.[2]

Possible acute and late-occurring side effects of brachytherapy are listed in Box 10.5 on page 190. See Chapter 11 for strategies to address nutrition-related side effects.

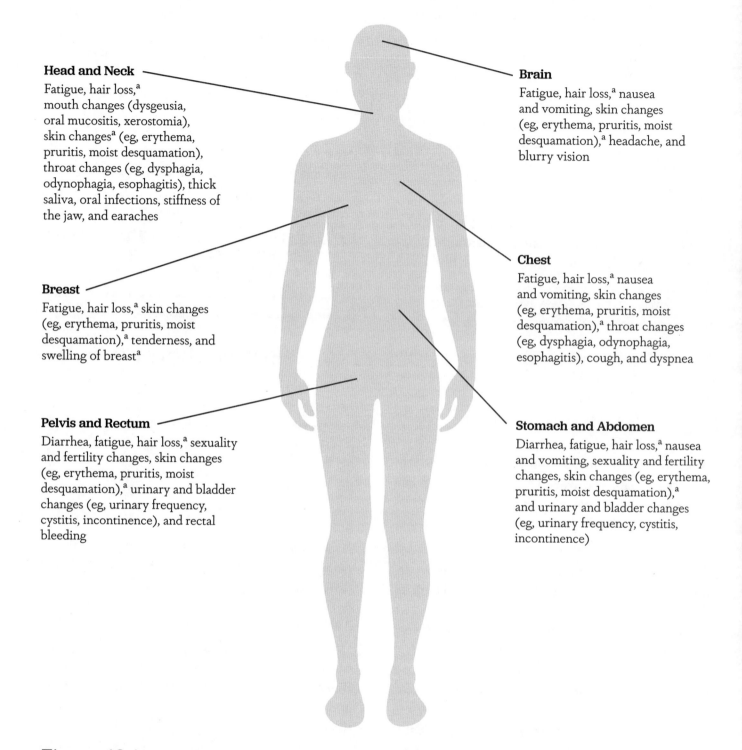

Head and Neck

Fatigue, hair loss,[a] mouth changes (dysgeusia, oral mucositis, xerostomia), skin changes[a] (eg, erythema, pruritis, moist desquamation), throat changes (eg, dysphagia, odynophagia, esophagitis), thick saliva, oral infections, stiffness of the jaw, and earaches

Brain

Fatigue, hair loss,[a] nausea and vomiting, skin changes (eg, erythema, pruritis, moist desquamation),[a] headache, and blurry vision

Breast

Fatigue, hair loss,[a] skin changes (eg, erythema, pruritis, moist desquamation),[a] tenderness, and swelling of breast[a]

Chest

Fatigue, hair loss,[a] nausea and vomiting, skin changes (eg, erythema, pruritis, moist desquamation),[a] throat changes (eg, dysphagia, odynophagia, esophagitis), cough, and dyspnea

Pelvis and Rectum

Diarrhea, fatigue, hair loss,[a] sexuality and fertility changes, skin changes (eg, erythema, pruritis, moist desquamation),[a] urinary and bladder changes (eg, urinary frequency, cystitis, incontinence), and rectal bleeding

Stomach and Abdomen

Diarrhea, fatigue, hair loss,[a] nausea and vomiting, sexuality and fertility changes, skin changes (eg, erythema, pruritis, moist desquamation),[a] and urinary and bladder changes (eg, urinary frequency, cystitis, incontinence)

Figure 10.1

Possible acute side effects of site-specific radiation therapy[2,9-11]

[a] In the treatment field.

Box 10.1

Possible Late Side Effects of Site-Specific Radiation Therapy[2,6,9-12]

Organ or body system treated	Late side effects
Brain	Headache, leukoencephalopathy (eg, cognitive impairment and changes in memory and attention), dementia
Bone	Damage to osteoblasts, osteopenia
Cardiovascular	Angina on exertion, pericarditis, cardiac enlargement, congestive heart failure
Esophagus	Esophageal stenosis, fibrosis, or necrosis
Gastrointestinal tract	Diarrhea, malabsorption, chronic enteritis or colitis, intestinal changes (eg, stricture, ulceration, obstruction, perforation, fistula), proctitis
Head and neck	Trismus, dental decay, permanent xerostomia, alterations in taste and smell, osteoradionecrosis, mucosal sensitivity
Lymphatics	Secondary lymphedema in irradiated area
Pulmonary	Dyspnea, cough, pneumonitis
Sexual organs	Changes in menstruation, symptoms of menopause, infertility, erectile dysfunction
Skin	Telangiectasias, pigmentation changes, atrophy, fibrosis
Urinary	Hematuria, cystitis
Other conditions	Development of secondary malignancies, cataracts (if eye in treatment area)

Box 10.2
Possible Side Effects of Total Body Irradiation[a,2,3,13]

Organ or body system affected	Acute side effects	Late side effects
Bone marrow	Anemia, neutropenia, pancytopenia, hemorrhage, infection	Secondary hematological cancers
Brain and central nervous system	Confusion, meningitis	Cognitive changes, memory loss
Gastrointestinal system	Xerostomia, mucositis, esophagitis, nausea, vomiting, diarrhea, electrolyte imbalance, acute graft-versus-host disease	Radiation enteritis, denudation of villi of small intestine, chronic graft-versus-host disease
Skin	Generalized erythema, hyperpigmentation	Fibrosis, delayed wound healing, increased risk for basal cell cancers
Other	Fatigue, fever, hair thinning or loss	Secondary malignancies, growth and development changes in children and adolescents, osteopenia, osteoporosis, infertility

[a] Used in combination with low- or high-dose conditioning chemotherapy.

Box 10.3
General Types of Brachytherapy Placement[2,4,8]

Type of brachytherapy placement	Description	Type of cancer
Interstitial	A radioactive source is placed into the tumor.	<ul><li>Breast</li><li>Gynecological</li><li>Head and neck</li><li>Lung</li><li>Prostate</li><li>Rectal</li></ul>
Intracavitary	A radioactive source is placed directly into a surgical or body cavity (eg, vagina or uterus) near a tumor.	<ul><li>Gynecological (eg, cervical and endometrial)</li><li>Head and neck</li></ul>
Contact	A radioactive source is placed on an external surface.	<ul><li>Skin</li></ul>

Box 10.4
Types of Brachytherapy by Duration[2,4,13]

Duration	Type and description	Examples
Temporary (radioactive source is implanted for a specific duration of time)	Low-dose-rate (LDR) brachytherapy is given in an inpatient setting using a protected, lead-shielded room. Radiation is delivered in a continuous, low-dose manner from a source over several days. The radiation source is held in place by an applicator.	An example of LDR therapy is the use of a tandem and ovoid applicator (the tandem is a small metal tube placed inside the uterus and the ovoid is placed on the side of the cervix) for the treatment of cervical cancer after EBRT has been completed. The length of time the applicator stays in place depends on the patient's specific cancer (generally 18 to 72 hours).
	Pulsed-dose-rate (PDR) brachytherapy combines the biological advantages of LDR brachytherapy and delivers radiation in short pulses to enhance treatment effectiveness. PDR brachytherapy provides advantages over LDR brachytherapy because it is a more precise application of the prescribed dose, treatment plans have greater reproducibility, and there is improved safety for staff. PDR brachytherapy takes into account tumor regression exposure to critical organs, such as the cervix.	Examples of PDR brachytherapy include use in breast reconstruction with flexible implants and gynecological, prostate, and many other tumors.
	High-dose-rate (HDR) brachytherapy is given either in one or several doses separated by at least 6 hours. In an outpatient setting, radioactive sources are placed remotely in the patient through a system of delivery tubes placed into or near a tumor. A computer-controlled remote after-loading machine is used to insert radiation sources.	A type of HDR for the treatment of breast cancer involves the interstitial placement of multiple catheters into the lumpectomy bed and surrounding margin. Treatment is reduced to 5 to 7 days instead of the 5 to 6 weeks required for EBRT.
Permanent (radioactive source is implanted permanently)	Permanent brachytherapy uses sealed sources of radiation material (radioactive seeds or pellets), which are inserted and permanently left in the tissue. Over time, the radioactivity of the seeds diminishes.	An example is the permanent placement of radioactive seeds containing iodine 125 or palladium 103 in the prostate gland for the treatment of prostate cancer.

Box 10.5
Possible Acute and Late-Occurring Side Effects of Brachytherapy[2,4,8]

Treatment site	Acute side effect	Late-occurring side effect
Breast	No known nutrition-related side effects	
Gynecological (eg, uterus, cervix, vagina)	■ Nausea ■ Diarrhea ■ Discomfort when urinating	■ Diarrhea ■ Bladder irritation
Esophagus	■ Esophagitis ■ Dysphagia ■ Odynophagia	■ Esophageal stenosis ■ Fibrosis, ulcerations
Prostate	■ Discomfort when urinating ■ Diarrhea ■ Cramping, bloating ■ Flatulence ■ Proctitis	■ Urinary stricture ■ Incontinence ■ Diarrhea
Tongue	■ Mucositis ■ Xerostomia ■ Taste alterations	■ Xerostomia ■ Mucosal fibrosis, ulcerations

Radiopharmaceutical Therapy

Radiopharmaceuticals are drugs that contain radioisotopes for systemic cancer treatment. These agents are grouped into three categories[2]:

■ radioimmunotherapy agents

■ radioactive substances

■ radiopharmaceuticals for relief of metastatic bone pain

Radioimmunotherapy Agents

Radioimmunotherapy agents are targeted therapies consisting of monoclonal antibodies combined with radioactive substances that deliver radiation therapy directly to cancer cells.[14] Action occurs when monoclonal antibodies bind to *CD20* receptor sites on the cancer cell surface and the radioisotope kills the cell.[11] This type of agent is currently used to treat B-cell lymphoma and follicular lymphoma. Other cancer indications are still under investigation. An example is ibritumomab tiuxetan (a combination of rituximab and yttrium 90).[13,14]

Acute side effects and nutritional impact include myelosuppression, infusion-related reactions, mild nausea and vomiting, diarrhea, decreased appetite, infection, cough, throat irritation, dyspnea, and generalized aches and pains. Possible late side effects include a risk for secondary malignancy.[12-15]

Radioactive Substances

This therapy uses radioactive materials such as radioactive iodine (RAI, also called iodine 131) to treat certain types of thyroid cancer. After part or all the thyroid gland is removed, iodine 131 is given to destroy the thyroid gland function, usually with minimal effect to other parts of the body. Thyroid ablation with iodine 131 involves a short hospital stay and then isolating the individual until the radiation dissipates to prevent exposing others to the radiation. Acute side effects include neck tenderness and swelling, nausea, vomiting, fatigue, salivary gland tenderness and swelling, taste changes, and xerostomia.[12] Long-term side effects include an increased risk for secondary malignancies.

Radioactive substances may also be used in palliative radiation therapy to relieve pain associated with symptomatic bone metastases caused by cancer. It consists of a type of radiopharmaceutical that can be used with or without other therapies (such as bisphosphates and taxane-based chemotherapy).[16] This therapy uses bone-targeted systemic radionuclide agents that bind to osteoblastic areas or skeletal metastatic lesions from the primary cancer. The emitted radiation shrinks the cancer, thereby relieving pain at the site of metastasis(es). One to three weeks often are required after treatment before a therapeutic effect is obtained. Examples of radiopharmaceuticals for metastatic bone pain include the following[2,15]:

- Strontium 89 (Mestastron) is given intravenously and is used to treat prostate cancer and advanced bone cancer and other cancers that have spread to the bone.

- Samaruim 153-lexidronam (Quadramet) emits radiation and is often used to treat bone pain caused by bone cancer.

- Radium R-223 dichloride (Xofigo) is used to treat prostate cancer that has spread to the bone but not to other organs.

Box 10.6 on page 192 lists the possible side effects of radiopharmaceuticals for metastatic bone pain. See Chapter 11 for strategies to address nutrition-related side effects.

Box 10.6
Possible Side Effects of Radiopharmaceuticals for Metastatic Bone Pain[2,3,13,17]

Agent	Indication	Acute side effects	Late-occurring side effects
Samarium 153 (Quadramet)	Pain relief for individuals with confirmed osteoblastic bone lesions that enhance on a radionuclide bone scan	■ Myelosuppression: anemia, thrombocytopenia, neutropenia ■ Nausea, vomiting ■ Neurological changes: dizziness, peripheral neuropathy	■ Risk of secondary malignancy
Strontium 89 (Metastron)	Pain relief for individuals with painful skeletal (bony) metastases	■ Myelosuppression: anemia, thrombocytopenia, neutropenia ■ Temporary increase in bone pain ■ Flushing	■ Risk of secondary malignancy
Radium 223 (Xofigo)	Treatment of castration-resistant prostate cancer, symptomatic bone metastases, and no known visceral metastatic disease	■ Myelosuppression: anemia, thrombocytopenia, neutropenia ■ Nausea, vomiting, diarrhea ■ Neurological changes: peripheral edema	

References

1. American Society for Radiation Oncology. CMS report on radiation therapy payment model charts path to value-based cancer care, says ASTRO. PR Newswire website. Accessed June 19, 2019. https://prnewswire.com/news-releases/cms-report-on-radiation-therapy-payment-model-charts-path-to-value-based-cancer-care-says-astro-300549456.html

2. Iwamoto RR, Haas ML, Gosselin TK. *Oncology Nursing Society's Manual for Radiation Oncology Nursing Practice and Education.* 4th ed. Oncology Nursing Society; 2012.

3. Vonkadich S. Overview of radiobiology. In: Washington CM, Leaver D, eds. *Principles and Practice of Radiation Therapy.* 3rd ed. Mosby; 2010:57-85.

4. Radiation therapy to treat cancer. National Cancer Institute website. Accessed June 19, 2019. https://cancer.gov/about-cancer/treatment/types/radiation-therapy

5. Miller KD, Siegel RL, Lin CC, et al. Cancer treatment and survivorship statistics, 2016. *CA Cancer J Clin.* 2016;66(4):271-289.

6. Newhauser WD, Berrington de Gonzalez A, Schulte R, Lee C. A review of radiotherapy-induced late effects research after advanced technology treatments. *Front Oncol.* 2016;6(13):1-11.

7. American Society for Clinical Oncology. Understanding radiation therapy. Cancer.Net website. Accessed June 19, 2019. www.cancer.net/navigating-cancer-care/how-cancer-treated/radiation-therapy/understanding-radiation-therapy

8. Wilkes GM, Barton-Burke, M, ed. Immunologic targeted therapy. In: *Oncology Nursing Drug Handbook.* Jones and Bartlett Learning; 2018:888-892.

9. Patient brochures. American Society for Radiation Oncology website. Accessed June 19, 2019. https://astro.org/Patient-Brochures.aspx

10. Yarbo CH, Wujcik D, Holmes Gobel B. *Cancer Symptom Management.* 4th ed. Jones and Bartlett Learning; 2014.

11. American Society for Clinical Oncology. Side effects of radiation therapy. Cancer.Net website. Accessed June 19, 2019. www.cancer.net/navigating-cancer-care/how-cancer-treated/radiation-therapy/side-effects-radiation-therapy

12. Preparing for transplant. Seattle Cancer Care Alliance website. Accessed on July 2, 2019. www.seattlecca.org/sites/default/files/page_content/2017-08/Preparing-for-Transplant-7-2017.pdf

13. Devlin PM, Stewart AJ, Cormack RA, Holloway CL. *Brachytherapy: Applications and Techniques.* 2nd ed. Demos Medical Publishing; 2016.

14. Polovich M, Olsen M, Lefebvre K. *Chemotherapy and Biotherapy Guidelines and Recommendations for Practice.* 4th ed. Oncology Nursing Society; 2014.

15. Radium 223 dichloride (Xofigo). Chemocare website. Accessed June 21, 2019. www.chemocare.com/chemotherapy/drug-info/radium-223-dichloride.aspx

16. Sartor O. Overview of samarium Sm 153 lexidronam in the treatment of painful metastatic bone disease. *Rev Urol.* 2004;6(suppl 10):S3-S12.

17. Zevalin. Chemocare website. Accessed June 21, 2019. www.chemocare.com/chemotherapy/drug-info/Zevalin.aspx

Chapter 11

Managing Nutrition Impact Symptoms of Cancer Treatment

Rhone M. Levin, MEd, RDN, CSO, LDN, FAND

Cancer and cancer treatment can precipitate complex symptoms, called nutrition impact symptoms, that negatively affect food intake, digestion, absorption, utilization of nutrients, and overall nutritional health.[1] These symptoms can reduce patients' quality of life and can result in malnutrition, which can be linked to suboptimal treatment outcomes.

Malnutrition and unintentional weight loss carry a negative prognostic significance for several treatment regimens. Many patients undergoing treatment report one or more nutrition impact symptoms that affect nutrition including anorexia, early satiety, constipation, diarrhea, malabsorption, dysphagia, mucositis, esophagitis, oral candidiasis, acid reflux, xerostomia, thick saliva, chemosensory alterations in taste and smell, and fatigue. Many of these symptoms can be prevented or minimized when identified early and when managed effectively through patient education, behavior modification, and appropriate use of medication. Effective management of nutrition impact symptoms has been shown to help maintain patients' nutritional status, protect quality of life, and support tolerance of treatment for most types of cancer.[1,2]

Tools for Assessing Nutrition Impact Symptoms

The routine assessment of nutrition impact symptoms is an essential component of quality cancer care. Many validated tools are available to help practitioners accurately characterize the presence, intensity, duration, and timing of nutrition impact symptoms throughout the cancer treatment cycle. Using patient-reported outcome measures gives clinicians valuable information to help reduce the side-effect burden of cancer treatment.[3]

An important component of patient care is accurately describing symptoms that affect nutrition and grading the severity of these symptoms. This promotes consistency in care and follow-up,

effective communication among the care team, and the ability to track outcomes for research purposes. The National Cancer Institute's Common Terminology Criteria for Adverse Events (CTCAE) grading system, which provides descriptive terminology for documenting and reporting adverse events (see Box 11.1 on page 196) including nutrition impact symptoms, is used by many oncology centers.[4]

Innovative technologies, such as patient symptom-tracker apps, can prompt patients to report symptoms in a timely manner, thus capturing their experience accurately. This information can be reported directly to the cancer center's electronic medical record and used to assist the multimodal team in providing relevant interventions.[5]

Medical Nutrition Therapy for Common Nutrition Impact Symptoms

Providing medical nutrition therapy (MNT) is a critical step in oncology nutrition care. Although nutrition interventions are an active area of research, evidence is currently lacking to guide registered dietitian nutritionists (RDNs) in the use of all oncology-related nutrition interventions.[6] Oncology RDNs must, therefore, consider all available evidence-based recommendations, including systematic reviews, randomized-controlled trials, cohort studies, case-controlled studies, case series, case reports, and expert opinion, including those available for other disciplines. The Academy of

Box 11.1
The National Cancer Institute's Common Terminology Criteria for Adverse Events: Grading System for Severity of Adverse Events [4]

Grade 1 Mild: asymptomatic or mild symptoms; clinical or diagnostic observations only; intervention not indicated

Grade 2 Moderate: minimal, local, or noninvasive intervention indicated; limiting age-appropriate instrumental activities of daily living (ADL)[a]

Grade 3 Severe or medically significant, but not immediately life-threatening: hospitalization or prolongation of hospitalization indicated; disabling; limiting self-care ADL[b]

Grade 4 Life-threatening consequences; urgent intervention indicated

Grade 5 Death related to adverse event

[a] Instrumental ADL refer to preparing meals, shopping for groceries or clothes, using the telephone, managing money, etc

[b] Self-care ADL refer to bathing, dressing and undressing, feeding self, using the toilet, taking medications, and not bedridden

Nutrition and Dietetics provides the Evidence Analysis Library oncology nutrition guidelines.[7] Other organizations with evidence-based oncology nutrition guidelines include the American Society for Parenteral and Enteral Nutrition,[8] the Clinical Oncology Society of Australia,[9] and the Oncology Nursing Society.[10]

The remainder of this chapter describes the following common nutritional impact symptoms of cancer therapy, along with their corresponding CTCAE severity grades, additional considerations, and MNT and pharmacotherapy interventions:

- anorexia and early satiety (Box 11.2)
- changes in taste and smell (see Box 11.3, pages 198 to 199)
- constipation (see Box 11.4, pages 200 to 201)
- diarrhea (see Box 11.5, pages 202 to 203)
- dysphagia (see Box 11.6, pages 204 to 205)
- fatigue (see Box 11.7, pages 206 to 207)
- malabsorption (see Box 11.8, pages 208 to 209)
- nausea and vomiting (see Box 11.9, pages 210 to 211)
- oral mucositis and esophagitis (see Box 11.10, pages 212 to 213)
- oral candidiasis (see Box 11.11, page 214)
- xerostomia (see Box 11.12, page 215)

Box 11.2
Anorexia and Early Satiety: Definition, Severity Grades, Considerations, and Interventions[4,11-14]

Definition	**Sample nutrition diagnosis/ PES[a] statement**	**Potential outcomes**
Anorexia is the involuntary loss of appetite or desire to eat, which may or may not be related to early satiety, which is the feeling of being full after eating or drinking a small amount.	Inadequate oral intake related to cancer anorexia and early satiety, as evidenced by consuming less than half of meals and weight loss of 2% in the past 2 weeks.	Inadequate energy intake, unintentional weight loss, sarcopenia, nutrient insufficiency and deficiency, dehydration, malnutrition

(continued)

[a] PES = problems, etiology, and signs and symptoms

Box 11.2
Anorexia and Early Satiety: Definition, Severity Grades, Considerations, and Interventions[4,11-14] *(continued)*

CTCAE[b] grade and description	
1	Loss of appetite without alteration in eating habits
2	Oral intake altered without significant weight loss or malnutrition; oral nutritional supplements indicated
3	Associated with significant weight loss or malnutrition (eg, inadequate oral energy and/or fluid intake); tube feeding or parenteral nutrition (PN) indicated
4	Life-threatening consequences; urgent intervention indicated
5	Death

Considerations

Evaluate for conditions and nutrition impact symptoms that may influence digestion (eg, slow gastric emptying, gastroparesis, constipation, obstruction, reflux).

Evaluate for use of medications that may slow gastric emptying and influence gastrointestinal (GI) function (eg, opioids, aluminum hydroxide antacids, histamine H2-receptor antagonists, proton pump inhibitor (PPI), sucralfate, interferon, levodopa, sedatives, antiemetic agents).

Evaluate patient's use of recommended symptom management strategies and medications, and explore with the patient any impediments to adherence.

Assess food and fluid intake quantitatively and qualitatively using diet history, food records, food-frequency instruments, and 24-hour recall.

Nutrition and behavioral interventions

Recommend that patients do the following:

- Eat small, frequent meals that include nutrient-dense foods and fluids.
- Schedule frequent small meals and snacks (six to eight times daily) and "eat by the clock," rather than waiting for appetite or hunger cues.
- Maximize intake at the time of day appetite is best.
- If eating is difficult, use oral nutrition supplements.
- Consume liquids between meals rather than with meals.
- Enhance nutrient density of food, as tolerated.
- Use foods that are easy to prepare and serve, to preserve energy.
- Keep convenience foods (eg, frozen meals, nutrition bars, nutrient-dense beverages) on hand.
- Approach eating as a part of overall treatment.
- Engage in light physical activity to help move food through the GI tract.

Pharmacotherapy

Antihistamines: cyproheptadine (Periactin), in children

Corticosteroids: dexamethasone (Decadron)

Progestational agents: medroxyprogesterone acetate (Provera); megestrol acetate (Megace)

Prokinetic agents: metoclopramide (Reglan)

Cannabinoids: dronabinol (Marinol); liquefied dronabinol (Syndros); nabilone (Cesamet)

Antidepressants: mirtazapine (Remeron): off-label use, should be used with caution and not taken concurrently or after recent use of monoamine oxidase inhibitor (MAOI) medications or diazepam

[b] CTCAE = Common Terminology Criteria for Adverse Events (from the National Cancer Institute)

Box 11.3

Changes in Taste and Smell: Definition, Severity Grades, Considerations, and Interventions[4,12,15-21]

Definition	Dysgeusia is change in the sense of taste. It can be experienced as a heightened sense of metallic, bitter, salty, or sweet taste. Hypogeusia is a reduction in taste and ability to smell. Ageusia and anosmia are the absence of taste and ability to smell, respectively.	**CTCAE[b] grade and description**

CTCAE[b] grade	description
1	Altered taste, but no change in diet
2	Altered taste with change in diet (eg, oral supplements); noxious or unpleasant taste; loss of taste

Sample nutrition diagnosis/ PES[a] statement	Limited food acceptance related to side effects of cancer treatment, as evidenced by dysgeusia and reduced food and beverage intake.
Potential outcomes	Decreased intake, nutrient insufficiency and deficiency, and unintentional weight loss

Considerations

Assess etiology of the changes in taste and smell. Chemotherapy-related alterations may be transient during the treatment cycle. Radiation-related changes may be progressive and more permanent.

Evaluate the oral cavity for candidiasis.

Encourage good oral hygiene.

Assess food and fluid intake, quantitatively and qualitatively, using diet history, food records, food-frequency instruments, and 24-hour recall.

Investigate which foods illicit the sense of dysgeusia or ageusia.

Identify which flavors the patient does perceive as accurate, pleasant, or tolerable, and modify food intake using these flavor profiles.

Pharmacotherapy

Cleansing rinse: Mix ¾ tsp salt and 1 tsp baking soda in 4 c of water. Rinse mouth with 1 c of mixture three or four times daily or as directed by physician.

Investigational products:

- Synsepalum dulcificum fruit supplements ("miracle fruit") may help reduce bitter, acidic, or metallic taste sensations.
- Herbal tea (Gymnema sylvestra), consumed before meals, may inhibit sweet taste.
- Zinc supplementation has not been proven to prevent loss of taste or change in taste in patients undergoing treatment for head and neck cancer.

(continued)

[a] PES = problems, etiology, signs and symptoms

[b] CTCAE = Common Terminology Criteria for Adverse Events (from the National Cancer Institute)

Box 11.3
Changes in Taste and Smell: Definition, Severity Grades, Considerations, and Interventions[4,12,15-21] *(continued)*

Nutrition and behavioral interventions

Recommend the following strategies to patients.

- If foods have little flavor or an "off" taste:
  - Opt for foods with fruity and salty flavors, as they often taste best.
  - Use marinades for meats to change the flavor.
  - Add herbs, spices, lemon, vinegar, pickles, or strongly flavored sauces and condiments to season foods.
  - Understand that hot ("spicy") seasonings, such as hot red pepper or hot sauce, may not make a difference, as heat is a sensation, not a flavor.

- To counter a bitter, acidic, or metallic taste:
  - Eat sweet fruits (watermelon, cantaloupe) alongside meals.
  - Drink sweet or sour beverages (eg, lemonade, apple juice, cranberry juice, sweet tea).
  - Use strongly flavored spices or seasonings, such as onion, garlic, or chili powder.
  - Use sugar-free lemon drops, gum, or mints to improve mouth taste.
  - Choose alternative protein sources, such as chicken, eggs, tofu, dairy foods, nuts, or beans.
  - Use bamboo or plastic silverware and chopsticks to reduce the sense of metal in the mouth.

- To counter a salty taste:
  - Choose foods that are naturally sweet.
  - Eat boiled food to reduce flavor.
  - Use low-sodium products or recipes.

- To counter an enhanced sweet taste:
  - Choose bland or sour flavors.
  - Dilute juices or serve over ice.
  - Choose vegetables rather than fruits.

- When smells are bothersome:
  - Eat food that is served at cold or room temperature (eg, smoothies, sandwiches, cottage cheese, yogurt, puddings, custards, nut butters, and fruit).
  - Avoid food with strong odors (eg, fish, onions, cabbage).
  - Avoid cooking areas during meal preparation.
  - Avoid lengthy cooking processes (eg, crockpot).
  - Avoid cooking areas during meal preparation. Ventilate cooking areas by using exhaust fans or opening windows.

Additional strategies:

- Advise the patient to make small, frequent attempts at oral intake and to schedule intake.
- Recommend the use of oral nutrition supplements if eating is difficult.
- Suggest using a cup with a lid and straw for cold and room-temperature beverages and soups to reduce exposure to flavors and odors.
- Encourage the patient to approach eating as a part of overall treatment.
- Educate the patient about the time frame of taste changes resulting from chemotherapy and radiation treatment, and the time frame for recovery of taste.

Box 11.4
Constipation: Definition, Severity Grades, Considerations, and Interventions[4,11,12,22]

		CTCAE[b] grade and description	
Definition	Constipation is characterized by irregular and infrequent or difficult bowel evacuation.	1	Occasional or intermittent symptoms; occasional use of stool softeners, laxatives, dietary modification, or enema
Sample nutrition diagnosis/ PES[a] statement	Altered gastrointestinal (GI) function related to side effects of chemotherapy medications, as evidenced by hard stool and infrequent bowel movements.	2	Persistent symptoms with regular use of laxatives or enemas; limiting instrumental activities of daily living (ADL)
Potential outcomes	Infrequent or hard-to-pass stools, pain, abdominal cramping, bloating, flatulence, early satiety, reflux, nausea, vomiting, impaction	3	Obstipation with manual evacuation indicated; limiting self-care ADL
		4	Life-threatening consequences; urgent intervention indicated
		5	Death

Considerations

Evaluate pattern of bowel habits and changes associated with treatment.

Evaluate frequency of bowel movement and volume and character of stool.

Evaluate for use of medications that may slow gastric emptying and influence GI function (eg, vinca alkaloids, opioids, aluminum hydroxide antacids, histamine H2-receptor antagonists, proton pump inhibitors, sucralfate, interferon, levodopa, sedatives, antiemetics).

Evaluate patient's use of recommended medications and bowel regimen for symptom management, and explore with the patient any impediments to adherence.

Assess food and fluid intake quantitatively and qualitatively using diet history, food records, food-frequency instruments, and 24-hour recall.

(continued)

[a] PES = problems, etiology, signs and symptoms

[b] CTCAE = Common Terminology Criteria for Adverse Events (from the National Cancer Institute)

Box 11.4
Constipation: Definition, Severity Grades, Considerations, and Interventions[4,11,12,22] *(continued)*

Nutrition and behavioral interventions	Pharmacotherapy

Nutrition and behavioral interventions

Recommend that patients do the following:

- Aim for a minimum of 64 to 80 oz (8 to 10 c) of fluid daily.

- Drink an additional 32 oz of fluid daily if using medicinal fibers.

- Consume adequate amount of dietary fiber (25 g/d for women and 38 g/d for men), increasing slowly as tolerated.

- Adopt a daily routine that includes the use of a hot beverage, hot cereal, or high-fiber food to stimulate bowel movements.

- Incorporate food-related probiotics or other supplements to help facilitate bowel movements.

- Engage in light activity or stretching to improve bowel regularity.

- With the addition of opioids, modify the bowel regimen: A combination of stimulant laxative plus stool softener is well tolerated.

- Schedule adequate bathroom time and privacy to facilitate bowel movements.

- Report if there has been no bowel movement for more than 3 days.

Educate patients about the following:

- the importance of adequate hydration, fiber intake, and total food intake on bowel regularity

- the effect of each medication on bowel function, and encourage bowel regimens that respond to the patient's experience (eg, increase in a step-wise fashion each day of no or inadequate bowel movement)

Pharmacotherapy

Insoluble food fiber: bran, flaxseed, wheat germ, inulin

Medicinal fibers: psyllium (Metamucil); wheat dextrin (Benefiber); carboxymethylcellulose (Trulance); methylcellulose (Citrucel); polycarbophil (FiberCon)

Stool softener: docusate (Colace, Surfak)

Lubricants: mineral oil

Osmotic laxatives: polyethylene glycol (MiraLAX); lactulose (Duphalac, Cadilose); magnesium hydroxide (Milk of Magnesia); magnesium citrate (Loso, Tridate)

Stimulant laxative agents: bisacodyl (Dulcolax, Correctol, Carter's pills); sennosides (Senokot, Ex-lax)

Opioid antagonist: methylnaltrexone bromide (Relistor); lubiprostone (Amitiza); naloxegol (Morantik); naldemedine (Symproic)

Herbals: probiotics, slippery elm, aloe juice, cascara sagrada

> *Caution:* Bacteremia is possible in immunocompromised patients. Avoid opening capsules of probiotics if a port is present.

Box 11.5
Diarrhea: Definition, Severity Grades, Considerations, and Interventions[4,11,23-25]

Definition	Diarrhea is an increase of three or more stools per day compared with usual, or an increase in liquidity of bowel movements.	**CTCAE[b] grade and description**	
		1	Increase of less than four stools per day over baseline; mild increase in ostomy output compared to baseline
Sample nutrition diagnosis/ PES[a] statement	Altered gastrointestinal (GI) function related to side effects of chemotherapy medications, as evidenced by hard stool and infrequent bowel movements.	2	Increase of four to six stools per day over baseline; moderate increase in ostomy output compared to baseline; limiting instrumental activities of daily living (ADL)
Potential outcomes	Frequent stools, dehydration, electrolyte imbalances, unintentional weight loss, fatigue, nutrient insufficiency and deficiency, malnutrition, skin irritation	3	Increase of seven or more stools per day over baseline; hospitalization indicated; severe increase in ostomy output compared to baseline; limiting self-care ADL
		4	Life-threatening consequences; urgent intervention indicated
		5	Death

Considerations

Assess etiology of the diarrhea: osmotic, malabsorptive, secretory, infectious or exudative, dysmotility-associated, chemotherapy-induced, or biotherapy-induced; radiation enteritis, GI mucositis, gut graft-versus-host disease (GVHD), or pancreatic insufficiency.

Evaluate pattern of bowel habits and changes associated with treatment.

Evaluate frequency of stooling, volume and consistency of stool, and associated symptoms (eg, nausea, flushing, diaphoresis, cramping, bloating, gassiness, foul odor).

Assess for risk factors indicating early and late dumping syndrome (eg, GI surgery).

Assess for secondary lactose intolerance and fat malabsorption.

Evaluate for treatments or use of medications or other substances that may speed gastric emptying and influence GI function (eg, chemotherapy irinotecan, VP-16 [etoposide], radiation therapy to the pelvis, antibiotics, prokinetic agents, stool softeners, laxatives, alcohol, caffeine, alcohol sugars, lactose, diet high in insoluble fiber).

Evaluate the patient's use of the recommended bowel regimen for symptom management strategies and medications, and work with the patient to resolve impediments to adherence.

Assess food and fluid intake quantitatively and qualitatively using diet history, food records, and food frequency questionnaire.

(continued)

[a] PES = problems, etiology, signs and symptoms

[b] CTCAE = Common Terminology Criteria for Adverse Events (from the National Cancer Institute)

Box 11.5
Diarrhea: Definition, Severity Grades, Considerations, and Interventions[4,11,23-25] *(continued)*

Nutrition and behavioral interventions	**Pharmacotherapy**
Recommend that patients do the following: - Eat small, frequent meals. - Achieve adequate hydration by drinking at least 8 to 10 c (64 to 80 oz) of fluid daily, adding 1 c (8 oz) for each loose bowel movement. Fluids include clear liquids and foods with high fluid content. - Eat a low-fat, low-insoluble-fiber, or low-lactose diet, or any combination thereof, if indicated. - Increase intake of soluble-fiber foods (eg, pectin, applesauce, bananas, oatmeal, potatoes, rice). - If gaseous or bloated, limit gas-forming foods (eg, cruciferous vegetables, legumes) and carbonation, avoid the use of straws, and avoid gum chewing. - Eliminate caffeine, alcohol, and highly spiced foods. - Avoid sorbitol or other products containing sugar-alcohol (eg, sugar-free gum and candy). Educate patients about the following: - consumption of electrolyte-containing foods and fluids - the use of oral rehydration salts (ORS) products and recipes, if appropriate - the use of lactase enzyme products and substitutions, if indicated	**Opioid receptor agonists:** loperamide (Imodium AD); dipheoxylate atropine (Lomotil) **Hormonal:** octreotide (Sandostatin) **Opioids:** anhydrous morphine (Paregoric), camphorated tincture of opium **Anti-inflammatory, anti-diarrheal:** bismuth subsalicylate (Pepto-Bismol); attapulgite (Kaopectate) **Bile acid sequestrant:** cholestyramine (Questran) **Anticholinergics:** diphenhydramine (Benadryl) **Medicinal Fibers:** psyllium (Metamucil); psyllium or calcium polycarbophil caplets (Konsyl); methylcellulose (Citrucel) **Preventive for gut radiotherapy:** amifostine (Ethyol) **Amino acids:** L-glutamine (may reduce duration but not severity); Enterade (a proprietary blend of amino acids) **Probiotics:** *Saccharomyces boulardii, Lactobacillus rhamnosus* GG ***Caution:*** Bacteremia is possible in immunocompromised patients. Avoid opening capsules of probiotics if a port is present.

Box 11.6
Dysphagia: Definition, Severity Grades, Considerations, and Interventions[4,11,12]

		CTCAE[b] grade and description	
Definition	Dysphagia is difficulty swallowing due to extrinsic compression of the esophagus, mechanical obstruction, neurological dysfunction, oral or esophageal mucositis, or infection.	1	Symptomatic, able to eat regular diet
		2	Symptomatic and altered eating or swallowing
Sample nutrition diagnosis/ PES[a] statement	Swallowing difficulty related to side effects of head and neck radiotherapy, as evidenced by abnormal swallow study and choking when eating.	3	Severely altered eating or swallowing; tube feeding, parenteral nutrition (PN), or hospitalization indicated
		4	Life-threatening consequences; urgent intervention indicated
Potential outcomes	Coughing, choking, feeling of "food getting stuck," odynophagia (pain while swallowing), aspiration, pneumonia, weight loss, nutrient insufficiencies and deficiencies, dehydration, and malnutrition	5	Death

Considerations

Assess etiology of the dysphagia.

Review swallow study results and speech-language pathologist (SLP) recommendations for safe eating and drinking.

Evaluate patient compliance with SLP recommendations for food, fluid textures, and consistencies.

Assess food and fluid intake quantitatively and qualitatively using diet history, food records, food-frequency instruments, and 24-hour recall.

(continued)

---

[a] PES = problems, etiology, signs and symptoms

[b] CTCAE = Common Terminology Criteria for Adverse Events (from the National Cancer Institute)

Box 11.6
Dysphagia: Definition, Severity Grades, Considerations, and Interventions[4,11,12] *(continued)*

Nutrition and behavioral interventions

Recommend that patients do the following:

- Alter food textures as directed by the SLP for safe swallowing.
- Use thickeners in liquids as directed by the SLP.
- Choose moist foods of a similar texture to help form a cohesive bolus in the mouth.
- Avoid dry foods and foods that separate into pieces (eg, rice, crackers).
- Moisten dry foods to ease bolus formation: Use gravies and sauces; dip bread into soups.
- Alternate a bite of solid food with a sip of liquid.
- Eat and drink while in an upright position.
- Avoid distractions and limit talking while eating.
- Avoid the use of straws that place food in the back of the mouth, unless recommended by the SLP.
- For odynophagia, use systemic pain medication or topical anesthetics, sprays, and lozenges.
- Practice chin-tuck swallowing and double swallowing to help food clear the pharynx.
- Practice verbalization after swallowing liquids to ensure clearing the pharynx.

Nutrition and behavioral interventions (continued)

Educate patients about the following:

- strategies to address quality-of-life concerns (eg, tolerable thickened water, coffee)
- strategies to address impediments to adherence
- which medications need to be taken in a cohesive food (eg, a spoonful of pudding or applesauce) or in a liquid form
- dysphagia guidelines based on the International Dysphagia Diet Standardisation Initiative (IDDSI) and resources
- the use of slurry textures

Pharmacotherapy

Topical anesthetics: lidocaine spray (Xylocaine)

Analgesia: opioids, various pain medications

Thickeners: commercial thickeners, such as Simply Thick gel; Thicken Right; Thicken Up; Thick & Easy; Thick It

Box 11.7
Fatigue: Definition, Severity Grades, Considerations, and Interventions[4,11,12,26]

		CTCAE[b] grade and description	
Definition	Fatigue refers to a lack of energy, tiredness, dizziness, and mental fuzziness possibly caused by anemia, inadequate energy or protein intake, weight loss, pain, medications, anticancer treatment, dehydration, or sleep disturbances.	1	Fatigue relieved by rest
		2	Fatigue not relieved by rest; limiting instrumental activities of daily living (ADL)
		3	Fatigue not relieved by rest, limiting self-care ADL
Sample nutrition diagnosis/ PES[a] statement	Impaired ability to prepare food and meals related to cancer treatment fatigue, as evidenced by infrequent meals and weight loss of 2% of usual weight over past 2 months.		
Potential outcomes	Decreased oral food and fluid intake, weight loss, weight gain, depression		

Considerations

Evaluate for anemias as a cause of lack of energy.

Evaluate hydration status.

Consider appropriateness of a multivitamin and mineral supplement.

Evaluate for unintentional weight loss and sarcopenia.

Assess actual food and fluid intake quantitatively and qualitatively using diet history, food records, food-frequency instruments, and 24-hour recall.

(continued)

[a] PES = problems, etiology, signs and symptoms

[b] CTCAE = Common Terminology Criteria for Adverse Events (from the National Cancer Institute)

Box 11.7
Fatigue: Definition, Severity Grades, Considerations, and Interventions[4,11,12,26] *(continued)*

Nutrition and behavioral interventions	Pharmacotherapy
Recommend that patients do the following: ■ Eat small, frequent meals and snacks. ■ Consider taking oral nutrition supplements to promote an adequate energy and nutrient intake. ■ Keep nonperishable snacks at the bedside (eg, granola bars or trail mix). ■ Plan a larger meal for when the appetite is best (eg, at breakfast time). ■ Consume soft, easy-to-chew foods if eating is difficult. ■ Consider using frozen meals, meal boxes, or grocery pick-up services. ■ Use easy-to-prepare meals, snacks, prepared foods, and energy-dense foods. ■ Save energy by limiting "duties or chores" as much as possible. ■ Continue to perform ADL and light activities. ■ Monitor weight weekly, report weight loss, and monitor hydration status. ■ Consider a physical therapy consult for muscle strengthening. ■ Avoid excessive daytime sleep, to help improve nighttime sleep quality.	Blood transfusions Erythropoietin given as epoetin alfa (Epogen, Procrit)

Box 11.8
Malabsorption: Definition, Severity Grades, Considerations, and Interventions[4,11,12,15-17]

Definition	Malabsorption decreases the ability to digest and absorb nutrients; it is possibly caused by chemotherapy, surgery, medications, medical conditions, or infections. Symptoms can include gas, bloating, gastrointestinal (GI) pain, and diarrhea.	**CTCAE[b] grade and description**	
		2	Altered diet; oral intervention indicated
		3	Inability to aliment adequately; parenteral nutrition (PN) indicated
		4	Life-threatening consequences; urgent intervention indicated
Sample nutrition diagnosis/ PES[a] statement	Altered GI function related to side effects of cancer treatment, as evidenced by steatorrhea and abnormal digestive enzyme studies.	5	Death
Potential outcomes	Abnormal digestive enzyme studies, steatorrhea, unintentional weight loss, dehydration, nutrient insufficiency and deficiency, malnutrition, and fatigue		

Considerations

Evaluate pattern of bowel habits and changes associated with surgery, and oncology diagnosis and treatment.

Evaluate frequency of stooling; volume, color, and consistency of stool; and associated symptoms (eg, nausea, flushing, diaphoresis, cramping, bloating, gassiness, foul odor).

Exocrine pancreatic insufficiency can occur following total or partial pancreatic resection, especially when followed by chemotherapy and radiation treatment. Monitor for symptoms of fat malabsorption throughout treatment of pancreatic cancer.

Check fecal elastase to evaluate level of exocrine pancreatic enzyme production.

Evaluate the patient's ability to manage the bowel regimen and use of pancreatic enzyme replacement therapy. Note the timing of enzyme use vs food and beverage intake. Titrate the dose upward until efficacy is achieved. Allow 1 to 2 weeks for each change in dosage. Work with the patient to address impediments to adherence.

Some pancreatic enzyme replacement therapies require concurrent use of a proton pump inhibitor (PPI) to maintain effectiveness.

The patient should not sprinkle or mix contents of enzyme capsules on dairy products or consume foods with a pH >4. If enzymes must be mixed into food, tell the patient to sprinkle them on applesauce immediately before eating a meal.

Assess for secondary lactose intolerance.

Assess actual food and fluid intake quantitatively and qualitatively, using diet history, food records, food-frequency instruments, and 24-hour recall.

(continued)

---

[a] PES = problems, etiology, signs and symptoms

[b] CTCAE = Common Terminology Criteria for Adverse Events (from the National Cancer Institute)

Box 11.8
Malabsorption: Definition, Severity Grades, Considerations, and Interventions[4,11,12,15-17] (continued)

Nutrition and behavioral interventions	Pharmacotherapy
For bloating and gas: Advise the patient to avoid swallowing air by limiting straw use; avoiding carbonated beverages and chewing gum; and eating slowly and chewing thoroughly, with the mouth closed.	Simethicone (Gas-X)
	Lactase enzyme (Lactaid)
	α-galactosidase (Beano)
For bloating, cramping, and gas from milk products: Advise the patient to follow a low-lactose diet and use of lactase-treated dairy products or lactase pills or drops. Suggest low-lactose alternatives.	**Probiotics (for gas, diarrhea):** *Saccharomyces boulardii, Lactobacillus rhamnosus* GG
	Caution: Bacteremia is possible in immunocompromised patients. Avoid opening capsules if a port is present.
For gas from vegetables: Advise the patient to avoid cruciferous vegetables, beans, and legumes or to take enzyme supplements with α-galactosidase and invertase (eg, Beano).	
For bulky, foul-smelling stools, or fatty stools:	Dosing per fat-gram content:
▪ Advise the patient to take pancreatic enzyme replacement therapy with fat-containing foods and beverages before the first bite and (if more than one capsule) halfway through the meal.	▪ Prescribe 500 to 1,000 lipase units per g of fat. ▪ Do not exceed 4,000 lipase units per g of fat. ▪ Do not exceed 2,500 lipase units per kg of body weight per meal, or 10,000 lipase units per kg of body weight per day.
▪ Recommend the use of medium-chain triglycerides to augment calorie intake, if needed.	Dosing per meal or snack: ▪ 20,000 to 75,000 lipase units per meal, and 5,000 to 50,000 lipase units per snack
▪ Educate the patient about the symptoms of fat malabsorption.	Dosing per kg of body weight:
▪ Educate the patient about the use of fat-gram counters or mobile nutrition apps to help track intake and assess enzyme adequacy.	▪ 500 lipase units per kg for meals, increasing as tolerated ▪ 250 lipase units per kg for snacks, increasing as tolerated
▪ Educate the patient about which foods and beverages do not require enzyme use.	
▪ Educate the patient on appropriate dosing of pancreatic enzymes.	

Box 11.9
Nausea and Vomiting: Definition, Severity Grades, Considerations, and Interventions[1,4,6,7,11,12,15,16,27-29]

Definition	Nausea is stomach distress and aversion to food with the urge to vomit or regurgitate the stomach contents.
Sample nutrition diagnosis/PES[a] statement	Altered gastrointestinal (GI) function related to chemotherapy-induced nausea and vomiting (CINV) as evidenced by frequent vomiting, reduced oral intake, and dehydration.
Potential outcomes	Dehydration, electrolyte and acid-base imbalances, nutrient insufficiency and deficiency, unintentional weight loss, aspiration, esophagitis, Mallory-Weiss syndrome, fractures, wound dehiscence, and potential withdrawal from antineoplastic treatment

Nausea

CTCAE[b] grade and description

1	Loss of appetite without alteration in eating habits
2	Oral intake decreased without significant weight loss, dehydration, or malnutrition
3	Inadequate oral energy or fluid intake; tube feeding, parenteral nutrition (PN), or hospitalization indicated

Vomiting

CTCAE[a] grade and description

1	Intervention not indicated
2	Outpatient intravenous (IV) hydration; medical intervention indicated
3	Tube feeding, PN, or hospitalization indicated
4	Life-threatening consequences
5	Death

Considerations

Assess the etiology of the nausea and vomiting: anticipatory (prior to chemotherapy); acute (24 hours after chemotherapy); delayed (1 to 7 days after chemotherapy); breakthrough (occurs despite prophylactic medications, requiring "rescue" medications); refractory (all medications have failed).

Evaluate the patient's ability to manage recommended antiemetic therapy, and work with patient to address impediments to adherence.

Assess for presence of constipation.

For radiotherapy-only treatment, assess for the site of radiation, field size, and total dose. Treatments that are high risk for inducing nausea include total body irradiation, upper abdominal radiotherapy, and craniospinal radiotherapy.

For chemotherapy, with or without radiotherapy, assess the emetogenic potential of the chemotherapy agents.

Evaluate the timing and patterns of nausea and emesis associated with the treatment cycle, medication use, and food and beverage intake.

Assess food and fluid intake, quantitatively and qualitatively, using diet history, food records, food-frequency instruments, and 24-hour recall.

(continued)

[a] PES = problems, etiology, signs and symptoms

[b] CTCAE = Common Terminology Criteria for Adverse Events (from the National Cancer Institute)

Box 11.9
Nausea and Vomiting: Definition, Severity Grades, Considerations, and Interventions[1,4,6,7,11,12,15,16,27-29] *(continued)*

Nutrition and behavioral interventions	Pharmacotherapy
Recommend that patients do the following: ■ Make small, frequent attempts at oral nutrition. ■ Choose bland, starchy foods and clear liquids, all served at room temperature. ■ Avoid greasy, high-fat foods and highly seasoned foods. ■ Consume liquids between meals rather than with meals. ■ Limit exposure to cooking odors by avoiding food preparation areas, and use exhaust fans or open windows. ■ Avoid or limit strong-smelling lotions, soaps, perfumes, and air fresheners. ■ Rest with the head elevated for 30 minutes after eating. ■ Time meals for when nausea medications are working their best. ■ Take pain medications with crackers or light food.	**For acute nausea and vomiting, serotonin antagonists (5-HT3 receptor antagonists):** ondansetron (Zofran); dolasetron (Anzemet); granisetron (Kytril); palonosetron (Aloxi); tropisetron (Navoban) **For delayed nausea and vomiting, dopamine antagonists, particularly phenothiazines:** prochlorperazine (Compazine), promethazine (Phenergan) **For delayed nausea and vomiting, neurokinin-1 (NK-1) receptor antagonists:** aprepitant or fosaprepitant (Emend); netupitant and palonsetron (Akynzeo); rolapitant (Varubi) **Benzamides:** metoclopramide (Reglan) **Cannabinoids:** dronabinol (Marinol); liquefied dronabinol (Syndros); nabilone (Cesamet) **Benzodiazapines:** lorazepam (Ativan); diazepam (Valium) **Corticosteroids:** dexamethasone (Decadron); prednisone **Combination medications for CINV prophylaxis:** a steroid plus a 5-HT3 receptor antagonist plus an NK-1 receptor antagonist, with or without a benzamide (eg, dexamethasone and ondansteron with aprepitant; possibly adding metoclopramide) **Investigational complementary therapies:** ginger tea, ginger ale, 0.5 to 1 g of ginger extract, acupressure bracelets, acupuncture, massage, transcutaneous electrical nerve stimulation, relaxation techniques, and self-hypnosis

Box 11.10
Oral Mucositis and Esophagitis: Definition, Severity Grades, Considerations, and Interventions[4,11,12,15-17, 29]

Definition	Mucositis and esophagitis are inflammations of the mouth or esophagus. Oral mucositis is characterized by painful mouth sores. Esophagitis is usually described as a painful, irritated throat or the feeling of a lump in the throat.
Sample nutrition diagnosis/ PES[a] statement	Inadequate oral intake related to mucositis and esophagitis resulting from chemotherapy, as evidenced by consuming less than half of meals and a diagnosis of dehydration.
Potential outcomes	Dehydration, unintentional weight loss, nutrient insufficiency and deficiency, and malnutrition

Mucositis

CTCAE[b] grade and description

1	Asymptomatic or mild symptoms; intervention not indicated
2	Moderate pain or ulcer that does not interfere with oral intake; modified diet indicated
3	Severe pain; interfering with oral intake
4	Life-threatening consequences; urgent intervention indicated
5	Death

Esophagitis

CTCAE[b] grade and description

1	Asymptomatic or mild symptoms; intervention not indicated
2	Symptomatic; altered eating or swallowing; oral supplements indicated
3	Severely altered eating or swallowing; tube feeding, parenteral nutrition (PN), or hospitalization indicated
4	Life-threatening consequences; urgent intervention indicated
5	Death

Considerations

Assess etiology of the mucositis and esophagitis: hematopoietic stem cell transplantation; chemotherapy-, biotherapy-, or radiation-induced; graft-versus-host disease (GVHD) of the gastrointestinal tract.

Evaluate for oral infections.

Evaluate the patient's ability to adopt recommended symptom-management strategies and medications, and work with the patient to address impediments to adherence.

Encourage good oral care using a soft toothbrush or toothette and woven dental floss.

Advise the patient to keep dentures clean and limit their use if they increase irritation.

(continued)

[a] PES = problems, etiology, signs and symptoms

[b] CTCAE = Common Terminology Criteria for Adverse Events (from the National Cancer Institute)

Box 11.10

Oral Mucositis and Esophagitis: Definition, Severity Grades, Considerations, and Interventions[4,11,12,15-17, 29] *(continued)*

Considerations *(continued)*

Advise avoiding alcohol ingestion and tobacco use.

Recommend the use of lip balm to moisten lips.

Assess food and fluid intake quantitatively and qualitatively using diet history, food records, food-frequency instruments, and 24-hour recall.

Nutrition and behavioral interventions	Pharmacotherapy
Prescribe cryotherapy (the therapeutic use of cold) during administration of fluorouracil (5-FU) bolus and high-dose melphalan chemotherapy. Have the patient consume ice chips, ice water, or a frozen ice pop for 30 minutes to reduce possible development of mucositis.	**Amino acids:** L-glutamine (may reduce severity of mucositis when used during chemoradiotherapy)
Recommend that patients to do the following:	**Topical anesthetics:** gels or rinses containing lidocaine, codeine, or morphine
■ Choose foods lower in acidity, and avoid tomato products, citrus juice, and pickled foods.	**Analgesia:** opioids, anti-inflammatory agents
■ Avoid strong seasoning and spices (eg, chilis, chili powder, curry, cloves, black pepper, and hot sauces).	**Topical anti-inflammatory gel:** gels containing dexamethasone
■ Moisten dry foods with sauces, gravy, or dressings, and dip dry breads in soups to moisten.	**Mucosal barriers and protectants:** zinc gluconate and taurine (Gel-X); adherent gel (Gelclair)
■ Choose soft foods (eg, cream soups, hot cereals, mashed potatoes, yogurt, eggs, tofu, and pudding).	**Soothing rinse:** Mix ¾ tsp salt and 1 tsp baking soda in 4 c of water. Rinse or gargle with 1 c of mixture three or four times daily or as directed by physician.
■ Serve foods at cool or room temperature.	**Anti-infective prophylaxis:** Rinse (orally), swish, and spit with a topical analgesic (eg, viscous lidocaine), an anti-inflammatory (diphenhydramine), and a coating agent (aluminum hydroxide and magnesium hydroxide suspension). Use three or four times daily or as directed by physician.
■ Prepare smoothies with low-acid fruits, such as melons, bananas, or peaches, and add yogurt, milk, or silken tofu.	
■ Limit carbonated beverages.	Mucositis may require antiviral prophylaxis medications.
■ Avoid alcohol-containing mouthwashes.	

Box 11.11
Oral Candidiasis: Definition, Severity Grades, Considerations, and Interventions[4,11,12,15-17,20-22,25]

Definition	Oral candidiasis is an opportunistic infection related to a suppressed immune status. It presents as irritated mucosa and white patches in the mouth, and causes taste alterations, sore mouth, and coated tongue.	

CTCAE[b] grade and description

1	Asymptomatic; local symptomatic management
2	Oral intervention indicated (eg, antifungal)
3	IV antifungal intervention indicated

Sample nutrition diagnosis/ PES[a] statement	Inadequate oral intake related to side effect of chemotherapy (presence of oral candidiasis), as evidenced by consuming less than half of usual meals, pain with chewing, and white coating on tongue.
Potential outcomes	Sore mouth and throat, taste changes, and decreased food intake

Considerations

Assess etiology of candidiasis: Oncology treatment may reduce blood counts, which makes patients susceptible to infections; note timing of infection within treatment cycle, hematopoietic transplant, and so on.

Evaluate patient's ability to tolerate oral intake, utilizing texture modification and pain management as needed.

Nutrition and behavioral interventions[11,20]

Recommend that patients to do the following:

- Practice effective oral hygiene, using saltwater rinses, and avoid mouthwashes that contain alcohol.
- Replace or sanitize toothbrushes, oral appliances, and dentures.
- Choose soft-textured, low-acid foods and beverages, and avoid carbonation.
- Consume active-culture yogurt several times daily.

Pharmacotherapy[11,12,20-22]

Polyene antifungal: nystatin (Mycostatin)

Azole antifungal: fluconazole (Diflucan)

Germicidal mouthwash: chlorhexidine gluconate (Peridex)

Probiotics: Use caution, as bacteremia is possible in immunocompromised patients. Avoid opening capsules of probiotics if a port is present.

Cleansing rinse: Mix ¾ tsp salt and 1 tsp baking soda in 4 c of water. Rinse mouth with 1 c of mixture three or four times daily or as directed by physician.

[a] PES = problems, etiology, signs and symptoms

[b] CTCAE = Common Terminology Criteria for Adverse Events (from the National Cancer Institute)

Box 11.12
Xerostomia: Definition, Severity Grades, Considerations, and Interventions[4,11,12,15-17]

		CTCAE[b] grade and description	
Definition	Xerostomia is abnormal dryness of the mouth that causes difficulty eating and swallowing, taste alterations, and thick and ropy saliva.	1	Symptomatic (eg, dry or thick saliva) without significant dietary alteration; unstimulated saliva flow >0.2 mL/min
Sample nutrition diagnosis/ PES[a] statement	Swallowing difficulty related to radiation treatment side effect (lack of saliva production), as evidenced by inability to consume dry breads and meats.	2	Moderate symptoms; oral intake alterations (eg, copious water, other lubricants, diet limited to purees and/or soft, moist foods); unstimulated saliva flow, 0.1 to 0.2 mL/min
Potential outcomes	Decreased oral intake, nutrient insufficiency and deficiency, dental decay, taste changes, avoidance of dry foods (including breads, meats, and items that are difficult to chew), and weight loss	3	Inability to adequately aliment orally; tube feeding or parenteral nutrition (PN) indicated; unstimulated saliva flow <0.1 mL/min

Considerations

Assess etiology of xerostomia: chemotherapy-induced changes may be transient; radiation-induced changes to the oral cavity typically occur in the second week of radiation therapy and may be permanent.

Encourage good oral hygiene.

Nutrition and behavioral interventions

Recommend that patients do the following:

- Eat small, frequent meals.
- Alternate bites and sips at meals.
- Add broth, gravies, and sauces to meals, and moisten dry foods in liquids.
- Sip liquids throughout the day; aim for 8 to 10 c of fluid daily. Carry a water bottle.
- Swish and spit using club soda or carbonated water.
- Use a humidifier at home to moisten the air.
- Practice good oral hygiene.
- Suck on hard candy, frozen grapes, or melon balls.
- Avoid mouthwash that contains alcohol.
- Avoid alcoholic beverages and tobacco products.

Pharmacotherapy

Mouth conditioners, artificial salivas: Biotene gel, liquid, or spray; BioXtra gel, spray, or tablets; Caphosol; Glandosane; Salivart; Xero-Lube; MouthKote; Xylimelts

Prophylaxis therapy: amifostine (Ethyol); pilocarpine (Salagen)

Cleansing rinse: Mix ¾ tsp salt and 1 tsp baking soda in 4 c of water. Rinse mouth with 1 c of mixture three or four times daily or as directed by physician.

[a] PES = problems, etiology, signs and symptoms

[b] CTCAE = Common Terminology Criteria for Adverse Events (from the National Cancer Institute)

References

1. Arends J, Bachmann P, Baracos V, et al. ESPEN guidelines on nutrition in cancer patients. *Clin Nutr*. 2017;36(1):11-48. doi:10.1016/j.clnu.2016.07.015

2. Tong H, Isenring E, Yates P. The prevalence of nutrition impact symptoms and their relationship to quality of life and clinical outcomes in medical oncology patients. *Support Care Cancer*. 2009;17(1):83-90. doi:10.1007/s00520-008-0472-7

3. Andrew IM, Waterfield K, Hildreth AJ, Kirkpatrick G, Hawkins C. Quantifying the impact of standardized assessment and symptom management tools on symptoms associated with cancer-induced anorexia cachexia syndrome. *Palliat Med*. 2009;23(8):680-688. doi:10.1177/0269216309106980

4. National Cancer Institute. Common Terminology Criteria for Adverse Events (CTCAE), Version 5.0. 2017. February 16, 2020. https://ctep.cancer.gov/protocolDevelopment/electronic_applications/docs/CTCAE_v5_Quick_Reference_5x7.pdf

5. Basch EM, Reeve BB, Mitchell SA, et al. Electronic toxicity monitoring and patient-reported outcomes. *Cancer J*. 2011;17(4):231-234. doi:10.1097/PPO.0b013e31822c28b3

6. Thompson KL, Elliott L, Fuchs-Tarlovsky V, Levin RM, Voss AC, Piemonte T. Oncology evidence-based nutrition practice guideline for adults. *J Acad Nutr Diet*. 2017;117(2):297-310. doi:10.1016/j.jand.2016.05.010

7. Academy of Nutrition and Dietetics Evidence Analysis Library. Oncology guideline. Accessed June 1, 2019. https://www.andeal.org/topic.cfm?menu=5291&cat=5066

8. Huhmann MB, August DA. Review of American Society for Parenteral and Enteral Nutrition (ASPEN) clinical guidelines for nutrition support in cancer patients: nutrition screening and assessment. *Nutr Clin Pract*. 2008;23(2):182-188. doi:10.1177/0884533608314530

9. Head and Neck Guideline Steering Committee. *Evidence-based practice guidelines for the nutritional management of adult patients with head and neck cancer*. Clinical Oncology Society of Australia. Accessed February 16, 2020. https://wiki.cancer.org.au/australia/COSA:Head_and_neck_cancer_nutrition_guidelines

10. Oncology Nursing Society. Symptom interventions and guidelines. Accessed February 16, 2020. www.ons.org/ons-guidelines

11. Oncology Nutrition Dietetic Practice Group. *Oncology Nutrition: Educational Handouts and Resources*. Academy of Nutrition and Dietetics; 2021.

12. PDQ Supportive and Palliative Care Editorial Board. *PDQ Nutrition in Cancer Care*. National Cancer Institute. Updated September 11, 2019. Accessed February 16, 2020. www.cancer.gov/about-cancer/treatment/side-effects/appetite-loss/nutrition-hp-pdq

13. Fearon K, Arends J, Baracos V. Understanding the mechanisms and treatment options in cancer cachexia. *Nat Rev Clin Oncol*. 2012;10(2):90-99. doi:10.1038/nrclinonc.2012.209

14. Couluris M, Mayer JLR, Freyer DR, Sandler E, Xu P, Krischer JP. The effect of cyproheptadine hydrochloride (Periactin) and megestrol acetate (Megace) on weight in children with cancer/treatment-related cachexia. *J Pediatr Hematol Oncol*. 2008;30(11):791-797. doi:10.1097/MPH.0b013e3181864a5e

15. Fieker A, Philpott J, Armand M. Enzyme replacement therapy for pancreatic insufficiency: present and future. *Clin Exp Gastroenterol*. 2011;4(1):55-73. doi:10.2147/CEG.S17634

16. Berry AJ. Pancreatic enzyme replacement therapy during pancreatic insufficiency. *Nutr Clin Pract*. 2014;29(3):312-321. doi:10.1177/0884533614527773

17. Petzel MQB, Hoffman L. Nutrition implications for long-term survivors of pancreatic cancer surgery. *Nutr Clin Pract*. 2017;32(5):588-598. doi:10.1177/0884533617722929

18. Rehwaldt M, Wickham R, Purl S, et al. Self-care strategies to cope with taste changes after chemotherapy. *Oncol Nurs Forum*. 2009;36(2):E47-56. doi:10.1188/09.ONF.E47-E56

19. Wilken MK, Satiroff BA. Pilot study of "miracle fruit" to improve food palatability for patients receiving chemotherapy. *Clin J Oncol Nurs*. 2012;16(5):E173-177. doi:10.1188/12.CJON.E173-E177

20. Saneja A, Sharma C, Aneja KR, Pahwa R. Gymnema sylvestre (gurmar): a review. *Der Pharm.* 2010;2(1):275-284. Accessed June 1, 2019. https://pdfs .semanticscholar.org /2495/8bd34b17f23b1e3e649fa 597eaee1510ff02.pdf?_ga=2.989 49214.11782604371569874851 -2079175024.1569874851

21. Lyckholm L, Heddinger SP, Parker G, et al. A randomized, placebo controlled trial of oral zinc for chemotherapy-related taste and smell disorders. *J Pain Palliat Care Pharmacother.* 2012;26(2):111-114. doi:10.3109 /15360288.2012.676618

22. Woolery M, Bisanz A, Lyons HF, et al. Putting Evidence into Practice: evidence-based interventions for the prevention and management of constipation in patients with cancer. *Clin J Oncol Nurs.* 2008;12(2):317-337. doi:10.1188/08 .CJON.317-337

23. Muehlbauer PM, Thorpe D, Davis A, Drabot R, Rawlings BL, Kiker E. Putting Evidence into Practice: evidence-based interventions to prevent, manage, and treat chemotherapy- and radiotherapy-induced diarrhea. *Clin J Oncol Nurs.* 2009;13(3):336-341. doi:10.1188/09.CJON.336-341

24. Stubbe CE, Valero M. Complementary strategies for the management of radiation therapy side effects. *J Adv Pract Oncol.* 2013;4(4):219-231. doi:10.6004 /jadpro.2013.4.4.3

25. Elad S, Raber-Durlacher JE, Brennan MT, et al. Basic oral care for hematology-oncology patients and hematopoietic stem cell transplantation recipients: a position paper from the joint task force of the Multinational Association of Supportive Care in Cancer/International Society of Oral Oncology (MASCC/ISOO) and the European Society for Blood and Marrow Transplantation (EBMT). *Support Care Cancer.* 2015;23(1):223-236. doi:10.1007/s00520-014-2378-x

26. Berger AM, Mooney K, Alvarez-Perez A, et al. Cancer-related fatigue, version 2.2015. *J Natl Compr Cancer Netw.* 2015;13(8):1012-1039. doi:10.6004 /jnccn.2015.0122

27. Roila F, Molassiotis A, Herrstedt J, et al. 2016 MASCC and ESMO guideline update for the prevention of chemotherapy- and radiotherapy-induced nausea and vomiting and of nausea and vomiting in advanced cancer patients. *Ann Oncol.* 2016;27(suppl 5):v119-v133. doi:10 .1093/annonc/mdw270

28. Einhorn LH, Rapoport B, Navari RM, Herrstedt J, Brames MJ. 2016 updated MASCC/ESMO consensus recommendations: prevention of nausea and vomiting following multiple-day chemotherapy, high-dose chemotherapy, and breakthrough nausea and vomiting. *Support Care Cancer.* 2017;25(1):303-308. doi:10.1007/s00520-016-3449-y

29. Lalla RV, Bowen J, Barasch A, et al. MASCC/ISOO clinical practice guidelines for the management of mucositis secondary to cancer therapy. *Cancer.* 2014;120(10):1453-1461. doi:10 .1002/cncr.28592

Chapter 12
Nutrition Support in the Oncology Setting

Amy Patton, RD, CSO, CNSC
Erin Williams, RD, CSO, CNSC

Malnutrition in the oncology population has been correlated with an increased risk of adverse outcomes, including mortality.[1] Incidence of malnutrition varies and is influenced by disease site. It can occur in as few as 30% of patients to as many as 85% of patients.[2,3] The inability to consume adequate oral nutrition can lead to weight loss and loss of lean body mass. This, in turn, may diminish response to treatment and increase risk for postoperative complications, incidence and severity of treatment-related side effects, and infection risk.[3]

Specialized nutrition support, including enteral nutrition (EN) and parenteral nutrition (PN), can be used when the oral feeding route is unavailable or not tolerated. Evidence is inconclusive as to whether specialized nutrition support stimulates tumor growth; therefore, these modalities should be limited to patients with clear clinical indications for nutrition support.[4-8] Primary indicators for nutrition support include mechanical or functional dysfunctions of the digestive tract, such as dysphagia, gastrointestinal (GI) obstruction, surgery to the head and neck region, or the inability to digest and absorb nutrients.[9,10] Nutrition support is not an appropriate routine adjunct to chemotherapy.[6]

This chapter examines the role of both EN and PN in the oncology population. General guidelines to promote successful use of these therapies, including the risks and benefits, are provided.

Enteral Nutrition

EN (also called tube feeding) provides nutrition directly into the GI system, bypassing the oral route. Feeding can be infused via nasogastric and nasoenteric tubes; tubes also can be inserted directly into the stomach and small intestine. A variety of EN formulas are commercially available.

Indications for Enteral Nutrition

EN support is most appropriate in patients receiving active anticancer treatment who are malnourished and who are expected to be unable to ingest or absorb adequate nutrients for more than 7 to 14 days. According to the American Society for Parenteral and Enteral Nutrition (ASPEN), patients undergoing major cancer operations do not benefit from routine use of EN.[6] Perioperative nutrition support may be beneficial in moderately or severely malnourished patients if administered for 7 to 14 days preoperatively, but the potential benefits must be weighed against potential risks and those of delayed surgical intervention.[6] EN may be a particularly vital part of treatment for those with head and neck cancer; other common diagnoses in which EN is especially beneficial include gastric, esophageal, and pancreatic malignancies. See Box 12.1 on page 220 for more information.

Enteral Nutrition for the Oncology Population

Unless contraindicated, EN is the preferred route of nutrition support over PN in oncology patients. EN uses first-pass metabolism in the liver, which can promote more efficient nutrient utilization and reduces the risk of bacterial translocation when compared with PN.[11]

Box 12.1
Oncology Specific Indications for Enteral Nutrition[5,12]

Clinical scenario	Potential oncology diagnosis or condition
Dysphagia	Esophageal cancer
	Head and neck cancers
	Side effects of radiation therapy, chemotherapy, and surgical resection
Esophageal obstruction	Esophageal cancer
Gastric outlet obstruction	Gastric or pancreatic cancer
Gastroparesis	Gastrointestinal malignancies
	Induced by medications
	Diabetes mellitus

EN also has a lower prevalence of infectious complications, reduction in length of stay in intensive care, and reductions in infectious morbidity, pneumonia, and central line infections. Other studies have found that EN can reduce hospital length of stay and lower the incidence of hyperglycemia.[9,13] Additionally, EN is more cost-effective than PN.[5]

Enteral Access Devices

Determining the appropriate enteral access device (EAD) for a patient requires consideration of the potential length of EN therapy as well as the patient's current and past medical and surgical conditions. EADs and considerations are outlined in Box 12.2.

Contraindications to Enteral Nutrition

There are both systemic and mechanical contraindications to EAD placement. Some examples of absolute contraindications include mechanical obstruction of the GI tract, active peritonitis, uncorrectable coagulopathy, and bowel ischemia.[17] Other conditions that may preclude placement of an EAD include recent GI bleeding, high-output GI fistula, hemodynamic instability, ascites, respiratory compromise, anatomic alterations, and a prognosis that is not consistent with need for artificial nutrition support.[14,15]

Enteral Nutrition Formulations

EN formulations vary in nutrient composition, energy and protein density, macronutrient sources, and water and fiber content. Some contain specialized nutrients (eg, glutamine, arginine, medium-chain triglycerides), but data on their routine use are limited.[5] Standard polymeric formulas, initiated at full strength, are appropriate for the majority of people with cancer. Some patients may require the addition of modular nutrients to enteral feedings. These are most often fiber and protein products, but lipid- and carbohydrate-based products also are used. Nearly all formulas are suitable for lactose intolerance and most are gluten-free, although they may contain other allergens, such as soy and milk

Box 12.2
Enteral Access Devices and Considerations[14,16,17]

Short-term access (up to 4 to 6 weeks)

Device	Placement	Special considerations and notations
Nasogastric tube, orogastric tube	Bedside Intraoperatively	Requires radiographic confirmation of catheter tip placement
Nasoduodenal, oroduodenal, nasojejunal, and orojejunal tubes	Bedside Intraoperative Image-guided Endoscopic	Requires radiographic confirmation of catheter tip placement Risk of catheter tip migration Requires infusion pump Possible increased reflux risk if tip proximal to ligament of Treitz

Long-term access (months to years)

Device	Placement	Special considerations and notations
Percutaneous endoscopic gastrostomy (PEG) tube, gastrostomy tube (G-tube)	Endoscopic Image-guided	Most common enteral access device
PEG-jejunostomy (PEG-J) tube	Endoscopic Image-guided	Risk of catheter tip migration and conversion to PEG Requires infusion pump Decreased risk for aspiration of gastric contents
Percutaneous endoscopic jejunostomy (PEJ) tube	Endoscopic Image-guided	Requires infusion pump Decreased risk for aspiration of gastric contents
Jejunostomy tube (J-tube)	Surgical	Requires infusion pump Decreased risk for aspiration of gastric contents
Low-profile button	Surgical (initial) Home or physician office (replacement)	Less obtrusive Extension sets needed for feeding administration

protein. Labels should be checked thoroughly and often, as manufacturers reformulate their products regularly. Detailed nutrient analysis, ingredient lists, and clinical indications can be found on manufacturers' websites. Box 12.3 summarizes the characteristics of common EN formulations.

Most EN formulations provide 70% to 85% of the body's required free water.[16] Additional hydration is needed for normal physiologic function and for patency of the feeding tube. Water flushes before and after giving medications, as well as between each medication, are needed. For patency, at least 30 mL of water at least every 4 hours during continuous feeds and before and after each intermittent feed is suggested.[5,14] Fluid needs may increase further when losses are high (eg, due to vomiting or large-volume diarrhea) and when certain emetogenic chemotherapeutic regimens are used (see Chapter 9). The nutrition assessment should identify the total fluid needs of each patient receiving EN.

Blenderized Tube Feedings

Oncology patients are increasingly interested in the use of blenderized tube feeding (BTF).[18] This may be due to perceived health benefits, special dietary preferences (eg, organic, vegan), or intolerances and allergies to ingredients in commercial EN formulas. Preparation of BTF can be labor intensive, may contribute to increased occurrence of tube occlusions due to viscosity, and poses the problem of uncertain nutritional value of homemade recipes.[15,19] Food safety, especially in immunocompromised cancer patients, remains a concern.[20] Use of safe food-handling techniques is imperative and includes discarding unused portions after 24 hours, limiting tube feeding hang time to 2 hours or less, and sanitizing blenders and other preparation tools after each use.[15]

There is a lack of published data on the efficacy of BTF, especially in oncology. Many factors must be considered before initiating BTF in a medically

stable patient, including the patient's tolerance to bolus feeds, the need for a gastrostomy tube (G-tube) larger than 14 Fr (French gauge) in diameter due to formula viscosity, availability of registered dietitian nutritionist (RDN) support, and a matured G-tube site. Resources needed include refrigeration, a high-quality blender, storage containers, clean water, multivitamins, and the ability to follow recipe instructions.[15,21]

In recent years, commercial BTF formulas have become available. See Box 12.3 for examples of manufacturers of these products. Some commercial BTF formulas are compatible with enteral feeding pumps, while others are for bolus use only per the manufacturer's specifications. For patients and caregivers wishing to prepare their own formulas, a recipe chart has been created by the University of Virginia Health System.[22] The chart presents a variety of BTF recipes ranging from 800 to 3,000 kilocalories per recipe. Other tools, such as the US Department of Agriculture's MyPlate, can also be used to create balanced menu plans.[23]

Initiation and Advancement of Enteral Feedings

The most appropriate feeding method depends on the location of the feeding tube, aspiration risk, GI status, and ability of the patient or caregiver to handle enteral feeding equipment. There are four primary methods of administration: bolus, intermittent (or gravity), cyclic, and continuous. Clinicians also may employ a combination of the methods. Syringe bolus feedings may be administered with a push technique, in which the plunger of the syringe is used. Bolus feedings may also be given via gravity, with the formula slowly flowing from the syringe into the tube. Syringe bolus feedings, either via push or gravity, are contraindicated with small-bowel feedings.[24] Table 12.1 on page 225 provides suggestions for the administration of enteral feedings. Feedings should be initiated with a full-strength formula. Some patients may benefit from a bolus feeding delivered by gravity.[14]

Complications of Enteral Nutrition

Metabolic aberrations, GI intolerance, enteral misconnections, mechanical or tube complications, microbial contamination, and drug-nutrient interactions can complicate EN.[25,26] Peristomal infection is the most common G-tube complication.[26]

Metabolic Complications

Refeeding syndrome can occur when malnourished patients are initially fed full-energy feeds or high-carbohydrate diets. It is potentially life threatening and is characterized by severe electrolyte abnormalities (eg, hypophosphatemia, hypokalemia, hypomagnesemia) and glucose and fluid shifts, which can result in fluid retention, cardiac dysfunction, and respiratory failure.[27,28] Conditions that increase the risk for refeeding syndrome include chronic malnutrition, prolonged

---

Box 12.3
Enteral Nutrition Formulations and Modular Nutrients[16]

Formulation	Characteristics	Manufacturers
Standard (polymeric)	Provides general nutritional needs Nutrient density varies from 1 to 2 kcal/mL Protein content varies from 14% to 25% of calories May contain fiber and prebiotics May be available at retail outlets	Abbott[a] Kate Farms[b] Nestlé Health Science[c] Trovita Health Science[d]
Semielemental (peptide-based)	For malabsorption, maldigestion, and feeding intolerance Nutrient density varies from 1 to 1.5 kcal/mL; some have higher content or ratio of medium-chain triglyceride (MCT) oil Peptide-based protein sources range from 16% to 25% of calories May contain fiber, prebiotics, arginine, omega-3 fatty acids	Abbott Kate Farms Nestlé Health Science
Elemental (monomeric)	For severely compromised gastrointestinal (GI) function Provides protein as 100% free amino acids Low in fat, with higher content or ratio of MCT oil	Nestlé Health Science
Commercially available blenderized tube feed	Formulated with real food ingredients May also contain more traditional ingredients Possibly suitable for those with food allergies	Abbott Functional Formularies[e] Kate Farms Nestlé Health Science Real Food Blends[f] Trovita Health Science

(continued)

[a] https://abbottnutrition.com
[b] www.katefarms.com
[c] www.nestlehealthscience.com
[d] https://trovitahealth.com

Box 12.3
Enteral Nutrition Formulations and Modular Nutrients[16] (continued)

Disease-specific formulations	Characteristics	Manufacturers
Diabetes	Reduced carbohydrate content May provide fiber May be higher in fat and protein	Abbott Nestlé Health Science
Renal disease	Reduced free water, sodium, potassium, phosphorus, and calcium Contains 1.8 to 2 kcal/mL Protein content varies from 7% to 18% of calories	Abbott Nestlé Health Science
Immune-modulating	May be higher in protein (peptide-based) and energy dense May contain arginine, glutamine, eicosapentaenoic acid (EPA), docosahexaenoic acid (DHA), and elevated amounts of vitamin C, vitamin E, and β carotene	Abbott Nestlé Health Science
Pulmonary	Nutrient density ~1.5 kcal/mL with reduced carbohydrate content Increased lipid content; protein content varies from 16% to 18% of calories May provide EPA, γ-linolenic acid (GLA), and added antioxidants	Abbott Nestlé Health Science

Modulars	Characteristics	Manufacturers	
Additives (fiber, protein, and others) to feeding that provide specific nutrients	Mixed with water and flushed into tube May increase risk for clogs and contamination	Fiber: ■ Global Health Products[g] ■ Medtrition[h] ■ Nestlé Health Science ■ Nutricia[i] Protein: ■ Abbott ■ Global Health Products	■ Nestlé Health Science ■ Medtrition ■ Nutricia Other: ■ Abbott ■ Medtrition ■ Nestlé Health Science ■ Nutricia

[e] www.functionalformularies.com
[f] www.realfoodblends.com
[g] https://globalhp.com

[h] www.medtrition.com
[i] www.nutricia.com

Table 12.1
Administration of Enteral Feeding[14,25,26]

Feeding method	Location of feeding tube	Delivery timing	Initiation rate	Advancement schedule	Equipment required
Syringe bolus	Gastric	~15 min	60-120 mL	Increase by 60-120 mL every 8-12 h (or every 1-2 feedings)	Catheter tip syringe
Intermittent (or gravity) drip	Gastric	~30-35 min	60-120 mL	Increase by 60-120 mL every 8-12 h (or every 1-2 feedings)	Gravity bags, pole
Cyclic	Gastric or small intestine	Often a 12- to 18-h infusion daily (<24 h)	10-40 mL/h	Increase by 10-20 mL/h every 8-12 h	Infusion pump with pole or backpack
Continuous	Gastric or small intestine	20- to 24-h infusion	10-40 mL/h	Increase by 10-20 mL/h every 4-24 h	Infusion pump with pole or backpack

hypocaloric feeding or fasting, taking nothing by mouth for more than 7 days, chronic alcoholism, and anorexia nervosa.

Appropriate monitoring and intravenous (IV) replacement of electrolytes with a plan for slow and gradual administration of EN is critical to avoid refeeding syndrome. Though a number of micronutrients play a role in refeeding syndrome, thiamin is considered to be the most important, as it is an essential coenzyme in the metabolism of carbohydrates. Additional thiamin supplementation may be of benefit to help prevent refeeding syndrome; 100 mg/d for 5 to 7 days can be used.[5,28] Once phosphorus, potassium, and magnesium levels have been restored to their normal ranges, EN should be initiated slowly.[30]

For those at risk for refeeding syndrome, EN should start with 25% of the patient's estimated energy needs and advance over 3 to 5 days to feeding goals.[30] The clinician should continue to monitor laboratory values, vital signs, and fluid balance until avoidance of refeeding syndrome has been assessed. Other metabolic complications of EN potential corrections are summarized in Box 12.4 on pages 226 to 227.

Gastrointestinal Complications

According to the 2016 guidelines for nutrition support therapy in adult critically ill patients from ASPEN and the Society of Critical Care Medicine, routine monitoring of gastric residual volumes (GRVs) for feeding tolerance is not recommended. GRV does not correlate with incidence of aspiration or pneumonia, and routine monitoring may lead to increased risk of EAD occlusion and inappropriate cessation of enteral feedings. These guidelines provide the recommendation to avoid holding enteral nutrition for a GRV of less than 500 mL in the absence of other signs of intolerance.[13] See Box 12.5 on pages 228 and 229 for how to assess for GI intolerance using physical symptoms.

Box 12.4

Metabolic Complications and Potential Corrections During Enteral Nutrition Therapy[27,28,31,32]

Dehydration

Possible causes:	Prevention or possible correction:
Inadequate free-water administration	Increase free water enterally or parenterally.
Fluid losses (emesis, diarrhea, drains, dialysis, fever)	Monitor fluid status and losses; monitor daily weights.
Concentrated formula	Change to a formula with higher free-water content.

Overhydration, volume overload

Possible causes:	Prevention or possible correction:
Excess fluid intake	Decrease free-water flushes; change to a lower-free-water formula.
Refeeding syndrome	Monitor fluid status and intake; monitor daily weights.

Hyperglycemia

Possible causes:	Prevention or possible correction:
Insulin resistance or diabetes mellitus	Change to a carbohydrate-controlled or fiber-containing formula.
Metabolic stress or sepsis	Recommend use of, or adjust dose of, insulin or oral hypoglycemic agents.
Steroids	

Hypernatremia

Possible causes:	Prevention or possible correction:
Inadequate free water	Increase free water to meet fluid needs.
Excess fluid losses (diuresis)	Monitor fluid status, fluid intake and output, and daily weights.

Hyponatremia

Possible causes:	Prevention or possible correction:
Water retention or fluid overload	Change to a lower-free-water formula; restrict fluids and free water.
Sodium losses (gastrointestinal)	Supplement with sodium.
Syndrome of inappropriate antidiuretic hormone (SIADH)	Restrict fluids and free water; induce diuresis.

(continued)

Box 12.4

Metabolic Complications and Potential Corrections During Enteral Nutrition Therapy[27,28,31,32] *(continued)*

Hyperkalemia

Possible causes:	Prevention or possible correction:
Metabolic acidosis	Correct acidosis; recheck serum potassium.
Excessive potassium intake	If possible, correct serum potassium before initiation of feedings. Reduce potassium intake from formula and oral diet; eliminate potassium from intravenous fluids.
Renal failure	Recommend medication therapy, such as potassium-binding resin, glucose, or insulin.

Hypokalemia

Possible causes:	Prevention or possible correction:
Refeeding syndrome	Decrease nutrition delivery to 25% of goal; replace potassium.
Excess gastrointestinal losses Diuretics or dialysis, insulin therapy	Replace potassium intravenously if serum levels are <3 mEq/L; replace potassium via enteral route if hypokalemia is mild.
Inadequate intake	Evaluate the need to change the formula.

Hyperphosphatemia

Possible causes:	Prevention or possible correction:
Kidney insufficiency or failure Tumor lysis syndrome	Consider changing to a lower-phosphorus formula; recommend phosphate binders.
Phosphate-containing antacids	Recommend a potential change in medications.

Hypophosphatemia

Possible causes:	Prevention or possible correction:
Refeeding syndrome	Decrease nutrition delivery to 25% of goal; replace phosphorus.
Insulin therapy	Replace phosphorus intravenously if severe; replace phosphorus via enteral route if mild.
Phosphate-binding antacids	Recommend discontinuation or adjustment of phosphate-binding antacids.

Box 12.5
Gastrointestinal Complications and Potential Corrections During Enteral Nutrition Therapy[13,26,32]

Aspiration, reflux (gastroesophageal reflux disease)

Possible causes:	Prevention or possible correction:
Flat head of bed	Elevate the head of bed 30° to 45°.
Incomplete closure of the lower esophageal sphincter	Use a small-bore enteral access device (EAD).
	Consider changing to a postpyloric EAD.
Large-volume feeding boluses	Provide continuous infusion.
Delayed gastric motility	Consider adding prokinetic agents.
	Consider changing to concentrated formula at a lower rate.
	Consider a fiber-free formula to enhance gastric emptying.

Nausea, vomiting, abdominal distention, bloating

Possible causes:	Prevention or possible correction:
Delayed gastric emptying	Use a continuous feeding method with a low-fat or isotonic formula or both.
Rapid infusion of feedings	Consider adding prokinetic agents.
	Consider changing to a postpyloric EAD.
	Minimize the use of narcotics, if possible.
	Consider a fiber-free formula to enhance gastric emptying.
	Provide antiemetics.
	Initiate feedings at a low rate and advance slowly.
	Check the EAD placement for possible migration.

Diarrhea

Possible causes:	Prevention or possible correction:
Medications	Evaluate the patient's use of hyperosmolar medications (sorbitol, magnesium-containing medications), laxatives, lactulose, and others.
Antibiotic-associated diarrhea	Evaluate the patient's usage of antibiotics.
	Provide antidiarrheals, if appropriate.
Infectious etiology	Check stool for *Clostridium difficile* or other infectious pathogens.

(continued)

Box 12.5
Gastrointestinal Complications and Potential Corrections During Enteral Nutrition Therapy[13,26,32] (continued)

Diarrhea (continued)

Possible causes:	Prevention or possible correction:
Bacterial contamination	Observe appropriate formula hang times; change tubing every 24 hours; use a closed system instead of either an open system or powdered, reconstituted formula.
Fiber-free formula or high-fiber formula	Consider changing the formula for different fiber content.
Malabsorption or steatorrhea	Consider changing to an elemental or semielemental formula.
	Adjust the formula selection to one with lower fat content or higher medium-chain triglyceride content.
	Consider adding pancreatic enzyme replacement therapy.

Constipation

Possible causes:	Prevention or possible correction:
Inadequate fluid intake	Increase free-water and fluid intake.
Inadequate or excessive fiber provision	Consider changing the formula to adjust fiber content.
Physical inactivity	Have the patient increase activity, if possible.
Medications	Minimize the use of narcotics, if possible.
	Recommend the addition of stool softeners or laxatives.
	Recommend a trial of prune juice.
Gastrointestinal obstruction, colonic dysmotility, ileus	Evaluate and address the underlying cause; may need to suspend EN until cause is determined.

Mechanical and Microbial Complications

Intraprocedural complications (eg, aspiration, hemorrhage, or perforation) are rare. Peristomal infection is the most common G-tube complication, and leakage around the site is also common but less recognized.[26] Clogged EAD are common, especially with small-diameter tubes (less than 8 to 10 Fr). Avoiding adding medications directly to enteral formula, limiting gastric residual checks, flushing the tube properly, and monitoring for potential interactions between the formula and medications may help prevent clogs. Water is preferred for irrigation; there is limited efficacy to other solutions, such as juice, carbonated beverages, and meat tenderizer.[33] Box 12.6 provides more information on managing EAD occlusions.

Tube dislocation prevalence varies based on the type of EAD and is a frequent complication with nasoenteric and oroenteric tubes. Securement of tubes along with routinely assessing for appropriate tube position can reduce the risk of complications associated with displacement. ASPEN's Safe Practices for Enteral Nutrition Therapy document outlines safe and effective methods for securing EADs.[17]

Medication Administration

As noted by ASPEN, most medications are not formulated to be administered through a feeding tube.[17] This can pose concerns when an EAD is the only available route for medication administration, as there is a risk of drug-nutrient interactions, drug-drug interactions, tube occlusions, and other adverse effects. In particular, extended or sustained release medications and enterically coated medications are not compatible with enteral feedings, because they should not be crushed. ASPEN's Safe Practices for Enteral Nutrition Therapy document is a good resource for addressing these concerns, and it provides some comprehensive

Box 12.6
Recommendations for Managing Clogged EADs[14,33,34]

Instill 5 mL of warm water as near to the clog as possible for up to 15 minutes.

Use a gentle push-pull motion with a 30- to 60-mL syringe plunger to help dislodge the clog and attempt to aspirate or flush with warm water.

A solution of pancrelipase mixed with sodium bicarbonate has also shown some efficacy with dissolving formula occlusions.

If unsuccessful, consider using a commercial unclogging device.

Commercially available decloggers, such as Clog Zapper and TubeClear, are not typically available at home and need to be used under medical supervision.

practice recommendations that practitioners can implement.[15] Box 12.7 also provides guidance on some of the more common EN-related medication interactions.

Although liquid medication preparations are often preferred for enteral administration, many liquid medications have osmolalities exceeding 1,000 mOsm/kg, and GI intolerances (eg, cramping, abdominal distention, and diarrhea) may occur following administration of hyperosmolar medications. Diluting the liquid medication with 10 to 30 mL of sterile water before administration may help reduce these effects. Inactive ingredients in liquid products, such as mannitol and sorbitol, may also pose a concern for GI-related side effects, particularly diarrhea.[35]

Patient Safety

For oncology patients who require EN, it can be a life-sustaining therapy, but it does come with the

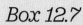

Box 12.7
Common Enteral Nutrition–Related Medication Concerns[35-39]

Medication	Specific medications not recommended for use in enteral access devices	Alternative medications for enteral access devices administration
Antidiarrheals Hydrolyzed guar gum can be used to thicken stool and is appropriate for administering via enteral access device (EAD) when mixed with water.	Cholestyramine (caution with small-bore tubes)	Loperamide liquid Diphenoxylate hydrochloride and atropine sulfate
Antiemetics Usually given before chemotherapy or with intravenous fluids Often given before meals or tube feeds Ondansetron ODT is absorbed in the stomach. If possible, have the patient dissolve the tablet in his or her mouth and swallow.	Aprepitant Ondansetron orally disintegrating tablet (ODT)	Intravenous fosaprepitant Lorazepam liquid Promethazine liquid Metoclopramide liquid Erythromycin liquid
Antibiotics	Fluoroquinolones (cirpofloxacin, levofloxacin)	No recommended alternatives
Appetite stimulants	Dronabinol	Megestrol acetate liquid Mirtazapine tablets Cyproheptadine tablets Dexamethasone Medroxyprogesterone
Pain medications Pain patches are available as well but are not always appropriate for patients with rapid weight loss due to altered drug levels in the blood.	Enteric-coated aspirin Morphine sulfate extended-release tablets Morphine sulfate sustained-release tablets Oxycodone	Morphine liquid Oxycodone liquid Acetaminophen and hydrocodone bitartrate Over-the-counter liquid medications such as ibuprofen or acetaminophen
Laxatives	Methylcellulose or psyllium Cholestyramine Bisacodyl tablets	Docusate liquid Senna Polyethylene glycol 3350 Lactulose Bisacodyl suppositories

(continued)

Box 12.7
Common Enteral Nutrition–Related Medication Concern[35-39] *(continued)*

Medication	Specific medications not recommended for use in enteral access devices	Alternative medications for enteral access devices administration
Histamine H2-receptor antagonists and proton pump inhibitor (PPIs) Mixing and administration instructions vary by brand and product type. Refer to package inserts or product websites for the most up-to-date information.	Pantoprazole tablets Rabeprazole tablets	Dexlansoprazole capsules and disintegrating tablet Esomeprazole capsule and packet Lansoprazole capsule and disintegrating tablet Omeprazole, Pantoprazole, Rabeprazole packet
Vitamins and supplements Liquid vitamins and minerals are often available.	Slow Mag K-Dur, Micro-K	
Other Sucralfate may bind to protein left in the feeding tube from formula.	Sucralfate	An appropriate PPI or H2 blocker formulation
For pancreatic enzyme replacement therapy, open the capsule and mix the contents into a small amount of applesauce if the oral route is available; otherwise, suspend the contents in water or nectar-thick juice. Do not administer in an alkaline food substance, such as yogurt.	Pancreatic enzyme replacement therapy capsules	

potential for adverse effects. Enteral tubing misconnections are a rare but potentially serious issue related to EN. They can occur when an enteral feeding device, such as a syringe or feeding bag, is connected to a nonenteral device, such as an IV line or ventilator tubing. As early as the 1970s, there were reports of enteral misconnections, but it was not until the Joint Commission addressed the issue in 2006 that discussions to change the design of enteral tubing began. In 2008, the International Organization for Standardization (ISO) began to develop standards for the design of enteral connectors. The first ISO-compliant enteral access connector is the ENFit connector. The ISO standards are recognized worldwide.[17]

The Global Enteral Device Supplier Association (GEDSA) is a nonprofit organization that was established in 2013 to help promote the safe delivery of enteral feedings. GEDSA has been working with regulatory agencies along with supply manufacturers to help promote patient safety by introducing new standards for health care tubing connectors. While there was a mandate in California to start the use of ENFit tubing in July 2016, there has been a lengthy transition period during which both the old and the new enteral products have been available. For updates on the current status of the transition and other tools to facilitate transition, see the GEDSA website (http://stayconnected.org/enteral-enfit).[40]

Home Enteral Nutrition

It is estimated that more than 437,000 people in the United States use home enteral nutrition (HEN), a dramatic increase over the past two decades.[41] Not all patients with cancer who rely on EN are candidates for HEN. The appropriateness of HEN must be evaluated. Candidates need access to running water for hand washing, electricity availability if a feeding pump is required, and adequate storage for formula and supplies.[41,42]

In the United States, home infusion companies or durable medical equipment (DME) companies supply feeding pumps, formula, and ancillary items needed to maintain the tube.[26] Whenever feasible, select a DME provider that has expertise in HEN reimbursement, 24-7 clinician availability, and a multidisciplinary team that includes an RDN.[42] As the required documentation of medical necessity for HEN can be extensive, coordination of care among the RDN, physician, nurse, speech therapist, and case manager is required. Community support, education, and outreach are provided by the Oley Foundation (https://oley.org).

Insurance Considerations

Coverage of HEN varies widely among commercial insurers and government-funded health insurance programs. Many insurers only cover supplies, leaving patients to cover the cost of the formula, and some policies exclude any coverage for HEN. Medicare Part B has clearly defined guidelines on coverage of HEN. According to the Medicare Coverage Database, HEN "is considered reasonable and necessary for a patient with a functioning gastrointestinal tract who, due to pathology to, or non-function of, the structures that normally permit food to reach the digestive tract, cannot maintain weight and strength commensurate with his or her general condition." It is also necessary to have documentation within the medical record that "the impairment will be of long and indefinite duration" for Medicare to cover HEN.[43] Patients with head and neck cancer who have undergone reconstructive surgery generally meet the coverage criteria, as may those with gastric and esophageal malignancies. Formulas used to supplement one's diet, whether oral or via tube, are not covered under Medicare Part B, nor are feedings used to manage malnutrition or anorexia. Additional justification is needed within the medical record to substantiate the need for a feeding pump or specialty formulas. Detailed criteria on Medicare coverage can be found in the Medicare Coverage Database (www.cms.gov/medicare-coverage-database).[43-46] Many DME companies also have print materials designed to help practitioners with the Medicare qualification process.

Home Regimens

Reimbursement of HEN needs to be considered when developing a HEN care plan. A patient's and his or her caregivers' willingness and ability to assist with feedings also must be evaluated, and a feeding regimen should take into account the patient's nutritional needs, tolerance, and lifestyle.[14,42]

Commercially prepared formulas are preferable to powders whenever possible, to limit bacterial contamination associated with the mixing of powdered formulas. If modulars are used, sanitary techniques for preparation must be reviewed with patients. Patients must also be instructed on the proper storage of formula, safe handling of syringes, and the need to examine the formula and supplies for damage, contamination, and expiration dates.[14] As with many inpatient facilities, DME providers may have a formulary that dictates which brand of formula is available.

Bolus, gravity, and pump feeds can all be administered in the home. Bolus feedings are the most simple and cost-effective method, but they carry an increased risk for aspiration, volume intolerance, and vomiting. Gravity-bag feedings may be used in the home in ambulatory patients who are intolerant to bolus feedings but do not want pump feedings. Ambulatory feeding pumps are available for home use, although each insurer may have its own guidelines for when pumps are covered. Pump feeds are often cycled to reduce the length of the feeding cycle. Insurers often require additional medical justification for coverage of feeding pumps in the home setting.

Tube clogs and feeding intolerance can occur in the home setting. See Box 12.4 on pages 226 to 227 for types and management of metabolic complications, and Box 12.5 on pages 228 and 229 for types and management of GI complications. Management of tube clogs can be complicated in the home setting because home nursing is not always an available option to help unclog the tube. Special care should be taken to ensure patients are properly instructed on tube flushing and medical administration to help minimize the risk of clogs. See Box 12.6 on page 230 for suggestions for managing tube occlusions.

Parenteral Nutrition

Parenteral nutrition is the IV infusion of nutrients. It can be a life-saving modality for people with cancer but should not be a routine adjunct to chemotherapy or considered standard to cancer care. There is a lack of high-quality data available to guide clinicians in selecting the best candidates for PN therapy in the oncology setting. Oncology outcomes data suggest that patients who cannot obtain 100% of their nutrition needs enterally, have an acceptable quality of life, and would die from malnutrition before tumor progression are appropriate candidates for PN therapy. There is no clear evidence that PN contributes to tumor growth in humans. Most of the data are derived from animal studies, and human outcomes data do not show deleterious effects of PN on oncology outcomes.[7]

Indications for Parenteral Nutrition

PN can benefit patients with moderate-to-severe malnutrition who have inadequate EN or oral intake for a prolonged period.[6] PN is more costly than EN and can result in mechanical, metabolic, and infectious complications. However, these risks can be minimized by appropriate patient selection and management of PN by a clinician trained in specialized nutrition support.[47] The routine use of PN in patients undergoing hematopoietic cell transplantation (HCT) is evolving, and more information can be found in Chapter 15.[7] Box 12.8 summarizes the ASPEN guidelines for the use of PN therapy and the corresponding common oncology-specific conditions.

Parenteral Nutrition Access

When PN support is indicated, the clinician must establish or recommend IV access. Central IV access via a central venous catheter (CVC) is required for total or central PN. Oncology patients often have established CVC access, allowing for CPN. However, a dedicated line or port used solely for PN is recommended, in order to reduce infectious complications.[48]

Central IV access positions the distal catheter tip in central vessels (distal superior vena cava or right atrium). CVCs are either tunneled or nontunneled. A peripherally inserted central catheter is a commonly placed CVC in the acute and home-care settings and may be kept in place for months to years. Tunneled catheters, such as Hickman and Broviac catheters, are associated with decreased infection risk, as the exit site and venipuncture sites are separated.[49] Many oncology patients have implanted ports for their chemotherapeutic regimens. In general, implanted ports demonstrate a significantly

Box 12.8
Oncology-Specific Indications for Parenteral Nutrition[7, 47]

Clinical scenario	Potential oncology diagnosis or condition
Paralytic or postoperative ileus	<ul><li>Abdominal debulking surgeries</li><li>Gastrointestinal (GI) cancers</li><li>Gynecological cancers</li><li>Hyperthermic intraperitoneal chemotherapy (HIPEC)</li></ul>
Malignant bowel obstruction	<ul><li>Ovarian or GI cancers</li><li>Peritoneal carcinomatosis</li><li>Peritoneal mesothelioma</li></ul>
High-output (>200 mL/d) distal GI fistula	<ul><li>GI cancers</li><li>Gynecological cancers</li><li>Radiation enteritis</li></ul>
Inability to tolerate enteral nutrition (EN) for >7 to 14 days	<ul><li>GI anastomotic or pancreatic leaks</li><li>Hematopoietic cell transplant (HCT) with grade 3 or 4 mucositis</li><li>Preoperative malnourished patients with inability to use GI tract for EN</li></ul>
Large-volume diarrhea or high-output ostomies refractory to medication management	<ul><li>GI malignancies</li><li>HCT with gut graft-versus-host disease (GVHD)</li><li>High-output ileostomies or colostomies related to chemotherapy or bowel surgery</li><li>Radiation enteritis</li><li>Significant GI resections</li></ul>

lower risk of infection in patients with cancer than tunneled catheters. However, ports require daily needle access for PN by a trained professional, and continuous access nullifies this infection-risk benefit. Regardless of the CVC chosen, infectious complications of central PN have been greatly reduced with the implementation of central line bundle practices.[50]

To provide peripheral parenteral nutrition (PPN), peripheral IV access is required. PPN should only be used to for a short time (5 days to 2 weeks) and is, therefore, infrequently indicated in the oncology setting. To minimize the risk of thrombophlebitis, a final concentration of PPN must be less than 900 mOsm/L, with a low dextrose concentration of 5% to 10% and a maximum amino acid concentration of 3%. Previous practices of rotating peripheral venous access sites every 48 to 72 hours to reduce the risk of thrombophlebitis are no longer recommended.[47,50]

Parenteral Nutrition Components

PN solutions consist of the macronutrients carbohydrate (dextrose), protein (amino acids), and fat (lipid emulsions), with an admixture of electrolytes, vitamins, and trace elements as well as additional fluid needed for adequate hydration.[51] Individual institutions or DME providers may determine fluid maximums per bag of PN. If necessary, additional IV fluids can be provided to the patient to optimize hydration.[52] Table 12.2 provides detailed dosing information for the adult patient receiving PN. Pediatric PN guidelines are covered in Chapter 13.

Dextrose is often the primary energy source in PN, with adequate amounts needed to support brain function and prevent gluconeogenesis. A minimum dose of 50 g/d is required to avoid ketone production.[53] However, excessive dextrose must be avoided to prevent hyperglycemia, excessive carbon dioxide production, and fatty liver.[52]

Amino acid solutions provide both essential and nonessential amino acids. Clinical status and renal function should be considered when selecting the most appropriate amino acid dosage for the oncology patient receiving PN. Parenteral glutamine supplementation may offer benefit in the HCT population, but no IV form is commercially available in the United States, and recent studies indicate lack of clear benefit in the critically ill population.[6,51]

IV fat emulsions (IVFEs) supply additional energy and are a source of essential fatty acids (omega-6 linoleic acid and omega-3 linolenic acid) to the patient receiving PN. PN provided without IVFE can result in clinical symptoms of essential fatty acid deficiency (EFAD), such as hair loss, scaly skin, abnormal liver function tests or liver dysfunction, dermatitis, and reduced growth. Furthermore, fat-free PN can promote hyperglycemia and nonketotic diabetic comas. Until recently, a soybean oil–based IVFE was the only IVFE product approved by the US Food and Drug Administration (FDA) for use in the United States. The high content of omega-6 fatty acids and phytoesterols in soybean oil–based IVFE is thought to contribute to PN-associated liver disease and infection risk.[54]

In 2016, the FDA approved the lipid injectable emulsion SMOFlipid (Fresenius Kabi), a mixed-oil source of IVFE for use in adults. It is composed of 30% soybean oil, 30% medium-chain triglycerides, 25% olive oil, and 15% fish oil. SMOFlipid contains higher levels of vitamin E than soybean oil-based IVFEs, providing 0.163 to 0.225 mg/mL of all-*rac*-α-tocopherol.[55] The Recommended Dietary Allowance (RDA) in adults for α-tocopherol (vitamin E) is 15 mg, with a tolerable upper limit of 1,000 mg/d.[56] There is concern that excessive supplementation of vitamin E and other antioxidants may reduce treatment benefit for the oncology patient.[57] SMOFlipid is unlikely to exceed the upper limit for vitamin E. For example, 1 g of SMOFlipid per kg of body weight for a 50-kg adult, combined with the 10 mg provided from the vitamin additives, would provide 50 to 66 mg of vitamin E.[51,55] Data on short-term use (<90 days) show that SMOFlipid results in significantly lower levels of the liver enzymes alanine aminotransferase and aspartate aminotransferase and lower levels of total bilirubin. However, longer-term trials are needed to determine if these findings improve clinical outcomes. SMOFlipid should be avoided with known hypersensitivities to soybean, fish, egg, or peanut protein.[51]

Omegaven (Fresenius Kabi), a 100% fish oil–based IVFE, has shown significant benefit for reversing or improving PN-associated liver disease in the pediatric population, as well as in some adult patients, and in 2018 became FDA-approved for use.[54] In addition, the low arachidonic acid and linoleic acid content may place patients at risk for EFAD.[51] To prevent this, ASPEN recommends that 1% to 2% of energy be derived from linoleic acid and 0.5% of energy from linolenic acid to prevent EFAD.[52]

Electrolyte doses added to the PN regimen vary widely depending on the patient's requirements. Table 12.3 lists the standard daily ranges for adults. Note that there are no standard dosing ranges for acetate and chloride; they are instead adjusted to maintain acid-base balance.[51] Oncology patients

Table 12.2
Macronutrients in Parenteral Nutrition Solutions for Adults[51,52,54,55]

Macronutrient	Dextrose	Amino acids	Lipids (intravenous fat emulsion, IVFE)
Concentration availability	2.5%-70%	3%-20%	Soybean oil: 20%, 30% SMOFlipid: 20% Omegaven: 10%
Energy provision (kcal/g)	3.4	4	10 (in 20% and 30% solutions) 11 (in 10% solutions)
Minimal daily requirement	100-150 g	0.8 g/kg of body weight (or individualized based on clinical need)	Soybean oil: 250 mL of 20% IVFE or 500 mL of 10% IVFE twice weekly; or 500 mL of 20% IVFE once weekly SMOFlipid: 63 mL for every 1,000 calories of parenteral nutrition (PN)
Optimal dosing range	To meet total daily energy goals[a]	0.8-1 g/kg of body weight (if medically stable) 1.2-2 g/kg of body weight (catabolism)	20%-30% of calories from fat, or 0.11 g/kg of body weight hourly
Maximum daily tolerance	7 g/kg of body weight, or 5 mg/kg of body weight per min for acutely ill patients or patients with poor glucose control	2.5 g/kg of body weight Individualized, based on patient tolerance	2.5 g/kg of body weight, or 60% of total energy (if medically stable)
Total daily energy goals[a]	20-30 kcal/kg of body weight (if medically stable) ~15 kcal/kg of body weight, or 2 mg/kg of body weight per minute for refeeding syndrome		
Total daily fluid needs[b]	30-40 mL/kg of body weight (if medically stable)		

[a] Energy goals are highly variable and should be based on the patient's individual nutrition goals and tolerance to nutrition therapy. Indirect calorimetry should be performed, when available, and used to determine the energy goal.

[b] Fluid restrictions or limitations may be needed for management of medical conditions, such as heart, liver, or kidney failure. Consider all sources of fluids, including intravenous fluids and medications.

Table 12.3
Standard Parenteral Electrolyte Requirements for Adults[48]

Electrolyte	Daily requirement
Sodium	1-2 mEq/kg of body weight
Potassium	1-2 mEq/kg of body weight
Acetate	As needed to maintain acid-base balance
Chloride	As needed to maintain acid-base balance
Calcium	10-15 mEq
Magnesium	8-20 mEq
Phosphorus	20-40 mmol

receiving PN may have excessive electrolyte losses related to their underlying diagnosis and treatment and to clinical conditions, such as high-output ileostomies, gastric fluid loss from a venting G-tube, or renal losses of electrolytes from platinum-based chemotherapy regimens. Close monitoring of laboratory values and a detailed review of physical symptoms are often necessary to appropriately adjust the PN regimen. Tables 12.4 and 12.5 present standard trace element additives and parenteral vitamin additives, respectively.

Vitamins and trace elements are added to the PN solution via commercially available products to prevent nutrient deficiencies. Multiple-element and single-element products can be used to tailor the PN to the individual patient's needs. Check with your institution or DME company on what products and doses are available. Current vitamin D content in PN multivitamin products is less than the RDA

Table 12.4
Standard Parenteral Trace Element Additives for Adults[51]

Trace element	Amount provided from daily dose of multi–trace element product[a]
Copper (cuprous chloride or cupric sulfate)	1.0-1.3 mg
Chromium (chromic chloride)	10-12 mcg
Manganese (manganese chloride or manganese sulfate)	270-500 mcg
Selenium (sodium selenite or selenious acid)	0-60 mcg
Zinc (zinc chloride or zinc sulfate)	3.0-6.5 mg
Iron (ferric chloride)	1.1 mg
Iodine (potassium iodide)	130 mcg
Molybdate (sodium molybdate dihydrate)	19 mcg
Fluoride (sodium fluoride)	950 mcg

[a] MTE-4 contains copper, chromium, manganese, and zinc. MTE-5 contains copper, chromium, manganese, zinc, and selenium. Addamel N contains all of the elements listed.

for this nutrient, and IV forms of vitamin D are not commercially available.[51] Additional oral supplementation or sun exposure to facilitate endogenous production of vitamin D is likely necessary, if possible. Iron is not routinely added to PN due to concerns for adverse reactions and incompatibility issues. The ferric iron causes breakdown of lipid emulsions, rendering fat-containing PN unsafe for use. Periodic IV iron is needed to avoid deficiency.[58] Multi–trace element products may contain excessive copper, manganese, and chromium, while some products do not contain selenium. ASPEN recommends using single-element products in place of multiple trace elements when appropriate for the patient's needs. PN product shortages are common in the United States, contributing to periodic lack of access to these products. ASPEN provides detailed guidelines and practice scenarios on managing the PN patient when shortages occur.[51]

Certain medications are compatible with PN and can be added directly to the formulation. These include histamine H2-receptor antagonists, such as famotidine, as well as insulin and heparin. Only regular human insulin is compatible with PN, and dosing requirements may be higher at the start of PN therapy, until the patient's clinical status stabilizes.[59] Oncology patients without diabetes mellitus may require insulin in the PN due to concurrent use

Table 12.5
Standard Parenteral Vitamin Additives for Adults[51]

Component	Dose (10 ml)
Vitamin A (retinol)	1 mg (3,300 USP[a] units)
Vitamin D (ergocalciferol or cholecalciferol)	5 mcg (200 USP units)
Vitamin E (DL-α tocopheryl acetate)	10 mg (10 USP units)
Vitamin K (phytonadione)	150 mcg
Thiamin	6 mg
Riboflavin 5-phosphate sodium	3.6 mg
Vitamin B6 (pyridoxine hydrochloride)	6 mg
Niacinamide	40 mg
Dexpanthenol (d-pantothenyl alcohol)	15 mg
Biotin	60 mcg
Folic acid	600 mcg
Vitamin B12 (cyanocobalamin)	5 mcg
Ascorbic acid	200 mg

[a] USP = United States Pharmacopeia

of medications, such as corticosteroids, or impaired glucose intolerance due to altered metabolism.[60] A knowledgeable clinician or defined protocols should be used to dose insulin in the PN to avoid serious complications. ASPEN recommends initial insulin dosing of 0.05 to 0.1 units per g of dextrose in the PN solution, or 0.15 to 0.2 units per g of dextrose for patients who are already hyperglycemic.[52]

PN is available for administration in two forms: two-in-one and total nutrient admixture (TNA), also known as three-in-one admixture. In a two-in-one solution, the IV lipid is administered as a separate "piggyback" infusion with a maximum hang time of 12 hours. A TNA system contains all three macronutrients in the same infusion, and lipids are added just prior to the infusion. The advantages of a TNA system are convenience and ease of administration; therefore, its use is common in the home setting. However, the lipids are less stable in TNA and do not allow the use of a bacteria-eliminating filter.[51]

Initiation of Parenteral Nutrition

PN should only be initiated in patients who are hemodynamically stable. Any metabolic derangements, such as significant hyperglycemia, electrolyte imbalances, or acid-base disorders, should be corrected before initiating PN.[47] To prevent hyperglycemia, PN should be initiated with approximately 150 to 200 g of dextrose (or 100 g for patients with poor glycemic control) for the first 24 hours. Typically, PN is initiated with a 24-hour continuous infusion. Once clinical tolerance has been established, a cyclic PN regimen of 12 to 16 hours a day can be considered.[52] Initiation of PN in the home setting is controversial and should be avoided in patients with diabetes mellitus, pulmonary disease, severe malnutrition, hyperemesis, and electrolyte disorders. Given the likelihood that the oncology patient has one or more of these conditions, PN initiation in the hospital setting is recommended.[47]

Monitoring of Parenteral Nutrition

Routine monitoring of laboratory data, physical exams, weights, oral intake and output, and physical signs and symptoms is critical when assessing a patient's tolerance to PN. The oncology patient often has multiple comorbidities and medical therapies that can affect tolerance to PN. A trained RDN can proactively manage the oncology patient's nutrition plan of care to prevent complications and optimize patient outcomes on PN. Box 12.9 provides monitoring guidelines for PN.

Complications of Parenteral Nutrition

Acute metabolic complications, such as hypertriglyceridemia and derangements in blood glucose, fluid, and electrolytes, are more common with PN than EN. Long-term complications can also include metabolic derangements, as well as micronutrient toxicities or deficiencies, organ dysfunction, and metabolic bone disease.[52] It is important to consider the contribution of the patient's underlying oncology diagnosis, stage, and metastatic spread, as it can confound laboratory data and physical signs and symptoms. Box 12.10 on pages 245 to 246 summarizes these complications and provides suggestions for their prevention and management.

Parenteral Nutrition in the Home Setting

Indications for home PN are generally the same as those for PN in the hospital, with some additional considerations for the oncology patient and for the home environment. Medicare reimbursement criteria should be met, including a nonfunctional GI tract or failed enteral trials and at least a 90-day need for PN therapy. These conditions must be documented in the medical record, or the patient could face high out-of-pocket costs.[47] Studies show that oncology patients with a high performance status (Karnofsky performance score >50) have improvements in quality of life and a longer survival rate on PN therapy.[47,61] Recent data also suggest that oncology patients on PN who require more than 2 L of fluid per day and more than 60 mmol of potassium per day had significantly decreased survival rates.[63]

Transitioning From Parenteral to Oral or Enteral Nutrition

Oral or enteral nutrition should be attempted when medically appropriate. Even a small dose of oral or enteral nutrition can reduce risk of GI mucosal atrophy and biliary sludge. As oral or enteral intake increases, the patient can be weaned off PN

Box 12.9
Suggested Monitoring of Patients on Parenteral Nutrition[52]

Parameter	At initiation of therapy (acute care)	During long-term therapy
Capillary glucose	Every 6 hours until patient is advanced to parenteral nutrition (PN) goal and as needed to maintain glucose at 140 to 180 mg/dL	Not routine; done as needed to coordinate with PN infusion cycle
Basic metabolic panel, phosphorus, magnesium	Daily, until patient is advanced to PN goal and stable; then one to two times per week	Weekly; then decrease frequency in stable patients
Complete blood count (CBC, with differential)	Baseline; then one to two times per week	Monthly; then decrease frequency in stable patients
Liver function: alanine aminotransferase (ALT), aspartate aminotransferase (AST), total bilirubin, international normalized ratio (INR)	Baseline; then weekly	Monthly; then decrease frequency in stable patients
Serum triglycerides	Baseline if patient is at risk for hypertriglyceridemia; then as needed	Not routine; done as needed
Iron studies, 25-hydroxyvitamin D	Not routine	Baseline; then every 3 to 6 months
Zinc, copper, selenium, manganese	Not routine	Baseline; then every 3 to 6 months
Weight	Daily	Daily
Total fluid intake and output	Daily until stable; then as needed	As needed

Box 12.10
Long-Term Complications From Parenteral Nutrition and Suggestions for Prevention and Management[52,62,63]

Hyperglycemia

Possible causes:	Suggested prevention and management:
Excessive carbohydrate in parenteral nutrition (PN)	Limit carbohydrate dose to 4 to 5 mg/kg of body weight per min, or 20 to 25 kcal/kg of body weight daily until blood glucose stabilizes.
Inadequate insulin dosing Impaired glucose tolerance	Add regular insulin to PN formulation.

Hypoglycemia

Possible causes:	Suggested prevention and management:
Excessive insulin dosing	Reduce subcutaneous insulin or insulin in PN.
Abrupt discontinuation of PN	Taper down PN over 1 to 2 hours prior to discontinuation.

Essential fatty acid deficiency

Possible causes:	Suggested prevention and management:
Inadequate fat in PN	See Table 12.2 for minimum PN fat requirements. Recommend a trial of topical skin application or oral ingestion of oils if PN fat is not tolerated.

Immunosupression

Possible causes:	Suggested prevention and management:
Soy-based intravenous (IV) lipid emulsions	Use alternative IV lipid formulations. Limit IV lipids in critically ill patients during the first week of PN therapy.
Overfeeding	Avoid overfeeding, particularly of dextrose.

(continued)

Box 12.10

Long-Term Complications From Parenteral Nutrition and Suggestions for Prevention and Management[52,62,63] *(continued)*

Hypertriglyceridemia

Possible causes:	Suggested prevention and management:
Dextrose overfeeding	See Table 12.2 for appropriate carbohydrate dosing.
Rapid infusion rate of IV lipid	Limit IV lipid infusion rate to less than 0.11 g/kg of body weight per hour.
	Limit daily IV lipid dose to less than 30% of total energy intake or 1 g/kg of body weight.
	Reduce dose of, or discontinue, IV lipid if serum triglycerides less than 400 mg/dL.

Azotemia

Possible causes:	Suggested prevention and management:
Excessive protein administration	Reduce amino acid dose.
Dehydration	Ensure adequate fluid in PN or provide additional IV fluids if needed.
Inadequate energy from nonprotein sources	Provide adequate nonprotein energy in PN.

Electrolyte derangements

Possible causes:	Suggested prevention and management:
Extrarenal losses from the following: ostomies; decompressing gastrostomy tubes; peritoneal, biliary, pancreatic, or pleural drains; nausea and vomiting	Replace renal or extrarenal fluid and electrolyte losses.
Renal losses from chemotherapeutic regimens	With SIADH, restrict fluid; consider increasing sodium concentration in PN.
Syndrome of inappropriate antidiuretic hormone (SIADH)	
Metabolic alkalosis	Adjust chloride-to-acetate ratio in PN.
Metabolic acidosis	
Refeeding syndrome	Limit dextrose when initiating PN; replete electrolytes separately from PN solution.

(continued)

Box 12.10
Long-Term Complications From Parenteral Nutrition and Suggestions for Prevention and Management[52,62,63] *(continued)*

Vitamin and mineral toxicities and deficiencies

Possible causes:	Suggested prevention and management[a]:
Excessive or inadequate dose in PN	Consider reducing the frequency of fat-soluble vitamin administration to twice weekly in patients with renal failure to avoid vitamin A toxicity.
	Empiric removal of manganese and copper during cholestasis.
	Periodic IV iron or blood transfusion for iron-deficient patients.
	Oral vitamin D supplementation, if tolerated.

Steatosis (hepatic fat accumulation)

Possible causes:	Suggested prevention and management:
Normal rise in aspartate aminotransferase (AST) and alanine aminotransferase (ALT) levels during the first 2 weeks of PN therapy	Monitor liver function tests (LFTs); serum values may normalize after 2 weeks on PN.
Overfeeding	Limit total energy intake and carbohydrates.

Cholestasis (impaired biliary secretion; total bilirubin >2 mg/dL)

Possible causes:	Suggested prevention and management:
Sepsis Ileal disease or resection Small intestinal bacterial overgrowth Malignant disease	Assess for and treat underlying contributing medical conditions.
Loss of enteric stimulation Short bowel syndrome	Encourage enteral intake or trickle tube feeding, as possible.
Duration of PN	Cycle PN over 12 to 16 hours.

Gallbladder sludge or stones

Possible causes:	Suggested prevention and management:
Impaired bile flow Lack of enteric stimulation	Encourage enteral intake or trickle tube feeding, as possible.

[a] See Box 12.9 for laboratory monitoring suggestions.

Box 12.10
Long-Term Complications From Parenteral Nutrition and Suggestions for Prevention and Management[52,62,63] *(continued)*

Metabolic bone disease

Possible causes:	Suggested prevention and management:
Vitamin D deficiency	Oral vitamin D repletion with ergocalciferol or cholecalciferol, if able.
	Encourage weight-bearing exercise, reduction in caffeine and alcohol intake, and smoking avoidance.
	Consider endocrinology referral for pharmacological management.
Inadequate calcium dosing or excessive urinary calcium losses	Provide 1 to 15 mEq of calcium gluconate in PN formulation.
	Avoid excessive protein in PN.
	Provide 20 to 40 mmol of phosphorus in PN.
	Maintain adequate magnesium and copper intake.
Chronic metabolic acidosis	Increase acetate to chloride ratio in PN.
Aluminum toxicity	Minimize aluminum contamination.

therapy. Once the patient is meeting 60% of his or her nutrition needs by the oral or enteral route, PN therapy can be safely discontinued.[64]

Nutrition Support in Palliative Care and End of Life

Palliative care is meant to improve pain and manage symptoms, and it can be provided in tandem with the oncology patient's cancer treatment. Hospice care is intended to provide comfort in place of treating the patient's disease. Financial coverage for PN varies among hospice providers. Nutrition support should be provided when it can improve the quality or quantity of life. However, it can contribute to medical complications and increase the burden on the patient at the end of life.[65] Further discussion is provided in Chapter 26.

References

1. Vigano A, Watanabe S, Bruera E. Anorexia and cachexia in advanced cancer patients. *Cancer Surv.* 1994;21:99-115.

2. Hébuterne X, Lemarié E, Michallet M, De Montreuil CB, Schneider SM, Goldwasser F. Prevalence of malnutrition and current use of nutrition support in patients with cancer. *JPEN J Parenter Enter Nutr.* 2014;38(2):196-204.

3. National Cancer Institute. Nutrition in cancer care (PDQ)–health professional version. Published 2017. Accessed November 22, 2017. https://cancer.gov/about-cancer/treatment/side-effects/appetite-loss/nutrition-hp-pdq

4. Bossola M, Pacelli F, Rosa F, Tortorelli A, Battista Doglietto G. Does nutrition support stimulate tumor growth in humans? *Nutr Clin Pract.* 2011;26(2):174-180.

5. Doley J, Phillips W. Overview of enteral nutrition. In: Mueller C, ed. *The ASPEN Adult Nutrition Support Core Curriculum.* 3rd ed. American Society for Parenteral and Enteral Nutrition; 2017: 213-226.

6. August D, Huhmann M, ASPEN Board of Directors. ASPEN clinical guidelines: nutrition support therapy during adult anticancer treatment and in hematopoietic cell transplantation. *JPEN J Parenter Enter Nutr.* 2009;33(5):472-500.

7. Bozzetti F, Arends J, Lundholm K, Micklewright A, Zurcher G, Muscaritoli M. ESPEN guidelines on parenteral nutrition: non-surgical oncology. *Clin Nutr.* 2009;28(4):445-454.

8. Braga M, Ljungqvist O, Soeters P, Fearson K, Weimann A. ESPEN guidelines on PN: surgery. *Clin Nutr.* 2009;28(4):378-386.

9. Huhmann MB, August DA. Perioperative nutrition support in cancer patients. *Nutr Clin Pract.* 2012;27(5):586-592.

10. Arends J, Bachmann P, Baracos V, et al. ESPEN guidelines on nutrition in cancer patients. *Clin Nutr.* 2017;36(1):11-48.

11. Barrett M, Demehri FR, Teitelbaum DH. Intestine, immunity, and parenteral nutrition in an era of preferred enteral feeding. *Curr Opin Clin Nutr Metab Care.* 2015;18(5):496-500.

12. Marian M, Mattox T, Williams V. Cancer. In: Mueller C, ed. *The ASPEN Adult Nutrition Support Core Curriculum.* 3rd ed. American Society for Parenteral and Enteral Nutrition; 2017:651-674.

13. McClave SA, Taylor BE, Martindale RG, et al. Guidelines for the provision and assessment of nutrition support therapy in the adult critically ill patient: Society of Critical Care Medicine (SCCM) and American Society for Parenteral and Enteral Nutrition (ASPEN). *JPEN J Parenter Enter Nutr.* 2016;40(2):159-211.

14. Merritt R. *The ASPEN Nutrition Support Practice Manual.* 2nd ed. American Society for Parenteral and Enteral Nutrition; 2005.

15. Boullata JI, Carrera AL, Harvey L, et al. ASPEN safe practices for enteral nutrition therapy. *JPEN J Parenter Enter Nutr.* 2017;41(1):15-103.

16. Academy of Nutrition and Dietetics. Nutrition Care Manual Formulary. Nutrition Care Manual website. Accessed September 2, 2020. www.nutritioncaremanual.org/formulary.cfm?ncm_category_id=16&ncm_heading

17. Krenitsky J. Gastric versus jejunal feeding: evidence or emotion? *Pract Gastroenterol.* 2006;42: 46-55.

18. Durfee SM, Adams SC, Arthur E, et al. ASPEN standards for nutrition support: home and alternate site care. *Nutr Clin Pract.* 2014;29(4):542-555.

19. Borghi R, et al. ILSI Task Force on enteral nutrition; estimated composition and costs of blenderized diets. *Nutr Hosp.* 2013;28(6):2033-2038.

20. Fessler T. Blenderized foods for home tube feeding: learn about the benefits, risks, and strategies for success. *Today's Dietitian.* 2015;17(1):30.

21. Escuro A. Blenderized tube feeding: suggested guidelines to clinicians. *Pract Gastroenterol.* Dec 2014;58-66.

22. Medicine Nutrition Support Team, University of Virginia Health System. Blenderized tube feeding recipes. University of Virginia School of Medicine website. Accessed September 2, 2020. https://med.virginia.edu/ginutrition/wp-content/uploads/sites/199/2014/06/BLENDERIZED_TUBE_FEEDING.pdf

23. US Department of Agriculture. MyPlate Plan. MyPlate website. Published 2018. Accessed September 2, 2020. https://myplate.gov/MyPlatePlan

24. Abbott Nutrition. *Best Practices for Managing Tube Feeding: A Nurse's Pocket Manual.* Abbott Laboratories; 2015. Accessed September 2, 2020. https://static.abbottnutrition.com/cms-prod/abbottnutrition-2016.com/img/M4619.005%Tube%Feeding%manual_tcm1411-57873.pdf

25. Bankhead R, Boullata J, Brantley S, et al. Enteral nutrition practice recommendations. *JPEN J Parenter Enteral Nutr.* 2009;33(2):122-167.

26. Boullata J, Carney L, Guenter P. *ASPEN Enteral Nutrition Handbook.* American Society for Parenteral and Enteral Nutrition; 2010.

27. Marinella MA. Refeeding syndrome: an important aspect of supportive oncology. *J Support Oncol.* 2009;7(1):11-16.

28. Mccray S, Parrish CR. Refeeding the malnourished patient: lessons learned. *Pract Gastroenterol.* 2016;40(9):56-66.

29. Parrish C, McCray S. Enteral feeding: dispelling myths. *Nutr Issues Pract Gastroenterol.* 2003;27(9):33-50.

30. Kraft MD, Btaiche IF, Sacks GS. Review of the refeeding syndrome. *Nutr Clin Pract.* 2005;20(6):625-633.

31. Cohn JN, Kowey PR, Whelton PK, Prisant LM. New guidelines for potassium replacement in clinical practice: a contemporary review by the National Council on Potassium in Clinical Practice. *Arch Intern Med.* 2000;160(16):2429-2436.

32. Malone A, Seres D, Lord L. Complications of enteral nutrition. In: Mueller C, ed. *The ASPEN Adult Nutrition Support Core Curriculum.* 3rd ed. American Society for Parenteral and Enteral Nutrition; 2017:265-283.

33. Fisher C, Blalock B. Clogged feeding tubes: a clinician's thorn. *Pract Gastroenterol.* 2014:38(3):16-22.

34. Charney P, Malone A, eds. *Academy of Nutrition and Dietetics Pocket Guide to Enteral Nutrition.* 2nd ed. Academy of Nutrition and Dietetics; 2013.

35. Beckwith MC, Feddema SS, Barton RG, Graves C. A guide to drug therapy in patients with enteral feeding tubes: dosage form selection and administration methods. *Hosp Pharm.* 2004;39(3):225–237.

36. Oral dosage forms that should not be crushed. Institute for Safe Medication Practices website. Published 2020. Accessed September 2, 2020. https://ismp.org/recommendations/do-not-crush

37. Enteral Parenteral Nutrition Support Committee. *Guidelines for the Administration of Drugs via Enteral Feeding Tubes.* Midlands Regional Hospital at Tullamore; 2009. Accessed September 2, 2020. https://scribd.com/doc/98100059/Guidelines-for-the-Adminstration-of-Drugs-via-Enteral-Feeding-Tubes

38. Ferrie S, Graham C, Hoyle M. Pancreatic enzyme supplementation for patients receiving enteral feeds. *Nutr Clin Pract.* 2011;26(3):349-351.

39. Russell, MK. Complications of enteral feedings. In: Charney P, Malone A, eds. *Pocket Guide to Enteral Nutrition.* 2nd ed. Academy of Nutrition and Dietetics; 2013:170-197.

40. GEDSA. PowerPoint slide show presented at: ENFit Advocacy Meeting; July 26, 2017; StayConnected website. Accessed September 2, 2020. http://stayconnected.org/wp-content/uploads/2017/08/ENFit-Advocacy-Meeting-uploadv2.pdf

41. Mundi MS. Prevalence of home parenteral and enteral nutrition in the United States. *Nutr Clin Pract.* 2017;32(6):799-805.

42. Konrad D, Mitchell R, Hendrickson E. Home nutrition support. In: Mueller C, ed. *The ASPEN Adult Nutrition Support Core Curriculum.* 3rd ed. American Society for Parenteral and Enteral Nutrition; 2017: 765-784.

43. National Coverage Determination (NCD) for Enteral and Parenteral Nutritional Therapy (180.2). Medicare Coverage Database. US Centers for Medicare and Medicaid Services; 2018. Accessed September 2, 2020. www.cms.gov/medicare-coverage-database/details/ncd details.aspx?NCDId=242&ncdver=1&DocID=180.2&SearchType=Advanced&bc=IAAAABAAAAAA&

44. Ojo O. The challenges of home enteral tube feeding: a global perspective. *Nutrients.* 2015;7(4):2524-2538.

45. Newton A, Barnadas G. Understanding Medicare coverage for home enteral nutrition: a case-based approach. *Pract Gastroenterol.* 2013;37: 10-24.

46. *Medicare Part B General Coverage Guidelines for Enteral Nutrition.* Nestlé Health Science; 2015. Accessed September 2, 2020. https://nestlehealthscience.us/asset-library/documents/reimbursement/medicare%part%b%guidelines%for%enteral%nutrition.pdf

47. Mirtallo J. Overview of parenteral nutrition. In: Mueller C, ed. *The ASPEN Adult Nutrition Support Core Curriculum.* 3rd ed. American Society for Parenteral and Enteral Nutrition; 2017:285-296.

48. Mirtallo J, Canada T, Johnson D, et al. Special report: safe practices for parenteral nutrition formulations. *JPEN J Parenter Enteral Nutr.* 2004;28(6):S39-S70.

49. Santacruz E, Mateo-Lobo R, Riveiro J, et al. Infectious complications in home parenteral nutrition: a long-term study with peripherally inserted central catheters, tunneled catheters, and ports. *Nutrition.* 2019;58:89-93.

50. Neal A, Drogan K. Parenteral access devices. In: Mueller C, ed. *The ASPEN Adult Nutrition Support Core Curriculum.* 3rd ed. American Society for Parenteral and Enteral Nutrition; 2017: 321-344.

51. Patel R. Parenteral nutrition formulations. In: Mueller C, ed. *The ASPEN Adult Nutrition Support Core Curriculum.* 3rd ed. American Society for Parenteral and Enteral Nutrition; 2017: 297-320.

52. Kumpf V, Gervasio J. Complications of parenteral nutrition. In: Mueller C, ed. *The ASPEN Adult Nutrition Support Core Curriculum.* 3rd ed. American Society for Parenteral and Enteral Nutrition; 2017: 345-360.

53. McDowe K, Ling P. Carbohydrates. In: Mueller C, ed. *The ASPEN Adult Nutrition Support Core Curriculum.* 3rd ed. American Society for Parenteral and Enteral Nutrition; 2017:41-55.

54. Mundi MS, Martindale RG, Hurt RT. Emergence of mixed-oil fat emulsions for use in parenteral nutrition. *JPEN J Parenter Enter Nutr.* 2017;41(1 suppl):3S-13S.

55. Smoflipid Package insert. Fresenius Kabi USA, LLC; 2016.

56. Vitamin E: fact sheet for professionals. Office of Dietary Supplements website. Updated July 31, 2020. September 2, 2020. https://ods.od.nih.gov/factsheets/VitaminE-HealthProfessional

57. Nakayama A, Alladin KP, Igbokwe O, White JD. Systematic review: generating evidence-based guidelines on the concurrent use of dietary antioxidants and chemotherapy or radiotherapy. *Cancer Invest.* 2011;29(10):655-667.

58. Hwa YL, Rashtak S, Kelly DG, Murray JA. Iron deficiency in long-term parenteral nutrition therapy. *JPEN J Parenter Enter Nutr.* 2016;40(6):869-876.

59. Canada T, Crill CM, Guenter P. Medication issues. In: Ayers P, Guenter P, Holcombe B, Plogsted S, eds. *ASPEN Parenteral Nutrition Handbook.* 2nd ed. American Society for Parenteral and Enteral Nutrition; 2014: 234-252.

60. Mantovani G, Madeddu C. Cancer cachexia: medical management. *Support Care Cancer.* 2010;18(1):1-9.

61. Canada T, Lord L. Fluids, electrolytes, and acid-base disorders. In: Mueller C, ed. *The ASPEN Adult Nutrition Support Core Curriculum.* 3rd ed. American Society for Parenteral and Enteral Nutrition; 2017: 113-137.

62. Keane N, Fragkos KC, Patel PS, et al. Performance status, prognostic scoring, and parenteral nutrition requirements predict survival in patients with advanced cancer receiving home parenteral nutrition. *Nutr Cancer.* 2018;70(1):73-82.

63. Lee V. Liver dysfunction associated with parenteral nutrition: What are the options? *Pract Gastroenterol.* 2006;30(12):49.

64. Canada T, Crill CM, Guenter P. Parenteral nutrition administration and monitoring. In: *ASPEN Parenteral Nutrition Handbook.* American Society for Parenteral and Enteral Nutrition; 2009:185-196.

65. Schwartz D, Barrocas A. Ethics and law. In: Mueller C, ed. *The ASPEN Adult Nutrition Support Core Curriculum.* 3rd ed. American Society for Parenteral and Enteral Nutrition; 2017: 785-804.

Chapter 13
Nutritional Management of the Pediatric Oncology Patient

Rachel Hill, RD, CSO, LD, CNSC

Nancy Sacks, MS, RD, LDN

Karen Ringwald-Smith, MS, RDN, LDN, FAND

Jennifer Caceres, MS, RD, CSP, LDN

Cancer is the leading cause of disease-related death in children aged 0 to 14 years in the United States.[1] Due to major advances in treatment of childhood cancers, 84% of children with cancer now survive 5 years or more, although survival rates can vary depending on the type of cancer and other factors.[2,3] For the year 2018, experts estimated that cancer would be diagnosed in 15,590 children and adolescents aged 0 to 19 years and that 1,925 children and adolescents would die from the disease.[4] Figure 13.1 illustrates the prevalence of various childhood cancers.

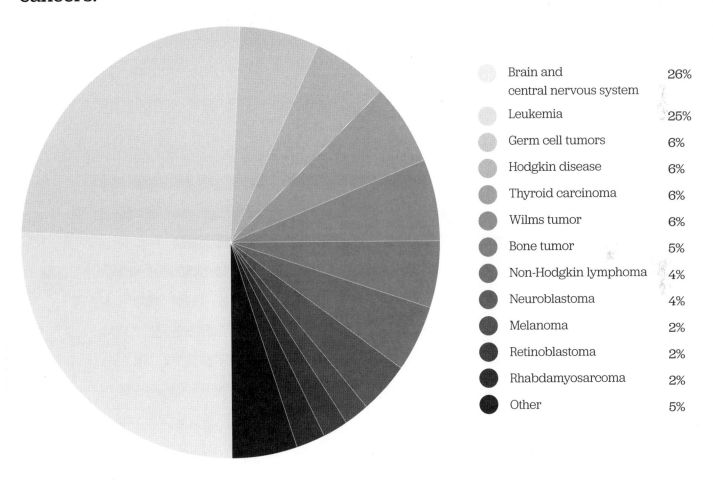

Brain and central nervous system	26%
Leukemia	25%
Germ cell tumors	6%
Hodgkin disease	6%
Thyroid carcinoma	6%
Wilms tumor	6%
Bone tumor	5%
Non-Hodgkin lymphoma	4%
Neuroblastoma	4%
Melanoma	2%
Retinoblastoma	2%
Rhabdamyosarcoma	2%
Other	5%

Figure 13.1
Distribution of childhood cancer diagnoses per year, United States

Based on a total of 15,590 childhood cancer diagnoses in children aged 0 to 19 years.

Adapted from Childhood cancer statistics. CureSearch for Children's Cancer website. Accessed September 14, 2020. https://curesearch.org/Childhood-Cancer-Statistic. See reference 4.

In 2017, there were approximately 465,000 survivors of childhood cancer (all persons in whom the disease was diagnosed at 0 to 19 years of age) in the United States.[5] The number of survivors continues to increase because both incidence and survival rates are increasing.[1,2] Figure 13.2 shows survival percentages for various diagnoses.[4]

Proper nutrition is essential for childhood growth and development. During oncology treatment, children are at greater risk than adults for malnutrition due to increased metabolic demands per kilogram of body weight and the need to maintain appropriate weight gain and linear growth throughout treatment. Cancer and its treatment often result in side effects that adversely affect nutritional status.[6,7] Lengthy treatment plans during crucial periods of a child's growth and development are particularly problematic, especially in young children and infants whose brains are rapidly developing.[7,8] This chapter reviews common pediatric cancer diagnoses, the impact of malnutrition on children with cancer, nutrition screening and assessment, and common nutrition interventions.

Childhood Cancers and Nutrition Side Effects

Comprehensive recommendations for the treatment of pediatric cancers are available from the Children's Oncology Group and the National Cancer Institute (see Box 13.1). Consult those recommendations for details regarding specific therapies. In the sections that follow, the side effects and nutrition impact symptoms (NIS) of various childhood cancers and their treatments are examined.

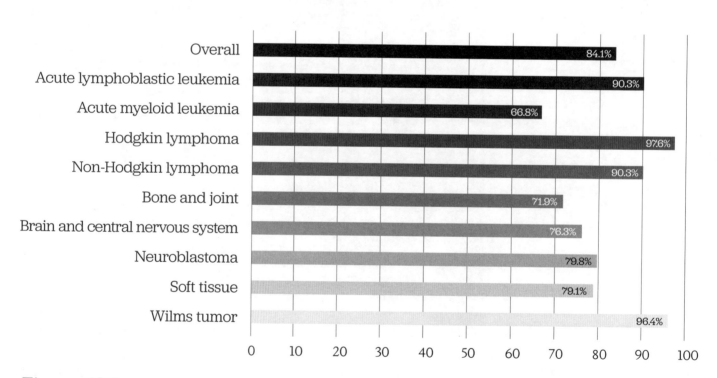

Figure 13.2

Percentage survival in childhood cancer patients by diagnosis, ages 0 to 19

Adapted from Childhood cancer statistics. CureSearch for Children's Cancer website. https://curesearch.org/Childhood-Cancer-Statistics. See reference 4.

Box 13.1

Childhood Cancer Resources

The Children's Oncology Group (COG). Patients and Families: COG Clinical Trial Summaries. https://childrensoncologygroup.org/index.php/patients-and-families

National Cancer Institute at the National Institutes of Health. Childhood Cancers. Treating Cancers. https://cancer.gov/types/childhood-cancers

Alphabetical List of PDQ Pediatric Cancer Treatment Summaries. https://cancer.gov/publications/pdq/information-summaries/pediatric-treatment

Acute Lymphoblastic Leukemia

Acute lymphoblastic leukemia (ALL) is a cancer of the blood and bone marrow; it is the most common childhood malignancy.[9] Malnutrition during therapy can affect disease response, infection risk, toxicities, and treatment delays. Box 13.2 on page 254 lists several of the most common nutrition-related side effects and NIS—and the associated drugs—for different treatment phases.[10]

Patients with ALL are at risk for developing obesity during the maintenance and continuation phases of treatment,[11] but this may be preventable. Studies indicate that early and regular intervention by a registered dietitian nutritionist (RDN) is essential for success.[12,13] Reduced bone mineral density may also be caused by treatment. Early relapses or refractory ALL may require hematopoietic cell transplantation (HCT) (see Chapter 15).[9]

Acute Myeloid Leukemia

Acute myeloid leukemia (AML) is the second most common type of childhood leukemia. It is treated initially with chemotherapy, but patients with high risk or relapsed disease may undergo HCT.[14]

Nutritional status at the time of diagnosis affects outcome. Patients with an unhealthy weight at the time of diagnosis, as indicated by a body mass index (BMI) below the 5th percentile or above the 85th percentile, have lower survival rates, often as a result of infection.[15] Patients with AML are particularly prone to anorexia, weight loss, nausea, vomiting, mucositis, and malnutrition due to the intensive chemotherapy regimen,[10] and they should be monitored closely and receive prompt intervention. Cardiomyopathy is a common late effect of treatment.[14]

Central Nervous System Tumors

Primary brain tumors may be benign or malignant. Box 13.3 on pages 255 to 256 provides an overview of pediatric central nervous system (CNS) tumors and corresponding nutritional considerations.[16-18]

Dysphagia is a potential complication for patients with posterior fossa brain tumors following tumor resection and for those with progressive disease that affects the cerebellum and brainstem areas.[19] At-risk patients should be evaluated by a speech therapist.

Long-term complications may include cognitive and motor-skill deficits, weight gain, central adiposity, or feeding difficulties.[20] Radiotherapy may disrupt ghrelin and leptin cues, causing excessive energy intake.[21] Central adiposity and fat mass are correlated with increased risk for cardiovascular complications.[22]

Hodgkin Lymphoma

Lymphoma is the third most common childhood cancer diagnosis. It is divided into two subgroups: Hodgkin lymphoma and non-Hodgkin lymphoma. Significant weight loss may be a presenting symptom in Hodgkin lymphoma and non-Hodgkin lymphoma.[23] Excellent supportive care during therapy for Hodgkin lymphoma often mitigates malnutrition risk; however, frequent steroid use may lead to unintentional weight gain.

Box 13.2
Acute Lymphoblastic Leukemia: Treatment Phases, Chemotherapy, and Side Effects[10,24]

Treatment phase	Chemotherapy (route)	Common nutrition-related side effects[a]
Remission induction	Vincristine (intavenous, IV) Steroids (oral) Asparaginase (IV) Daunorubicin (IV) Cytarabine (intrathecal, IT)	Constipation, jaw pain Increased appetite, weight gain Drug-induced hyperglycemia, pancreatitis,[b] anorexia, nausea and vomiting, mucositis
Consolidation	Cyclophosphamide (IV) Cytarabine (IV and/or IT) Mercaptopurine (oral) Vincristine (IV) Pegasparaginase (IV) Methotrexate (IT)	Anorexia Nausea and vomiting Mouth sores Constipation, jaw pain Pancreatitis
Interim maintenance	Methotrexate (IV, high-dose) Methotrexate (IT) Vincristine (IV) Mercaptopurine (oral)	Mucositis and mouth sores Decreased appetite Constipation, jaw pain
Delayed intensification	Vincristine (IV) Steroids (oral) Doxorubicin (IV) Methotrexate (IT) Pegasparaginase (IV) Cyclophosphamide (IV) Cytarabine (IV and/or IT) Thioguanine	Constipation, jaw pain Increased appetite, weight gain Anorexia, mucositis Drug-induced hyperglycemia Pancreatitis Nausea and vomiting
Maintenance and continuation	Steroids (oral) Mercaptopurine (low-dose, oral) Methotrexate (low-dose, oral or IT) Vincristine (IV)	Increased appetite, weight gain

[a] This is not a comprehensive list. Please see Chapter 9 for more details.

[b] Pancreatitis is commonly caused by asparaginase; steroids and 6-mercaptopurine also may contribute. Risk factors include age >10 years and prior history of pancreatitis. See reference 24.

Box 13.3
Categories of Central Nervous System Tumors and Nutritional Considerations[17-19]

Astrocytoma

Possible tumor site:
Any area of the central nervous system (CNS)

Nutritional considerations:
Anorexia due to chemotherapy and radiotherapy

Medical treatment options:
New (low-grade): Surgery and observation; occasionally chemotherapy

Recurrent or progressive (low-grade): Chemotherapy (typically carboplatin-based or vinblastine), radiotherapy, or both

New (high-grade): Surgery with chemotherapy, radiotherapy, or both

Recurrent (high-grade): Palliative care; also surgery, high-dose chemotherapy, targeted therapy, and sometimes radiotherapy in unique cases

Brainstem glioma

Possible tumor site:
Diffuse intrinsic pontine glioma (DIPG): pons; focal lesions: usually medulla or midbrain

Nutritional considerations:
Difficulty chewing or swallowing and rapid weight gain with steroids

Medical treatment options:
New (DIPG): Radiation; chemotherapy (only for infants)

Recurrent: Palliative care; sometimes repeat radiotherapy

New and recurrent (focal lesions): Surgery, with or without chemotherapy or radiotherapy (or both); observation; targeted therapy

Embryonal tumor: atypical teratoid/rhabdoid tumor

Possible tumor site:
Anywhere in the CNS, but most commonly posterior fossa (in about half of cases)

Nutritional considerations:
Taste changes and anorexia.

Medical treatment options:
New: Surgery, radiotherapy, aggressive multiagent chemotherapy, high-dose chemotherapy with stem cell rescue

Recurrent: Palliative care; no standard

Embryonal tumor: medulloblastoma

Possible tumor site:
Posterior fossa; malignant tumor with rapid growth and potential for metastasis within the CNS

Nutritional considerations:
Dysphagia and anorexia

Medical treatment options:
New: Surgery with chemotherapy and radiotherapy

Recurrent: Palliative care; no standard; involves same as with new diagnosis, possibly high-dose chemotherapy with stem cell rescue

(continued)

Though overall survival nears 95%, late effects of treatment pose significant risks for survivors.[24] Mediastinal radiation can cause abnormal thyroid, heart, and lung function; anthracyclines further increase cardiovascular risks.[24] Survivors also have an increased risk for secondary cancers: most commonly breast, thyroid, and skin cancers.[24] In addition, childhood lymphoma survivors may have decreased lean body mass and increased body fat after treatment.[25]

Non-Hodgkin Lymphoma

Non-Hodgkin lymphoma (NHL) encompasses all childhood lymphomas that are not Hodgkin lymphoma. The four most common subtypes are precursor lymphoblastic lymphoma, Burkitt or Burkitt-like lymphoma, diffuse large B-cell lymphoma, and anaplastic large cell lymphoma.[26]

Common NIS include nausea, vomiting, anorexia, and constipation.[10] Fluid retention and hyperglycemia may result from steroid use. Mucositis and diarrhea are less common but can significantly affect nutritional status if they occur.[10] Due to the increased risk for NIS during NHL treatment, patients with NHL should be monitored closely throughout treatment and provided with intervention to alleviate symptoms and prevent malnutrition when possible.

Survivors of NHL are at risk for anthracycline-induced cardiomyopathy and secondary malignancies.[26] Obesity, hypertension, impaired mobility, and reduced strength also are potential posttreatment effects.[27]

Neuroblastoma

Neuroblastoma is the most common solid tumor in children and is often diagnosed in the first year of life.[28,29] Neuroblastoma commonly arises from cells in the sympathetic nervous system. Infants less than 6 months of age often present with the lowest-risk disease, and many of these patients are simply observed. Older children often present with more aggressive and often metastatic disease at the time of diagnosis, and intensive treatment is required; this often includes myeloablative chemotherapy with subsequent allogeneic stem cell rescue.[30]

Malnutrition at the time of diagnosis has been reported in as many as 20% to 50% of cases.[31] This often persists throughout treatment due to the acute NIS that are often associated with neuroblastoma treatment, including nausea, vomiting, taste changes, anorexia, and abdominal discomfort. However, literature has established that this risk is not the result of increases in energy expenditure at the time of diagnosis or during treatment.[32] Late effects may include underweight status, decreased growth and development (after HCT), musculoskeletal complications, neurological complications, and endocrine complications.[33]

Rhabdomyosarcoma

Rhabdomyosarcoma is a soft tissue tumor. It often occurs in the head and neck area, genitourinary tract, extremities, and occasionally in the trunk.[34] Short-term treatment effects may include anorexia, constipation, and jaw pain.[10] Patients with high-risk disease (such as metastatic or alveolar subtype) may undergo more intensive therapy and be at greater risk for developing malnutrition.[34]

Late effects may include small bowel obstruction, esophageal strictures, renal tubular dysfunction, and secondary malignancies. Radiotherapy to the head and neck may result in dental problems and growth hormone deficiency. Lower-risk patients may be given lower doses of radiation and certain chemotherapy agents to decrease secondary cancer risk.[34]

Wilms Tumor

Wilms tumor is the most common kidney malignancy in children. Patients often present with a large abdominal mass and sometimes with hypertension.[35] Malnutrition at the time of diagnosis may be caused by anorexia and early satiety from the growing tumor. Mid-upper arm circumference (MUAC) may provide a better assessment of malnutrition risk than weight or BMI alone, due to tumor weight.[36-38]

Surgery, chemotherapy, and sometimes radiotherapy (for higher-risk disease) are used to treat Wilms tumor.[35] Side effects of Wilms tumor chemotherapy include constipation, jaw pain, nausea, vomiting, and anorexia.[10] Whole abdomen or flank radiotherapy may increase risk for radiation enteritis.[35] Late effects of treatment may include cardiotoxicity and secondary malignancies. End-stage renal disease occurs occasionally in patients with bilateral disease.[35]

Osteosarcoma

Osteosarcoma is the most common bone tumor in pediatric patients. It typically occurs in the extremities during periods of rapid growth. Pain is the most common presenting symptom. Treatment includes chemotherapy and complete resection, if possible. Surgery may involve amputation or limb-salvage surgery; the latter may aid in preserving functional status.[39] Common NIS of chemotherapy for osteosarcoma include nausea, vomiting, anorexia, hypomagnesemia, metallic taste changes, and mucositis.[10] Malnutrition is exacerbated by treatment, with the incidence of underweight status increasing from 7.8% at the time of diagnosis to 36.1% a year later.[40] Common late effects include cardiotoxicity and nephrotoxicity.[39]

Ewing Sarcoma

Ewing sarcoma is the second most common bone tumor in children and adolescents. Although it can occur in almost any bone or soft tissue, it most often presents in the lower extremities, pelvis, and chest wall.[41] A small, retrospective study demonstrated that an abnormal BMI at the time of diagnosis (whether the patient is underweight, overweight, or obese) is associated with poorer response at the time of surgical resection,[42] which is prognostically significant.[41] Progressive malnutrition during treatment may result in an underweight status increasing from 12.9% at time of diagnosis to 31.6% a year later.[40]

Treatment includes chemotherapy and either surgery or radiation for local control.[41] The NIS of chemotherapy include nausea, vomiting, anorexia, and weight loss.[10] Surgery and radiotherapy may significantly affect functional status, mobility, and growth. Pelvic radiation may cause enteritis, obstruction, or perforation.[41]

Hepatoblastoma

Hepatoblastoma is the most common liver malignancy in children, usually occurring before age 3 years. Risk factors include prematurity (birth wt <1,500 g) and familial cancer syndromes.[43] Malnutrition at the time of diagnosis may be related to anorexia caused by the abdominal tumor growth. MUAC measurements can be useful in identifying malnutrition, which may be masked by a normal weight due to the added weight of the tumor.[36,44]

Treatment for hepatoblastoma includes chemotherapy and complete resection, if possible.[43] Chemotherapy for hepatoblastoma may cause anorexia, nausea, vomiting, mucositis, diarrhea, renal toxicity, and electrolyte wasting.[10]

Selected Novel Therapies and Associated Nutrition Side Effects

Chimeric antigen receptor (CAR) T-cell therapy was approved for the treatment of children and adolescents with relapsed or refractory B-cell ALL.[45] Infusion of CAR T-cells can cause cytokine release syndrome, which can include fever, nausea, vomiting, vascular leakage, renal complications, and seizures.[46]

Hyperthermic intraperitoneal chemotherapy (HIPEC) is an approach to treating extensive peritoneal disease and involves administering heated chemotherapy agents directly into the peritoneal cavity.[47] A retrospective study of the first 50 HIPEC procedures suggested that HIPEC may be most effective for patients with desmoplastic small round-cell tumors.[48] Postoperatively, patients may require enteral nutrition (EN) or parenteral nutrition (PN) support because of the difficulty of feeding after extensive debulking surgery[49,50]; occasionally, a feeding tube is placed at the time of the procedure.[51]

Malnutrition Prevalence and Outcomes in Childhood Cancer

Children with cancer are prone to nutritional status disturbances. Malnutrition is reported to occur in 5% to 21.5% of patients at the time of cancer diagnosis, and those with solid tumors are at the greatest risk.[52,53] During treatment, malnutrition incidence increases to 65%.[54] Malnutrition and obesity at diagnosis and throughout treatment are associated with poorer survival.[16,54-57] Additionally, malnutrition is associated with increased treatment toxicity, increased infection risk, loss of lean body mass, decreased functional status, and poorer quality of life.[55-61]

A systematic review suggests that obesity affects between 8% to 78% of childhood cancer patients.[54] Despite the ambiguity of this large range, it is obvious from the literature that obesity in children with cancer, especially following treatment, warrants significant attention.[12-14,22,62] Moreover, research indicates that childhood cancer patients and survivors of childhood cancer experience significant changes in body composition, namely increased fat mass and decreased lean mass.[58,62-65] This suggests that even patients and survivors with a healthy BMI may be at increased risk for metabolic derangements.

Box 13.4 summarizes risk factors to help identify pediatric oncology patients who are at high nutritional risk due to malnutrition.

Consensus criteria for diagnosing pediatric malnutrition that were developed in 2014 (see Table 13.1 on page 260)[67] can also be used for pediatric patients with cancer. This population is prone to inadequate weight gain and significant weight loss. MUAC may be particularly helpful in identifying malnutrition in children with large solid tumors or significant hepatosplenomegaly.[36,38,44] z Scores are used to express how many standard deviations a child's measurements deviate from the mean (eg, a BMI-for-age z score of less than -1 indicates that a child's BMI z score is less than the mean for age by at least 1 full standard deviation).[68]

Box 13.4
Risk Factors for Malnutrition in Pediatric Patients With Cancer[66]

Low nutritional risk	High nutritional risk
Nonmetastatic tumors	Depletion of body stores at diagnosis
Favorable prognosis at diagnosis	Advanced disease at diagnosis
Advanced diseases in remission during maintenance treatment	Solid tumor with unfavorable histology (eg, Wilms tumor)
	Stages III and IV neuroblastoma, especially with unfavorable biology
	Advanced stage at diagnosis
	Medulloblastoma and other high-grade brain tumors
	Complications after diagnosis
	Acute leukemias during induction
	Multiply relapsed leukemia
	Stem cell transplantation, especially with graft-versus-host disease

---

Table 13.1
Pediatric Malnutrition Consensus Criteria

Primary Indicators When a Single Data Point Is Available			
	Mild malnutrition	Moderate malnutrition	Severe malnutrition
Weight-for-height z score	–1 to –1.9	–2 to –2.9	–3 or less
Body mass index-for-age z score	–1 to –1.9	–2 to –2.9	–3 or less
Length/height-for-age z score	No data	No data	–3 or less
Mid-upper arm circumference z score	–1 to –1.9	–2 to –2.9	–3 or less

Primary Indicators When Two or More Data Points Are Available			
	Mild malnutrition	Moderate malnutrition	Severe malnutrition
Weight gain velocity (<2 years of age)	<75% of expected weight gain for age	<50% of expected weight gain for age	<25% of expected weight gain for age
Weight loss (2-20 years of age)	5% of usual weight	7.5% of usual weight	10% of usual weight
Deceleration in weight-for-length or body mass index z score	Decline of 1 z score	Decline of 2 z score	Decline of 3 z score
Inadequate nutrient intake	51%-75% of estimated energy and protein needs	26%-50% of estimated energy and protein needs	≤25% of estimated energy and protein needs

Adapted with permission from Becker PJ, Nieman Carney L, Corkins MR, et al. *J Acad Nutr Diet.* 2014; 114(12):1988-2000. See reference 67.

Nutrition Screening in Childhood Cancer

Although there is increasing awareness about over- and undernutrition in childhood cancer patients and survivors,[53-55] malnutrition continues to be underrecognized and unmonitored in many pediatric oncology centers.[69-71] Every child diagnosed with cancer should be screened for malnutrition and receive a nutrition assessment at diagnosis, along with a periodic reassessment of nutritional status during and after treatment.[60]

Early identification is essential for the prevention of malnutrition and its complications during cancer treatment. Currently, only one validated tool exists for identifying children at the greatest risk for malnutrition: the nutrition screening tool for childhood cancer (SCAN).[72] Using a quick and simple process, SCAN helps clinicians identify patients who are currently undernourished, or are at high risk for becoming malnourished, based on their current nutritional status and symptoms (see Figure 13.3).

Nutrition Screening Tool for Childhood Cancer (SCAN)

Question	Points
Does the patient have a high-risk cancer?	1
Is the patient currently undergoing intensive treatment?	1
Does the patient have any symptoms relating to the gastrointestinal tract?	2
Has the patient had poor intake over the past week?	2
Has the patient had any weight loss over the past month?	2
Does the patient show signs of undernutrition?	2
Total	__ / 10

Score indication:
≥3 At risk of malnturiton: Refer to a dietitian for further assessment.

Figure 13.3
Nutrition screening tool for childhood cancer (SCAN) for identifying patients at high risk for malnutrition

Adapted with permission from Murphy AJ, White M, Viani K, Mosby TT. Evaluation of the nutrition screening tool for childhood cancer (SCAN). *Clin Nutr.* 2016;35(1):219-224. doi:10.1016/j.clnu.2015.02.009. See reference 72.

Nutrition Assessment in Childhood Cancer

Once a child is identified as being at high risk for malnutrition, an appropriate assessment should be conducted (see Box 13.5 for suggested assessment parameters), and patient and family education should begin. Although the Pediatric Subjective Global Nutrition Assessment is not specific to pediatric oncology, it has been validated for use in hospitalized pediatric patients.[73-75]

Children With Amputations

Some children with cancer, particularly those with osteosarcoma or Ewing sarcoma,[39,41] may require amputation. When assessing these patients for nutritional status, adjusted values for weight, BMI, and ideal body weight (IBW) should be used. These values are calculated using the equations shown in Box 13.6 on page 265 and the estimated percentages of total body weight lost with each amputation, as provided in Table 13.2.

Estimating Nutrition Requirements

Energy

The best method for determining the energy requirements of pediatric patients with cancer remains controversial, mainly because energy demands vary based on disease, clinical status, treatment intensity, nutritional status, and activity level. Predictive energy equations may overestimate the needs of pediatric oncology patients.[76] In one study in which energy requirements were evaluated using indirect calorimetry (IC) in 16 pediatric cancer patients (50% with solid tumors), researchers found that requirements were not significantly different compared to healthy controls.[77] This study highlights the need for future studies to identify the best method for determining energy needs and identifying factors that may alter

Table 13.2

Estimated Percentage of Total Body Weight of Missing Limbs for Various Amputation Levels[80]

Level of amputation	Estimated percentage of total body weight
Foot	1.30
Below-knee	3.26
Above-knee	9.96
Hemipelvectomy or hip disarticulation	11.83
Shoulder Disarticulation	5.00
Above-elbow	3.55
Below-elbow	1.45
Hand	0.70

energy requirements in this population. RDNs should reassess their patients' energy needs, based on intake and anthropometric trends, regularly.

The gold standard for assessing resting energy expenditure (REE) is IC, when it is available. Because few RDNs will have IC available to use in all patients, the estimated energy requirement (EER) equations can be used (see Table 13.3 on page 265) in its place.[78] RDNs should use their clinical judgment to adjust EER based on a patient's individual clinical and nutritional status, as well as on physical activity (see Table 13.4 on page 265).

In critically ill patients, the World Health Organization equation for REE can be used to estimate energy needs (see Table 13.5, on page 266).[79-81] The REE represents the energy needed to sustain vital organ function, and it should be adjusted by stress factors, as needed. RDNs should closely monitor acutely ill pediatric oncology patients and reassess their energy needs (such as with changes

Box 13.5
Recommended Assessment Parameters for Pediatric Oncology Patients[7,66,67,82-84]

Anthropometric measurements

For patients with amputations, calculate adjusted weight (see the section on amputations in this chapter).

Growth charts	Use the 2006 World Health Organization growth charts[a] (0 to 24 months) and the 2000 Centers for Disease Control and Prevention growth charts (2 to 20 years).[b]
Weight	Use admission weight if recent weight gain is due to intravenous fluid provision with chemotherapy; track weight changes from recent weights and overall weight trends since diagnosis (growth velocity or percentage weight loss).
Length or height	Investigate z scores more than ±2. Monitor linear growth in young children undergoing treatment.
Weight-for-length or body mass index (BMI)	Investigate z scores less than −1, and work to increase weight unless stable with patient's ongoing trends.
Mid-upper arm circumference (MUAC)	MUAC helps to identify baseline malnutrition and distinguish between weight loss due to true malnutrition and weight loss due to decreased tumor burden following initial treatment.
	MUAC is particularly helpful in patients with large tumors, hepatosplenomegaly, or altered fluid status.
MUAC and triceps skinfold thickness	Consider this measurement if necessary using available tools; the clinician may also assess arm muscle and arm fat during the physical assessment.
	Body composition using dual-energy x-ray absorptiometry (DXA) or bioelectrical impedance often indicates inadequate muscle mass and excess body fat.

Biochemical Data

Complete blood count (CBC)	The CBC most often reflects changes due to chemotherapy rather than nutritional status.
Absolute neutrophil count (ANC)	The ANC indicates the ability to fight infection and often affects how the patient feels and eats.
Glucose level	Monitor glucose when steroids are used, particularly in patients at high risk for insulin resistance (based on factors such as obesity, ethnicity, family history); insulin may be indicated to prevent rapid weight loss.
Ferritin level	Ferritin is often falsely elevated due to inflammation.

(continued)

[a] www.who.int/childgrowth/standards/Technical_report.pdf

[b] www.cdc.gov/growthcharts/clinical_charts.htm

Box 13.5

Recommended Assessment Parameters for Pediatric Oncology Patients[7,66,67,82-84]
(continued)

Biochemical data *(continued)*

Vitamin D level	Patients are frequently deficient in vitamin D; consider supplementation due to this nutrient's importance for bone health and immune health.
Lipase level	Patients may develop pancreatitis from chemotherapy agents, including steroids or asparaginase.

Clinical and medical history

- Assess history for medical conditions or personal circumstances that may affect baseline nutritional status.
- Inquire about family history of diet-related chronic illnesses (diabetes, heart disease, cancer, osteoporosis).
- Assess current medical status for neutropenia, fever, and infection.

- Individuals with Down syndrome are at greater risk for developing leukemia. Consider baseline feeding practices and likelihood of maintaining these practices throughout treatment when assessing risk.
- Review cancer treatment and anticipated nutrition-related side effects (see condition-specific sections).

Dietary and activity assessment

Assess the patient for the following:

- total dietary intake (quality and quantity), including intake from nutrition support if applicable
- use of dietary supplements

- baseline and recent physical activity level
- treatment side effects, including anorexia, hyperphagia, nausea, or vomiting

Nutrition-focused physical findings

Assess the patient for the following:

- fluid status: edema, ascites, hydration status
- presence of hepatosplenomegaly (leukemia) or large solid tumors (neuroblastoma, Wilms tumor, and hepatoblastoma)
- gastrointestinal tract issues: mucositis; esophagitis; reflux; enteritis or colitis; gas, diarrhea, or constipation; pancreatitis

- skin condition: dry skin, skin integrity, wounds
- muscle condition: temporalis, deltoid, quadriceps, interosseous hand muscles
- fat: orbital fat, subcutaneous fat, fat around triceps or biceps, central adiposity

Box 13.6
Equations for Adjusting Body Weight for Amputations

Adjusted weight (kg)=

$$\frac{\text{Actual weight (kg) x 100}}{(100-\% \text{ body weight of amputated limb})}$$

Adjusted body mass index (BMI, in kg/m^2)=

$$\frac{\text{Adjusted weight (kg)}}{\text{height (m)}^2}$$

Adjusted ideal body weight (IBW, in kg)=

$$\frac{\text{IBW (kg) x 100}}{(100-\% \text{ body weight of amputated limb})}$$

Table 13.3
Estimated Energy Requirement Equations for Pediatrics[78]

Age	Sex	Estimated Energy Requirements (kcal)=total energy expenditure+energy deposition
0-3 mo	Male or female	$(89 \times \text{weight in kg} - 100) + 175$
4-6 mo	Male or female	$(89 \times \text{weight in kg} - 100) + 56$
7-12 mo	Male or female	$(89 \times \text{weight in kg} - 100) + 22$
13-36 mo	Male or female	$(89 \times \text{weight in kg} - 100) + 20$
3-8 y	Male	$88.5 - (61.9 \times \text{age in years}) + \text{physical activity factor} \times (26.7 \times \text{weight in kg} + 903 \times \text{height in meters}) + 20$
	Female	$135.3 - (30.8 \times \text{age in years}) + \text{physical activity factor} \times (10 \times \text{weight in kg} + 394 \times \text{height in meters}) + 20$
9-18 y	Male	$88.5 - (61.9 \times \text{age in years}) + \text{physical activity factor} \times (26.7 \times \text{weight in kg} + 903 \times \text{height in meters}) + 25$
	Female	$135.3 - (30.8 \times \text{age in years}) + \text{physical activity factor} \times (10 \times \text{weight in kg} + 394 \times \text{height in meters}) + 25$

Table 13.4
Physical Activity Factors for Estimated Energy Requirement Equations[78]

Physical activity level	Male (3-18 years)	Female (3-18 years)
Sedentary	1.0	1.0
Low active	1.13	1.16
Active	1.26	1.31
Very active	1.42	1.56

in respiratory status) throughout the illness.[7] The Schofield equation may also be used in critically ill pediatric oncology patients.[87,88]

For cancer survivors, the EER equation may significantly overestimate energy needs (by as much as 491 kcal/d in a study comparing survivors that had received cranial radiation therapy versus those who did not).[21] Recent studies have shown that many childhood cancer survivors have reduced lean body mass,[58,64] and this may partially account for differences in energy expenditure compared with healthy peers.[89,90] Considering this and an increased risk for obesity reported in this population,[91] RDNs should be involved in survivorship care to monitor anthropometrics and to educate patients about appropriate energy intake and physical activity in order to promote a healthy weight, rebuild lean body mass, and optimize energy expenditure.

Protein

Adequate protein is fundamental for proper growth and development in children. No data exist regarding specific protein needs for pediatric cancer patients. However, practitioners can assume that a minimum of the Recommended Dietary Allowance (RDA) for protein is required, increasing as needed to account for metabolic stress (see Table 13.6).[78] Protein needs for children increase during and after significant illness, stress, infection, fever, mucositis, steroid courses, and even diarrhea.[92] Additional protein also is needed for wound healing and tissue repair following surgery, radiation, and chemotherapy. Pediatric cancer patients or survivors who are stable and not affected by any of these stressors may be sufficiently nourished by the RDA for protein. Patients affected by any of these factors may have protein needs as high as 150% to 200% of the RDA.[93]

Adequate protein status depends not only on protein intake but also on energy intake. If total energy intake is inadequate in the setting of stress, protein is metabolized.[78,93] Inadequate energy intake occurs regularly during cancer treatment, and this could be partially responsible for the altered body composition found in many children with cancer and survivors of childhood cancer.[58,62-65] In a study of 115 pediatric cancer patients, an average of 181% of the RDA for protein was consumed, but energy intake was inadequate and the patients still experienced wasting.[81] RDNs should assist patients in meeting energy and protein needs to prevent muscle and fat wasting during treatment.

Table 13.5
Resting Energy Expenditure Equations for Critically Ill Children[84-86]

Age	Male	Female
<1 y	Use Estimated Energy Requirement equation.	Use Estimated Energy Requirement equation.
1-3 y	$60.9 \times$ weight in kg -54	$61.0 \times$ weight in kg -51
3-10 y	$22.7 \times$ weight in kg $+495$	$22.5 \times$ weight in kg $+499$
10-18 y	$17.5 \times$ weight in kg $+651$	$12.2 \times$ weight in kg $+746$
18-30 y	$15.3 \times$ weight in kg $+679$	$14.7 \times$ weight in kg $+496$

Oncology Nutrition *for* Clinical Practice

Survivors of childhood cancer may have lower lean body mass.[58,62-65] Boland and colleagues[65] evaluated the relationship between protein intake and lean muscle mass in survivors of childhood ALL compared with healthy controls. Although protein intake between the two groups was similar, ALL survivors had lower lean muscle mass compared with controls. Importantly, the cancer survivors participated in resistance-training exercise less often than their healthy peers. The authors predicted that an additional 1 g of protein per kg of body weight per day plus increased resistance training may improve lean muscle mass by about 3%.[65] This highlights not only the importance of adequate protein intake but also the essential role physical activity plays in rebuilding healthy lean body mass after treatment.[94]

Fluid

The Holliday-Segar method (see Box 13.7) should be used to estimate maintenance fluid needs for pediatric patients with cancer, adjusting as needed for electrolyte imbalances, organ dysfunction, or treatment side effects that may affect fluid needs (eg, mucositis, diarrhea, vomiting, fever, increased

Table 13.6
Estimating Protein Needs in Pediatric Patients With Cancer[83,93]

Age	RDA[a] (g/kg)	Stressed (RDA × 1.5 to 2) (g/kg)
0-6 mo[a]	1.52	2.3-3.0
7-12 mo	1.20	1.8-2.4
1-3 y	1.05	1.6-2.1
4-13 y	0.95	1.4-1.9
14-18 y	0.85	1.3-1.7

[a] RDA = Recommended Dietary Allowance
[b] Adequate Intake is used in this age group.

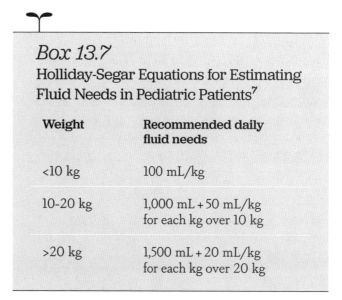

Box 13.7
Holliday-Segar Equations for Estimating Fluid Needs in Pediatric Patients[7]

Weight	Recommended daily fluid needs
<10 kg	100 mL/kg
10-20 kg	1,000 mL + 50 mL/kg for each kg over 10 kg
>20 kg	1,500 mL + 20 mL/kg for each kg over 20 kg

salivation).[7] Patients receiving PN and EN should receive maintenance requirements, unless clinically contraindicated.[7] Additional fluids often accompany chemotherapy, per treatment protocols, and may exceed daily needs.

Micronutrients

Micronutrient goals for pediatric cancer patients should meet the RDA for all micronutrients, unless a deficiency is identified. Because research repeatedly reports inadequate calcium intake and low vitamin D levels in patients with childhood cancers, we discuss these in more detail here.[95,96]

Calcium Studies indicate that pediatric cancer patients often do not meet the Adequate Intakes for calcium.[97,98] This poses a significant risk to bone health in an already-vulnerable population. RDNs should counsel patients on meeting age-appropriate RDAs (see Table 13.7 on page 268) through dietary sources and supplementation, as needed.

Vitamin D Vitamin D insufficiency is a common issue in pediatric oncology, but whether or not these patients are at greater risk than the general population is debatable.[78,99] Vitamin D deficiency in children with cancer may be due to malabsorption, decreased sun exposure, inadequate intake, exclusive breastfeeding, obesity, or drug-nutrient

Table 13.7
Daily Adequate Intake Levels for Calcium[97]

Age	Male	Female
0-6 mo	200 mg	200 mg
7-12 mo	260 mg	260 mg
1-3 y	700 mg	700 mg
4-8 y	1,000 mg	1,000 mg
9-13 y	1,300 mg	1,300 mg
14-18 y	1,300 mg	1,300 mg
19-50 y	1,000 mg	1,000 mg

Table 13.8
Suggested Vitamin D Status Definitions for Pediatric Patients with Cancer[106]

25-hydroxyvitamin D level (ng/mL)	Vitamin D status
30-100	Sufficient
20-29	Insufficient
<20	Deficient

Table 13.9
Recommended Dietary Allowances for Vitamin D[97]

Age	Male	Female
0-12 mo	400 IU	400 IU
1-18 y	600 IU	600 IU

interactions. The adverse impact of vitamin D insufficiency on intestinal calcium absorption, bone mineral density, and osteoporosis risk is well known,[100] but emerging evidence supports a relationship between vitamin D and the immune system, including but not limited to low levels of 25-hydroxyvitamin D being associated with increased *Clostridium difficile* and *Staphylococcus aureus* infections and recurrences.[101,102]

A plethora of evidence suggests that survivors of childhood cancer also are at risk for vitamin D deficiency, and Zhang and colleagues[96] demonstrated that only 4% of ALL survivors met vitamin D requirements. Regular monitoring and supplementation is encouraged.[95,103-105] The Institute of Medicine (now the Health and Medicine Division of the National Academies of Sciences, Engineering, and Medicine) has suggested that serum 25-hydroxyvitamin D levels above 20 ng/mL are likely sufficient in children[97]; however, the Endocrine Society recommends a minimum level of 30 ng/mL.[100] For pediatric cancer patients and survivors, a serum 25-hydroxyvitamin D level of 30 ng/mL may be a more appropriate minimum goal (see Table 13.8). If levels are normal, patients should aim to meet the age-appropriate RDA for vitamin D (see Table 13.9).[97]

Nutrition Interventions and Support

RDNs have a variety of clinical tools for optimizing the nutritional status of their pediatric patients with cancer. Some concerns can be corrected with targeted nutrition education, while others may require additional interventions, such as oral nutrition supplements, appetite stimulants, and nutrition support.

Oral nutrition supplements are a viable way to increase energy, protein, vitamin, and mineral intake, thereby helping children with cancer meet their nutritional needs.[7,60] Selecting the appropriate supplement requires a detailed review of the child's medical history and treatment plan, pertinent medications, nutritional status, organ function, and taste and smell alterations.[60,69,107]

Appetite stimulants include several medications (see Box 13.8) used to improve intake during treatment of childhood cancer.[9,97-102]

EN may be necessary when oral intake is inadequate. Although many patients requiring EN will require it for more than 3 months, the decision of which feeding device to place (nasoenteric tube versus surgically placed gastrostomy tube) should be discussed by the team to minimize postsurgical complications.[51,114,115] Current research indicates that EN can be safely tolerated and can help minimize weight loss.[114,115] However, the surgical placement of feeding tubes in pediatric oncology patients is not without risk, and the medical team and family should determine the best option for the child after considering the anticipated duration of the EN requirement and the risks and benefits of nasoenteric placement versus surgical placement. Patients who may require enteral feeding access should be closely monitored.

PN should be provided for patients who require nutrition support and do not have a functioning

Box 13.8
Appetite Stimulants Commonly Used in Pediatric Oncology[7,108-113]

Medication	Dosing[a]	Comments
Cyproheptadine (Periactin)	Children aged 2 to 6 years: 0.25 mg/kg/d or 8 mg/m²/d or 2 mg two to three times daily; maximum of 12 mg/d Children aged 7 to 14 years: 4 mg two to three times daily; maximum of 16 mg/d Adolescents aged less than 14 years: Refer to adult dosing	Divide total dose into two to three daily doses. Some clinicians use this as a first choice. Side effects include drowsiness and dry mouth.
Dronabinol (Marinol)	2.5 mg twice daily Increase as needed up to the maximum dosage of 20 mg/d in divided doses	Typically used in adolescents and adults. Side effects include improved nausea and euphoria.
Megestrol acetate (Megace)	Titrate dosage to response; decrease dosage by 50% if weight gain is excessive Children (tablets or 40 mg/mL suspension): 7.5 to 10 mg/kg/d in one to four divided doses; not to exceed 800 mg/d or 15 mg/kg/d Adolescents and adults (tablets or 40 mg/mL suspension): 800 mg/d in one to four divided doses; doses of 400 to 800 mg/d have been clinically effective Megace ES: 625 mg once daily	Side effects include increased fat mass, mood changes, hyperglycemia, hyperlipidemia, deep vein thrombosis, and adrenal suppression.

[a] Dosing information obtained from the St. Jude Children's Research Hospital Medication Formulary; 2020.

gut (eg, due to intractable vomiting or diarrhea, severe mucositis, ileus, neutropenic colitis or typhlitis, gastrointestinal hemorrhage, or pneumatosis intestinalis). PN should be used only when medically necessary, as it can lead to increased risk for infectious and metabolic complications.[7,108]

Discussing nutrition support options with patients and their families early and at multiple points throughout the treatment cycle can help improve communication and decision-making, and it is a key step that RDNs can take in collaboration with health care teams. For example, for patients who will undergo very intensive chemotherapy, it may be prudent to discuss EN support as an anticipated supportive measure that the child will need during his or her treatment, similar to the need for a central line for chemotherapy administration. Montgomery and colleagues[116] showed that nurses often initiate the conversation within the first month of diagnosis, while physicians initiate discussion only after noting changes in a patient's nutritional status. Providers have reported that patients and families can be more resistant when discussing EN than PN, but a pilot study in Australia showed that decision aid providing information about various nutrition methods and the importance of nutrition during pediatric oncology treatment is useful.[116,117] Of 31 parents surveyed, 90% reported improved understanding of the purpose, risks, and benefits of nutrition support.[117] This study reveals an opportunity for the RDN to collaborate with the health care team to develop a standardized approach for discussing nutrition support options with patients and families early and at multiple intervals throughout treatment for improved communication and decision-making.

Summary

Children with cancer have unique needs throughout the care continuum. Patient needs vary based on age, diagnosis, treatment plan, prognosis, and NIS. RDNs working with pediatric oncology patients and their families should work closely with the medical team and develop a working knowledge of treatment plans so that prompt, proactive nutrition intervention can be provided to maintain optimal nutritional status throughout treatment.

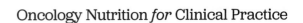

References

1. Childhood cancers. National Cancer Institute website. Updated August 28, 2020. Accessed September 15, 2020. https://cancer.gov/types/childhood-cancers

2. Cancer in children. American Cancer Society website. Updated August 24, 2020. Accessed September 15, 2020. www.cancer.org/cancer/cancer-in-children/key-statistics.html

3. Siegel R, Miller K, Jemal A. Cancer statistics. *CA Cancer J Clin.* 2017;67(1):7-30.

4. Childhood cancer statistics. CureSearch for Children's Cancer website. Accessed September 15, 2020. https://curesearch.org/childhood-cancer-statistics

5. Howlader N, Noone AM, Krapcho M, et al, eds. SEER cancer statistics review, 1975–2017, National Cancer Institute. Surveillance, Epidemiology, and End Results Program website. Updated January 1, 2017. Accessed September 15, 2020. https://seer.cancer.gov/csr/1975_2017/results_merged/sect_29_childhood_cancer_iccc.pdf#search=childhood%20survivors

6. Ladas EJ, Sacks N, Meacham L, et al. A multidisciplinary review of nutrition considerations in the pediatric oncology population: a perspective from Children's Oncology Group. *Nutr Clin Pract.* 2005;20(4):377-393. doi:10.1177/0115426505020004377

7. Sacks N, Henry D, White-Collins A, et al. Oncology, hematopoietic transplant, gastrointestinal supportive care medications and survivorship. In: Corkins M, Balint J, Bobo E, Plogsted S, Yaworski J, eds. *The ASPEN Pediatric Nutrition Support Core Curriculum.* 2nd ed. American Society for Parenteral and Enteral Nutrition; 2015:459-494.

8. Ilhan I, Sari N, Yesil S, Eren T, Tacyildiz N. Anthropometrics and biochemical assessment of nutritional status in pediatric cancer patients. *Pediatr Hematol Oncol.* 2015;32(6):415-422.

9. Rabin K, Gramatges M, Margolin J, Poplack D. Acute lymphoblastic leukemia. In: Pizzo PA, Poplack DG, eds. *Principles and Practice of Pediatric Oncology.* 7th ed. Wolters Kluwer; 2015:463-497.

10. Chemotherapy drugs and drugs often used during chemotherapy. Chemocare website. Published 2018. Accessed January 27, 2018. http://chemocare.com/chemotherapy/drug-info/default.aspx

11. Zhang F, Parsons S. Obesity in childhood cancer survivors: call for early weight management. *Adv Nutr.* 2015;6(5):611-619.

12. Hill R, Hamby T, Bashore L, et al. Early nutrition intervention attenuates weight gain for pediatric acute lymphoblastic leukemia patients in maintenance therapy. *J Pediatr Hematol Oncol.* 2017;40(2):104-110.

13. Li R, Donnella H, Knouse P, et al. A randomized nutrition counseling intervention in pediatric leukemia patients receiving steroids results in reduced caloric intake. *Pediatr Blood Cancer.* 2017;64(2):374-380.

14. Arceci R, Meshinchi S. Acute myeloid leukemia and myelodysplastic syndromes. In: Pizzo PA, Poplack DG, eds. *Principles and Practice of Pediatric Oncology.* 7th ed. Wolters Kluwer; 2015:498-544.

15. Inaba H, Surprise HC, Pounds S, et al. Effect of body mass index on the outcome of children with acute myeloid leukemia. *Cancer.* 2012;118(23):5989-5996. doi:10.1002/cncr.27640

16. Brain cancer. National Cancer Institute website. Accessed September 15, 2020. https://cancer.gov/types/brain

17. Chi S, Zimmerman M, Yao X, et al. Intensive multimodality treatment for children with newly diagnosed CNS atypical teratoid rhabdoid tumor. *J Clin Oncol.* 2009;27(3):385-389.

18. Tekautz T, Fuller C, Blaney S, et al. Atypical teratoid/rhabdoid tumors (ATRT): improved survival in children 3 years of age and older with radiation therapy and high-dose alkylator-based chemotherapy. *J Clin Oncol.* 2005;23(7):1491-1499.

19. Park D, Chun M, Lee S, Song Y. Comparison of swallowing functions between brain tumor and stroke patients. *Ann Rehabil Med.* 2013;37(5):633-641.

20. Margelisch K, Studer M, Ritter B, Steinlin M, Leibundgut K, Heinks T. Cognitive dysfunction in children with brain tumors at diagnosis. *Pediatr Blood Cancer.* 2015;62(10):1805-1812.

21. Zhang F, Roberts SB, Parsons SK, et al. Low levels of energy expenditure in childhood cancer survivors. *J Pediatr Hematol Oncol.* 2015;37(3):232-236. doi:10.1097/MPH.0000000000000250

22. Wang K, de Souza R, Fleming A, et al. Adiposity in childhood brain tumors: a report from the Canadian Study of Determinants of Endometabolic Health in Children (Can DECIDE Study). *Sci Rep.* 2017;22(7):45078.

23. Metzger M, Krasin M, Choi J, Hudson M. Hodgkin lymphoma. In: Pizzo PA, Poplack DG, eds. *Principles and Practice of Pediatric Oncology.* 7th ed. Wolters Kluwer; 2015:568-586.

24. Combination chemotherapy in treating young patients with newly diagnosed high-risk B acute lymphoblastic leukemia and Ph-like TKI sensitive mutations. ClinicalTrials.gov identifier: NCT01406756. Accessed February 22. 2021. https://clinicaltrials.gov/ct2/show/NCT01406756

25. Nysom K, Holm K, Michaelsen K, Hertz H, Muller J, Molgaard C. Degree of fatness after treatment of malignant lymphoma in childhood. *Med Pediatr Oncol.* 2003;40(4):239-243.

26. Allen C, Kamdar K, Bollard C, Gross T. Malignant non-Hodgkin lymphomas in children. In: Pizzo PA, Poplack DG, eds. *Principles and Practice of Pediatric Oncology.* 7th ed. Wolters Kluwer; 2015:587-603.

27. Ehrhardt M, Sandlund J, Zhang N, et al. Late outcomes of adult survivors of childhood non-Hodgkin lymphoma: a report from the St. Jude Lifetime Cohort Study. *Pediatr Blood Cancer.* 2017;64(6). Epub ahead of print. doi:10.1002/pbc.26338

28. Goodman M, Gurney J, Smith M, Olshan A. Sympathetic nervous system tumors. In: Ries LA, Smith MA, Gurney JG, et al, eds. *Cancer Incidence and Survival Among Children and Adolescents: United States SEER Program, 1975–1995.* National Cancer Institute; 1999:35.

29. Gurney J, Ross J, Wall D, Bleyer W, Severson R, Robison L. Infant cancer in the U.S. *J Pediatr Hematol Oncol.* 1997;19(5):428-432.

30. Brodeur G, Hogarty M, Bagatell R, Mosse Y, Maris J. Neuroblastoma. In: Pizzo P, Poplack DG, eds. *Principles and Practice of Pediatric Oncology.* 7th ed. Wolters Kluwer; 2015:772-797.

31. Small A, Thwe L, Byrne J, et al. Neuroblastoma, body mass index, and survival. *Medicine (Baltimore).* 2015;94(14):e713.

32. Green G, Weitzman S, Pencharz P. Resting energy expenditure in children newly diagnosed with stage IV neuroblastoma. *Pediatr Res.* 2008;63(3):332-336.

33. Laverdière C, Liu Q, Yasui Y, et al. Long-term outcomes in survivors of neuroblastoma: a report from the Childhood Cancer Survivor Study. *J Natl Cancer Inst.* 2009;101(16):1131-1140.

34. Wexler L, Skapek S, Helman L. Rhabdomyosarcoma. In: Pizzo PA, Poplack DG, eds. *Principles and Practice of Pediatric Oncology.* 7th ed. Wolters Kluwer; 2015:855-876.

35. Fernandez C, Geller J, Ehrlich P, Hill D, Kalapurakal J, Dome J. Renal tumors. In: Pizzo PA, Poplack DG, eds. *Principles and Practice of Pediatric Oncology.* 7th ed. Wolters Kluwer; 2015:753-771.

36. Barr R, Collins L, Nayiager T, et al. Nutritional status at diagnosis in children with cancer. 2. An assessment by arm anthropometry. *J Pediatr Hematol Oncol.* 2011;33(3):e101-e104.

37. Sala A, Rossi E, Antillon F, et al. Nutritional status at diagnosis is related to clinical outcomes in children and adolescents with cancer: a perspective from Central America. *Eur J Cancer.* 2012;48(2):243-252. doi:10.1016/j.ejca.2011.06.006

38. Lifson L, Hadley G, Wiles N, Pillay K. Nutritional status of children with Wilms' tumour on admission to a South African hospital and its influence on outcome. *Pediatr Blood Cancer*. 2017;64(7). Epub ahead of print. doi: 10.1002/pbc.26382

39. Gorlick R, Janeway K, Marina N. Osteosarcoma. In: Pizzo PA, Poplack DG, eds. *Principles and Practice of Pediatric Oncology*. 7th ed. Wolters Kluwer; 2015:877-898.

40. Tenardi R, Frühwald M, Jürgen's H, Hertroijs D, Bauer J. Nutritional status of children and young adults with Ewing sarcoma and osteosarcoma at diagnosis and during multimodality therapy. *Pediatr Blood Cancer*. 2012;59(4):621-626.

41. Hawkins D, Brennan B, Bölling, T, et al. Ewing sarcoma. In: Pizzo PA, Poplack DG, eds. *Principles and Practice of Pediatric Oncology*. 7th ed. Wolters Kluwer; 2015:855-876.

42. Goldstein G, Shemesh E, Frenkel T, Jacobson J, Toren A. Abnormal body mass index at diagnosis in patients with Ewing sarcoma is associated with inferior tumor necrosis. *Pediatr Blood Cancer*. 2015;62(11):1892-1896.

43. Meyes R, Trobaugh-Lotrario A, Malogolowkin M, Katzenstein H, López-Terrada D, Finegold M. Liver tumors. In: Pizzo PA, Poplack DG, eds. *Principles and Practice of Pediatric Oncology*. 7th ed. Wolters Kluwer; 2015:726-752.

44. Shah P, Jhaveri U, Idhate T, Dhingra S, Arolkar P, Arora B. Nutritional status at presentation, comparison of assessment tools, and importance of arm anthropometry in children with cancer in India. *Indian J Cancer*. 2015;52(2):210-215.

45. Lee D, Wayne A, Huynh V, et al. ZUMA-4 preliminary results: phase 1 study of KTE-C19 chimeric antigen receptor T cell therapy in pediatric and adolescent patients (pts) with relapsed/refractory acute lymphoblastic leukemia (R/R ALL). *Ann Oncol*. 2017;28(suppl 5).

46. Fitzgerald J, Weiss S, Maude S, et al. Cytokine release syndrome after chimeric antigen receptor t cell therapy for acute lymphoblastic leukemia. *Crit Care Med*. 2017;45(2):e124-e131.

47. Hyperthermic intraperitoneal chemotherapy. MD Anderson website. Published 2019. Accessed April 19, 2019. https://mdanderson.org/treatment-options/hyperthermic-intraperitoneal-chemotherapy.html

48. Hayes-Jordan A, Green H, Lin H, et al. Cytoreductive surgery and hyperthermic intraperitoneal chemotherapy (HIPEC) for children, adolescents, and young adults: the first 50 cases. *Ann Surg Oncol*. 2015;22(5):1726-1732.

49. Vashi P, Gupta D, Lammersfeld C, et al. The relationship between baseline nutritional status with subsequent parenteral nutrition and clinical outcomes in cancer patients undergoing hyperthermic intraperitoneal chemotherapy. *Nutr J*. 2013;12(118). doi:10.1186/1475-2891-12-118

50. Swain D, Yates A, Mohamed F, et al. Do patients undergoing cytoreductive surgery and HIPEC for peritoneal malignancy need parenteral nutrition? *Pleura Peritoneum*. 2018;3(4):2018-0123. doi:10.1515/pp-2018-0123

51. Hamilton E, Curtin T, Slack R, et al. Surgical feeding tubes in pediatric and adolescent cancer patients. *J Pediatr Hematol Oncol*. 2017;39(7):e342-e348.

52. Połubok J, Malczewska A, Rąpała M, et al. Nutritional status at the moment of diagnosis in childhood cancer patients. *Pediatr Endocrinol Diabetes Metab*. 2017;23(2):77-82.

53. Zimmermann K, Ammann RA, Kuehni CE, De Geest S, Cignacco E. Malnutrition in pediatric patients with cancer at diagnosis and throughout therapy: a multicenter cohort study. *Pediatr Blood Cancer*. 2013;60(4):642-649. doi:10.1002/pbc.24409

54. Iniesta R, Paciarotti I, Brougham M, McKenzie J, Wilson D. Effects of pediatric cancer and its treatment on nutritional status: a systematic review. *Nutr Rev*. 2015;73(5):276-295.

55. Loeffen EAH, Brinksma A, Tissing WJE. Clinical implications of malnutrition in children with cancer. *Support Care Cancer.* 2015;23(1):143-150. doi:10.1007/s00520-015-2800-z

56. Orgel E, Sposto R, Malvar J, et al. Impact on survival and toxicity by duration of weight extremes during treatment for pediatric acute lymphoblastic leukemia: a report from the Children's Oncology Group. *J Clin Oncol.* 2014;32(13):1331-1337.

57. den Hoed MAH, Pluijm SMF, de Groot-Kruseman HA, et al. The negative impact of being underweight and weight loss on survival of children with acute lymphoblastic leukemia. *Haematologica.* 2015;100(1):62-69. doi:10.3324/haematol.2014.110668

58. Murphy A, White M, Elliott S, Lockwood L, Hallahan A, Davies P. Body composition of children with cancer during treatment and in survivorship. *Am J Clin Nutr.* 2015;102(4):891-896.

59. Brinksma A, Sanderman R, Roodbol P, et al. Malnutrition is associated with worse health-related quality of life in children with cancer. *Support Care Cancer.* 2015;23(10):3043-3052.

60. Ballal S, Bechard L, Duggan C. Nutritional supportive care. In: Pizzo PA, Poplack DG, eds. *Principles and Practice of Pediatric Oncology.* 7th ed. Wolters Kluwer; 2015:1058-1066.

61. Gokcebay D, Emir S, Bayhan T, Demir H, Gunduz M, Tunc B. Assessment of nutritional status in children with cancer and effectiveness of oral nutritional supplements. *J Pediatr Hematol Oncol.* 2015;32(6):423-432.

62. Wang K-W, Fleming A, Johnston DL, et al. Overweight, obesity and adiposity in survivors of childhood brain tumours: a systematic review and meta-analysis. *Clin Obes.* 2017;8(1):55-67. doi:10.1111/cob.12224

63. Brinksma A, Roodbol PF, Sulkers E, et al. Changes in nutritional status in childhood cancer patients: a prospective cohort study. *Clin Nutr.* 2015;34(1):66-73. doi:10.1016/j.clnu.2014.01.013

64. Marriott C, Beaumont L, Farncombe T, et al. Body composition in long-term survivors of acute lymphoblastic leukemia diagnosed in childhood and adolescence: a focus on sarcopenic obesity. *Cancer.* 2018;124(6):1225-1231.

65. Boland A, Gibson T, Lu L, et al. Dietary protein intake and lean muscle mass in survivors of childhood acute lymphoblastic leukemia: report from the St. Jude Lifetime Cohort Study. *Phys Ther.* 2016;96(7):1029-1038.

66. Bauer J, Jürgens H, Frühwald MC. Important aspects of nutrition in children with cancer. *Adv Nutr.* 2011;2(2):67-77. doi:10.3945/an.110.000141

67. Becker P, Nieman Carney L, Corkins M, et al. Consensus statement of the Academy of Nutrition and Dietetics/American Society for Parenteral and Enteral Nutrition: indicators recommended for the identification and documentation of pediatric malnutrition (undernutrition). *J Acad Nutr Diet.* 2014;114(12):1988-2000.

68. Mehta NM, Corkins MR, Lyman B, et al. Defining pediatric malnutrition: a paradigm shift toward etiology-related definitions. *J Parenter Enter Nutr.* 2013;37(4):460-481. doi:10.1177/0148607113479972

69. Murphy A, Mosby T, Rogers P, Cohen J, Ladas E. An international survey of nutritional practices in low- and middle-income countries: a report from the International Society of Pediatric Oncology (SIOP) PODC Nutrition Working Group. *Eur J Clin Nutr.* 2014;68(12):1341-1345.

70. Ladas E, Sacks N, Meacham L, et al. A multidisciplinary review of nutrition considerations in the pediatric oncology population: a perspective from children's oncology group. *Nutr Clin Pract.* 2005;20(4):377-393.

71. Selwood K, Ward E, Gibson F. Assessment and management of nutritional challenges in children's cancer care: a survey of current practice in the United Kingdom. *Eur J Oncol Nurs.* 2010;14(5):439-446.

72. Murphy AJ, White M, Viani K, Mosby TT. Evaluation of the nutrition screening tool for childhood cancer (SCAN). *Clin Nutr*. 2016;35(1):219-224. doi:10.1016/j.clnu.2015.02.009

73. Academy of Nutrition and Dietetics. Pediatric Nutrition Care Manual: oncology nutritional indicators. Nutrition Care Manual website. Accessed March 12, 2020. https://nutritioncaremanual.org/topic.cfm?ncm_category_id=13&lv1=144629&lv2=273744&ncm_toc_id=273744&ncm_heading=Nutrition%20Care%20home%20page

74. Secker D, Jeejeebhoy K. Subjective global nutritional assessment for children. *Am J Clin Nutr*. 2007;85(4):1083-1089.

75. Secker DJ, Jeejeebhoy KN. How to perform Subjective Global Nutritional Assessment in children. *J Acad Nutr Diet*. 2012;112(3):424-431. doi:10.1016/j.jada.2011.08.039

76. Brinksma A, Roodbol P, Sulkers E, Al E. Finding the right balance: an evaluation of the adequacy of energy and protein intake in childhood cancer patients. *Clin Nutr*. 2015;34(2):284-290.

77. Galati P, Resende C, Salomao R, Scridelli C, Tone L, Monteiro J. Accurate determination of energy needs in children and adolescents with cancer. *Nutr Cancer*. 2011;63(2):306-313.

78. Dietary reference intakes for energy, carbohydrate, fiber, fat, fatty acids, cholesterol, protein, and amino acids (macronutrients). Institute of Medicine. 2005. Dietary Reference Intakes for Energy, Fatty Acids, Cholesterol, Protein and Amino Acids. The National Academies Press. doi:10.17226/10490

79. Hunt K, Charuhas Macris P. Nutrition assessment and management of the child with cancer. *Nutr Focus*. January/February 2009:1-8.

80. Sacks N, Ringwald-Smith, K, Hale G. Nutritional support. In: Altman A, ed. *Supportive Care of Children with Cancer: Current Therapy and Guidelines from the Children's Oncology Group*. 3rd ed. Johns Hopkins University Press; 2004:243-261.

81. Mehta N, Skillman H, Irving S, et al. Guidelines for the provision and assessment of nutrition support therapy in the pediatric critically ill patient: Society of Critical Care Medicine and American Society for Parenteral and Enteral Nutrition. *Pediatr Crit Care Med*. 2017;18(7):675-715.

82. Raja RA, Schmiegelow K, Frandsen TL. Asparaginase-associated pancreatitis in children. *Br J Haematol*. 2012;159(1):18-27. doi:10.1111/bjh.12016

83. Denton CC, Rawlins YA, Oberley MJ, Bhojwani D, Orgel E. Predictors of hepatotoxicity and pancreatitis in children and adolescents with acute lymphoblastic leukemia treated according to contemporary regimens. *Pediatr Blood Cancer*. 2018;65(3). Epub ahead of print. doi:10.1002/pbc.26891

84. Helou M, Ning Y, Yang S, et al. Vitamin D deficiency in children with cancer. *J Clin Oncol*. 2014;36(3):212-217.

85. Himes JH. New equation to estimate body mass index in amputees. *J Amer Diet Assoc*. 1995;95(6):646.

86. About body mass index (BMI). Amputee Coalition website. Published 2018. Accessed January 27, 2020. https://amputee-coalition.org/limb-loss-resource-center/resources-filtered/resources-by-topic/healthy-living/about-bmi

87. American Academy of Pediatrics Committee on Nutrition. Energy. In: Kleinman RD, Greer FR, eds. *Pediatric Nutrition*. 8th ed. American Academy of Pediatrics; 2019:431-448.

88. Schofield WN, Schofield C, James WPT. Basal metabolic rate-review and prediction, together with annotated bibliography of source material. *Hum Nutr Clin Nutr*. 1985;39C(suppl 1):1-96.

89. Bosy-Westphal A, Schautz B, Lagerpusch M, et al. Effect of weight loss and regain on adipose tissue distribution, composition of lean mass, and resting energy expenditure in young overweight and obese adults. *Int J Obes*. 2013;37(10):1371-1377.

90. Breene R, Williams R, Hartle J, Gattens M, Acerini C, Murray M. Auxological changes in UK survivors of childhood acute lymphoblastic leukaemia treated without cranial irradiation. *Br J Cancer*. 2011;104(5):746-749.

91. Withycombe J, Post-White J, Meza J, et al. Weight patterns in children with higher risk ALL: a report from the Children's Oncology Group (COG) for CCG 1961. *Pediatr Blood Cancer*. 2009;53(7):1249-1254.

92. American Academy of Pediatrics Committee on Nutrition. Protein. In: Kleinman RD, Greer FR, eds. *Pediatric Nutrition*. 8th ed. American Academy of Pediatrics; 2019:449-480.

93. American Academy of Pediatrics Committee on Nutrition. Nutritional management of children with cancer. In: Kleinman RD, Greer FR, eds. *Pediatric Nutrition*. 8th ed. American Academy of Pediatrics; 2019:1151-1168.

94. Zhang F, Saltzman E, Must A, Parsons S. Do childhood cancer survivors meet the diet and physical activity guidelines? A review of guidelines and literature. *Int J Child Heal Nutr*. 2012;1(1):44-58. doi:10.6000/1929-4247.2012.01.01.06

95. Modan-Moses D, Pinhas-Hamiel O, Munitz-Shenkar D, Temam V, Kanety H, Toren A. Vitamin D status in pediatric patients with a history of malignancy. *Pediatr Res*. 2012;72(6):620-624. doi:10.1038/pr.2012.131

96. Zhang F, Saltzman E, Kelly, MJ, et al. Comparison of childhood cancer survivors nutritional intake with US dietary guidelines. *Pediatr Blood Cancer*. 2015;62(8):1461-1467.

97. Institute of Medicine Committee to Review Dietary Reference Intakes for Vitamin D and Calcium. *Dietary Reference Intakes for Calcium and Vitamin D*. Ross AC, Taylor CL, Yaktine AL, Del Valle HB, eds. National Academies Press; 2011.

98. Sinha A, Avery P, Turner S, Bailey S, Cheetham T. Vitamin D status in paediatric patients with cancer. *Pediatr Blood Cancer*. 2011;57(4):597-608.

99. Iniesta R, Rush R, Paciarotti I, et al. Systematic review and meta-analysis: prevalence and possible causes of vitamin D deficiency and insufficiency in pediatric cancer patients. *Clin Nutr*. 2016;36(1):95-108.

100. Holick M, Brinkley N, Bischoff-Ferrari H, et al. Evaluation, treatment and prevention of vitamin D deficiency: an Endocrine Society clinical practice guideline. *J Clin Endocrinol Metab*. 2011;96(7):1911-1930.

101. Furuya-Kanamori L, Wangdi K, Yakob L, et al. 25-Hydroxyvitamin D concentrations and *Clostridium difficile* infection: a meta-analysis. *JPEN J Parenter Enter Nutr*. 2017;41(5):890-895.

102. Wang JW, Hogan PG, Hunstad DA, Fritz SA. Vitamin D sufficiency and *Staphylococcus aureus* infection in children. *Pediatr Infect Dis J*. 2015;34(5):544-545.

103. Rosen GP, Beebe KL, Shaibi GQ. Vitamin D levels differ by cancer diagnosis and decline over time in survivors of childhood cancer. *Pediatr Blood Cancer*. 2013;60(6):949-952. doi:10.1002/pbc.24349

104. Choudhary A, Chou J, Heller G, Sklar C. Prevalence of vitamin D insufficiency in survivors of childhood cancer. *Pediatr Blood Cancer*. 2013;60(7):1237-1239. doi:10.1002/pbc.24403

105. Neville K, Walker J, Cohn R, Cowell C, White C. The prevalence of vitamin D deficiency is higher in adult survivors of childhood cancer. *Clin Endocrinol*. 2015;82(5):657-662.

106. Lee JY, So T-Y, Thackray J. A review on vitamin D deficiency treatment in pediatric patients. *J Pediatr Pharmacol Ther*. 2013;18(4):277-291. doi:10.5863/1551-6776-18.4.277

107. Cohen J, Laing D, Wilkes F, Chan A, Gabriel M, Cohn R. Taste and smell dysfunction in childhood cancer survivors. *Appetite.* 2014;75:135-140.

108. Yavuzsen T, Davis M, Walsh D, LeGrand S, Lagman R. Systematic review of the treatment of cancer-associated anorexia and weight loss. *J Clin Oncol.* 2005;23(33):8500-8511.

109. Baracos V, Martin L, Korc M, Guttridge D, Fearon K. Cancer-associated cachexia. *Nat Rev Dis Prim.* 2018;4:17105. doi:10.1038/nrdp.2017.105

110. Gullett N, Mazurak V, Hebbar G, Ziegler T. Nutritional interventions for cancer-induced cachexia. *Curr Probl Cancer.* 2011;35(2):58-90.

111. Cuvelier G, Baker T, Peddie E, et al. A randomized, double–blind, placebo–controlled clinical trial of megestrol acetate as an appetite stimulant in children with weight loss due to cancer and/or cancer therapy. *Pediatr Blood Cancer.* 2014;61(4):672-679.

112. Jatoi A, Windschitl H, Loprinzi C, et al. Dronabinol versus megestrol acetate versus combination therapy for cancer-associated anorexia: a North Central Cancer Treatment Group study. *J Clin Oncol.* 2002;20(2):567-573.

113. Couluris M, Mayer J, Freyer D, Sandler E, Xu P, Krischer J. The effect of cyproheptadine hydrochloride (Periactin) and megestrol acetate (Megace) on weight in children with cancer/treatment-related cachexia. *J Pediatr Hematol Oncol.* 2008;30(11):791-797.

114. Fernandez-Pineda I, Sandoval J, Jones R, et al. Gastrostomy complications in pediatric cancer patients: a retrospective single-institution review. *Pediatr Blood Cancer.* 2016;63(7):1250-1253.

115. Schmitt F, Caldari D, Corradini N, et al. Tolerance and efficacy of preventive gastrostomy feeding in pediatric oncology. *Pediatr Blood Cancer.* 2012;59(5):874-880. doi:10.1002/pbc.24161

116. Montgomery K, Belongia M, Schulta C, Mulberry M, Nugent M, Simpson P. Health care providers' perceptions of nutrition support in pediatric oncology and hematopoietic stem cell transplant patients. *J Pediatr Oncol Nurs.* 2015;33(4):265-272.

117. Sajeev M, Cohen J, Wakefield C, Fardell J, Cohn R. Decision aid for nutrition support in pediatric oncology: a pilot study. *JPEN J Parenter Enter Nutr.* 2015;33(4):265-272.

Chapter 14
Medical Nutrition Therapy for Hematologic Malignancies

Alicia Gilmore, MS, RD, CSO, LD
Kelli Oldham, MS, RDN, CSO, LDN

The group of cancers known as hematologic malignancies includes several diverse diseases. These cancers arise from hematopoietic and lymphoid tissues and can affect the production (hematopoiesis) and function of blood cells. The normal process of blood cell development is interrupted by uncontrolled growth of abnormal cells, which can prevent healthy cells from carrying on their regular functions, such as fighting infection, forming blood clots, and carrying oxygen to other cells.[1]

Approximately 10% of cancers diagnosed in the United States are leukemia, lymphoma, or multiple myeloma. Overall survival rate varies by diagnosis, and approximately 9.4% of cancer deaths in the United States are expected to be caused by these three blood cancers in 2020.[2]

Risk Factors for Hematologic Malignancies

Risk factors for hematologic malignancy are similar among the different types, although some specific factors are associated with specific types. General risk factors include[1,3-10]:

- age greater than 65 years (except for Hodgkin lymphoma, which can also occur between the ages of 20 and 39 years);
- exposure to environmental toxins (including benzene and Agent Orange);
- family history of blood disorders;
- smoking;
- White race (except for multiple myeloma, which occurs more frequently in Black persons);
- exposure to high-dose radiation;
- inherited genetic syndromes;
- male sex;
- previous chemotherapies; and
- autoimmune diseases, certain viral infections, and a weakened immune system.

The Role of Body Mass Index and Weight

The World Cancer Research Fund International and the American Institute for Cancer Research completed a meta-analysis of many large published prospective studies and found that a higher body mass index (BMI) in adulthood and in early adulthood (aged 18 to 21 years) is associated with an increased risk of Hodgkin and non-Hodgkin lymphomas, acute myeloid leukemia, chronic myeloid leukemia, chronic lymphocytic leukemia, and multiple myeloma.[11] Research has shown that within non-Hodgkin lymphoma, the subgroup of diffuse large B-cell lymphoma was found to be most consistently positively associated with all anthropometric factors except for waist circumference. In regard to non-Hodgkin lymphoma specifically, BMI and weight in early adulthood may be more relevant than current BMI and weight. This finding would support the importance of maintaining a healthy weight from the start of early of adulthood to possibly prevent the development of non-Hodgkin lymphoma.[12]

The Cancer Prevention Study II (CPS-II) revealed a positive association between BMI and risk of myeloid leukemia which was further strengthened by another meta-analysis of 10 published prospective studies between the years 2004 and 2013.[13,14] The CPS-II found that overweight and obesity were associated with a 36% and 43%

higher risk of myeloid leukemia than normal BMI, respectively. Each subtype studied, including acute myeloid leukemia, chronic myeloid leukemia, and myelodysplastic syndrome, were found to have positive associations for BMI.[13]

In the 2016 International Agency for Research on Cancer consensus report on body fatness and cancer risk, multiple myeloma was the only hematologic subgroup found for which there is sufficient evidence that lack of body fatness lowers cancer risk.[15]

Types of Hematologic Malignancies

Numerous types of hematologic malignancies are known. Figure 14.1 shows the three main types of disease and several subtypes.

Leukemia

Leukemia is caused mainly by increased production of white blood cells (WBCs), although some leukemias can originate in other blood cells.[4] The large production of abnormal WBCs impairs the body's ability to fight infection and to produce new red blood cells (RBCs) and platelets. The four main types of leukemia are:

- acute lymphoblastic leukemia (ALL);
- acute myeloid leukemia (AML);
- chronic lymphocytic leukemia (CLL); and
- chronic myeloid leukemia (CML).

General signs and symptoms for leukemias include bone or joint pain, decreased appetite, enlarged lymph nodes, fatigue, fever, multiple or lingering infections, night sweats, shortness of breath, signs of bleeding (eg, petechiae or increased bruising), abdominal swelling, weight loss, anemia, shortness of breath, and splenomegaly.

Lymphoma

Lymphoma begins in the lymphatic system. The lymphatic system is made up of lymph nodes, vessels, and organs, and it fights infection and disease in the body. Lymphocytes, a type of WBC, are carried in the lymph and are distributed throughout the body via lymphatic vessels. Because the lymph is present throughout the body, lymphoma can originate at multiple sites.[16] There are two main types of lymphomas: Hodgkin and non-Hodgkin.

Hodgkin lymphoma (HL) accounted for 0.5% of new cancer cases between 2008 and 2014.[17,18] Signs and symptoms of HL include cough or chest pain, fatigue, fever, itching, night sweats, swelling in the lymph nodes, and weight loss.

Non-Hodgkin lymphoma (NHL) is more prevalent than HL and accounted for 4.3% of all new cancer cases from 2008 to 2014.[17,18] It includes more than 60 different subtypes, each classified according to the type of WBC involved (natural killer cells, T-cells, and B-cells). Some subtypes are fast-growing, while others are slow-growing. The most common types of NHL are diffuse large B-cell lymphoma (DLBCL), which is fast-growing, and follicular lymphoma, which is slow-growing.[1,16,19] Of the NHL subtypes that affect B-cells, DLBCL accounts for 30% of all NHL diagnoses, while follicular lymphoma accounts for roughly 20% of all cases, making it the second most common B-cell lymphoma[20]; and double-hit DLBCL is an aggressive subtype that accounts for about 5% of all cases. General signs and symptoms for NHL include abdominal swelling, fatigue, fever, night sweats, pain, skin rash or itchy skin, swelling in the lymph nodes, trouble breathing, and weight loss.[20,21]

Plasma Cell Neoplasms

Plasma cell neoplasms are conditions in which plasma cells develop from B-cells in the bone marrow in response to infection from bacteria

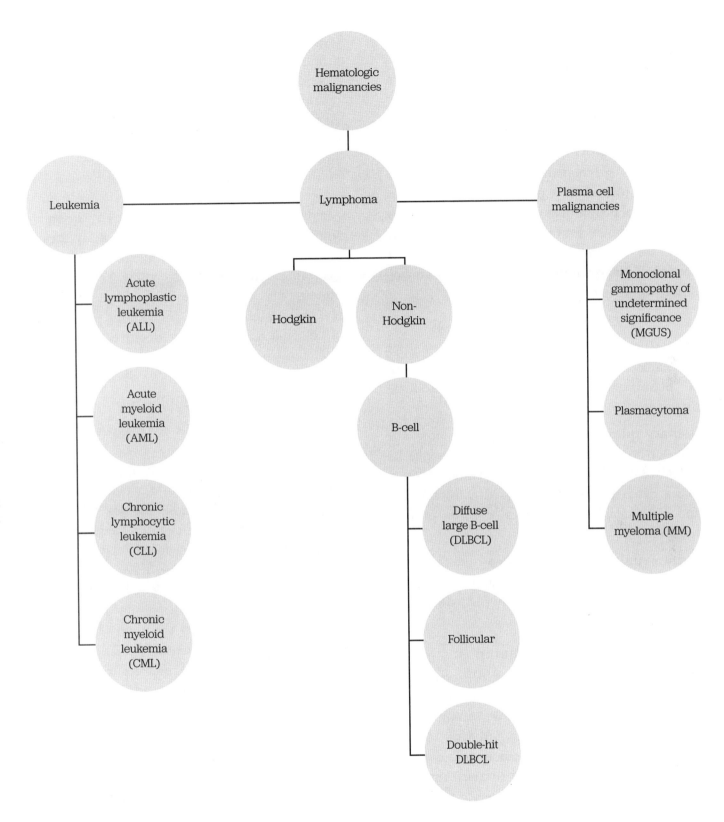

Figure 14.1
Hematologic malignancy types

and viruses. The plasma cells produce antibodies to fight the infection. Some plasma cell neoplasms are benign; others are malignant. There are several types of plasma cell neoplasm.

Monoclonal Gammopathy of Undetermined Significance

Monoclonal gammopathy of undetermined significance (MGUS) is a precancerous disease that affects 3% of people over the age of 50 years.[22] Most cases are benign; however, up to 25% of MGUS diagnoses convert to multiple myeloma or to another B-cell–related disorder, including amyloidosis, lymphoma, or macroglobulinemia.[22]

Plasmacytomas

Plasmacytomas usually form a tumor of abnormal plasma cells in one location. There are two types of plasmacytoma: isolated (or solitary) and extramedullary.[23,24]

Solitary plasmacytomas are uncommon and make up no more than 6% of plasma cell neoplasms. They are most often found in the bone.[24] Solitary plasmacytomas are usually treated with radiation, and some may require surgical excision prior to radiation[23,24]

Extramedullary plasmacytomas are found in the soft tissue, most often in the upper respiratory tract.[23] These are most commonly treated with surgical excision.[24]

Multiple Myeloma

Multiple myeloma (MM) affects 90% of those in whom plasma cell neoplasm is diagnosed. It affects multiple areas of the body, most commonly the spine, skull, long bones, and ribs.[25] Myeloma plasma cells produce an antibody protein called monoclonal immunoglobulin (or M protein) that does not fight infection and is superfluous to the body.[26] M proteins can build up in the blood and urine, causing possible damage to the kidneys and other organs.[25] MM is differentiated by the M protein produced.[26] Immunoglobulin G (IgG) MM is the most common form. Signs and symptoms for MM include anemia, bone pain, bones that break easily, elevated serum creatinine, fatigue, frequent infections, hypercalcemia, trouble breathing, weakness, and weight loss.

Amyloidosis

Amyloidosis is rare disease caused by insoluble amyloid proteins being deposited in body organs, commonly the kidneys, heart, nervous system, and gastrointestinal tract.[5,27] Over time, the abnormal protein build-up in tissues leads to organ dysfunction and death. Although amyloidosis is not a type of cancer, it may be associated with certain plasma cell neoplasms, like MM.[27,28]

Diagnosis

Hematologic malignancies are diagnosed using a variety of methods, including physical exam, bone marrow aspirate and biopsy, imaging, and serum blood analysis. An accurate diagnosis drives the best treatment plan for these diseases.[29] A peripheral blood smear is sufficient to diagnose some malignancies, but more in-depth analysis of bone marrow aspirate, blood serum draws, or imaging is required to diagnose others.[4,16] A high level of M protein in blood or urine is diagnostic for MM.[29] The higher the M protein level, the more advanced the disease.[30] Computed tomography (CT), magnetic resonance imaging (MRI), and positron emission tomography (PET) are used to assess if the disease has metastasized. Some disease subtypes are diagnosed using other tests, such as colonoscopy for mantle cell lymphoma, or upper and lower gastrointestinal (GI) endoscopy for mucosa-associated lymphoid tissue lymphoma.[2]

Staging and Classification

The staging and classification system for hematologic cancers is unique to this group of cancers, and the system varies among the different types. The TNM staging system (see Chapter 1) is not used because hematologic cancers normally do not form solid tumors. Stages of leukemia are commonly characterized by blood cell counts and by the accumulation of leukemia cells in other organs, such as the liver or spleen. Both HL and NHL are staged using the Lugano Classification System, in which the staging level is based on the number and location of cancerous lymph nodes, whether the cancerous lymph nodes are on one or both sides of the diaphragm, and whether the disease has metastasized outside the lymphatic system.[22-24,26]

Treatment

Treatment for hematologic malignancies includes systemic therapies, such as chemotherapy or other anticancer agents, radiotherapy, surgery, and sometimes high-dose chemotherapy followed by a hematopoietic cell transplantation (HCT).[29] Responses to treatment vary based on the type of cancer; however, cytogenetic abnormalities associated with each type are becoming crucial factors for identifying the best treatment to produce the best prognosis.[31] With an improved understanding of the various types of lymphoma, leukemia, and MM, specific treatments continue to emerge. It is now clear that every type of hematologic cancer is complex and unique, and each requires a specialized approach to ensure an optimal outcome.[29] General treatment regimens are summarized here. Refer to the National Comprehensive Cancer Network (NCCN) guidelines in oncology for the individual malignancies (available on the NCCN website at www.nccn.org/professionals/physician _gls/default.aspx) for details of specific therapies

for each disease. See Chapters 9 and 10 for information regarding treatment side effects, and Chapter 11 for details on managing nutrition impact symptoms. Chapter 15 covers medical nutrition therapy for patients undergoing HCT.

Treatment for Acute Myeloid Leukemia

Chemotherapy remains the standard treatment for AML, if the patient is able to tolerate it. Targeted therapies are also being used. Because AML is found throughout the blood, use of radiotherapy is limited, but it can be used to shrink myeloid sarcoma or when the disease has metastasized to the brain. AML treatment is divided into two phases: induction therapy and consolidation (postremission) therapy.[32] Induction therapy is designed to establish complete remission. Efficacy of the induction therapy is evaluated using a bone marrow aspirate and biopsy 14 to 21 days after therapy initiation.[33] Sometimes two rounds of induction treatment are required to ensure remission. Because AML almost always reoccurs without further treatment, consolidation therapy is typically given. The timing of this second induction course in persistent AML is controversial.[34] Persistent disease after two courses of induction therapy is considered to be an induction failure. Treatment for relapsed or refractory AML could include salvage chemotherapy, a clinical trial, or HCT.[33,34] Allogeneic HCT may be effective in 25% to 30% of patients with induction failure.[33]

Consolidation therapy aims to destroy leukemia cells that survived induction chemotherapy but are undetectable by medical tests.[33,35] The three main options for consolidation therapy are chemotherapy, autologous HCT, and allogeneic HCT. HCT is the best current treatment to prevent a recurrence of AML and presently the only cure, but a transplant is associated with high treatment-related morbidity and mortality, especially in older patients, and not everyone is a candidate.[32,36] Newer treatments, such as the introduction of kinase inhibitors and demethylating agents in clinical trials, given after intense consolidation therapy, are providing more targeted approaches.[37]

Treatment for Acute Lymphoblastic Leukemia

Treatment for ALL also includes different stages. Treatment generally spans years and includes induction, consolidation, and long-term maintenance therapies. The goal of induction therapy is to achieve complete remission. Many of the same medications used for induction therapy are used for consolidation therapy and are given for a few months. High-risk patients may undergo allogeneic HCT.[38] Radiation is not commonly used unless ALL has spread to the central nervous system (CNS).[39]

Treatment for Chronic Myeloid Leukemia

Treatment for CML depends on the disease phase: chronic, accelerated, or blastic. Standard treatment in the chronic phase includes targeted tyrosine kinase inhibitors (TKIs). If CML advances to the accelerated phase, the goal is to keep it from progressing to the blastic phase. A clinical trial is typically the standard treatment for accelerated CML, followed by TKIs as a second option. Once the blastic phase is reached, allogeneic HCT is needed. The induction chemotherapy used is similar to the chemotherapy used to treat pretransplant AML, with the addition of a TKI.[40,41]

Treatment for Chronic Lymphocytic Leukemia

Although many patients live a long time with CLL, it is difficult to cure. Immediate treatment is not always indicated, and the disease can be monitored.[42] Various treatments are used including chemotherapy, monoclonal antibodies, and targeted therapies.[42,43] If the CLL is high risk, HCT may be suggested.[43] Localized radiotherapy may be used if the spleen is enlarged or if there are swollen lymph nodes in a part of the body. If CLL is present in very high amounts within the cells, leukapheresis may be needed before chemotherapy to improve the effectiveness of the chemotherapy.[42]

If the patient does not respond to initial treatment or if the patient's CLL relapses, targeted therapy and monoclonal antibodies are commonly used, alone or in combination. Chemotherapy also may be an option. An HCT may be needed for patients with high-risk CLL and is an option for patients with relapsed or refractory CLL who respond well to second-line treatment.[43]

Treatment for Multiple Myeloma

Treatment for MM includes a variety of regimens. Standard systemic first-line therapy includes alkylating agents, immunomodulatory drugs, and proteasome inhibitors commonly used with the addition of steroids to achieve complete remission. Radiation is typically used for symptom management of bone pain.[44,45] Patients who achieve at least a very good partial remission after four to six cycles of induction therapy proceed to an autologous HCT per current NCCN guidelines for MM. High-dose melphalan is currently the most widely used conditioning regimen for autologous HCT for patents with MM.[46]

Treatment for Non-Hodgkin Lymphoma

Treatment for NHL depends on the type and stage of the lymphoma. Many times, a combination of medications is used, but the number and dosage of the drugs along with the length of therapy will vary. NHL treatment commonly includes chemotherapy, targeted therapy, immunotherapy, or radiation, alone or in combination. Intrathecal chemotherapy is used to treat lymphoma that has reached the CNS.[47]

Radiation can be used as the primary treatment for early stages of NHL because NHL tumors respond very well to radiation.[48] Radiation is most often given to patients with localized lymphoma or to patients with a large lymph node. It can also provide symptom relief in patients with advanced disease.[49]

Within immunotherapy, monoclonal antibodies and chimeric antigen receptor (CAR) T-cell therapy are being used to treat NHL. Specific target antigens include CD20, CD52, and CD30. CAR T-cell therapy involves the collection of a patient's T cells. The T cells are then altered in a laboratory to have specific receptors designed to seek out lymphoma cells once replaced in a patient's blood.[50]

Consolidation therapy with an autologous or allogeneic HCT with or without radiation may sometimes be used to treat refractory or relapsed lymphomas.[50,51]

Treatment for Hodgkin Lymphoma

Treatment for HL is similar to that for NHL but normally includes different drug combinations. Chemotherapy, radiation, and surgery are the three standard therapies used to treat HL. Early, favorable HL is treated with combination chemotherapy, combination chemotherapy with radiation to cancer-involving sites, or radiation alone to affected areas or the mantle area (neck, chest, armpits). Treatment of early, unfavorable HL may include combination chemotherapy or combination chemotherapy with radiation. Advanced HL is normally treated with combination chemotherapy. Recurrent HL treatment can be a combination of any of the aforementioned treatments but may also include a clinical trial.[52]

HCT is not a first-line treatment for HL, but it may be needed for patients who have progressive or relapsed lymphoma following treatment.[52]

Treatment for Indolent Lymphoma

Indolent lymphoma, a slowly progressing subtype of NHL, does not need treatment if patients are asymptomatic. Instead, watchful waiting includes regular physical examinations, imaging tests, and laboratory evaluations. Treatment with chemotherapy, immunotherapy, or targeted therapy is started if symptoms develop or tests indicate the cancer is growing.[51]

Chimeric Antigen Receptor T-Cell Therapy

CAR T-cell therapy is an emerging treatment modality displaying significant success in treating patients with hematologic malignancies, including large B-cell lymphoma and B-cell-precursor ALL.[53] Studies observed specific toxicities, including cytokine release syndrome and CAR T-cell therapy-related neurotoxicity, which typically present within the first days of infusion.[54,55] Manifestations of cytokine release syndrome include fevers, hypotension, hypoxia, end-organ dysfunction, cytopenias, coagulopathy, and hemophagocytic lymphohistiocytosis.[56]

Nutrition Assessment

Studies have shown that the prevalence of malnutrition among patients with hematologic cancers ranges from 27% to 50.4%.[57-60] In one study, 15% of patients with AML presented with undernutrition at the time of hospital admission and 9.5% of patients had a weight loss exceeding 5%. Undernutrition increased to 17% after induction chemotherapy.[61] The PREDyCES study, one of the largest multicenter studies of malnutrition in hospitalized patients, showed that 23% of oncology patients admitted were at risk of malnutrition on admission; this figure increased to 36.8% within the hematologic malignancy subgroup.[62]

Tumor-related malnutrition is possible with some lymphomas and with amyloidosis. The majority of nutrition impact symptoms of hematologic cancers are associated with treatment or with the patient's physiological response to the disease.[63,64] The disease itself can lead to malnutrition as well.[63] Chemotherapy, immunotherapy, and radiation therapy can commonly result in nutrition impact symptoms, such as frequent hospitalizations, GI symptoms, fatigue, depression, anxiety, and pain. These side effects are all considered risks for malnutrition during cancer treatment.[65,66] Research has also shown that undernutrition in patients with hematologic cancers is a risk factor for infectious complications.[67]

Malnutrition Screening

Early malnutrition screening can increase the percentage of patients who meet nutrient requirements during treatment and can help avoid declines in nutritional status. Ongoing follow-up is needed because nutritional status is likely to be affected if the disease is resistant to initial treatment and requires additional highly toxic treatments.[60,68] In one study of patients admitted with a variety of hematologic malignancies, the Malnutrition Screening Tool (MST) indicated a positive score for 37.8% of the patients.[60] Following an initial nutrition assessment completed by a registered dietitian nutritionist (RDN), 90.8% of the patients with a positive MST score were found to be malnourished, and 54.1% were considered to be moderately or severely malnourished. This represents a 25% rate of malnutrition in the total hematologic malignancy population screened at admission. This study showed that the initiation of a nutritional protocol within hematologic inpatients can lead to better detection of malnutrition and improve the process of therapeutic decisions. After the nutrition intervention, less than 25% of the malnourished patients needed oral supplementation. Also, upon reassessment after 1 week, there was a 21.7% increase in the percentage of patients who met their energy and protein needs.[60]

The patient-generated subjective global assessment (PG-SGA) has been found to be effective in assessing nutritional risk in patients with ALL. Studies have shown that average PG-SGA scores in high-risk patients with acute leukemia were significantly higher, indicating that nutritional status might be associated with risk category.[69] Patients with AML have been found to have higher PG-SGA scores than patients with ALL, with one explanation being the difference in induction treatment regimens.[70] Cytarabine, which is known to cause toxicities (eg, infection, fever, GI disorders, or stomatitis) is commonly included in the chemotherapy regimen for patients with AML. Also, myeloid hematopoietic cells are uncontrolled and grow rapidly in AML, which could decrease the levels of neutrophils, erythrocytes, and platelets, resulting in infection, anemia, and hemorrhage.[69] Each of these side effects can contribute to poor appetite, leading to less food intake and weight loss in patients with AML. BMI was also found to be higher in patients with ALL on day 21 of induction treatment. One study predicted that the use of prednisone in the ALL treatment protocol may have prevented these patients from excessive weight loss and inflammation.[70]

Similar results have been found in patients with MM. In one study, a higher PG-SGA score before chemotherapy was associated with reduced survival.[71] Research has revealed that early screening for malnutrition and nutritional interventions improves overall energy and protein intake in this population.[72] See Chapter 4 for additional information on nutrition screening.

Nutrition Assessment

The complete nutrition assessment may look different depending on the type of hematologic malignancy. Many solid tumors tend to share similar trajectories of illness, whereas hematologic malignancies can demonstrate more heterogeneity and, therefore, present varying nutritional needs. Some hematologic cancers are indolent, making them more manageable with specific disease-directed treatment of comparatively low intensity (eg, CLL, follicular lymphoma); others, such as AML and DLBCL, are more aggressive and require more-toxic, higher-risk therapies that increase nutrition-related risks.[73] Nutrition comorbidities, such as renal disease, type 2 diabetes, steroid-induced hyperglycemia, lipid changes, and osteoporosis, are also common within hematologic malignancies and should be evaluated and considered when completing a nutrition assessment. See Chapter 5 for additional details regarding assessment of nutritional needs.

Nutrition Problems and Interventions

Nutrition Status Before Hematopoetic Cell Transplantation

The maintenance or achievement of adequate nutrition status during induction therapy is important because of the known impacts of pretransplant nutrition status on outcomes after HCT. Research has shown that pretransplant nutrition status affects overall outcome, including length of hospital stay.[57] Patients undergoing bone marrow transplantation should receive a routine nutrition assessment pretransplantation.[57,74] Nutrition status before HCT can be affected by the patient's disease status, time of last chemotherapy, infections, and appetite. Weight loss of 10% or more in the 6 months before HCT has been found to negatively affect transplant outcomes.[57,75] A

meta-analysis of 26 studies (total of 32,683 patients) involving subjects diagnosed with hematologic malignancies and treated with HCT showed that patients with lower BMI had worse overall survival and event-free survival than patients with normal BMI. In this same study, improved overall survival was experienced by overweight or obese patients compared with underweight patients.[74]

Chemotherapy-Induced Nausea and Vomiting

Chemotherapy-induced nausea and vomiting (CINV) is a very common side effect of AML due to the use of several particular chemotherapies. Standard frontline chemotherapy for AML consists of cytarabine, given as a 7-day continuous infusion, plus 3 days of an anthracycline, most commonly daunorubicin. This regimen is typically administered on an inpatient basis.[76] Daunorubicin at this dose is regarded as a moderately emetogenic drug, whereas cytarabine is only mildly emetogenic at the doses used.[77] Compared to patients with solid tumors, patients with hematologic tumors are more commonly younger, which increases their risk of CINV. Currently, there are no collective international guidelines for combating CINV in these patients.[78] See Chapter 11 for information regarding the management of CINV.

Bone Health

Nutrition assessment and intervention for patients with MM should include a focus on bone health, as bone disease is a major cause of morbidity and mortality in this population.[79] Up to 80% of patients with MM will have osteolytic bone lesions at the time of diagnosis, and 60% can expect to develop pathologic fractures over the course of their disease.[80,81] It has been estimated that 75% of patients with MM have osteopenia or osteoporosis.[81]

Currently, only general recommendations exist regarding diet and supplementation for the protection of bone health in patients with MM.[82] RDNs should stress consumption of a well-balanced diet that includes sources of calcium and vitamin D. The National Osteoporosis Foundation (NOF) recommends supplementing with vitamin D and calcium if patients are unable to meet their needs through diet, particularly if patients are receiving bisphosphate therapy.[83] NOF follows the guidelines set by the Institute of Medicine (IOM; now the Health and Medicine Division of the National Academies of Sciences, Engineering, and Medicine). The IOM recommendations state that men aged 50 to 70 years should consume 1,000 mg of calcium per day and that women aged 51 years and older and men aged 71 years and older should consume 1,200 mg of calcium per day. A calcium supplement should be taken to meet these requirements if diet alone is not sufficient. NOF recommends an intake of vitamin D of 400 to 800 IU/d for adults aged less than 50 years, and 800 to 1,000 IU/d for adults aged 50 years and older (higher than the IOM recommendation) through diet plus supplementation. NOF also encourages weight-bearing and weight-strengthening exercises as the patient is able.[82,83] Patients with hypercalcemia or renal insufficiency should not take calcium supplements.[82]

Sarcopenia

A few studies have examined the effect of sarcopenia on the clinical outcome of patients with lymphoma. One study found a statistically significant and independent association of sarcopenia with higher nonrelapse mortality, more complications, and more days spent in the hospital (in men and women) after autologous HCT in patients with both HL and NHL.[84] A study specific to DLBCL found that sarcopenia is a strong and independent prognostic factor in elderly patients with DLBCL who have been treated with chemotherapy plus rituximab. In this study, less lean body mass was found to correlate with an increased risk of not completing the planned treatment and an increased frequency of having a more advanced disease and poorer performance status. Sarcopenia was found to be predictive of progression-free survival and overall survival independent of albuminemia, BMI, or revised International Prognostic Index in a study involving patients over the age of 70 years.[85]

With the known negative impacts of sarcopenia in patients with lymphoma, nutrition intervention should place considerable emphasis on the maintenance or gain of muscle mass. Physical activity or performance status can further lead to loss of lean body mass; therefore, it is recommended by the European Society for Clinical Nutrition and Metabolism that nutrition and physical therapy be combined.[86] These studies indicate the importance of making body composition part of the nutrition assessment in order to guide nutrition interventions. There should be specific measurements to determine muscle and fat reserves. Specific measurements can be provided through dual-energy x-ray absorptiometry, anthropometry, CT scans at lumbar level 3, or bioimpedance analysis.[87]

Serum Vitamin D Status

Vitamin D affects cellular differentiation, proliferation, apoptosis, and angiogenesis, and has recently been studied as a modifiable prognostic factor in many cancers.[88] Although more research is required, recent studies suggest that vitamin D deficiency is associated with poorer prognosis, higher rates of relapse, significantly longer hospital stays, and decreased rate of remission in patients with hematologic malignancies, including HL, myelodysplastic syndromes, NHL, MM, and leukemia.[89-93]

Low levels of 25-hydroxyvitamin D in patients with AML were found to be associated with worse outcomes in one study. In this study, patients with AML who had an *FLT3* gene mutation were even more likely to have low vitamin D levels, and patients with AML and normal vitamin D levels rarely had this mutation. More research is needed to determine if supplementing with vitamin D would improve outcomes for patients with AML.[90]

Vitamin D insufficiency at the time of CLL diagnosis is associated with a decreased time to the initiation of treatment, according to one study.[94] Another study revealed that supplementation with vitamin D in patients with CLL appears to be safe; however, whether it actually alters cancer prognosis remains to be determined.[95]

Multiple recent studies have found a high incidence of vitamin D deficiency and insufficiency in patients with MM.[91,96,97] This insufficiency should be of particular concern in MM diagnoses because skeletal complications are a chief cause of morbidity, and there is clear evidence that vitamin D plays a significant role in skeletal metabolism.[91,96,98] Also, patients with chronic renal disease have been found to be at higher risk of vitamin D deficiency, even at very early stages.[98] However, even a higher vitamin D supplementation (>1,000 IU/d) does not appear to be enough for MM patients. Additionally, a study demonstrated the difficulties with correcting existing deficits, with the majority of patients not achieving sufficient long-term 25-hydroxyvitamin D levels during follow-up.[97]

Although a causal relationship has not yet been firmly established, there is some research demonstrating that vitamin D supplementation might improve patient outcomes in patients with DLBCL who are receiving rituximab. One such study demonstrated that vitamin D supplementation led to significantly better event-free survival in patients receiving conventional rituximab-containing chemotherapy for their DLBCL.[99] Another study showed that low 25-hydroxyvitamin D3 serum levels were associated with a worse outcome in elderly patients with DLBCL.[100] This finding was found in patients with follicular lymphoma as well.[101]

A meta-analysis of randomized controlled trials of vitamin D supplementation and total cancer incidence and mortality found that vitamin D supplementation significantly reduced total cancer mortality but did not reduce total cancer incidence.[102] A meta-analysis specific to colon cancer found similar results, while another study did not support an association between supplemental calcium or vitamin D-3 (or both) taken for 3 to 5 years and risk of recurrent colorectal adenoma.[103,104] More research specific to hematologic cancers is needed to determine if vitamin D supplementation in patients who are deficient in this nutrient is associated with improved outcomes because no large-scale trial of vitamin D supplementation has yet confirmed such a causal relation with cancer incidence.[105]

RDNs can play an active role in advocating for the evaluation of all patients with hematologic malignancies for vitamin D deficiency and recommending supplementation as needed. There are currently no established guidelines for vitamin D screening in patients with cancer, but it is important, as a clinician, to be aware that cancer patients are predisposed toward vitamin D deficiency because of such factors as insufficient dietary intake, malnutrition, and limited sun exposure and physical activity owing to fatigue and a poor performance status.[106] The American Cancer Society recommends a diet including foods rich in vitamin D, with a goal of meeting the patient's age-specific Recommended Dietary Allowance (RDA) in order to maximize bone health and muscle function. The RDA for vitamin D for persons aged 1 to 70 years is 600 IU/d; and for adults older than 70 years, it is 800 IU/d.[103] It is not currently known if the established RDA is enough to provide all of the potential nonskeletal health benefits associated with vitamin D. The Endocrine Society recommends a maintenance tolerable upper limit of vitamin D of 4,000 IU/d for everyone over 8 years of age, and this should not be exceeded without medical supervision.[107]

Renal Disease

Both acute and chronic renal insufficiencies are common in patients with MM. As many as 50% of people in whom MM is diagnosed have an elevated creatinine level.[70] Acute kidney injury (AKI) is common, at least with an initial MM diagnosis, and nutritional needs and recommendations may need to be tailored. AKI in patients with MM can occur as a result of protein build-up that leads to glomeruli blockage (light-chain cast nephropathy), volume depletion, hypercalcemia, or tumor lysis syndrome.[108,109] Specific macronutrient and micronutrient recommendations for patients with kidney disease may vary throughout treatment, and RDNs should provide routine follow-up assessments to address necessary changes. The Academy of Nutrition and Dietetics strongly recommends that the RDN monitor the nutritional status of patients with chronic kidney disease (CKD) every 1 to 3 months, and more frequently if there is inadequate nutrient intake, protein-energy malnutrition, mineral and electrolyte disorders, or the presence of an illness that may worsen nutritional status.[110] It has been estimated that within 1.2 years of diagnosis of MM, 61% of patients develop renal impairment and 50% develop CKD.[111] As mentioned in the diagnosis section, renal failure is one of the components used to diagnosis MM.[112]

Nutrition recommendations vary based on the level of renal disease and use of dialysis.[112] Malnutrition is a common side effect of renal disease, but research has demonstrated that nutrition interventions can reduce the risk for malnutrition as well as other common symptoms, such as muscle wasting (sarcopenia), hypertension, fatigue, nausea, and overall poor quality of life.[87] The National Kidney Foundation's Kidney Disease Outcomes Quality Initiative created the initial recommendations for nutrition in CKD.[109] The general guidelines of the National Institute of Diabetes and Digestive and Kidney Diseases are as follows[113]:

- Limit sodium intake to less than 2,300 mg/d.
- Eat adequate but not excessive protein. For early kidney disease, limit portion sizes to one serving per meal. Advanced stages with dialysis require a protein-rich diet. Compare to the Adequate Intake for protein of 0.8 g per kg of body weight per day.
- Choose heart-healthy foods to reduce the risk of cardiovascular events.
- Restrict phosphorus if elevated.
- Restrict potassium if elevated.

A full nutrition assessment should be performed on all patients with renal disease. The assessment should include a nutrition-focused physical examination along with assessments of micronutrient status and overall dietary intake. Vitamin B6, vitamin K, selenium, zinc, and vitamin C are all examples of micronutrients at risk for patients with CKD. Supplementation with a renal-specific multivitamin with minerals may improve mortality risk if oral nutrition intake is not sufficient.[112-117] Because a renal diet can be so restrictive, it is recommended that RDNs create individualized meal plans that are feasible, sustainable, and suited for a patient's needs, preferences, and overall quality of life.[118]

Amyloidosis

Amyloidosis is associated with certain blood cancers, such as MM, and can lead to specific nutrition issues, depending on which organs are affected. Common organs affected include the heart, kidneys, liver, and GI tract. Amyloidosis could impair nutrition status, especially if GI involvement is present. Although research is limited and includes only small sample sizes, studies have shown that as much as one quarter of outpatients with primary amyloidosis (AL amyloidosis) may be malnourished.[119] Research has also demonstrated that malnutrition is an independent predictor of survival for AL amyloidosis, and a deterioration of nutritional status negatively affects quality of life in these patients.[119-122] Nutritional counseling in patients with AL amyloidosis was shown to be useful in helping patients maintain body weight, effective in improving energy intake, and associated with better survival.[123]

GI manifestations of systemic amyloidosis may include pain and bloating, nausea, early satiety, weight loss, reflux, diarrhea, constipation, bleeding, and dysphagia. Amyloid deposition within the GI tract can impair the structure and function of the GI tract, which can lead to resistant digestion and gastroparesis, among other symptoms. GI manifestations of amyloidosis can occur in the mouth, esophagus, stomach, small intestine, and colon. Liver involvement is also common; an estimated 70% of patients with amyloidosis are found to have hepatomegaly and elevated alkaline phosphatase levels.[124]

Amyloidosis located in the mouth commonly presents as macroglossia. This causes problems with swallowing and chewing, along with speech issues. The inability to close the mouth and involvement of the salivary glands can lead to xerostomia. If the tongue is enlarged enough, this can result in obstruction of the upper airway. Common nutrition-related symptoms include weight loss and dysgeusia.[124]

Nutrition interventions should aim to alleviate specific GI symptoms (see Chapter 11), such as the possible need for nutritional and vitamin supplementation if malabsorption is present and also diet-related treatment for diarrhea or possible obstruction.[125,126]

Symptoms of cardiac amyloidosis may include anorexia, dysphagia, dysgeusia, vomiting, diarrhea, malabsorption, and weight loss.[119] Renal involvement is one of the most common sites in AL amyloidosis, with clinically evident renal disease estimated in 48% to 82% of patients. Patients with the renal amyloidosis can develop severe hypertension and volume overload. For this reason, nutrition counseling on dietary salt and fluid restriction is recommended as an important component of the management of edema.[127]

Hyperglycemia

During cancer treatment, hyperglycemia can result not only from a preexisting history of diabetes but also from steroid-induced hyperglycemia. Steroids, specifically dexamethasone and prednisone, are part of several treatment regimens for lymphoma, leukemia, and MM. In a study of adults with AML, a history of type 2 diabetes was associated with an increased risk for 30-day mortality, even after controlling for other factors such as age and comorbidities.[128]

Hypertriglyceridemia

Although rare, this can occur in patients with ALL who receive a pediatric regimen that includes PEG-L-asparaginase. Dietary intervention should be considered a first-line treatment and should include decreasing total fat intake (<10% to 15% of total energy intake) and choosing complex carbohydrates that are higher in dietary fiber. Patients with obesity or diabetes should be carefully monitored for the occurrence of hypertriglyceridemia.[129,130]

Body Composition and Body Mass Index

In a large study in patients with AML, obesity prior to induction chemotherapy treatment (ie, at the time of diagnosis) was found to be positively associated with higher responses to treatment. Although an increased BMI was associated with higher response rates and lower rates of resistance to chemotherapy, there was no impact on survival, treatment-related deaths, or toxicities.[131] Because obesity is associated with an increased risk of comorbidities, such as diabetes and heart disease, these findings were surprising because obesity has also been found to lead to more toxicities.[132]

Survivorship

Long-term effects of hematologic malignancies and its treatments can precipitate the following problems that warrant long-term dietary follow-up.

Cardiovascular Events

A study of 46,829 survivors of HL and 14,764 survivors of NHL showed an increased risk for fatal cardiovascular events in lymphoma survivors (compared with the general population) who were treated with anthracycline-containing chemotherapy regimens (eg, AVBD, BEACOPP) and radiotherapy to the chest area.[133,134] The majority of the excess cardiac risk is not realized until 10 years after exposure, and the risk remains significantly elevated for at least 25 years. The presence of cardiovascular disease risk factors not associated with cancer treatment are additive to this elevated risk.[135] Numerous studies have shown that smoking, hypertension, dyslipidemia, and diabetes can pose additional risk to HL survivors; therefore, this group should be targeted for cardiovascular screening and prevention campaigns.[133-140] One study recommends that all survivors of HL be educated regarding the risk of late effects and advised to practice a healthy lifestyle that includes maintaining a healthy weight through diet and exercise.[135] The American Heart Association recommends the following dietary interventions to help prevent cardiovascular disease[141]:

■ Balance energy intake and physical activity to achieve or maintain a healthy body weight. Exercise for at least 30 minutes on most days (60 minutes for adults trying to lose weight and for children).

■ Consume a diet rich in vegetables and fruits, especially carrots, peaches, and berries because of their high nutrient content.

■ Choose whole grain, high-fiber foods.

■ Consume fish, especially oily fish, at least twice a week.

■ Limit intake of saturated and *trans* fats and cholesterol. Consume less than 7% of energy as saturated fat and less than 1% as *trans* fat, and consume less than 300 mg of cholesterol per day.

■ Minimize intake of beverages and foods with added sugars.

■ Choose and prepare foods with little or no salt. Consume no more than 2.3 g of sodium daily.

■ Consume alcohol in moderation, if at all. Men should limit their alcohol intake to no more than two drinks per day, and women to no more than one. Alcoholic drinks should be consumed with meals.

Osteoporosis

Bone changes commonly occur in patients with MM, due to increased osteoclast and decreased osteoblast activity, which can lead to fractures. Risk for osteoporosis and bone loss is further increased by the long-term use of corticosteroids in MM treatment regimens.[142] Bone health should be reinforced for all MM patients. Although many patients receive bisphosphonate therapy, calcium and vitamin D supplementation also are recommended. Calcium supplements should be used with caution in patients with renal insufficiency.[108] The National Kidney Foundation recommends that the total dose of elemental calcium provided by calcium-based phosphate binders not exceed 1,500 mg/d and the total intake of elemental calcium (including dietary calcium) not exceed 2,000 mg/d in patients who have stage 3 through 5 CKD.[109]

Glucose Intolerance

Studies show that survivors of hematologic malignancies have an increased risk for developing type 2 diabetes, particularly if treatment has included HCT or radiotherapy.[143-145] Diabetes, particularly steroid-induced hyperglycemia, may be associated with poor clinical outcomes in patients with MM.[145] In survivors of HL specifically, radiation to the para-aortic lymph nodes or pancreatic tail has been found to increase the risk of developing type 2 diabetes mellitus. The direct cause of developing type 2 diabetes following radiation in HL to the pancreatic area is not currently known[144]; therefore, medical nutrition therapy provided by the RDN should address glucose intolerance. The Academy of Nutrition and Dietetics evidence-based nutrition practice guidelines include the following recommendations for patients with type 2 diabetes[146,147]:

- Recognize that a variety of eating patterns (combinations of different foods or food groups) are acceptable for the management of diabetes.

- Individualize the nutrition prescription for macronutrients.

- Encourage the intake of fiber and whole grain foods.

- Encourage moderate-intensity physical activity as tolerated.

- If the patient is prescribed medication, educate him or her on potential food and drug interactions and nutrition-related adverse effects.

- Counsel the patient based on established, well-defined behavior changes.

- Consider the patient's personal preferences (eg, tradition, culture, religion, health beliefs and goals, economics) and metabolic goals when recommending one eating pattern over another.

Summary

Hematologic malignancies are varied, and treatment for these diseases can be complex and ongoing. Early screening and nutrition intervention may prevent malnutrition in these patients. Besides the common side effects of chemotherapy and radiation, the RDN should be aware of disease-specific side effects that may warrant more involved medical nutrition therapy. It is important for the RDN to be aware of long-term side effects from these treatments, and ongoing follow-up is necessary for this population.

Because the treatments provided have long-term nutrition-related side effects that influence the health of survivors, the RDN should continue to assess this population and provide interventions as warranted years into survivorship. Related to the research demonstrating the possible increased risk of developing certain hematologic malignancies based on BMI, RDNs may also play a key role in the prevention and risk of recurrence. Adherence to the American Cancer Society guidelines on weight, nutrition, and physical activity has been found to reduce risk of total cancer incidence and mortality among older nonsmoking adults.[148]

Sample PES Statements
for Hematologic Malignancies

Intake domain: Inadequate energy intake related to decreased ability to consume sufficient energy due to side effects of cancer therapy, as evidenced by chemotherapy-induced nausea and vomiting, weight loss of 3% in the past month, and a dietary intake of <75% of estimated needs.

Clinical domain: Moderate, chronic, disease-related, or condition-related malnutrition related to anorexia and early satiety, as evidenced by a weight loss of 5% in the past month and dietary intake of <75% of estimated needs in the past month.

Behavioral-environmental domain: Food- and nutrition-related knowledge deficit related to lack of prior exposure to immunosuppressive food safety precautions, as evidenced by reported consumption of raw and unprocessed foods such as fish and nuts.

References

1. Blood cancers (for patients). American Society of Hematology website. Accessed October 29, 2020. https://hematology.org /Patients/Cancers

2. Facts and statistics. Leukemia and Lymphoma Society website. Accessed October 29, 2020. www .lls.org/facts-and-statistics/facts -and-statistics-overview/facts-and -statistics

3. Cancer facts and figures 2020. American Cancer Society website. Accessed November 3, 2020. www.cancer.org/content /dam/cancer-org/research /cancer-facts-and-statistics /annual-cancer-facts-and-figures /2020/cancer-facts-and-figures -2020.pdf

4. Leukemia. American Cancer Society website. Accessed October 29, 2020. www.cancer .org/cancer/leukemia.html

5. What is multiple myeloma? American Cancer Society website. Accessed October 29, 2020. www.cancer.org/cancer /multiple-myeloma/about/what-is -multiple-myeloma.html

6. Cancer stat facts. National Cancer Institute Surveillance, Epidemiology, and End Results Program website. Accessed October 29, 2020. https://seer .cancer.gov/statfacts

7. American Society of Clinical Oncology. Lymphoma-Hodgkin: risk factors. Cancer.Net website. Updated April 2019. Accessed October 29, 2020. www.cancer .net/cancer-types/lymphoma -hodgkin/risk-factors

8. American Society of Clinical Oncology. Leukemia—acute lymphocytic—ALL. Cancer. Net website. Accessed October 29, 2020. www.cancer.net /cancer-types/leukemia-acute -lymphocytic-all

9. American Society of Clinical Oncology. Leukemia—acute myeloid—AML. Cancer.Net website. Accessed October 29, 2020. www.cancer.net /cancer-types/leukemia -acute-myeloid-aml

10. Multiple myeloma. American Cancer Society website. Accessed October 29, 2020. https:// cancer.org/cancer/multiple -myeloma.html

11. Abar L, Sobiecki JG, Cariolou M, et al. Body size and obesity during adulthood, and risk of lympho-haematopoietic cancers: an update of the WCRF-AICR systematic review of published prospective studies. *Ann Oncol.* 2014;30(4):528-541. doi:10.1093 /annonc/mdz045

12. Hidayat K, Li HJ, Shi BM. Anthropometric factors and non-Hodgkin's lymphoma risk: systematic review and meta-analysis of prospective studies. *Crit Rev Oncol Hematol.* 2018;129:113-123. doi:10.1016/j .critrevonc.2018.05.018

13. Calle EE, Rodriguez C, Jacobs EJ, et al. The American Cancer Society Cancer Prevention Study II Nutrition Cohort: rationale, study design, and baseline characteristics. *Cancer.* 2002;94(9):2490-2501.

14. Teras LR, Patel AV, Carter BD, Rees-Punia E, McCullough ML, Gapstur SM. Anthropometric factors and risk of myeloid leukaemias and myelodysplastic syndromes: a prospective study and meta-analysis. *Br J Haematol.* 2019;186(2):243-254. doi:10.1111 /bjh.15904

15. Lauby-Secretan B, Scoccianti C, Loomis D, Grosse Y, Bianchini F, Straif K. Body fatness and cancer—viewpoint of the IARC Working Group. *N Eng J Med.* 2016;375(8):794-798. doi:10.1056 /NEJMsr1606602

16. Lymphoma. American Cancer Society website. Accessed October 29, 2020. www.cancer .org/cancer/lymphoma.html

17. Cancer stat facts: non-Hodgkin lymphoma. National Cancer Institute Surveillance, Epidemiology, and End Results Program website. Accessed October 29, 2020. https://seer .cancer.gov/statfacts/html /nhl.html

18. Cancer stat facts: Hodgkin lymphoma. National Cancer Institute Surveillance, Epidemiology, and End Results Program website. Accessed October 29, 2020. https://seer .cancer.gov/statfacts/html /hodg.html

19. Thumallapally N, Meshref A, Mousa M, Terjanian T. Solitary plasmacytoma: population-based analysis of survival trends and effect of various treatment modalities in the USA. *BMC Cancer*. 2017;17:13. doi:10.1186/s12885-016-3015-5

20. American Society of Clinical Oncology. Lymphoma—non-Hodgkin: subtypes. Cancer.Net website. Accessed October 29, 2020. www.cancer.net/cancer-types/lymphoma-non-hodgkin/subtypes

21. Zhang Y, Dai Y, Zheng T, Ma S. Risk factors of non-Hodgkin lymphoma. *Expert Opin Med Diagn*. 2011;5(6):539-550. doi:10.1517/17530059.2011.618185

22. Berenson JR. Monoclonal gammopathy of undetermined significance (MGUS). Merck Manual website, professional version. Accessed August 17, 2018. www.merckmanuals.com/professional/hematology-and-oncology/plasma-cell-disorders/monoclonal-gammopathy-of-undetermined-significance-mgus

23. Plasma cell neoplasms (including multiple myeloma)—health professional version. National Cancer Institute website. Accessed October 29, 2020. www.cancer.gov/types/myeloma/hp

24. American Society of Clinical Oncology. Leukemia—chronic lymphocytic—CLL. Cancer.Net website. Accessed October 29, 2020. www.cancer.net/cancer-types/leukemia-chronic-lymphocytic-cll

25. American Society of Clinical Oncology. Multiple myeloma: stages. Cancer.Net website. Accessed October 29, 2020. www.cancer.net/cancer-types/multiple-myeloma/stages

26. Myeloma. Leukemia and Lymphoma Society website. Accessed October 29, 2020. www.lls.org/disease-information/myeloma

27. Baker KR, Rice L. The amyloidosis: clinical features, diagnosis and treatment. *Methodist DeBakey Cardiovasc J*. 2012;8(3):3-7. doi:10.14797/mdcj-8-3-3

28. National Cancer Institute. Plasma cell neoplasms (including multiple myeloma) treatment (PDQ)–health professional version. Updated October 22, 2020. Accessed October 29, 2020. www.cancer.gov/types/myeloma/hp/myeloma-treatment-pdq

29. Berenson JR. Multiple myeloma: pathophysiology. Merck Manual website, professional version. Accessed May 31, 2019. www.merckmanuals.com/professional/hematology-and-oncology/plasma-cell-disorders/multiple-myeloma#v976233

30. Olsen M. Overview of hematological malignancies. In: Olsen M, Zitella LJ, eds. *Hematologic Malignancies in Adults*. Oncology Nursing Society; 2013:1-17.

31. Prakash G, Kaur A, Malhotra P, et al. Current role of genetics in hematologic malignancies. *Indian J Hematol Blood Transfus*. 2016;32(1):18-31. doi:10.1007/s12288-015-0584-4

32. American Society of Clinical Oncology. Leukemia—acute myeloid—AML: treatment options. Cancer.Net website. October 29, 2020. www.cancer.net/cancer-types/leukemia-acute-myeloid-aml/treatment-options

33. O'Donnell MR, Tallman MS, Abboud CN, et al. Acute myeloid leukemia. *J Natl Compr Canc Netw*. 2017;15(7):926-957.

34. National Comprehensive Cancer Network. *NCCN Clinical Practice Guidelines in Oncology (NCCN Guidelines): Acute Myeloid Leukemia*. Version 2.2018. National Comprehensive Cancer Network; 2018. Accessed August 22, 2018. www.nccn.org/professionals/physician_gls/pdf/aml.pdf

35. Larson RA. Post-remission therapy for acute myeloid leukemia in younger adults. UpToDate website. Accessed January 2, 2018. www.uptodate.com/contents/post-remission-therapy-for-acute-myeloid-leukemia-in-younger-adults

36. Dombret H, Gardin C. An update of current treatments for adult acute myeloid leukemia. *Blood*. 2016;127(1):53-61. doi:10.1182/blood-2015-08-604520

37. Schlenk, RF. Post-remission therapy for acute myeloid leukemia. *Haemetalogia.* 2014;99(11):1663-1670. doi:10.3324/haematol.2014.114611

38. Typical treatment of acute lymphocytic leukemia (ALL). American Cancer Society website. Updated October 17, 2018. Accessed October 29, 2020. www.cancer.org/cancer/acute-lymphocytic-leukemia/treating/typical-treatment.html

39. Terwilliger T, Abdul-Hay M. Acute lymphoblastic leukemia: a comprehensive review and 2017 update. *Blood Cancer J.* 2017;7(6):e577. doi:10.1038/bcj.2017.53

40. National Comprehensive Cancer Network. *NCCN Clinical Practice Guidelines in Oncology (NCCN Guidelines): Chronic Myeloid Leukemia.* Version 2.2018. National Comprehensive Cancer Network; 2018. Accessed August 22, 2018. www.nccn.org/professionals/physician_gls/pdf/cml.pdf

41. American Society of Clinical Oncology. Leukemia—chronic myeloid—CML: types of treatment. Cancer.Net website. October 29, 2020. www.cancer.net/cancer-types/leukemia-chronic-myeloid-cll/treatment-options

42. Typical treatment of chronic lymphocytic leukemia. American Cancer Society website. Updated April 22, 2020. Accessed October 29, 2020. www.cancer.org/cancer/chronic-lymphocytic-leukemia/treating/treatment-by-risk-group.html

43. American Society of Clinical Oncology. Leukemia—chronic lymphocytic—CLL: types of treatment. Cancer.Net website. Accessed October 29, 2020. www.cancer.net/cancer-types/leukemia-chronic-lymphocytic-cll/types-treatment

44. American Society of Clinical Oncology. Multiple myeloma: types of treatment. Cancer.Net website. Accessed October 29, 2020. www.cancer.net/cancer-types/multiple-myeloma/treatment-options

45. Standard treatments. Multiple Myeloma Research Foundation website. Accessed October 29, 2020. https://themmrf.org/multiple-myeloma/treatment-options/standard-treatments

46. Melphalan (Alkeran). International Myeloma Foundation website. Accessed May 1, 2019. https://myeloma.org/treatment/current-fda-approved-medications/melphalan-alkeran

47. Chemotherapy for non-Hodgkin lymphoma. American Cancer Society website. Updated August 1, 2018. Accessed February 18, 2019. www.cancer.org/cancer/non-hodgkin-lymphoma/treating/chemotherapy.html

48. Immunotherapy for non-Hodgkin lymphoma. American Cancer Society website. Updated August 1, 2018. Accessed February 18, 2019. www.cancer.org/cancer/non-hodgkin-lymphoma/treating/immunotherapy.html

49. Radiation therapy for non-Hodgkin lymphoma. American Cancer Society website. Updated November 30, 2018. Accessed February 18, 2019. www.cancer.org/cancer/non-hodgkin-lymphoma/treating/radiation-therapy.html

50. American Society of Clinical Oncology. Lymphoma—non-Hodgkin: treatment options. Cancer.Net website. Accessed February 18, 2019. https://cancer.net/cancer-types/lymphoma-non-hodgkin/treatment-options

51. High-dose chemotherapy and stem cell transplant for non-Hodgkin lymphoma. American Cancer Society website. Updated August 1, 2018. Accessed February 18, 2019. www.cancer.org/cancer/non-hodgkin-lymphoma/treating/bone-marrow-stem-cell.html

52. American Society of Clinical Oncology. Lymphoma—Hodgkin: types of treatment. Cancer.Net website. Accessed February 18, 2019. www.cancer.net/cancer-types/lymphoma-hodgkin/types-treatment

53. Boyiadzis MM, Dhodapkar MV, Brentjens RJ, et al. Chimeric antigen receptor (CAR) T therapies for the treatment of hematologic malignancies: clinical perspective and significance. *J Immunother Cancer.* 2018;6(1):137. doi:10.1186/s40425-018-0460-5

54. Bonifant CL, Jackson HJ, Brentjens RJ, Curran KJ. Toxicity and management in CAR T-cell therapy. *Mol Ther Oncolytics.* 2016;3:16011. doi:10.1038/mto.2016.11

55. Maude SL, Frey N, Shaw PA, et al. Chimeric antigen receptor T cells for sustained remissions in leukemia. *N Engl J Med.* 2014;371(16):1507-1517. doi:10.1056/NEJMoa1407222

56. Brudno JN, Kochenderfer JN. Recent advances in CAR T-cell toxicity: mechanisms, manifestations and management. *Blood Rev.* 2019;34:45-55. doi:10.1016/j.blre.2018.11.002

57. Horsley P, Bauer J, Gallagher B. Poor nutritional status prior to peripheral blood stem cell transplantation is associated with increased length of hospital stay. *Bone Marrow Transplant.* 2005;35(11):1113-1116. doi:10.1038/sj.bmt.1704963

58. Baltazar Luna E, Omaña Guzmán LI, Ortiz Hernández L, Ñamendis-Silva SA, De Nicola Delfin L. Estado nutricional en pacientes de primer ingreso a hospitalización del Servicio de Hematología del Instituto Nacional de Cancerología. *Nutr Hosp.* 2013;28(3):1259-1265. doi:10.3305/nh.2013.28.4.6484

59. Calleja Fernandez A, Pintor de la Maza B, Vidal Casariego A, et al. Food intake and nutritional status influence outcomes in hospitalized hematology-oncology patients. *Nutr Hosp.* 2015;31(6):2598-2605. doi:10.3305/nh.2015.31.6.8674

60. Villar-Taibo R, Calleja-Fernandez A, Vidal-Casariego A, et al. A short nutritional intervention in a cohort of hematological inpatients improves energy and protein intake and stabilizes nutritional status. *Nutr Hosp.* 2016;33(6):1347-1353. doi:10.20960/nh.794

61. Deluche E, Girault S, Jesus P, et al. Assessment of the nutritional status of adult patients with acute myeloid leukemia during induction chemotherapy. *Nutrition.* 2017;41:120-125. doi:10.1016/j.nut.2017.04.011

62. Álvarez-Hernández J, Planas Vila M, León-Sanz M, et al. Prevalence and costs of malnutrition in hospitalized patients; the PREDyCES Study. *Nutr Hosp.* 2012;27(4):1049-1059. doi:10.3305/nh.2012.27.4.5986

63. Gómez-Candela C, Canales Albendea MA, Palma Milla S, et al. Nutritional intervention in oncohematological patient. *Nutr Hosp.* 2012;27(3):669-680. doi:10.3305/nh.2012.27.3.5863

64. Kumar, NB. Assessment of malnutrition and nutritional therapy approaches in cancer patients. In: *Nutritional Management of Cancer Treatment Effects.* Springer-Verlag; 2012:7-41. doi:10.1007/978-3-642-27233-2

65. Gómez-Candela C, Luengo LM, Cos AI, et al. Subjective global assessment in neoplastic patients. *Nutr Hosp.* 2003;18(6):353-357.

66. Waitzberg DL, Caiaffa WT, Correia MI. Hospital malnutrition: the Brazilian national survey (IBRANUTRI): a study of 4000 patients. *Nutrition.* 2001;17(7–8):573-580. doi:10.1016/s0899-9007(01)00573-1

67. Schneider SM, Veyres P, Pivot X, et al. Malnutrition is an independent factor associated with nosocomial infections. *Br J Nutr.* 2004;92(1):105-111. doi:10.1079/BJN20041152

68. Santarpia L, Contaldo F, Pasanisi F. Nutritional screening and early treatment of malnutrition in cancer patients. *J Cachexia Sarcopenia Muscle.* 2011;2(1):27-35. doi:10.1007/s13539-011-0022-x

69. Li J, Wang C, Liu X, et al. Severe malnutrition evaluated by patient-generated subjective global assessment results in poor outcome among adult patients with acute leukemia: a retrospective cohort study. *Medicine (Baltimore).* 2018;97(3):e9663. doi:10.1097/MD.0000000000009663

70. Esfahani A, Ghoreishi Z, Abedi Miran M, et al. Nutritional assessment of patients with acute leukemia during induction chemotherapy: association with hospital outcomes. *Leuk Lymphoma*. 2014;55(8): 1743-1750. doi:10.3109 /10428194.2013.853766

71. Kim HS, Lee JY, Lim SH, et al. Patient-Generated Subjective Global Assessment as a prognosis tool in patients with multiple myeloma. *Nutrition*. 2017;36:67-71. doi:10.1016/j.nut.2016.06.009

72. Gangadharan A, Choi SE, Hassan A, et al. Protein calorie malnutrition, nutritional intervention and personalized cancer care. *Oncotarget*. 2017;8(14):24009–24030. doi:10 .18632/oncotarget.15103

73. Hochman MJ, Yu Y, Wolf SP, Samsa GP, Kamal AH, LeBlanc TW. Comparing the palliative care needs of patients with hematologic and solid malignancies. *J Pain Symptom Manage*. 2018;55(1):82–88.e1. doi:10.1016/j.jpainsymman.2017 .08.030

74. Raynard B, Nitenberg G, Gory-Delabaere G, et al. Summary of the standards, options and recommendations for nutritional support in patients undergoing bone marrow transplantation. *Br J Cancer*. 2003;89(suppl 1): S101-S106. doi:10.1038/sj.bjc .6601091

75. Krawczyk J, Kraj L, Korta T, Wiktor-Jedrzejczak W. Nutritional status of hematological patients before hematopoietic stem cell transplantation and in early posttransplantation period. *Nutr Cancer*. 2017;69(8):1205-1210. doi:10.1080/01635581.2017 .1367937

76. Brandwein JM, Seki JT, Atenafu EG, et al. A phase II open-label study of aprepitant as anti-emetic prophylaxis in patients with acute myeloid leukemia (AML) undergoing induction chemotherapy. *Support Care Cancer*. 2019;27(6):2295-2300. doi:10.1007/s00520-018-4515-4

77. Roila F, Molassiotis A, Herrstedt J, et al. 2016 MASCC and ESMO guideline update for the prevention of chemotherapy- and radiotherapy-induced nausea and vomiting and of nausea and vomiting in advanced cancer patients. *Ann Oncol*. 2016;27(suppl 5):119–133. doi:10 .1093/annonc/mdw270

78. Matsumaru A, Tsutsumi Y, Ito S. Comparative investigation of the anti-emetic effects of granisetron and palonosetron during the treatment of acute myeloid leukemia. *Mol Clin Oncol*. 2017;7(4):629–632. doi:10.3892 /mco.2017.1350

79. Coleman, RE. Clinical features of metastatic bone disease and risk of skeletal morbidity. *Clin Cancer Res*. 2006;12(20):6243s-6249s. doi:10.1158/1078-0432.CCRz -06-0931

80. Palumbo A, Anderson K. Multiple myeloma. *N Engl J Med*. 2011;364:1046-1060. doi:10.1056 /NEJMra1011442

81. Melton LJ, Kyle RA, Achenbach SJ, Oberg AL, Rajkumar SV. Fracture risk with multiple myeloma: a population-based study. *J Bone Miner Res*. 2005;20(3):487-493. doi:10.1359/JBMR.041131

82. Miceli TS, Colson K, Faiman BM, Miller K, Tariman JD. Maintaining bone health in patients with multiple myeloma: survivorship care plan of the International Myeloma Foundation Nurse Leadership Board. *Clin J Oncol Nurs*. 2011;Aug15:9-23. doi:10.1188 /11.S1.CJON.9-23

83. Cosman F, Jan de Buer S, LeBoff MS, et al. Clinician's guide to prevention and treatment of osteoporosis. *Osteoporos Int*. 2014;25(10):2359-2381. doi:10 .1007/s00198-014-2794-2

84. Caram MV, Bellile EL, Englesbe MJ, et al. Sarcopenia is associated with autologous transplant-related outcomes in patients with lymphoma. *Leuk Lymphoma*. 2015;56(10):2855-2862. doi:10 .3109/10428194.2015.1014359

85. Camus V, Lanic H, Kraut J, et al. Prognostic impact of fat tissue loss and cachexia assessed by computed tomography scan in elderly patients with diffuse large B-cell lymphoma treated with immunochemotherapy. *Eur J Haematol*. 2014;93(1):9-18. doi:10.1111/ejh.12285

86. Arends J, Bachmann P, Baracos V, et al. ESPEN guidelines on nutrition in cancer patients. *Clin Nutr.* 2017;36(1):11-48. doi:10.1016/j.clnu.2016.07.015

87. Fearon K, Strasser F, Anker SD, et al. Definition and classification of cancer cachexia: an international consensus. *Lancet Oncol.* 2011;12(5):489-495. doi:10.1016/S1470-2045(10)70218-7

88. Wang W, Li G, He X, et al. Serum 25-hydroxyvitamin D levels and prognosis in hematological malignancies: a systematic review and meta-analysis. *Cell Physiol Biochem.* 2015;35(5):1999-2005. doi:10.1159/000374007

89. Tracy SI, Maurer MJ, Witzig TE, et al. Vitamin D insufficiency is associated with an increased risk of early clinical failure in follicular lymphoma. *Blood Cancer J.* 2017;7(8):e595. doi:10.1038/bcj.2017.70

90. Sfeir JG, Drake MT, LaPlant BR, et al. Validation of a vitamin D replacement strategy in vitamin D-insufficient patients with lymphoma or chronic lymphocytic leukemia. *Blood Cancer J.* 2017;7(2):e526. doi:10.1038/bcj.2017.9

91. Ng AC, Kumar SK, Rajkumar SV, Drake MT. Impact of vitamin D deficiency on the clinical presentation and prognosis of patients with newly diagnosed multiple myeloma. *Am J Hematol.* 2009;84(7):397-400. doi:10.1002/ajh.21412

92. Thomas X, Ghelghoum Y, Fanari N, Cannas G. Serum 25-hydroxyvitamin D levels are associated with prognosis in hematological malignancies. *Hematology.* 2011;16(5):278-283. doi:10.1179/102453311X13085644679908

93. Radujkovic A, Schnitzler P, Ho AD, Dreger P, Luft T. Low serum vitamin D levels are associated with shorter survival after first-line azacitidine treatment in patients with myelodysplastic syndrome and secondary oligoblasitc acute myeloid leukemia. *Clin Nutr.* 2017;36(2):542-551. doi:10.1016/j.clnu.2016.01.021

94. Lee, HJ, Muindi JR, Tan W, et al. Low 25(OH) vitamin D3 levels are associated with adverse outcome in newly diagnosed, intensively treated adult acute myeloid leukemia. *Cancer.* 2014;120(4):521-529. doi:10.1002/cncr.28368

95. Shanafelt TD, Drake MT, Maurer MJ, et al. Vitamin D insufficiency and prognosis in chronic lymphocytic leukemia. *Blood.* 2011;117(5):1492-1498. doi:10.1182/blood-2010-07-295683

96. Badros A, Goloubeva O, Terpos E, et al. Prevalence and significance of vitamin D deficiency in multiple myeloma patients. *Br J Haematol.* 2008;142(3):492–494. doi:10.1111/j.1365-2141.2008.07214.x

97. Lauter B, Schmidt-Wolf IG. Prevalence, supplementation, and impact of vitamin D deficiency in multiple myeloma patients. *Cancer Invest.* 2015;33(10):505-509. doi:10.3109/07357907.2015.1081690

98. Polly P, Tan TC. The role of vitamin D in skeletal and cardiac muscle function. *Front Physiol.* 2014;5:145. doi:10.3389/fphys.2014.00145

99. Hohaus S, Tisi MC, Bellesi S, et al. Vitamin D deficiency and supplementation in patients with aggressive B-cell lymphomas treated with immunochemotherapy. *Cancer Med.* 2018;7(1):270-281. doi:10.1002/cam4.1166

100. Bittenbring JT, Neumann F, Altmann B, et al. Vitamin D deficiency impairs rituximab-mediated cellular cytotoxicity and outcome of patients with diffuse large B-cell lymphoma treated with but not without rituximab. *J Clin Oncol.* 2014;32(29):3242-3248. doi:10.1200/JCO.2013.53.4537

101. Kelly JL, Salles G, Goldman B, et al. Low serum vitamin D levels are associated with inferior survival in follicular lymphoma: a prospective evaluation in SWOG and LYSA studies. *J Clin Oncol.* 2015;33(13):1482-1490. doi:10.1200/JCO.2014.57.5092

102. Keum N, Lee DH, Greenwood DC, Manson JE, Giovannucci E. Vitamin D supplements and total cancer incidence and mortality: a meta-analysis of randomized controlled trials. *Ann Oncol.* 2019;30(5):733-743. doi:10.1093/annonc/mdz059

103. Calderwood AH, Baron JA, Mott LA, et al. No evidence for posttreatment effects of vitamin D and calcium supplementation on risk of colorectal adenomas in a randomized trial. *Cancer Prev Res (Phila).* 2019;12(5):295-304. doi:10.1158/1940-6207.CAPR-19-0023

104. Savoie MB, Paciorek A, Zhang L, et al. Vitamin D levels in patients with colorectal cancer before and after treatment initiation. *J Gastrointest Cancer.* 2018 (July 30). Epub ahead of print. doi:10.1007/s12029-018-0147-7

105. Simon, S. Are you getting enough vitamin D? American Cancer Society website. Published March 5, 2019. Accessed March 6, 2019. www.cancer.org/latest-news/are-you-getting-enough-vitamin-d.html

106. Alkan A, Köksoy EB. Vitamin D deficiency in cancer patients and predictors for screening (D-ONC study). *Curr Probl Cancer.* 2019 (January 17). doi:10.1016/j.currproblcancer.2018.12.008

107. Holick MF, Binkley NC, Bischoff-Ferrari HA, et al. Evaluation, treatment, and prevention of vitamin D deficiency: an Endocrine Society clinical practice guideline. *J Clin Endocrinol Metab.* 2011;96(7):1911–1930. doi:10.1210/jc.2011-0385

108. Terpos E, Morgan G, Dimopoulos MA, et al. International Myeloma Working Group recommendations for the treatment of multiple myeloma-related bone disease. *J Clin Oncol.* 2013;31(18):2347-2357. doi:10.1200/JCO.2012.47.7901

109. National Kidney Foundation Kidney Disease Outcomes Quality Initiative (NKF KDOQI). KDOQI clinical practice guidelines for bone metabolism and disease in chronic kidney disease: Guideline 5. Use of phosphate binders in CKD. National Kidney Foundation website. Published 2003. Accessed October 11, 2018. http://kidneyfoundation.cachefly.net/professionals/KDOQI/guidelines_bone/guide5.htm

110. Academy of Nutrition and Dietetics. Chronic kidney disease. CKD: executive summary of recommendations (2010). Academy of Nutrition and Dietetics Evidence Analysis Library website. Accessed June 1, 2019. https://andeal.org/topic.cfm?cat=3929

111. Bhowmilk D, Qian Y, Bond TC, et al. Prevalence of renal impairment in patients with multiple myeloma: analysis of real-world database. *Value in Health.* 2016;19(3):A141. doi:10.1016/j.jval.2016.03.2006

112. Leung N, Nasr SH. Myeloma-related kidney disease. *Adv Chronic Kidney Dis.* 2014;21(1):36–47. doi:10.1053/j.ackd.2013.08.009

113. Eating right for chronic kidney disease. National Institute of Diabetes and Digestive and Kidney Diseases website. Accessed March 6, 2019. https://niddk.nih.gov/health-information/kidney-disease/chronic-kidney-disease-ckd/eating-nutrition

114. Druml W, Joannidis M, John S, et al. Metabolic management and nutrition in critically ill patients with renal dysfunction [in German]. *Med Klin Intensivmed Notfmed.* 2018;113(5):393. doi:10.1007/s00063-018-0427-9

115. Anderson CA, Nguyen HA, Rifkin DE. Nutrition interventions in chronic kidney disease. *Med Clin North Am.* 2016;100(6):1265-1283. doi:10.1016/j.mcna.2016.06.008

116. Steiber AL. Chronic kidney disease: considerations for nutrition interventions. *JPEN J Parenter Enteral Nutr.* 2014;38(4):418-26. doi:10.1177/0148607114527315

117. Steiber AL, Kopple JD. Vitamin status and needs for people with stages 3–5 chronic kidney disease. *J Ren Nutr.* 2011;21(5):355-368. doi:10.1053/j.jrn.2010.12.004

118. Andreucci VE, Fissell RB, Bragg-Gresham JL, et al. Dialysis Outcomes and Practice Patterns Study (DOPPS) data on medications in hemodialysis patients *Am J Kidney Dis.* 2004;44(5)(suppl 2):61-67. doi:10.1053/j.ajkd.2004.08.013

119. Sattianayagam PT, Lane T, Fox Z, et al. A prospective study of nutritional status in immunoglobulin light chain amyloidosis. *Haematologica.* 2013;98(1):136-140. doi:10.3324/haematol.2012.070359

120. Palladini G, Hegenbart U, Milani P, et al. A staging system for renal outcome and early markers of renal response to chemotherapy in AL amyloidosis. *Blood.* 2014;124(15):2325-2332. doi:10.1182/blood-2014-04-570010

121. Caccialanza R, Palladini G, Klersy C, et al. Nutritional status independently affects quality of life of patients with systemic immunoglobulin light-chain (AL) amyloidosis. *Ann Hematol.* 2012;91(3):399-406. doi:10.1007/s00277-011-1309-x

122. Caccialanza R, Palladini G, Klersy C, et al. Malnutrition at diagnosis predicts mortality in patients with systemic immunoglobulin light-chain amyloidosis independently of cardiac stage and response to treatment. *JPEN J Parenter Eternal Nutr.* 2014;38(7):891-894. doi:10.1177/0148607113501328

123. Caccialanza R, Palladini G, Cereda E, et al. Nutritional counseling improves quality of life and preserves body weight in systemic immunoglobulin light-chain (AL) amyloidosis. *Nutrition.* 2015;31(10):1228-1234. doi:10.1016/j.nut.2015.04.011

124. Caccialanza R, Palladini G, Klersy C, et al. Nutritional status of outpatients with systemic immunoglobulin light-chain amyloidosis 1. *Am J Clin Nutr.* 2006;83(2):350-354. doi:10.1093/ajcn/83.2.350

125. Rowe K, Pankow J, Nehme F, Salyers W. Gastrointestinal amyloidosis: review of the literature. *Cureus.* 2017;9(5):e1228. doi:10.7759/cureus.1228

126. Dember LM. Amyloidosis-associated kidney disease. *J Am Soc Nephrol.* 2006;17(12):3458-3471. doi:10.1681/asn.2006050460

127. Syed U, Ching Companioni RA, Alkhawam H, Walfish A. Amyloidosis of the gastrointestinal tract and the liver: clinical context, diagnosis and management. *Eur J Gastroenterol Hepatol.* 2016;28(10):1109-1121. doi:10.1097/MEG.0000000000000695

128. Tawfik B, Pardee T, Isom S, et al. Comorbidity, age and mortality among adults treated intensively for acute myeloid leukemia (AML). *J Geriatr Oncol.* 2016;7(1):24-31. doi:10.1016/j.jgo.2015.10.182

129. Galindo RJ, Yoon J, Devoe C, Myers AK. PEG-asparaginase induced severe hypertriglyceridemia. *Arch Endocrinol Metab.* 2016;60(2):173-177. doi:10.1590/2359-3997000000068

130. Tong WH, Pieters R, de Groot-Kruseman HA, et al. The toxicity of very prolonged courses of PEGasparaginase or *Erwinia* asparaginase in relation to asparaginase activity, with a special focus on dyslipidemia. *Haematologica.* 2014;99(11):1716-1721. doi:10.3324/haematol.2014.109413

131. Medeiros BC, Othus M, Estey EH, Fang M, Appelbaum FR. Impact of body-mass index on the outcome of adult patients with acute myeloid leukemia. *Haematologica.* 2012;97(9):1401-1404. doi:10.3324/haematol.2011.056390

132. Wang YC, McPherson K, Marsh T, Gortmaker SL, Brown M. Health and economic burden of the projected obesity trends in the USA and the UK. *Lancet.* 2011;378(9793):815-825. doi:10.1016/S0140-6736(11)60814-3

133. Boyne DJ, Mickle AT, Brenner DR, et al. Long-term risk of cardiovascular mortality in lymphoma survivors: a systematic review and meta-analysis. *Cancer Med.* 2018;7(9):4801-4813. doi:10.1002/cam4.1572

134. Al-Kindi SG, Abu-Zeinah GF, Kim CH, et al. Trends and disparities in cardiovascular mortality among survivors of Hodgkin lymphoma. *Clin Lymphoma Myeloma Leuk.* 2015;15(12):748-752. doi:10.1016/j.clml.2015.07.638

135. Thompson CA, Mauck K, Havyer R, Bhagra A, Kalsi H, Hayes SN. Care of the adult Hodgkin lymphoma survivor. *Am J Med.* 2011;124(12):1106-1112. doi:10.1016/j.amjmed.2011.05.020

136. Aleman BM, van den Belt-Dusebout AW, Klokman WJ, Van't Veer MB, Bartelink H, van Leeuwen FE. Long-term cause-specific mortality of patients treated for Hodgkin's disease. *J Clin Oncol.* 2003;21(18):3431-3439. doi:10.1200/JCO.2003.07.131

137. Heidenreich PA, Schnittger I, Strauss HW, et al. Screening for coronary artery disease after mediastinal irradiation for Hodgkin's disease. *J Clin Oncol.* 2007;25(1):43-49. doi:10.1200/JCO.2006.07.0805

138. Meacham LR, Chow EJ, Ness KK, et al. Cardiovascular risk factors in adult survivors of pediatric cancer—a report from the Childhood Cancer Survivor Study. *Cancer Epidemiol Biomarkers Prev.* 2010;19(1):170-181. doi:10.1158/1055-9965.EPI-09-0555

139. Hequet O, Le QH, Moullet I, et al. Subclinical late cardiomyopathy after doxorubicin therapy for lymphoma in adults. *J Clin Oncol.* 2004;22(10):1864-1871. doi:10.1200/JCO.2004.06.033

140. Hull MC, Morris CG, Pepine CJ, Mendenhall NP. Valvular dysfunction and carotid, subclavian, and coronary artery disease in survivors of Hodgkin lymphoma treated with radiation therapy. *JAMA.* 2003;290(21):2831-2837. doi:10.1001/jama.290.21.2831

141. The American Heart Association diet and lifestyle recommendations. American Heart Association website. Last reviewed August 15, 2015. Accessed June 1, 2019. www.heart.org/en/healthy-living/healthy-eating/eat-smart/nutrition-basics/aha-diet-and-lifestyle-recommendations

142. Zhang L, Mager DE. Systems modeling of bortezomib and dexamethasone combinatorial effects on bone homeostasis in multiple myeloma patients. *J Pharm Sci.* 2019;108(1):732-740. doi:10.1016/j.xphs.2018.11.024

143. Gebauer J, Fick EM, Waldmann A, et al. Self-reported endocrine late effects in adults treated for brain tumours, Hodgkin and non-Hodgkin lymphoma: a registry based study in Northern Germany. *Eur J Endocrinol.* 2015;173(2):139-148. doi:10.1530/EJE-15-0174

144. van Nimwegen FA, Schaapveld M, Janus CP, et al. Risk of diabetes mellitus in long-term survivors of Hodgkin lymphoma. *J Clin Oncol.* 2014;32(29):3257-3263. doi:10.1200/JCO.2013.54.4379

145. Wu W, Merriman K, Nabaah A, et al. The association of diabetes and anti-diabetic medications with clinical outcomes in multiple myeloma. *Br J Cancer.* 2014;111(3):628-636. doi:10.1038/bjc.2014.307

146. Academy of Nutrition and Dietetics. Diabetes type 1 and 2. DM: executive summary of recommendations (2015). Academy of Nutrition and Dietetics Evidence Analysis Library website. Accessed June 1, 2019. https://andeal.org/topic.cfm?menu=5305&cat=5596

147. Academy of Nutrition and Dietetics. Diabetes type 1 and 2. Recommendations summary. DM: individualize nutrition prescription (2015). Academy of Nutrition and Dietetics Evidence Analysis Library website. Accessed June 1, 2019. https://andeal.org/template.cfm?template=guide_summary&key=4425

148. McCullough ML, Patel AV, Kushi LH, et al. Following cancer prevention guidelines reduces risk of cancer, cardiovascular disease and all-cause mortality. *Cancer Epidemiol Biomarkers Prev.* 2011;20(6):1089-1097. doi:10.1158/1055-9965.EPI-10-1173

Chapter 15
Medical Nutrition Therapy for Hematopoietic Cell Transplantation

Katie Harper, MS, RD, CNSC, CSO
Kerry K. McMillen, MS, RD, CSO, FAND

Hematopoietic cell transplantation (HCT) is an established therapeutic modality for select hematologic malignancies and solid tumors. It also is a treatment for certain nonmalignant conditions, such as bone marrow disorders, immunodeficiency syndromes, and inborn errors of metabolism.[1] Stem cells are obtained from bone marrow, peripheral blood, or umbilical cord blood. The objective of HCT is to replace malignant or defective marrow in order to restore normal hematopoiesis and immune system function.[2]

The HCT process includes the collection of cells, with the source varying dependent on the type of transplant, followed by administration of a conditioning regimen intended to kill remaining cancer cells, weaken the immune system, and prevent the body from rejecting the new stem cells. Once the conditioning regimen is completed, the stem cells, known as the graft, are infused into the patient. Finally, in a stage known as engraftment, the transplanted stem cells begin homing to the patient's marrow and produce blood cells of all types. Engraftment is first evident when new white blood cells, red blood cells, and platelets begin to appear in the patient's blood.

More than 65,000 transplants are performed worldwide annually; the one millionth HCT was performed in 2013.[3] Patient survival varies greatly and depends on the type of malignancy and stage of disease, donor type, graft source, patient age, and intensity of conditioning therapy. In recent years, there has been a steady increase in the survival rate due to improved techniques in donor matching, as well as to advances in supportive care and infection control.[4] There are more than 100,000 survivors of HCT worldwide, and that number is estimated to increase fivefold by 2030.[3]

Types of Hematopoietic Cell Transplantation

There are three types of HCT:

- Autologous HCT uses the patient's own hematopoietic stem cells, which are collected before the conditioning regimen. Following the conditioning regimen, the patient's graft is reinfused to restore hematopoiesis. Autologous HCT is primarily used to treat multiple myeloma, non-Hodgkin lymphoma (NHL), and Hodgkin lymphoma (HL).[2]

- Syngeneic HCT uses hematopoietic stem cells from an identical twin sibling donor.[2]

- Allogeneic HCT uses hematopoietic stem cells from a donor who is fully or closely matched. It is used mainly for the treatment of acute and chronic leukemias, NHL, and marrow diseases, such as severe aplastic anemia, myelodysplastic syndrome, and myeloproliferative diseases.[2] Donor types include the following[5]:

- matched related donor
- matched unrelated donor
- mismatched unrelated donor
- half-matched related donor (haploidentical)
- umbilical cord blood

Conditioning Regimens

The preparative regimen, also known as conditioning, includes either cytotoxic chemotherapy, total body irradiation (TBI), or both, administered before the stem cell infusion.[6] The goal of conditioning is to provide immunoablation to prevent graft rejection and to reduce tumor burden. Conditioning regimens vary in intensity and are chosen based on the patient's disease and other factors, such as age and comorbidities. Standard conditioning regimens have not been established and can vary by institution. Conditioning regimens are categorized into three types according to the intensity of the regimen[6]:

■ High-dose, or myeloablative, regimens: These include a combination of chemotherapy agents that ablate bone marrow hematopoiesis and do not allow for autologous reconstitution; therefore, the patient requires stem cell infusion to rebuild bone marrow.

■ Nonmyeloablative regimens: These use chemotherapy that causes minimal cytopenias; therefore, the patient does not require stem cell infusion.

■ Reduced intensity conditioning (RIC): This type of regimen uses less intensive chemotherapy or TBI (or both) that causes prolonged cytopenias, resulting in the patient requiring stem cell infusion.

Both RIC and nonmyeloablative regimens involve less bone marrow suppression and organ toxicity compared with myeloablative (high-dose chemotherapy) regimens.[5,6] These lower-dose regimens rely more on the graft-versus-tumor (GVT) effect—a response in which the infused graft stem cells attack and kill remaining cancer cells that were not killed by the lower chemotherapy doses—to eradicate disease.[6] They are used in patients who are older, have been heavily pretreated, or who have comorbidities and are unable to tolerate myeloablative

conditioning.[5,6] Figure 15.1 illustrates a range of conditioning regimens and their toxicities, intensities, and reliance on the GVT effect—from nonmyeloablative regimens, which are the lowest-intensity with the lowest toxicity, to myeloablative regimens, which are the highest-intensity with the highest toxicity.[7]

Side Effects of Conditioning Regimens

Side effects of conditioning regimens can vary with the intensity of the regimen and can negatively affect the patient's nutritional status. More intense conditioning regimens cause a more significant impact on nutritional intake. High-dose or myeloablative conditioning regimens have the highest toxicity profiles, followed by RIC and nonmyeloablative.[6] Medical nutrition therapy (MNT) is required during this time due to gastrointestinal (GI) toxicities that lead to decreased oral intake and impaired nutrient utilization coupled with increased nutrient requirements.[8] After the stem cell infusion (referred to as day 0), the patient often is neutropenic for 2 to 3 weeks until engraftment. When a patient's cells start to engraft, the white blood cell count and absolute neutrophil count slowly begin to increase.[9]

Table 15.1 on page 308 shows the average time to neutrophil engraftment, based on the type and source of stem cells. Complete immune function does not return for months after transplantation.

Nutrition Assessment

Initial and serial nutrition assessments are recommended for all patients undergoing HCT. An initial comprehensive nutrition assessment before HCT (baseline assessment) identifies patients at high nutrition risk who might require nutrition intervention prior to transplantation. Frequent, serial nutrition assessments throughout the HCT process are essential because of the toxicities associated with conditioning regimens and the complications

Increasing Requirement of GVT Effect

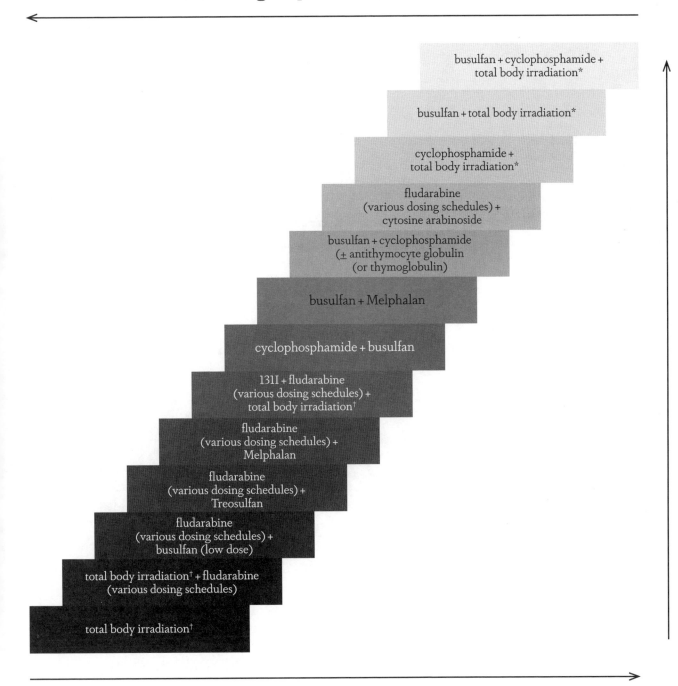

Intensity

Figure 15.1
Selected conditioning regimens of differing dose intensities

*High-dose TBI (800-1320 cGy)   †Low-dose TBI (200-400 cGy)

Adapted with permission from Deeg HJ, Sandmier BM. Who is fit for allogeneic stem cell transplant? *Blood*. 2010;116: 4762-4770. See reference 7.

Table 15.1
Average Time Until Neutrophil Engraftment by Type of Transplant[5,6,9,10]

Type of transplant	Average days to engraftment
Autologous	10-12
Allogeneic	
Matched related donor (MRD) and matched unrelated donor (MUD) with peripheral blood	14-16
Haploidentical	
MRD and MUD with bone marrow	19-21
Umbilical cord blood	21

associated with HCT, such as graft-versus-host disease (GVHD), that affect nutritional status.[11]

The baseline pretransplant nutrition assessment may include data obtained from patient-generated questionnaires, a validated malnutrition screening tool, the medical record, and a nutrition-focused physical exam. Box 15.1 describes the components of the baseline nutrition assessment.

Nutrient and Fluid Requirements

Studies assessing energy requirements for children and adults undergoing HCT are limited, especially in patients with obesity. Research shows that more than 50% of pediatric patients undergoing HCT had suboptimal nutritional status before transplantation. Suboptimal nutrition before HCT was associated with negative prognostic factors leading to delayed engraftment and posttransplant complications.[12] Protein requirements increase to promote tissue repair and to minimize the loss of lean muscle mass. Based on current research, indirect calorimetry (IC) is the gold standard for assessing nutritional needs.[13,14] If IC is not available, clinical judgment should be used along with ongoing nutrition reassessment to monitor for signs of overfeeding and underfeeding. See Chapter 5 for more details on nutrient needs. Box 15.2 on pages 310 to 312 lists the daily nutrient and fluid requirements for patients undergoing HCT.[13-19]

Nutrition Problems and Interventions

Immunocompromised State

Oral feeding is recommended for patients with a functional GI tract. Although several studies have examined the relationship between diet and risk for infection, the protective benefit of "low-microbial," "antimicrobial," and "neutropenic" diets in fighting infection has not been established.[11] Recent studies have indicated that the use of these restrictive diets in the HCT population is not supported by evidence.[20-22] A large, single-center study found that common bacterial foodborne infections were rare within 1 year of HCT in patients who followed a diet designed for immunosuppressed patients.[23]

Box 15.3 on page 313 shows dietary guidelines for immunocompromised patients following HCT. To date, there have been no randomized controlled trials to evaluate the length of time that patients should follow these dietary guidelines following engraftment and the duration of immunosuppressive medication therapy. To minimize the risk for

Oncology Nutrition *for* Clinical Practice

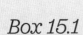

Box 15.1
Baseline Nutrition Assessment Before Hematopoietic Cell Transplantation[1]

Component	Assessment data	Examples and notes (eg, rationale)	
Nutrition history	Oral and gastrointestinal (GI) symptoms	Dysgeusia or hypogeusia	Heartburn or reflux
		Xerostomia	Nausea and vomiting
		Dysphagia or odynophagia	Early satiety
		Dental health	Anorexia
		Oral aversions	Altered bowel habits
		Mucositis or esophagitis	
	Current diet	Include any special diets	
	Food allergies or intolerances	Identify known foods to avoid post-hematopoietic cell transplantation (HCT); update the medical record	
	Supplement use	Vitamin, mineral, and herbal supplements; include dosage	
	Other modalities	Use of integrative medicine therapies	
		Note that the use of nonconventional therapies (eg, herbals, dietary supplements, and megavitamin therapy) may alter the effectiveness of chemotherapy, radiotherapy, and other medications.	
	Nutrition support interventions	Current or past interventions (eg, parenteral nutrition, enteral nutrition, intraveous fluids)	
	Age-associated specifics for infants and young children	Breast-fed or formula-fed (if formula-fed, determine type and concentration)	
		Stage of eating development (eg, cup vs bottle; puree vs solids)	
Medical history	Medical history with specific effects on nutritional status	Past oral and GI surgeries	
		Comorbidities (eg, diabetes mellitus, cardiovascular disease)	
		Pain status and use of narcotics	
Anthropometric measurements	Baseline height and weight	Use to determine body surface area and calculate medication doses and fluid requirements	
	Arm anthropometry	Indicator of somatic muscle protein and adipose reserves	
	Hand grip strength	Marker of nutritional status	
	Age-associated specifics for infants up to 24 months	Recumbent length and occipital frontal circumference; plot on the Centers for Disease Control and Prevention growth charts	
		Provides a baseline for serial measurements throughout HCT	

(continued)

Box 15.1
Baseline Nutrition Assessment Before Hematopoietic Cell Transplantation[1] *(continued)*

Component	Assessment data	Examples and notes (eg, rationale)
Physical activity	Typical exercise pattern	
Biochemical indices	Baseline values	Obtain the following and use to recommend changes in nutrient and fluid requirements during HCT, especially if there are changes in organ function: ■ electrolytes ■ glucose ■ renal function ■ liver function ■ blood lipids ■ ferritin ■ 25-hydroxyvitamin D

Box 15.2
Daily Nutrient Requirements During Hematopoietic Cell Transplantation[8,13-18]

Energy

Daily requirement for children:

Aged 0 to 6 years	Basal metabolic rate × 1.6 to 1.8
Aged 7 to 14 years	Basal metabolic rate × 1.4 to 1.6
Aged 15 to 18 years	Basal metabolic rate × 1.5 to 1.6
Daily Requirement for Adults:	Basal metabolic rate × 1.3 to 1.5, or 25 to 30 kcal per kg of body weight

Increase during the immediate posttransplant period because of metabolic stress induced by the preparative regimen, fever, or infections.

Decrease during engraftment; absence of metabolic complications.[a]

(continued)

[a] See Chapter 5 for considerations in obese patients.

Box 15.2
Daily Nutrient Requirements During Hematopoietic Cell Transplantation[8,13-18] *(continued)*

Protein

Daily requirement for children:

Aged 0 to 12 months	3.0 g/kg of body weight
Aged 1 to 6 years	2.5 g/kg of body weight
Aged 7 to 10 years	2.4 g/kg of body weight
Aged 11 to 14 years	2.0 g/kg of body weight
Aged 15 to 18 years	1.8 g/kg of body weight

Daily Requirement for Adults:	1.5 g/kg of body weight
	If obese (body mass index ≥30): 2 to 2.5 g/kg of ideal body weight

Increase during the immediate posttransplant period; during corticosteroid treatment; during continuous renal replacement therapy (CRRT).

Decrease in presence of renal or hepatic dysfunction.

Carbohydrate

Requirement is 50% to 60% of total daily energy intake.

Modify oral intake when insulin is required.

Decrease in the presence of preexisting diabetes or hyperglycemia, lower parenteral nutrition (PN) dextrose concentration.

Fat

Minimum dose: 6% to 8% of total daily energy intake

Maximum dose: 40% of total daily energy intake

Increase when providing lower PN dextrose concentrations.

Decrease if hyperlipidemia.

(continued)

Box 15.2
Daily Nutrient Requirements During Hematopoietic Cell Transplantation[8,13-18] *(continued)*

Fluids

If body weight is 1 to 10 kg: 100 mL per kg of body weight per day

If body weight is 11 to 20 kg: 1,000 mL + 50 mL for every kg over 10 kg of body weight daily

If body weight is less than 20 kg: 1,500 mL + 20 mL for every kg over 20 kg of body weight daily

Increase during fever; excessive gastrointestinal losses; hypermetabolism; high-output renal failure; nephrotoxic medications.

Decrease if compromised organ function; iatrogenic fluid overload.

Vitamins

Oral: after PN is discontinued, oral vitamin-mineral supplement without iron

Parenteral: follow ASPEN guidelines [b]

Discontinue extra vitamin C during presence of elevated serum ferritin (>1,000 mcg/L) to decrease oxidative damage from release of free iron

Trace minerals and electrolytes

Parenteral: ASPEN guidelines [b]

Oral: after PN is discontinued, oral vitamin-mineral supplement without iron

Increase calcium during corticosteroid therapy or with osteoporosis. Increase zinc with large-volume diarrhea: 1 mg per 100 mL of stool output. Electrolyte needs may be higher with food-drug interactions.

Eliminate copper and manganese from PN in presence of hepatic dysfunction. Iron supplementation is contraindicated.

[b] Refer to the *The ASPEN Adult Nutrition Support Core Curriculum* for more information. See reference 19.

foodborne infections, the emerging practice is to emphasize strict adherence to food safety guidelines and to avoid high-risk foods.[11] Further studies are needed to assess this in clinical practice.

Impact of Body Weight on Outcomes

Recent studies indicate that pre-HCT weight affects clinical outcome of HCT in adults. An underweight status prior to HCT is a risk factor for poor overall survival, due to increased risk for relapse, while obesity increases the risk for nonrelapse mortality.[25,26]

Studies in pediatric patients undergoing HCT also found decreased survival associated with a high BMI and low muscle reserves before transplantation.[27,28] Baumgartner and colleagues[29] found that a more pronounced weight loss during HCT (>7% versus <2%) was associated with an increased risk for bacterial and fungal infections. In addition,

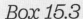

Box 15.3
Dietary Guidelines for Immunosuppressed Patients Following Hematopoietic Cell Transplantation[24]

Immunosuppression increases susceptibility to foodborne illness. Dietary guidelines for immunosuppressed patients are intended to minimize the introduction of pathogenic organisms into the gastrointestinal (GI) tract by food while maximizing healthy food options. These guidelines should be coupled with evidence-based food safety recommendations to ensure proper food preparation and storage in the home and hospital kitchen. High-risk foods identified as potential sources of organisms known to cause infection in immunosuppressed patients are restricted.

In general, patients who have undergone autologous hematopoietic cell transplantation (HCT) should follow the diet for the first 3 months after transplantation. Patients who have undergone allogeneic HCT should follow the diet until immunosuppressive therapy (eg, cyclosporine, tacrolimus, or prednisone) is discontinued. Duration of the diet may vary by health care facility.

Food restrictions

Immunosuppressed patients should avoid the following foods after HCT:

- raw and undercooked meat (including game), fish, shellfish, poultry, eggs, sausage, and bacon

- raw tofu, unless pasteurized or aseptically packaged

- lunch meats (including salami, bologna, hot dogs, and ham) unless heated until steaming

- refrigerated smoked seafood typically labeled as lox, kippered, nova-style, smoked, or fish jerky (unless contained in a cooked dish); pickled fish

- unpasteurized milk and raw milk products, unpasteurized cheese, and unpasteurized yogurt

- blue-veined cheeses, including blue, Gorgonzola, Roquefort, and Stilton

- uncooked soft cheeses, including Brie, Camembert, feta, and farmer

- Mexican-style soft cheeses, including queso blanco and queso fresco

- cheeses containing chili peppers or other uncooked vegetables

- fresh salad dressings (stored in the grocer's refrigerated case) containing raw eggs or contraindicated cheeses

- unwashed raw or frozen fruits and vegetables and those with visible mold; all raw vegetable sprouts (alfalfa, mung bean, and all others)

- unpasteurized commercial fruit and vegetable juices

- well water, unless boiled for 15 to 20 minutes and consumed within 48 hours of boiling

---

malnourished HCT recipients had a longer length of hospital stay than well-nourished HCT recipients.[29,30] Fuji and colleagues[25] showed that the risk for GVHD increased in overweight individuals compared with normal-weight groups. Another study found that obese persons with higher baseline levels of proinflammatory cytokines were associated with an increased risk for developing GVHD.[26]

Oral and Gastrointestinal Complications

Oral and GI manifestations are frequent complications of HCT. Chapter 11 describes dietary interventions for common nutrition sequelae of HCT (eg, nausea, mucositis, and early satiety). GI toxicities associated with the conditioning regimen typically start to diminish as engraftment begins, at which point the patient can begin increasing oral intake.

Mucositis

Mucositis occurs in up to 80% of patients undergoing myeloablative conditioning regimens. The patients with the most severe mucositis are typically those receiving a regimen that includes TBI (12 to 14 Gy) or high-dose etoposide or melphalan. Patients who receive methotrexate as GVHD prophylaxis after stem cell infusion also tend to develop severe mucosistis. Cryotherapy—the placement of ice chips in the mouth during infusion—with melphalan helps reduce mucositis by decreasing blood flow and exposure to chemotherapy.[31]

Several studies examining the role of glutamine supplementation during HCT have found that supplementation decreased the severity and duration of mucositis, the incidence of infections, and GVHD.[11,32-34] However, glutamine also may increase the risk for relapse of the malignancy.[32-34] In critically ill patients with renal dysfunction, glutamine was found to be detrimental,[31] and current available evidence does not support the role of glutamine supplementation in HCT recipients.[11] Larger, well-designed studies examining the appropriate timing, duration, and long-term effects of glutamine on outcome are needed before recommendations can be made.[32]

Sinusoidal Obstructive Syndrome

Sinusoidal obstructive syndrome (SOS) occurs when the effects of chemotherapy cause sinusoidal endothelial and hepatocyte damage that triggers a cascade of events leading to narrowing and occlusion of hepatic venules, fibrosis, and hepatocyte necrosis. This, in turn, causes decreased hepatic outflow, portal hypertension, ascites, and hepatomegaly, and can lead to multiorgan failure and death. SOS usually occurs within the first few weeks of HCT.[35]

The incidence of SOS varies widely from 0% to 60%, based on the type of transplant, diagnostic criteria used, and population risk factors. Severe SOS may occur in up to 40% of patients and is associated with a mortality rate exceeding 80%. Medical management of SOS includes diuresis, sodium restriction, renal replacement therapy (hemodialysis or continuous renal replacement therapy), pain management, and use of defibrotide.[36]

Hyperglycemia

Hyperglycemia is a frequent post-HCT complication caused by medications (especially prednisone), the use of parenteral nutrition (PN), and metabolic alterations that occur in the early phase of recovery.[37,38] If hyperglycemia occurs during the neutropenic period of HCT, it may lead to delayed neutrophil recovery and impaired neutrophil function, increase the risk for infection, prolong the engraftment time, and increase the risk for acute GVHD.[37-39] Independent risk factors associated with hyperglycemia within the first 10 days following HCT include a body mass index (BMI) of more than 25, preexisting insulin resistance, use of tacrolimus or glucocorticoids, a myeloablative conditioning regimen, and PN. One study has shown that the use of PN increased the risk for hyperglycemia in HCT patients fourfold compared with the risk in patients who did not receive PN.[37] Fuji and colleagues[38] found that the incidence of grades III (severe) and IV (very severe) GVHD was higher in patients who developed hyperglycemia (blood glucose >150 mg/dL) during the neutropenic phase.

Renal Impairment

Renal impairment may be related to chemotherapeutic agents, TBI, nephrotoxic medications (eg, antibiotics and calcineurin inhibitors), SOS, intravascular volume depletion, and sepsis.[1] Nutrition intervention during renal compromise includes maximizing nutrition support within the fluid allowance, correcting electrolyte imbalances, and maintaining sufficient intravascular volume.[40] During continuous renal replacement therapy, protein and vitamin needs are altered as shown in Box 15.2 on page 312.[1,15,16]

Infection

Infection is a major source of morbidity and mortality for patients receiving HCT. Bloodstream infections, pneumonia, and GI infections, including typhlitis and *Clostridium difficile*, are the most common infections during HCT. Treatment includes antibiotic, antiviral, and antifungal agents, which may induce oral and GI symptoms that affect nutritional status. Parenteral nutrition (PN) may be an independent risk factor for developing multidrug-resistant bloodstream infections during HCT; however, judicious use of PN and increased use of enteral nutrition (EN) when the patient is unable to meet his or her nutritional needs orally may be a strategy for reducing bloodstream infections.[41]

GI infections often present similarly to diarrhea, abdominal pain, nausea, and vomiting; thus, the source of infection needs to be determined before developing MNT interventions. Typhlitis, also known as neutropenic enterocolitis, is treated with antibiotics; and, if severe, gut rest with the potential need for PN is warranted. Milder cases of typhlitis may be treated conservatively with a bland diet and adequate hydration. In cases of *C. difficile* infection, antidiarrheal medications should be avoided, and the focus should be on MNT for diarrhea management.[42]

About half of all patients undergoing HCT develop clinically significant cytomegalovirus (CMV) within the first 100 days following HCT. CMV infection can affect multiple organs and lead to pneumonia, gastroenteritis, retinitis, and central nervous system involvement. It also precipitates the following nutrition impact symptoms[43]:

- CMV enteritis: nonspecific GI issues that can lead to ulcerations anywhere along the GI tract; diagnosed via endoscopy with a biopsy to rule out other causes of acute diarrhea (eg, GVHD) if tests for infectious diarrhea are negative

- CMV gastritis: often causes severe epigastric pain

- CMV esophagitis: can present as odynophagia and dysphagia

- CMV colitis: may lead to diarrhea, abdominal pain, anorexia, and fever

MNT for colitis depends on the location of CMV and associated symptoms; see Chapter 11 for symptom management strategies. Medical treatment for CMV includes intravenous ganciclovir, which can affect electrolytes, and cidofovir (Vistide) or foscarnet (Foscavir), which can affect renal function.[42]

Acute Graft-Versus-Host Disease

GVHD is a T-cell mediated immunologic reaction of engrafted lymphoid cells against the host tissues. It remains one of the most daunting complications associated with allogeneic HCT and is associated with significant morbidity and mortality.[44] The risk for GVHD increases as the donor source is less matched; thus, unrelated donors and mismatched donors pose increased risk.

Acute GVHD typically occurs within the first 100 days; however, it can appear after 100 days if it is persistent, reoccurs, or is late-onset acute. Major organs affected include the skin (75%), liver (20%), and GI tract (50%).[44]

Although less common, GVHD can occur after autologous HCT, with a reported incidence of approximately 5% to 20%.[45] Auto-GVHD is usually less severe than allogeneic GVHD, and it can be one of the manifestations of engraftment syndrome with the release of inflammatory cytokines and infiltration of autoreactive T cells into affected tissue.[46] The majority of patients with auto-GVHD respond well to treatment with corticosteroids without evidence of recurrence.[46]

Chronic GVHD develops later after HCT and is addressed in the section Survivorship later in this chapter.

Clinical manifestations of gut GVHD include the following:

- nausea
- vomiting
- anorexia
- food intolerance
- abdominal pain
- voluminous diarrhea and cramping if the lower GI tract is involved

Symptoms can last for weeks to months, even with treatment, and can lead to malnutrition and significant weight loss in 14% to 43% of patients. Underlying causes for these symptoms include villous atrophy, mucosal ulcerations, secretory dysfunction, osmotic factors, rapid passage, and pancreatic insufficiency. Intestinal protein losses and fat malabsorption are also characteristic of intestinal GVHD.[44]

Diarrhea associated with GVHD has an elevated protein content, which can sometimes give stool a rope-like appearance.[47] Loss of gut protein often precedes symptoms. Decreases in serum albumin of greater than or equal to 0.5 g/dL may be a useful marker of impending lower-gut GVHD.[47,48]

Measures to prevent or to treat GVHD include pre-HCT donor selection with human leukocyte antigen matching and post-HCT multidrug immunosuppressive therapies (see Box 15.4).[47] One study has shown that prophylaxis with ursodiol (a naturally occurring bile acid) significantly reduced patients' risk for hyperbilirubinemia, severe acute GVHD, liver GVHD, and intestinal GVHD with no adverse effects observed.[49]

Nutrition Support
Enteral Nutrition

Historically, EN was not routinely used in HCT because studies supporting its use were limited and there were concerns about EN intolerance associated with GI toxicities from conditioning regimens. The American Society for Parental and Enteral Nutrition (ASPEN) and the European Society for Clinical Nutrition and Metabolism (ESPEN) now recommend EN as first-line nutrition support during HCT for patients who are malnourished or who have inadequate intake that is expected to be prolonged.[11,52] The benefits of EN support include maintenance of mucosal gut integrity with stimulation of mucosal repair, decreased incidence of hyperglycemia, maintenance of normal gut barrier function, decreased risk of infection, and decreased cost.[15,53]

Recent research has highlighted the importance of bacteria, particularly the gut microbiota, in HCT outcome and in GVHD development.[54,55] It is likely that some changes in the microbiota observed during HCT and GVHD may be due to insufficient nutrients in the gut required to maintain a balanced flora, especially with longer exposure to PN.[54,56] Given the emerging data regarding the gut microbiome as a key component of the human immune system and its link to reduced GVHD, efforts to maintain adequate nutrient intake via oral feeding or EN are encouraged.[54] This suggests that oral or enteral feeding, alone or in combination, as opposed to parenteral feeding, may exert a beneficial effect on intestinal flora after HCT and perhaps accelerate patient recovery.[54,56]

EN should be considered for patients who are:

- undergoing allogeneic HCT and have a functional GI tract[8,57];
- malnourished before autologous and allogeneic HCT;

Box 15.4

Therapies for the Prevention and Treatment of Graft-Versus-Host Disease[1,49-51]

Therapy	Gastrointestinal and oral side effects	Other side effects and nutrition considerations
Beclomethasone dipropionate	Dysgeusia Oral candidiasis	
Budesonide	Xerostomia	
Calcineurin inhibitors (cyclosporine, tacrolimus)	Nausea Vomiting	Hypomagnesemia Hyperkalemia Renal insufficiency Food-drug interaction (with grapefruit, bergamot, bitter orange, pomegranate)
Methotrexate	Nausea Vomiting Anorexia Mucositis Diarrhea	Renal and hepatic changes
Mycophenolate mofetil	Diarrhea Constipation Abdominal pain Nausea	Interaction with dietary calcium and with magnesium and iron supplements Should be taken on an empty stomach
Sirolimus		Hypertriglyceridemia
Prednisone	Dyspepsia Hyperphagia	Insulin resistance Hyperglycemia Edema Hypokalemia Hypophosphatemia Hyperlipidemia Skeletal muscle catabolism Osteoporosis Growth retardation in children

(continued)

Box 15.4
Therapies for the Prevention and Treatment of Graft-Versus-Host Disease[1,49-51] *(continued)*

Therapy	Gastrointestinal and oral side effects	Other side effects and nutrition considerations
Extracorporeal photopheresis		Hypocalcemia Intravenous fluid may be needed to maintain adequate hydration status May not be possible with significant hypertriglyceridemia (lipemic serum blocks ultraviolet light)
Psoralen and ultraviolet irradiation	Nausea	Hepatotoxicity
Ruxolitinib		Weight gain Abnormalities in lipid metabolism
Ursodiol	Nausea Vomiting Diarrhea Dyspepsia	

- unable to meet estimated energy and protein needs for a prolonged period after engraftment or in association with chronic GVHD[52]; or

- discharged to home following HCT but have not yet established adequate oral intake.[11,52,57]

EN should be continued until the patient is able to meet the majority of nutrition needs orally.

Parenteral Nutrition

Historically, PN was the standard of care for HCT recipients because the many adverse effects of regimen-related toxicities limited tolerance to oral feedings or to EN. Early studies found that PN support during HCT was associated with improved visceral protein status and maintenance of body weight, as well as decreased mortality, improved overall survival, and increased time to relapse.[58-60] Since the introduction of RIC and nonmyeloablative conditioning regimens, PN is no longer considered standard supportive care for HCT, because many of these regimens are associated with fewer oral and GI toxicities compared with myeloablative regimens.[61,62]

PN is associated with a greater risk of hyperglycemia, infection, increased need for antifungal medications, volume overload, and delayed platelet engraftment.[40,57,60,63] Shortening the time of exposure to PN is likely advantageous for the HCT patient. Increased infection rates associated with PN are thought to be related to increased bacterial translocation that occurs when there is a lack of gut stimulation due to absence of oral or enteral nutrition and increased intestinal permeability during HCT.[63]

ESPEN guidelines state that PN should only be used in patients with the following conditions[11,60]:

- severe mucositis (>grade 3)
- ileus
- intractable vomiting
- GVHD with more than 1 L of stool per day
- inability to place a nasogastric tube
- significant intolerance to EN

PN should be discontinued as soon as the engraftment has occurred, the patient is able to consume adequate nutrition orally or enterally and the excessive stool from GVHD is controlled.[8,52] Box 15.5 outlines the indications for PN in GVHD and the diet progression as symptoms improve.

Enteral Nutrition Compared to Parenteral Nutrition

Studies comparing EN to PN in adult and pediatric populations show EN demonstrates protective benefits for many important factors in HCT. In both populations, EN was found to have better overall survival, improved platelet engraftment, and decreased acute GVHD.[57,63] Additionally, the adult population showed improved neutrophil engraftment, and the pediatric group showed decreased nonrelapse mortality and decreased length of stay with EN. Although EN is preferred, some patients might have poor tolerance to EN, and PN may, therefore, be indicated. PN may also be considered for patients unable to advance to EN due to intolerance symptoms, such as diarrhea, vomiting, early satiety, and feeding tube dislodgement. Other indications for PN may include refusal of feeding tube placement and acute intestinal GVHD of grades III to IV.[40,57,63]

Monitoring Nutrition Support

Daily monitoring of the patient's medical condition, nutritional status, blood chemistries, and treatment-related symptoms is necessary, as changes in these factors might require modifications in nutrient and fluid support. During the early posttransplant period (from conditioning through the neutropenic phase), the patient's weight and total intake and output volumes should be monitored daily throughout the hospital stay. Oral and intravenous energy, protein, and fluid intake levels should also be evaluated daily so appropriate nutrition support can be provided. When oral feedings or EN support

---

Box 15.5
Dietary Progression for Gastrointestinal Symptoms in Graft-Versus-Host Disease[1]

Phase 1: Bowel rest

Clinical symptoms	Diet	Symptoms of diet intolerance
Gastrointestinal (GI) cramping Large-volume, watery diarrhea >500 mL/d Depressed serum albumin Severely reduced transit time Small bowel obstruction or diminished bowel sounds Nausea and vomiting	Oral: nothing by mouth (npo) Intravenous (IV): meet energy and protein requirements	N/A

(continued)

Box 15.5
Dietary Progression for Gastrointestinal Symptoms in Graft-Versus-Host Disease[1] (continued)

Phase 2: Introduction of oral feeding

Clinical symptoms	Diet	Symptoms of diet intolerance
Minimal GI cramping Diarrhea <500 mL/d Improved transit time Infrequent nausea and vomiting	Oral: isotonic, low-residue, low-lactose fluids IV: as for phase 1	Increased stool volume or diarrhea Increased emesis Increased abdominal cramping

Phase 3: Introduction of solids

Clinical symptoms	Diet	Symptoms of diet intolerance
Minimal or no GI cramping Formed stool	Oral: allow introduction of solid foods containing minimal lactose, low fiber, low fat, low total acidity, no gastric irritants IV: as for phase 1	As in phase 2

Phase 4: Expansion of diet

Clinical symptoms	Diet	Symptoms of diet intolerance
Minimal or no GI cramping Formed stool	Oral: add foods containing minimal lactose, low fiber, low total acidity, no gastric irritants; if stools indicate fat malabsorption, prescribe a low-fat diet IV: as needed to meet nutrition requirements	As in phase 2

Phase 5: Resumption of regular diet

Clinical symptoms	Diet	Symptoms of diet intolerance
No GI cramping Normal stool Normal transit time Normal serum albumin	Oral: progress to regular diet; allow acid foods with meals, fiber-containing foods, lactose-containing foods; order of addition will vary, depending on individual tolerances and preferences; patients without steatorrhea should have fat restriction slowly liberalized IV: discontinue when oral intake meets nutrient needs	As in phase 2

is instituted, it is necessary to monitor the patient's oral and GI tolerance.

Survivorship

Chronic Graft-Versus-Host Disease

Difficulty eating and malnutrition are often significant issues for patients with chronic GVHD and are associated with nausea, vomiting, diarrhea, mouth pain, dysphagia, dysgeusia, xerostomia, anorexia, early satiety, and weight loss. Box 15.6 on page 322 identifies medical nutrition therapy strategies for common nutrition impact symptoms associated with chronic GVHD. Malnutrition is a significant complication for patients with chronic GVHD and is associated with GI, lung, and mouth manifestations, as well as impaired functional status and reduced quality of life.[64]

Bone Disease

Bone disease (osteoporosis) is a recognized complication of HCT. Prevalence is as high as 50%, as early as 1 year after transplantation.[65,66] Chemotherapy, TBI exposure, calcineurin inhibitors, and glucocorticoids all contribute to bone loss. Nutrition intervention to ensure adequate calcium and vitamin D intake is recommended in order to prevent and manage bone disease. Calcium requirements vary by patient age, and vitamin D needs are typically based on serum vitamin D levels. Additional recommendations for maintaining or improving bone density after HCT include regular weight-bearing and muscle-strengthening exercises and bisphosphonate therapy.[67,68]

Vitamin D Deficiency and Insufficiency

Vitamin D deficiency and insufficiency are common following HCT in both adults and children.[69,70]

Recent studies have examined the relationship between vitamin D status pre-HCT and vitamin D supplementation, and the impact on post-HCT outcomes and GVHD. Emerging data suggest a potential benefit of vitamin D supplementation in reducing chronic GVHD, due to vitamin D's immunoregulatory properties in certain genotypes.[71] Further studies are needed to determine the clinical impact and outcomes in HCT of both pre-HCT vitamin D status and of supplementation recommendations.[72,73]

Growth and Development

Growth and development in children undergoing HCT should be assessed regularly. Decreased growth velocity, growth hormone deficiency, and delayed onset of puberty occur frequently in children who have had HCT.[74] When abnormal endocrine function is detected, initiation of appropriate hormone therapy may improve growth and development.

Metabolic Syndrome

Metabolic syndrome is prevalent in both adult and pediatric transplant survivors. It can occur soon after HCT, and studies have found high incidences at 1 and 5 years after transplantation.[75,76] Markers of metabolic syndrome are found as early as 80 days post-HCT and have been shown to be predictive of metabolic syndrome at 1 year after HCT.[77]

Cardiometabolic Changes

Cardiometabolic changes, including central adiposity, hypertension, insulin resistance, and dyslipidemia, show a statistically significant difference in incidence among survivors of HCT for acute myeloid leukemia in childhood compared with controls ($P = .02$).[82] Pediatric HCT survivors are more likely to develop diabetes and hypertension than the general population and should be monitored throughout adulthood.[78,79] Referral to a

Box 15.6
Nutrition Impact Symptoms of Chronic Graft-Versus-Host Disease and Recommended Medical Nutrition Therapies[81-8]

Oral

Nutrition impact symptom	Increased sensitivity
	Xerostomia
	Dysphagia (due to esophageal webbing or stricture)
Manifestations	Affects ability to chew and to swallow food properly
	Reduced variety of foods in diet
Medical nutrition therapy	For dysphagia, refer to a speech pathologist for swallowing evaluation
	Esophageal dilatation for severe symptoms
	Gastrostomy tube for enteral nutrition if oral or esophageal symptoms preclude adequate calorie-protein intake for weight maintenance and support

Gastrointestinal

Nutrition impact symptom	Abnormal intestinal mucosa
	Intestinal bile salt deficiency
	Pancreatic enzyme insufficiency or atrophy
	Bacterial overgrowth
Manifestations	Diarrhea
	Nutrient malabsorption
Medical nutrition therapy	Screening tests (fecal elastase or serum trypsinogen) to confirm fat malabsorption
	Oral pancreatic enzyme replacement therapy
	Dietary fat restriction
	Supplementation with products containing medium-chain triglycerides

Pulmonary

Nutrition impact symptom	Pulmonary insufficiency
Manifestations	Increased metabolic demands leading to increased energy requirement to prevent weight loss and debilitation
Medical nutrition therapy	Monitor nutritional status closely

registered dietitian nutritionist (RDN) for nutritional counseling to address contributing dietary factors to metabolic syndrome is appropriate for both pediatric and adult populations.

Iron Overload

Iron overload, most commonly related to multiple red blood cell transfusions, is frequently observed after transplantation.[85] For this reason, iron supplementation and iron-containing multivitamins are contraindicated during HCT.[52]

Emerging Treatment Modalities

Chimeric antigen receptor (CAR) T-cell therapies are an emerging treatment modality displaying significant success in treating patients with hematologic malignancies, such as diffuse large B-cell lymphoma and precursor B-cell acute lymphoblastic leukemia.[86] Studies have observed specific toxicities, including cytokine release syndrome (CRS) and CAR T-cell therapy–related neurotoxicity, which typically present within the first days of CAR T-cell infusion.[87,88] Manifestations of CRS include fevers, hypotension, hypoxia, end organ dysfunction, cytopenias, coagulopathy, and hemophagocytic lymphohistiocytosis.[89]

Guidelines for toxicity management vary among treatment centers but typically include supportive care plus immunosuppression with tocilizumab or corticosteroids administered for severe toxicity.[89]

Summary

HCT is a medically complex treatment modality that results in multiple acute and long-term nutritional challenges. The RDN is an integral member of the multidisciplinary team that will recommend and implement nutrition intervention strategies, including nutrition support, for this complex population. Ongoing nutrition assessment and monitoring is essential for the best outcome in this highly challenging and ever-changing therapeutic modality.

Sample PES Statements
for Hematopoietic Cell Transplantation

Intake domain: Inadequate oral intake related to decreased ability to consume sufficient energy due to side effects of cancer therapy, as evidenced by a calorie count indicating an intake of <50% of estimated needs, mucositis, and nausea.

Clinical domain: Severe, acute disease- or injury-related malnutrition related to decreased ability to consume sufficient energy due to side effects of cancer therapy, as evidenced by a weight loss of 3% in the past week, intake <50% of estimated needs in the past 5 days, mucositis, nausea, and vomiting.

Behavioral-environmental domain: Food- and nutrition-related knowledge deficit related to lack of prior exposure to information, as evidenced by reported consumption of unwashed raw fruits and vegetables and undercooked eggs.

References

1. Macris P, McMillen K. Nutrition support of the hematopoietic cell transplant recipient. In: Forman S, Negrin R, Antin J, Appelbaum F, eds. *Thomas' Hematopoietic Cell Transplantation: Stem Cell Transplantation.* 2 vols. 5th ed. Wiley-Blackwell; 2016:1216-1224.

2. Tierney KD. Hematopoietic cell transplantation. In: Olsen M, Zitella LJ, eds. *Hematologic Malignancies in Adults.* Oncology Nursing Society; 2013:499-530.

3. Battiwalla M, Hashmi S, Majhail N, Pavletic S, Savani BN, Shelburne N. National Institutes of Health Hematopoietic Cell Transplantation Late Effects Initiative: developing recommendations to improve survivorship and long-term outcomes. *Biol Blood Marrow Transplant.* 2017;23(1):6-9.

4. Patel S, Rybicki LA, Corrigan D, et al. Prognostic factors for mortality among day +100 survivors after allogeneic hematopoietic cell transplantation. *Biol Blood Marrow Transplant.* 2018;24(5):1029-1034.

5. Kekre N, Antin J. Hematopoietic stem cell transplantation donor sources in the 21st century: choosing the ideal donor when a perfect match does not exist. *Blood.* 2014;124(3):334-343.

6. Gyurkocza B, Sandmaier B. Conditioning regimens for hematopoietic cell transplantation: one size does not fit all. *Blood.* 2014;124(3):344-353.

7. Deeg HJ, Sandmier BM. Who is fit for allogeneic stem cell transplant? *Blood.* 2010;116(23):4762-4770.

8. Marian M, Mattox T, Williams V. Cancer. In: Muller CM, ed. *The ASPEN Adult Nutrition Support Core Curriculum.* 3rd ed. American Society for Parenteral and Enteral Nutrition; 2017:651-670.

9. Holtick, U, Albrecht M, Chemnitz JM, et al. Bone marrow versus peripheral blood allogeneic haematopoietic stem cell transplantation for haematological malignancies in adults. *Cochrane Database Syst Rev.* 2014;(4):CD010189.

10. Shaughnessy P, Uberti J, Devine S, et al. Plerixafor and G-CSF for autologous stem cell mobilization in patients with NHL, Hodgkin's lymphoma and multiple myeloma: results from the expanded access program. *Bone Marrow Transplant.* 2013;48(6):777–781.

11. Arends J, Bachmann P, Baracos V, et al. ESPEN guidelines on nutrition in cancer patients. *Clin Nutr.* 2017;36(1):11-48.

12. White M, Murphy AJ, Hastings Y, et al. Nutritional status and energy expenditure in children pre-bone-marrow-transplant. *Bone Marrow Transplant.* 2005;35(8):775-779.

13. Charuhas PM, Lipkin A, et al. Hematopoietic stem cell transplantation. In: Merritt RJ, ed. *The A.S.P.E.N. Nutrition Support Practice Manual.* 2nd ed. American Society for Parenteral and Enteral Nutrition; 2005: 666-662.

14. McClave S, Taylor B, Marinadale R, et al. Guidelines for the provision and assessment of nutrition support therapy in the adult critically ill patient: Society of Critical Care Medicine (SCCM) and American Society for Parenteral and Enteral Nutrition (A.S.P.E.N.). *JPEN J Parenter Enteral Nutr.* 2016;40(2):159-211.

15. Lipkin C, Lenssen P, Dickson BJ. Nutrition issues in hematopoietic stem cell transplantation: state of the art. *Nutr Clin Pract.* 2005;20(4):423-439.

16. Mirtallo J, Canada T, Johnson D, et al; Task Force for the Revision of Safe Practices for Parenteral Nutrition. Safe practices for parenteral nutrition. *JPEN J Parenter Enteral Nutr.* 2004;28(6):S39-S70.

17. Hematopoietic Stem Cell Transplant. In: *Pediatric Nutrition Care Manual.* Accessed October 29, 2020. www.nutritioncaremanual.org/topic.cfm?ncm_toc_id=144782

18. Choban P, Dickerson R, Malone A, Worthington P, Compher C. A.S.P.E.N. clinical guidelines: nutrition support of hospitalized adult patients with obesity. *JPEN J Parenter Enteral Nutr.* 2013;37(6):714-744.

19. Patel R. Parenteral Nutrition Formulations. In: Muller CM, ed. *The ASPEN Adult Nutrition Support Core Curriculum*. 3rd ed. American Society for Parenteral and Enteral Nutrition; 2017:303.

20. Trifilio S, Helenowski I, Giel M, et al. Questioning the role of a neutropenic diet following hematopoietic stem cell transplantation. *Biol Blood Marrow Transpl*. 2012;18 (9):1385-1390.

21. Van Dalen EC, Mank A, Leclercq E, et al. Low bacterial diet versus control diet to prevent infection in cancer patients treated with chemotherapy causing episodes. *Cochrane Database Syst Rev*. 2016;(4):CD006247.

22. Moody K, Finlay J, Mancuso C, Charlson M. Feasibility and safety of a pilot randomized trial of infection rate: neutropenic diet versus standard food safety guidelines. *J Pediatr Hematol Oncol*. 2006;28(3):126-133.

23. Boyle NM, Podczervinski S, Jordan K, et al. Bacterial foodborne infections after hematopoietic cell transplantation. *Biol Blood Marrow Transplant*. 2014;20(11):1856-1861.

24. Seattle Cancer Care Alliance. Diet Guidelines for Immunosuppressed Patients. Accessed October 29, 2020. www.seattlecca.org/PDF/diet -guidelines-immunosuppressed

25. Fuji S, Tadano K, Mori T, et al. Impact of pretransplant body mass index on the clinical outcome after allogeneic hematopoietic SCT. *Bone Marrow Transplant*. 2014;49(12):1505-1512.

26. Gleimer M, Li L, Paczesny S, et al. Baseline body mass index among children and adults undergoing allogeneic hematopoietic cell transplantation: clinical characteristics and outcomes. *Bone Marrow Transplant*. 2015;(3):402-410.

27. White M, Murphy A, Hallahan A, et al. Survival in overweight and underweight children undergoing hematopoietic stem cell transplant. *Eur J Clin Nutr*. 2012;66(10):1120-1123.

28. Hoffmeister P, Storer B, Macris P. Body mass index and arm anthropometry predict outcomes after pediatric allogeneic hematopoietic cell transplantation for hematologic malignancies. *Biol Blood Marrow Transplant*. 2013;19(7):1081-1086.

29. Baumgartner A, Zueger N, Bargetzi A, et al. Association of nutritional parameters with clinical outcomes in patients with acute myeloid leukemia undergoing hematopoietic stem cell transplantation. *Ann Nutr Metab*. 2016;69(2):89-98.

30. Horsley P, Bauer J, Gallagher B. Poor nutritional status prior to peripheral blood stem cell transplantation is associated with increased length of hospital stay. *Bone Marrow Transplant*. 2005;35(11):1113-1116.

31. Lalla RV, Bowen J, Barasch A. MASCC/ISOO clinical practice guidelines for the management of mucositis secondary to cancer therapy. *Cancer*. 2014;120(10):1453-1461.

32. Crowther M, Avenell A, Culligan DJ. Systemic review and meta-analyses of studies of glutamine supplementation in haematopoietic stem cell transplantation. *Bone Marrow Transplant*. 2009;44(7):413-425.

33. Pytlik R, Benes P, Patorkova M, et al. Standard parenteral alanyl-glutamine dipeptide supplementation is not beneficial in autologous transplant patients: a randomized, double-blind, placebo controlled study. *Bone Marrow Transplant*. 2002;30(12):953-961.

34. Sykorova A, Horacek J, Zak P, et al. A randomized, double blind comparative study of prophylactic parenteral nutritional support with or without glutamine in autologous stem cell transplantation for hematological malignancies— three years' follow-up. *Neoplasma*. 2005;52(6)476-482.

35. Hopps SA, Borders EB, Hagemann TM. Prophylaxis and treatment recommendations for sinusoidal obstruction syndrome in adult and pediatric patients undergoing hematopoietic stem cell transplant: a review of the literature. *J Oncol Pharm Practice*. 2016;23(3):496-510.

36. Richardson P, Smith AR, Triplett BM, et al. Earlier defibrotide initiation post-diagnosis of veno-occlusive disease/sinusoidal obstruction syndrome improves D+100 survival following haematopoietic stem cell transplantation. *Br J Haematol.* 2017;178(1):112-118.

37. Verdi Shumacher M, Moreira Faulhaber GA. Nutritional status and hyperglycemia in the peritransplant period: a review of associations with parenteral nutrition and clinical outcomes. *Rev Bras Hematol Hemoter.* 2017;39(2):155-162.

38. Fuji S, Einsele H, Svani BP, Kapp M. Systematic nutritional support in allogeneic hematopoietic stem cell transplant recipients. *Biol Blood Marrow Transplant.* 2015;21(10):1707-1713.

39. Fuji S, Kim S, Mori S, et al. Hyperglycemia during the neutropenic period is associated with a poor outcome in patients undergoing myeloablative allogeneic hematopoietic stem cell transplantation. *Transplantation.* 2007;84(7):814-820.

40. Guieze R, Lemal R, Cabrespine A, et al. Enteral versus parenteral nutritional support in allogeneic haematopoietic stem-cell transplantation. *Clin Nutr.* 2014;33(3):533-538.

41. Ferreira AM, Moreira F, Guimaraes T, et al. Epidemiology, risk factors and outcomes of multi-drug-resistant bloodstream infections in haematopoietic stem cell transplant recipients: importance of previous gut colonization. *J Hosp Infect.* 2018;100(1):83-91.

42. Schmidt-Hieber M, Bierwirth J, Buchheid T, et al. Diagnosis and management of gastrointestinal complications in adult cancer patients: 2017 updated evidence-based guidelines of the Infectious Diseases Working Party (AGIHO) of the German Society of Hematology and Medical Oncology (DGHO). *Ann Hematol.* 2018;97(1):31-49.

43. Bhat V, Joshi A, Sarode R, Chavan P. Cytomegalovirus infection in the bone marrow transplant patient. *World J Transplant.* 2015;5(4):287-290.

44. Van der Meij BS, de Graaf P, Wierdsma NJ, et al. Nutritional support in patients with GVHD of the digestive tract: state of the art. *Bone Marrow Transplant.* 2013;48(4):474-482.

45. Goddard D, Ruben B, Mathes E, et al. A case of severe cutaneous, GI and liver GVHD in a patient with multiple myeloma, status-post-second auto-SCT. *Bone Marrow Transplant.* 2010;45(2):409–411.

46. Hammami M, Talkin R, Al-Taee A, et al. Autologous graft-versus-host disease of the gastrointestinal tract in patients with multiple myeloma and hematopoietic stem cell transplantation. *Gastroenterology Res.* 2018;11(1):52-57.

47. Rezvani A, Storer B, Storb R, et al. Decreased serum albumin as a biomarker for severe acute graft-versus-host disease after reduced-intensity allogeneic hematopoietic cell transplantation. *Biol Blood Marrow Transplant.* 2011;17(11):1594-1601.

48. McDonald G. How I treat acute graft-versus-host disease of the gastrointestinal tract and the liver. *Blood.* 2016;127(12):1544-1550.

49. Ruutu, T, Juvonen E, Remberger M, et al. Improved survival with ursodeoxycholic acid prophylaxis in allogeneic stem cell transplantation: long-term follow-up of a randomized study. *Bio Blood Marrow Transplant.* 2014;20(1):135-138.

50. Khandelwal P, Teusink-Cross A, Davies S, et al. Ruxolitinib as salvage therapy in steroid-refractory acute graft-versus-host disease in pediatric hematopoietic stem cell transplant patients. *Biol Blood Marrow Transplant.* 2017;23(7):1122-1127.

51. Vainchenker W, Leroy E, Gilles L, et al. JAK inhibitors for the treatment of myeloproliferative neoplasms and other disorders. *F1000Res.* 2018;7:82.

52. August DA, Huhmann MB; American Society for Parenteral and Enteral Nutrition (A.S.P.E.N.) Board of Directors. A.S.P.E.N. clinical guidelines: nutrition support therapy during adult anticancer treatment and in hematopoietic cell transplantation. *JPEN J Parenter Enteral Nutr.* 2009;33(5):472-500.

53. Thompson JL, Duffy J. Nutrition support challenges in hematopoietic stem cell transplant patients. *Nutr Clin Pract.* 2008;23(5):533-546.

54. Staffas A, Burgos da Silva M, van den Brink MRM. The intestinal microbiota in allogeneic hematopoietic cell transplant and graft-versus-host disease. *Blood.* 2017;129(8): 927-933.

55. Shono Y, van den Brink MRM. Gut microbiota injury in allogeneic haematopoietic stem cell transplantation. *Nat Rev Cancer.* 2018;18(5):283-295.

56. Jeng RR, Taur Y, Delvin S. Intestinal *Blautia* is associated with reduced death from graft-versus-host disease. *Biol Blood Marrow Transplant.* 2015;21(8):1373–1383.

57. Gonzales F, Bruno B, Alarcón Fuentes M, et al. Better early outcome with enteral rather than parenteral nutrition in children undergoing MAC allo-SCT. *Clin Nutr.* 2017;37(6 pt A):2113-2121.

58. Uderzo C, Rovelli A, Bonomi M, et al. Total parenteral nutrition and nutritional assessment in leukaemic children undergoing bone marrow transplantation. *Eur J Cancer.* 1991;27(6):758-762.

59. Yokoyama S, Fujimoto T, Mitomi T, et al. Use of total parenteral nutrition in pediatric bone marrow transplantation. *Nutrition.* 1989;5(1):27-30.

60. Baumgartner A, Bargetzi A, Zueger N, et al. Revisiting nutritional support for allogeneic hematologic stem cell transplantation—a systematic review. *Bone Marrow Transplant.* 2017;52(4):506-513.

61. Diaconescu R, Flowers CR, Storer B, et al. Morbidity and mortality with nonmyeloablative compared with myeloablative conditioning before hematopoietic cell transplantation from HLA-matched related donors. *Blood.* 2004;104(5):1550-1558.

62. Topcuoglu P, Arat M, Ozcan M, et al. Case-matched comparison with standard versus reduced intensity conditioning regimen in chronic myeloid leukemia patients. *Ann Hematol.* 2012;91(4):577-586.

63. Seguy D, Duhamel A, Rekeb MB, et al. Better outcome of patients undergoing enteral tube feeding after myeloablative conditioning for allogeneic stem cell transplantation. *Transplantation.* 2012;94(3):287-294.

64. Bassim C, Fassuk G, Dibbub N, et al. Malnutrition in patients with chronic GVHD. *Bone Marrow Transplant.* 2014;49(10): 1300-1306.

65. Tauchmanova L, Colao A, Lombardi G, et al. Bone loss and its management in long-term survivors from allogeneic stem cell transplantation. *J Clin Endocrinol Metab.* 2007;92(12):4536-4545.

66. Yao S, McCarthy P, Dunford L, et al. High prevalence of early-onset osteopenia/osteoporosis after allogeneic stem cell transplantation and improvement after bisphosphonate therapy. *Bone Marrow Transplant.* 2008;41(4):393-398.

67. McClune B, Majhail N, Flowers M. Bone loss and avascular necrosis of bone after hematopoietic cell transplantation. *Semin Hematol.* 2012;49(1):59-65.

68. Carpenter P, Hoffmeister P, Chesnut C, et al. Bisphosphonate therapy for reduced bone mineral density in children with chronic graft-versus-host disease. *Biol Blood Marrow Transplant.* 2007;13(6):683-690.

69. Urbain P, Ihorst G, Biesalski H, et al. Course of serum 25-hydroxyvitamin D_3 status and its influencing factors in adults undergoing allogeneic hematopoietic cell transplantation. *Ann Hematol.* 2012;91(5):759-766.

70. Duncan C, Vrooman L, Apfelbaum E, et al. 25-hydroxy vitamin D deficiency following pediatric hematopoietic stem cell transplant. *Biol Blood Marrow Transplant.* 2011;17(5):749-753.

71. Carrillo-Cruz E, García-Lozano J, Márquez-Malaver F, et al. Vitamin D modifies the incidence of graft-versus-host disease after allogeneic stem cell transplantation depending on the vitamin D receptor (VDR) polymorphisms. *Clin Cancer Res.* 2019;25(15):4616-4623.

72. von Bahr L, Blennow O. Increased incidence of chronic GvHD and CMV disease in patients with vitamin D deficiency before allogeneic stem cell transplantation. *Bone Marrow Transplant.* 2015;50(9):1217-1223.

73. Hansson M, Norlin A, Omazic B, et al. Vitamin D levels affect outcome in pediatric hematopoietic stem cell transplantation. *Biol Blood Marrow Transplant.* 2014;20(10):1537-1543.

74. Sanders JE. Growth and development after hematopoietic cell transplant in children. *Bone Marrow Transplant.* 2008;41(2):223-227.

75. Majhail N, Flowers M, Ness K, et al. High prevalence of metabolic syndrome after allogeneic hematopoietic cell transplantation. *Bone Marrow Transplant.* 2009;43(1):49-54.

76. Annaloro C, Usardi P, Airaghi L, et al. Prevalence of metabolic syndrome in long-term survivors of hematopoietic stem cell transplantation. *Bone Marrow Transplant.* 2008;41(9):797-804.

77. McMillen K, Schmidt E, Storer B, et al. Metabolic syndrome appears early after hematopoietic cell transplantation. *Metab Syndr Relat Disord.* 2014;12(7):367-371.

78. Chow E, Simmons J, Roth C, et al. Increased cardiometabolic traits in pediatric survivors of acute lymphoblastic leukemia treated with total body irradiation. *Biol Blood Marrow Transplant.* 2010;16(12):1674-1681.

79. Hoffmeister P, Storer B, Sanders J. Diabetes mellitus in long-term survivors of pediatric hematopoietic cell transplantation. *J Pediatr Hematol Oncol.* 2004;26(2):81-90.

80. Hoffmeister P, Hingorani S, Storer B, et al. Hypertension in long-term survivors of pediatric hematopoietic cell transplantation. *Biol Blood Marrow Transplant.* 2010;16(4):515-524.

81. Elsaadany BA, Ahmed EM, Aghbary SMH. Efficacy and safety of topical corticosteroids for management of oral chronic graft versus host disease. *Int J Dent.* 2017;2017:article ID 1908768. doi:10.1155/2017/1908768

82. Kida A, McDonald G. Gastrointestinal, hepatobiliary, pancreatic, and iron-related diseases in long-term survivors of allogeneic hematopoietic cell transplantation. *Semin Hematol.* 2012;49(1):43-58.

83. Stern JM. Nutritional assessment and management of malabsorption in the hematopoietic stem cell transplant patient. *J Am Diet Assoc.* 2002;102(12):1812-1815.

84. Nakasone H, Ito A, Endo H, et al. Pancreatic atrophy is associated with gastrointestinal chronic GVHD following allogeneic PBSC transplantation. *Bone Marrow Transplant.* 2010;45(3):590-592.

85. Trottier B, Burns L, DeFor T, et al. Association of iron overload with allogeneic hematopoietic cell transplantation outcomes: a prospective cohort study using R2-MRI–measured liver iron content. *Blood.* 2013;122(9):1678-1684.

86. Boyiadzis MM, Dhodapkar MV, Brentjens RJ, et al. Chimeric antigen receptor (CAR) T therapies for the treatment of hematologic malignancies: clinical perspective and significance. *J Immunother Cancer.* 2018;6(1):137.

87. Bonifant CL, Jackson HJ, Brentjens RJ, et al. Toxicity and management in CAR T-cell therapy. *Mol Ther Oncolytics.* 2016;3:16011. doi:10.1038/mto.2016.11

88. Maude S, Frey N, Shaw PA, et al. Chimeric antigen receptor T cells for sustained remissions in leukemia. *N Engl J Med.* 2014;371(16):1507-1517.

89. Brudno J, Kochenderfer J. Recent advances in CAR T-cell toxicity: mechanisms, manifestations and management. *Blood Rev.* 2019;34:45-55.

Chapter 16
Medical Nutrition Therapy for Primary Brain Tumors

Michelle Bratton, RDN, CSO

Ally F. Gottfried, MFN, RDN, CSO, LD

Kristen Miller, MS, RD, CSP, CLEC

Lindsay Rypkema, RD, CSP, CLEC

Tumors in the brain emanate from a combination of aberrant cell growth and abnormal cell death and can be malignant or benign. Unlike benign tumors in other areas of the body, those located in different areas of the brain can be disabling or life threatening due to pressure on and destruction of normal brain tissue.[1] Benign tumors can also become malignant, likely as a result of rapid growth. Because benign tumors can be equally as serious as malignant tumors, the term *brain tumor*, rather than *brain cancer*, is used to describe this group of conditions.[1,2]

Tumors can occur in any part of the brain. See Figure 16.1 on page 332 for normal brain anatomy. There are two main categories of brain tumors:

- Primary—There are more than 120 different types of primary brain tumor (PBT).[3] Tumors are classified by histology and grade (grades 1 to 4, I to IV, or G1 through G4; see Chapter 1). G4 tumors are high-grade tumors that reproduce rapidly, often invading normal brain tissue, developing new blood vessels, and resulting in areas of necrosis, but they rarely spread (metastasize) to other areas of the body. The World Health Organization (WHO) 2016 classification for brain and central nervous system tumors includes molecular genetic features, such as mutations, to improve prognostic value and possibly guide patient management.[4] PBTs are the subject of this chapter.

- Secondary (metastatic)—These are tumors that have spread to the brain from other types of cancers, such as lung, breast, kidney, and blood cancers. Treatment options differ for metastatic brain tumors, depending largely on where the cancer originated.[2] Health care providers, including registered dietitian nutritionists (RDNs), can help reinforce this important concept for patients.

Risk Factors

Radiation exposure is the largest risk factor for PBT development; however, most PBTs have no apparent cause. Dietary factors may influence incidence, although the data are inconclusive. A 2002 case-control study showed no association between consumption of cured meat and risk for PBTs,[5] whereas a 2003 meta-analysis showed an increased risk with cured-meat consumption.[6] Several studies have shown an inverse relationship between PBT risk and specific foods, including fish,[7] coffee and tea,[8] beans,[5] and dark yellow vegetables.[5] Larger case-control studies of healthy dietary patterns, such as the European Prospective Investigation into Cancer and Nutrition (EPIC),[8] Dietary Approaches to Stop Hypertension (DASH),[9] and the Index for Nutritional Quality (ie, diets high in fiber, fruits and vegetables, low-fat milk, and nuts, and low in total fat, saturated fat, and red meat),[10] also show a similar inverse relationship; as the quality of the diet increases, incidence decreases.

Incidence and Diagnosis

The incidence of malignant primary brain tumors is 6.5 per 100,000.[11] The lifetime risk of being diagnosed with a tumor of the brain or nervous system is 0.6% (based on data from 2012 to 2014). Incidence has declined 2% per year for the 10 years ranging from 2007 to 2016, and 5-year survival rate

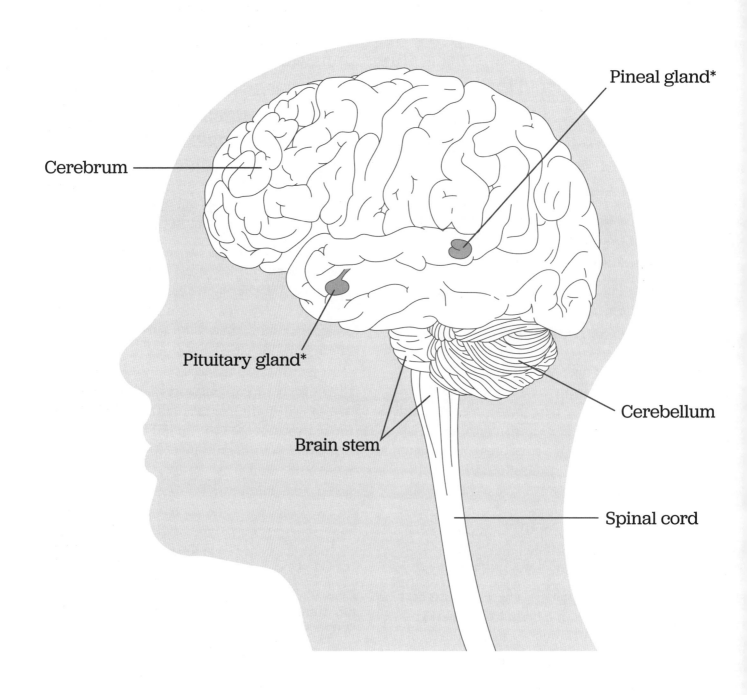

Cerebrum

Pineal gland*

Pituitary gland*

Brain stem

Cerebellum

Spinal cord

Figure 16.1
Major parts of the brain

* Pituitary gland and pineal grands are deep inside the brain.

is 32.9%.[12] Anaplastic astrocytomas and glioblastomas account for 38% of primary brain tumors, and meningiomas account for 27% of the total.[2] Brain tumors can increase intracranial pressure, which can lead to symptoms such as headache, nausea, vomiting, blurred vision, balance problems, personality changes, and seizures. If a brain tumor is suspected, the physician will order magnetic resonance imaging or a computed tomography scan. Once a tumor is identified, a biopsy may be performed to determine its type.

Treatment

Treatment varies according to the tumor type but often includes surgery, radiotherapy, and chemotherapy. Surgery often may be curative for low-grade tumors, while higher-grade tumors require adjuvant radiotherapy and chemotherapy.[13] Loss of appetite, fatigue, nausea, vomiting, alopecia, and hypogeusia are the most common side effects reported by patients undergoing brain radiotherapy.[13-15] Box 16.1 on page 334 lists chemotherapy agents often used in this population and their associated nutrition impact symptoms. For comprehensive recommendations and details of specific therapies, see *NCCN Clinical Practice Guidelines in Oncology (NCCN Guidelines): Central Nervous System Cancers*.[16] Seizure activity is common in patients with brain tumors, and preferred antiepileptic drugs (also shown in Box 16.1 on page 334) are those that avoid interference with chemotherapy agents.[17]

Tumor-treating fields—low-intensity, alternating electric fields that disrupt cancer cell division—are a relatively new treatment modality used in addition to chemotherapy. Tumor-treating field devices are worn on the head, and the electrical fields pulse through the scalp and provide a low-intensity alternating electric field therapy to disrupt cell division.[15,16]

Nutrition Assessment

The prevalence of malnutrition in patients with PBT is relatively low (17.6%) compared to its prevalence in those with gastrointestinal, lung, and head and neck malignancies.[18] The most common nutrition impact symptoms identified by malnourished patients meeting the subjective global assessment (SGA) criteria for categories SGA-B and SGA-C are weight loss, nausea, vomiting, headache, dysphagia, and fatigue.[19]

Two studies in 2016 and 2017 showed that patients with poor survival and high-grade gliomas also had low prognostic nutritional indexes (PNIs). The PNI is derived from total lymphocyte count and serum albumin concentration: a lower PNI indicates decreased lymphocytes or albumin, or both. In the 2017 study of patients diagnosed with WHO grade III and IV gliomas, those with a higher PNI had better progression-free survival and overall survival than those with a lower PNI.[20] The 2016 study showed that overall survival and efficacy of adjuvant treatment was improved in patients with a higher PNI. Although the authors of this study recommended the correction of nutrition and immune status in patients with glioblastoma as a means of optimizing outcomes,[21] the PNI has not been validated as a screening or assessment tool for oncology patients.[22] The use of serum hepatic proteins to identify malnutrition is not recommended (see Chapter 4).

Nutrition Problems and Interventions

Hyperglycemia

Patients with PBT frequently receive dexamethasone to decrease peritumoral edema and radiotherapy-related side effects.[23] Increased serum glucose associated with dexamethasone is caused by a combination of insulin resistance, promotion of hepatic glucose production, and decreased insulin

Box 16.1

Nutrition Impact Symptoms Associated With Treatment Medications Used for Primary Brain Tumors[13,16,17]

Drug	Type	Nutrition impact symptoms and precautions
Temozolomide (Temodar)	Chemotherapy	Nausea, vomiting, constipation, fatigue Take on an empty stomach
Procarbazine (Matulane)	Chemotherapy	Nausea, vomiting, anorexia, stomatitis Avoid alcohol Avoid tyramine-rich foods
Lomustine (CCNU, CeeNU)	Chemotherapy	Nausea, vomiting, anorexia, stomatitis Avoid alcohol
Vincristine (Oncovin)	Chemotherapy	Constipation, weight loss, nausea, vomiting Avoid alcohol
Irinotecan (Camptosar)	Chemotherapy	Diarrhea, anorexia, nausea, vomiting
Carmustine (Gliadel wafer)	Chemotherapy	Nausea, vomiting
Bevacizumab (Avastin)	Targeted therapy	Anorexia, stomatitis, nausea, vomiting, constipation, diarrhea
Levetiracetam (Keppra)	Antiepileptic	Diarrhea, fatigue, anorexia
Lacosamide (Vimpat)	Antiepileptic	Nausea
Lamotrigine (Lamictal)	Antiepileptic	Nausea, dyspepsia, constipation
Valproate (Depakote)	Antiepileptic	Diarrhea, change in appetite, weight gain or weight loss, constipation
Dexamethasone (Decadron)	Glucocorticoid	Increased appetite, hyperglycemia, muscle weakness, impaired wound healing

secretion from the islet cells.[23] Several studies[24-27] have identified an inverse relationship between hyperglycemia and survival in this population; however, intensive glucose management and its potential effect on survival has not been studied in these patients and is not a common treatment goal, possibly due to the poor prognosis associated with high-grade PBTs. Patients are less likely to be at risk for long-term diabetic complications, and providers may associate intensive management with decreased quality of life. Increased appetite and weight gain are also side effects of dexamethasone. Depending on the patient's disease state, MNT may be indicated to address these issues.

Ketogenic Diet

The ketogenic diet (KD) is a high-fat, low-carbohydrate, adequate-protein diet that is increasingly used as an adjuvant therapy to standard chemotherapy and radiotherapy in patients with PBT, although it is not the standard of care.[28] Prior to implementation of the KD, appropriateness should be evaluated by the multi-disciplinary care team and patient input should be considered.

In the 1950s, Otto Warburg observed that most cancer cells rely on an increased glycolysis for energy, rather than mitochondrial-based oxidative phosphorylation, regardless of oxygen availability.[29] This observation, known as the Warburg effect, gave way to the theory that changing the brain's energy source from glucose to ketone bodies can induce oxidative stress within cancer cells, leading to apoptosis.

Many *in vitro* and *in vivo* studies have examined the use of the KD as a component of cancer treatment. In one meta-analysis of *in vivo* studies, eight of nine studies (89%) supported the theory that the KD is protective against cancer, and seven of eight studies (88%) showed that it may slow cancer progression.[30] The tumor types studied were prostate, brain, colon, gastric, and metastatic cancers. A comprehensive review of oncology studies in adults concluded there is potential for antineoplastic effects among humans[31]; however, current human studies lack control groups and have methodological limitations, conflicting results, and small sample sizes. Although animal models have demonstrated promising results, well-designed human clinical trials are required to determine efficacy in humans.

The safety and feasibility of the KD in patients undergoing cancer treatment has been well reported.[32-36] To ensure safety, the medical team must assess for potential contraindications prior to initiating the KD (see Box 16.2).[37,38] The diet is contraindicated if a patient has a metabolic condition, such as primary carnitine deficiency, carnitine palmitoyltransferase I or II deficiency, carnitine-acylcarnitine translocase deficiency, β-oxidation defects, pyruvate carboxylase deficiency, and porphyria.[39] Because there is a potential for further

---

Box 16.2
Screening and Monitoring for the Ketogenic Diet[37,38]

What to monitor	When to monitor
Serum acylcarnitine profile, urine organic acids, serum amino acids, lactate, ammonia	Before starting diet, to rule out metabolic conditions and contraindications
Urine ketones	Daily at first; if stable, can decrease monitoring
Complete blood count, comprehensive metabolic panel, phosphorus, fasting lipids, free and total carnitine, serum ketones, 25-hydroxyvitamin D	One month after initiation and then every 3 months
Zinc, selenium, magnesium	Every 6 months
Bone mineral density	As needed
Weight	Routine

---

weight loss while following a restrictive diet such as the KD, malnutrition also may be a contraindication. Steroids alone are not a contraindication to the KD; however, ketone levels may be lower in patients receiving steroids. The KD was shown to be effective when started concurrently with radiation for brain cancer.[31,40]

Types of Ketogenic Diets

The classic KD has been in use since the 1920s as a component of treatment for intractable epilepsy. The classic diet is often started during inpatient admission, due to the need for close monitoring. The content of meals and snacks is determined by ratio—namely, the ratio of fat (in grams) to carbohydrate plus protein (also both in grams):

$$\text{fat (g)} : [\text{carbohydrate (g)} + \text{protein (g)}]$$

Ratios such as 3:1 and 4:1 are often used to achieve ketosis.[41] With a ketogenic ratio of 3:1, 87% of energy is derived from fat (based on 9 kcal/g). With a diet that follows a 4:1 ratio, 90% of energy is derived from fat. Recipe ingredients are provided in grams and must be carefully weighed on a scale.

For patients who can consume foods orally, common fat sources include heavy whipping cream, avocado, butter, oil, and sour cream. All-in-one meals (eg, soup, stew, or pizza) should ensure the goal ratio is met, particularly when patients are unable to consume all of their meal. Patients receiving enteral feeding are good candidates for the classic KD; goal ratios can be more consistently achieved with enteral feeding, as there are fewer variables compared to an oral diet. Commercial ketogenic formulas, such as KetoCal (Nutricia) and KetoVie (Cambrooke), are available in 3:1 and 4:1 ratios.

The modified Atkins diet, a type of KD, allows for liberalization of carbohydrate and a reduction of fat (65% to 82% of calories). This diet is started as an outpatient and is a more flexible option than the classic ketogenic diet for oral intake. Daily carbohydrate goals are typically 10 to 20 g/d, and ketogenic ratios of 1:1 or 2:1 are often achieved.[39,41] Instead of weighing all food items on a gram scale, patients use food labels to count their net intake of carbohydrate (total grams of carbohydrate consumed minus grams of fiber consumed).

Implementing the Ketogenic Diet

Following the KD may be overwhelming for patients undergoing cancer treatment. The RDN plays a vital role in equipping patients and families with ample tools, resources, and education to ensure success. To ensure successful hospitalizations, the RDN needs to create ketogenic hospital menus, as well as educate hospital staff (physicians, pharmacists, ancillary providers, nurses, and kitchen staff) about the KD. See Box 16.3 for a list of additional dietitian roles and responsibilities during implementation and monitoring of the KD.

Additional training is beneficial for RDNs to help them manage the KD and create a successful KD program. Several resources, including training seminars, are presented in Box 16.4 on page 338.

When creating an oncology ketogenic program, consider forming institution-wide guidelines that can be referenced by all inpatient and outpatient staff, such as the following[37-39]:

1. Evaluate for potential contraindications (see Box 16.2 on page 335).

2. Create initiation and weaning protocols.

3. Build order sets in the electronic medical record for initiation and readmissions.

4. Create educational materials and hospital menus for patients.

5. Monitor laboratory values (see Box 16.2).

6. Manage side effects (see Box 16.5 on pages 338 to 339).

7. Create sick-day guidelines.

8. Collaborate with the pharmacy to avoid dextrose in intravenous fluids and medications.

Box 16.3
Responsibilities for Implementation and Monitoring of the Ketogenic Diet

Classic ketogenic diet	Modified Atkins diet
Assess patient and caregiver abilities to adhere to guidelines associated with a regimented diet.	Assess patient and caregiver abilities to adhere to guidelines associated with a regimented diet.
Determine the appropriate energy and macronutrient goals.	Determine the appropriate energy and macronutrient goals.
Create recipes using the KetoDietCalculator provided by the Charlie Foundation for Ketogenic Therapies (https://ketodietcalculator.org).	Provide online, print, and smartphone application resources for recipes. Examples include the ruled.me website (www.ruled.me), *The Modified Keto Cookbook* by Dawn Marie Martenz with Beth Zupec-Kania (Springer, 2015), and the Cronometer mobile app (https://cronometer.com).
Educate the patient and caregivers during inpatient admission about the use of the gram scale, label reading, and sick-day guidelines for acute illnesses, which could include managing vomiting due to chemotherapy or radiation, and at-home monitoring.	Educate the patient and caregivers on an outpatient basis about how to read food labels, determine net carbohydrate intake, analyze recipes, and do at-home monitoring.
Communicate frequently and adjust recipes to maintain the patient's weight and ketosis.	Communicate frequently and analyze the patient's intake to provide diet recommendations, which could include decreasing carbohydrate or protein (or both) or increasing fat to maintain weight and ketosis.
Order routine laboratory monitoring.[a]	Order routine laboratory monitoring.[a]

[a] See Box 16.1.

A long-term monitoring plan is an essential part of an oncology KD program (see Box 16.2), and the RDN and multidisciplinary medical team must continuously evaluate the patient for potential side effects (as outlined in Box 16.5). A lack of provider and staff acceptance and understanding of the KD can be a potential barrier; therefore, ongoing staff education is crucial after implementing an oncology KD program.

Survivorship
Caregiver Support

The burden of PBT includes poor long-term survival, cognitive impairment, seizures, paralysis, permanent neurological damage, and personality changes, any of which can present considerable strain both on patients and their caregivers.[42] Because the focus is usually on the patient, the emotional burden of caregiving often goes unnoticed and unsupported. Box 16.6 on page 341 provides practical suggestions for caregivers to help them lessen the strain.[43]

Many side effects from brain surgery, chemotherapy, and radiation are similar to those experienced by patients with traumatic head injury. Using suggestions and ideas developed from this patient population can help patients, families, and caregivers. The neurocognitive effects of PBT, especially when tumors are frontal in location, can have a significant impact on all cognitive function. Clinicians should always take this into account

Box 16.4
Ketogenic Diet: Resources for Professionals

Resource	Description
The Charlie Foundation for Ketogenic Therapies https://charliefoundation.org	Website
Ketogenic Training Seminar sponsored by the Charlie Foundation for Ketogenic Therapies https://charliefoundation.org/request-training https://charliefoundation.org/resources Email: ketogenicseminars@wi.rr.com	On-site training and materials
Cambrooke Keto Resource: Professional Training in Ketogenic Therapy https://www.ketovie.com/clinical-resources/training Email: info@ketovie.com	On-site or virtual training

Box 16.5
Managing Potential Side Effects of the Ketogenic Diet[37-40]

Potential side effect	Prevention and treatment measures
Inadequate oral intake	Make recipe modifications and suggestions.
Constipation	Incorporate vegetables. Add a medium-chain triglyceride supplement to the diet. Ensure adequate fluid intake. Consider medications, such as laxatives.
Nausea and vomiting	Maximize the antiemetic regimen if symptoms are associated with treatment. Consider a decrease in the diet ratio. Monitor and treat excessive ketosis, metabolic acidosis, and hypoglycemia.
Weight loss	Increase energy intake as needed. Increase protein as needed. Decrease the diet ratio if needed.

(continued)

Box 16.5
Managing Potential Side Effects of the Ketogenic Diet[37-40] *(continued)*

Potential side effect	Prevention and treatment measures
Acidosis	Ensure adequate hydration.
	Evaluate for excessive ketosis.
	Ensure adequate phosphorus.
	Initiate a bicarbonate or citrate supplement.
Hyperlipidemia	Educate the patient about healthy fat sources.
	Reduce the diet ratio.
	Consider carnitine therapy.
	Supplement with long-chain omega-3 fatty acids, such as eicosapentaenoic or docosahexaenoic acid.
Carnitine deficiency	Monitor carnitine level closely.
	Supplement as needed.
Vitamin or mineral deficiency	Consider prophylactic use of a carbohydrate-free multivitamin with calcium (depending on the chemotherapy regimen).
Pancreatitis	Monitor lipid levels closely.
	Check amylase and lipase if concerned.
	Start carnitine if necessary.
	Reduce the diet ratio if needed.
Osteoporosis	Ensure adequate calcium, vitamin D, magnesium, and phosphorus.
	Prevent or correct acidosis.
	Encourage weight-bearing activity, as tolerated.
Kidney stones	Ensure adequate hydration.
	Prevent or correct acidosis.
	Supplement with oral citrates.
Decreased quality of life	Communicate openly, particularly with patients with refractory diseases.
	Ensure a caregiver commitment.
	Consider liberalization or discontinuation of the diet due to caregiver burden.

when creating interventions and relaying them to patients and caregivers. Some of the more challenging neurocognitive changes include memory loss, impaired reasoning and processing, attention deficits, and problems with the ability to sequence or perform multiple tasks at one time. Tools such as menus and food diaries should be considered to help the patient with meal planning and self-monitoring. Role changes might occur within the family dynamic that can require caregivers to assume new responsibilities for which they are untrained or unprepared.

In addition to the nutrition impact symptoms already discussed, patients also can experience depression and fatigue, which can have an adverse effect on appetite and intake. Unusual eating behaviors can develop, leading to undereating or overeating or to repetitive desires to eat the same foods every day in the same or large amounts.[42,43] Box 16.7 provides some strategies for addressing common meal and nutrition issues experienced by patients with PBT.

General Mealtime Strategies

RDNs are in a unique position to provide meal planning and guidance to caregivers. In addition to the suggestions in Box 16.7, RDNs should make food-choice suggestions that address the texture, consistency, and taste of foods. They can also recommend shopping, cooking, and community resources for food provisions. Remind caregivers that there are many aspects to supporting a loved one undergoing medical treatment of the brain. Time spent preparing and sharing meals in the kitchen can improve social connections and relationships, dexterity, confidence, and understanding for patients. The use of all five senses helps activate different parts of the brain. Smelling fresh herbs, tasting sauces, touching dried beans or grains, and choosing a variety of colors and textures at the market also helps stimulate the brain. Muscles tend to remember things the mind has forgotten. For

example, a patient might not remember how to bake his or her famous cookies, but when presented with a lump of dough, one might be surprised at how quickly that person begins rolling out the dough. Recommend the purchase of bagged salads that are easy to open and put in a serving dish so that there is no need to use sharp knives while cutting up vegetables. To better differentiate serving spaces, it can be helpful to use different colors on the kitchen table (eg, white plates against a red tablecloth or other tactics to help patients remember what they are supposed to do).

There are other strategies caregivers can use to help patients experiencing memory loss and decreased cognitive function, which affect overall quality of life. Use wordplay, such as rhyming, to help the patient remember words and objects. Encourage plenty of rest and quiet; overstimulation can be tiring. Dedicate one drawer in a central location (kitchen) for keys, phones, and other important items so that the patient has only one place to remember to look. Have one brightly colored book to record appointments. Keep a list of important phone numbers on the refrigerator door in bold lettering. Recognize that cognitive function may be better at certain times of day, usually earlier in the day. Schedule important conversations or decision-making for that time. Purchase appliances that turn off automatically. Use timers or alarms as reminders of important tasks. Limit access to sharp knives or utensils that require fine motor skills and that might harm the patient. Put away kitchen chemicals that might not be recognized as hazardous.

Summary

PBTs, especially those of a high grade, can be difficult to manage and patients may face a poor prognosis. It is essential for the patient to maintain adequate nutrition during treatment. The RDN can function as a member of the care team to provide early intervention that can benefit the

Box 16.6
Recommendations for Caregivers of Patients With Primary Brain Tumor

Set realistic goals and take breaks during the day.

Have a "backup" person who can take over as caregiver if needed.

If people offer to bring food, ask for small portions in freezer containers; or ask for help with grocery shopping.

Serve the patient foods that are easy to eat with a spoon, such as finger foods, sandwiches, and soft foods that are easy to chew.

Keep a notebook to help schedule the patient's meal and snack times.

Keep a nutrition log to record the patient's food and fluid intake.

Keep a pill organizer box.

Box 16.7
Mealtime Strategies for Patients With Primary Brain Tumors

Challenges that affect nutrition for patients with primary brain tumor	Strategies
Inability to recognize appetite cues; forgetting meal times or when ate last meal	Schedule and plan meal times. Write a simple daily menu to help the patient remember what was served at the last meal.
Fatigue, too tired to prepare a meal; excessive sleeping limits time to eat meals	Use a clock, phone, or computer alarm to remind the patient of the need to eat. Suggest "meals on a tray" in a favorite chair and the use of drink containers with a lid and straw to reduce the risk of spills.
Decreased ability to distinguish between hot and cold foods and beverages	Use red mugs and cups for hot beverages and blue mugs and cups for cold beverages.
Loss of coordination and finer motor skills; difficulty holding eating utensils	Use a lipped bowl or plate with an edge. Use spoons for utensils. Serve finger foods that are easy to handle and coordinate. (The registered dietitian nutritionist should refer the patient to occupational therapy as needed.)
Decreased taste perception	Use fresh herbs and spices liberally. Use FASS (fat, acid, salty, sweet) techniques to enhance flavors and increase taste acuity. Keep foods moist.
Distractions at and during mealtime	Keep the eating table clear of clutter. Put a brightly colored place mat or special chair where you want the patient to sit.
Dehydration because of forgetting to drink or diminished thirst acuity	Maintain a cup with a lid and straw nearby. Use a variety of hot and cold beverages. Keep foods moist.
Inability to follow steps, making it difficult to complete meal-related tasks (eg, forgetting to take meals out of the refrigerator to eat; inability to gather meal components and then follow the steps to put them together)	Keep a short, simple checklist of daily reminders for activities and include mealtime reminders. Include check boxes for the patient to check when a task has been completed. (This list can also include appointment reminders and activities of daily living, such as dental care and personal hygiene.) Limit multistep instructions, or write out each step for the patient to follow. Guide the patient to attempt one step at a time and avoid distractions.

patient and caregiver, offering guidance and strategies to address the multiple physical and cognitive issues that may be present in the patient. The RDN can also evaluate the advisability of new and novel nutrition therapies; therefore, it is essential for the RDN to stay abreast of current literature.

Sample PES Statements
for Primary Brain Tumors

Intake domain: Inadequate oral intake related to chemotherapy-induced nausea, as evidenced by unintentional weight loss of 3% in 1 month.

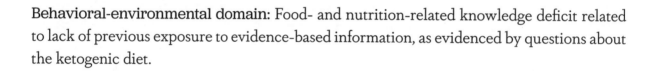

Behavioral-environmental domain: Food- and nutrition-related knowledge deficit related to lack of previous exposure to evidence-based information, as evidenced by questions about the ketogenic diet.

References

1. About brain and spinal cord tumors in adults. American Cancer Society website. Accessed October 29, 2020. www.cancer.org/cancer/brain-spinal-cord-tumors-adults/about.html

2. Brain Tumors—Health Professional Version. National Cancer Institute website. Accessed October 29, 2020. www.cancer.gov/types/brain/hp

3. Brain tumor types. American Brain Tumor Association website. Accessed October 29, 2020. www.abta.org/about-brain-tumors/brain-tumor-diagnosis/brain-tumor-types

4. Louis D, Perry A, Reifenberger G, et al. The 2016 World Health Organization classification of tumors of the central nervous system: a summary. *Acta Neuropathol*. 2016;131(6):803-820.

5. Chen H, Ward M, Tucker K, et al. Diet and risk of adult glioma in eastern Nebraska, United States. *Cancer Causes Control*. 2002;13(7):647-655.

6. Huncharek M, Kupelnick B, Wheeler L. Dietary cured meat and the risk of adult glioma: a meta-analysis of nine observational studies. *J Environ Pathol Toxicol Oncol*. 2003; 22(2):129-137.

7. Lian W, Wang R, Xing B, Yao Y. Fish intake and the risk of brain tumor: a meta-analysis with systematic review. *Nutr J*. 2017;16(1):1.

8. Michaud D, Gallo V, Schlehofer B, et al. Coffee and tea intake and risk of brain tumors in the European Prospective Investigation into Cancer and Nutrition (EPIC) cohort study. *Am J Clin Nutr*. 2010;92(5):1145-1150.

9. Benisi-Kohansal S, Shayanfar M, Mohammad-Shirazi M, et al. Adherence to the Dietary Approaches to Stop Hypertension-style diet in relation to glioma: a case-control study. *Br J Nutr*. 2016;115(6):1108-1116.

10. Shayanfar M, Vahid F, Faghfoori Z, Davoodi S, Goodarzi R. The association between Index of Nutritional Quality (INQ) and glioma and evaluation of nutrient intakes of these patients: a case-control study. *Nutr Cancer*. 2017;70:213-220.

11. Brain and other nervous system. American Cancer Society Cancer Statistics Center website. Accessed March 20, 2020. https://cancerstatisticscenter.cancer.org/#!/cancer-site/Brain%20and%20other%20nervous%20system

12. Cancer stat facts: brain and other nervous system cancer. National Cancer Institute Surveillance, Epidemiology, and End Results Program website. Accessed March 20, 2020. https://seer.cancer.gov/statfacts/html/brain.html

13. Page M, Fedoroff A. Central nervous system malignancies. In: Newton S, Hickey M, Marrs J, eds. *Mosby's Oncology Nursing Advisor: A Comprehensive Guide to Clinical Practice*. Mosby Elsevier; 2009:40-44.

14. Bitterlich C, Vordermark D. Analysis of health-related quality of life in patients with brain tumors prior and subsequent to radiotherapy. *Oncol Lett*. 2017;14(2):1841-1846.

15. McFaline-Figueroa J, Lee E. Brain tumors. *Am J of Med*. 2018;131(8):874-882. doi:10.1016/j.amjmed.2017.12.039

16. National Comprehensive Cancer Network. *NCCN Clinical Practice Guidelines in Oncology (NCCN Guidelines): Central Nervous System Cancers*. Version 3.2020. National Comprehensive Cancer Network; 2020. Accessed March 11, 2020. www.nccn.org/professionals/physician_gls/pdf/cns.pdf

17. Chemotherapy drugs and drugs often used during chemotherapy. Chemocare website. Accessed October 29, 2020. http://chemocare.com/chemotherapy/drug-info/default.aspx

18. Grant B, Byron J. Nutritional implications in chemotherapy. In: Elliott L, Molseed L, McCallum PD, eds., with Grant B, technical ed. *Medical Nutrition Therapy in Oncology*. 2nd ed. American Dietetic Association; 2006:72-87.

19. McCall M, Leone A, Cusimano M. Nutritional status and body composition of adult patients with brain tumours awaiting surgical resection. *Can J Diet Pract Res*. 2014;75(3):148-151. doi:10.3148/cjdpr-2014-007

20. He Z, Ke C, Al-Nahari F, et al. Low preoperative prognostic nutritional index predicts poor survival in patients with newly diagnosed high-grade gliomas. *J Neurooncol*. 2017;132:239-247. do:10.1007/s11060-016-2361-0

21. Zhou X, Dong H, Yang Y, et al. Significance of the prognostic nutritional index in patients with glioblastoma: a retrospective study. *Clin Neurol Neurosurg*. 2016;151:86-91. doi:10.1016/j.clineuro.2016.10.014

22. Thompson KL, Elliott L, Fuchs-Tarlovsky V, Levin RM, Voss AC, Piemonte T. Oncology evidence-based nutrition practice guideline for adults. *J Acad Nutr Diet*. 2017:117(2):297-310.

23. Hempen C, Weiss E, Hess C. Dexamethasone treatment in patients with brain metastases and primary brain tumors: do the benefits outweigh the side-effects? *Support Care Cancer*. 2002;10(4):322-328.

24. Oyer D, Shah A, Bettenhausen S. How to manage steroid diabetes in the patient with cancer. *J Support Oncol*. 2006;4(9):479-483.

25. Derr R, Ye X, Islas M, Desideri S, Saudek C, Grossman S. Association between hyperglycemia and survival in patients with newly diagnosed glioblastoma. *J Clin Oncol*. 2009;27(7):1082-1086.

26. Tieu M, Lovblom L, McNamara M, et al. Impact of glycemia on survival of glioblastoma patients treated with radiation and temozolomide. *J Neurooncol*. 2015;124(1):119-126.

27. Chaichana K, McGirt M, Woodworth G, et al. Persistent outpatient hyperglycemia is independently associated with survival, recurrence and malignant degeneration following surgery for hemispheric low grade gliomas. *Neurol Res*. 2010;32(4):442-448.

28. Reardon CH, Zienius K, Wood S, Grant R, Williams M. Ketogenic diet for primary brain and spinal cord tumours. *Cochrane Database Syst Rev*. 2017;(6):CD012690.

29. Warburg O. On the origin of cancer cells. *Science*. 1956;123(3191):309-314.

30. Lv M, Zhu A, Wang H, Wang F, Guan W. Roles of caloric restriction, ketogenic diet and intermittent fasting during initiation, progression and metastasis of cancer in animal models: a systematic review and meta-analysis. *PLoS ONE*. 2014;9(12):e115147.

31. Oliveira CLP, Mattingly S, Schirrmacher R, Sawyer MB, Fine EJ, Prado CM. A nutritional perspective of ketogenic diet in cancer: a narrative review. *J Acad Nutr Diet*. 2018;118(4):668-688.

32. Champ CE, Palmer JD, Volek JS, et al. Targeting metabolism with a ketogenic diet during the treatment of glioblastoma multiforme. *J Neurooncol*. 2014;117(1):125-131.

33. Tan-Shalaby JL, Carrick J, Edinger K, et al. Modified Atkins diet in advanced malignancies—final results of a safety and feasibility trial within the Veterans Affairs Pittsburgh Healthcare System. *Nutr Metab.* 2016;13:52.

34. Schmidt M, Pfetzer N, Schwab M, Strauss I, Kämmerer U. Effects of a ketogenic diet on the quality of life in 16 patients with advanced cancer: a pilot trial. *Nutr Metab (Lond).* 2011;8(1):54.

35. Fine EJ, Segal-Isaacson CJ, Feinman RD, et al. Targeting insulin inhibition as a metabolic therapy in advanced cancer: a pilot safety and feasibility dietary trial in 10 patients. *Nutrition.* 2010;28(10):1028-1035.

36. Breitkreutz R, Tesdal K, Jentschura D, Haas O, Leweling H, Hom E. Effects of a high-fat diet on body composition in cancer patients receiving chemotherapy: a randomized controlled study. *Wien Klin Wochenschr.* 2005;117(19–20):685-692.

37. Kossoff EH, Turner Z, Doerrer S, Cervenka MC, Henry BJ. *Ketogenic Diet and Modified Atkins Diet: Treatments for Epilepsy and Other Disorders.* 6th ed. Demos Medical Publishing; 2016.

38. Lee P, Kossoff E. Dietary treatments of epilepsy: management guidelines for the general practitioner. *Epilepsy Behav.* 2011;21(2):115-121.

39. Abdelwahab MG, Fenton KE, Preul MC, et al. The ketogenic diet is an effective adjuvant to radiation therapy for the treatment of malignant glioma. *PLoS One.* 2012;7(5):e36197.

40. Kossoff E, Zupec-Kannia B, Ballaban-Gill K, et al. Optimal clinical management of children receiving dietary therapies for epilepsy: updated recommendations of the International Ketogenic Diet Study Group. *Epilepsia Open.* 2018;3(2):175-192.

41. Charlie Foundation for Ketogenic Therapies. Accessed March 19, 2020. https://charliefoundation.org/diet-plans/

42. Ford E, Catt S, Chalmers A, Fallowfield L. Systematic review of supportive care needs in patients with primary malignant brain tumors. *Neuro Oncol.* 2012;14(4):392-404.

43. Schubart J, Kinzie M, Farace E. Caring for the brain tumor patient: family caregiver burden and unmet needs. *Neuro Oncol.* 2008;10(10):61-72.

Chapter 17
Medical Nutrition Therapy for Breast Cancer

Laura Brown, MS, RD, CSO, CNSC

Breast cancer is the most commonly diagnosed cancer in the United States. Approximately 12.9% of women will be diagnosed with breast cancer in their lifetime. The National Cancer Institute estimated that in 2020, there would be 276,480 new cases of breast cancer diagnosed in women. Five-year survival rates for women with breast cancer are relatively high, especially compared with those for other cancers.[1]

If the disease is diagnosed early, the 5-year survival rate for stage I breast cancer is 98.9%. Due to this high survival rate, an estimated 3,577,264 women in the United States were living with breast cancer in 2017.[1] Breast cancer in males is much less prevalent. Recent data suggest only 1 in 1,000 men will be diagnosed with breast cancer.[2] The American Cancer Society (ACS) identifies modifiable and nonmodifiable risk factors for breast cancer.[3] These risk factors are summarized in Box 17.1.

Breast cancer can occur in male and female breast tissue. There are several types of breast cancer, almost all of which are carcinomas that begin in ductal or lobular cells. Ductal carcinoma in situ (DCIS) is a condition in which abnormal cells replace normal epithelial cells in the ducts of the breast. DCIS is a noninvasive cancer, as it has not extended into the stroma; however, it can progress to invasive cancer. Cancer cells that have metastasized to surrounding breast tissues are called infiltrative, or invasive, breast cancer.[2] See Figure 17.1 on page 348 for illustrations of DCIS and invasive breast cancer.

Breast cancer prognosis is largely determined by staging, which evaluates the extent of the cancer. To complete staging for breast cancer, a mammogram, clinical breast exam, ultrasound, magnetic resonance imaging, lumpectomy, and biopsy may be required. Prognostic biomarkers include estrogen receptor (ER) and progesterone receptor (PR) expression, human epidermal growth factor receptor 2 (HER2) status, histological grading (including tubule formation and mitotic rate), and a multigene assay recurrence score best known by the assay's brand name, Oncotype DX (Genomic Health).

Box 17.1
Modifiable and Nonmodifiable Risk Factors for Breast Cancer[3]

Modifiable risk factors	Nonmodifiable risk factors
Alcohol consumption	Inherited genes (including *BRCA1* and *BRCA2*)
Overweight and obesity	Race and ethnicity (especially Ashkenazi Jewish)
Low levels of physical activity	Having dense breast tissues
Use of oral contraceptives for birth control	Having onset of menarche before age 12 years
Use of hormone replacement therapy	Reaching menopause after the age of 55 years
Childbearing and breastfeeding	Receiving radiation to the chest

Ductal Carcinoma in Situ (DCIS)

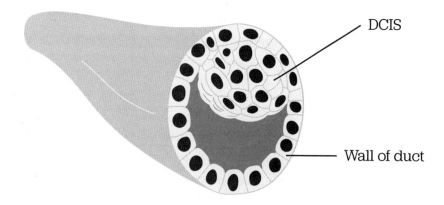

DCIS

Wall of duct

Invasive Breast Cancer

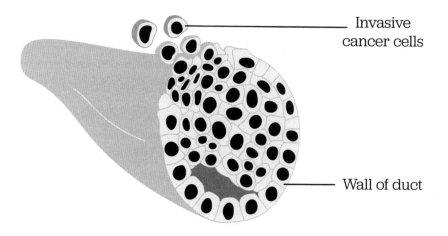

Invasive
cancer cells

Wall of duct

Figure 17.1
Types of breast cancer

Adapted from the National Cancer Institute. Breast cancer ductal carcinoma in situ. Visuals Online. https://visualsonline.cancer
.gov/details.cfm?imageid=4353

Adapted from the National Cancer Institute. Invasive breast cancer. Visuals Online. https://visualsonline.cancer.gov/details.cfm
?imageid=4352

Treatment

Treatment for breast cancer depends largely on staging criteria, biomarkers, histologic grade, patient preferences, and menopausal status. Refer to the *NCCN Clinical Practice Guidelines in Oncology (NCCN Guidelines): Breast Cancer* for details of specific therapies.[4] Treatments include surgery, systemic therapy, or radiation therapy individually or in combination.

Surgery

Surgery can include breast-conserving therapy or mastectomy or lymph node biopsy or dissection. Options may include[5]:

- **Sentinel lymph node biopsy:** This procedure removes and tests the first lymph node to which breast cancer would likely spread. If this sentinel lymph node tests positive for carcinoma involvement, additional lymph nodes may be removed.

- **Axillary lymph node dissection:** This procedure removes more axillary (armpit) lymph nodes than are removed in a sentinel lymph node biopsy.

- **Breast-conserving surgery:** In this type of surgery, also known as a partial mastectomy or lumpectomy, cancerous tissue and a surgical margin are removed.

- **Total mastectomy:** Total mastectomy is the surgical removal of the entire breast.

- **Modified radical mastectomy:** This is the removal of the entire breast, plus additional lymph nodes under the arm.

- **Radical mastectomy:** In a radical mastectomy, the entire breast, lymph nodes, and underlying chest muscles are removed.

- **Contralateral prophylactic mastectomy:** This is a bilateral mastectomy for women who choose to have an unaffected breast surgically removed.

- **Ovarian ablation:** This option involves permanent ovarian ablation through an oophorectomy (surgical removal of the ovaries).

Systemic Therapy

Depending on tumor characteristics, adjuvant systemic therapy may be used in addition to surgery. This may include, separately or in combination, chemotherapy, targeted therapy, or endocrine therapy. Refer to Box 17.2 on page 350 for therapeutic drug classes commonly used in breast cancer patients and to chapter 9 for details on these therapies. Endocrine therapy (also called hormone therapy) attempts to decrease estrogen levels or block the effects of estrogen on breast cancer cells. It usually is offered to patients with hormone receptor–positive cancer, such as ER-positive (ER+) breast cancer. HER2-targeted therapy is available for HER2-positive cancers. Refer to the NCCN guidelines for Breast Cancer for details of specific therapies.[5]

Nutrition Assessment

The general goals of nutrition care in patients with breast cancer are to:

- address any nutrition impact symptoms resulting from the disease and its treatment;

- support the patient's goals while providing evidence-based care;

- limit unintentional weight loss during treatment to less than 1 to 2 pounds per week; and

- encourage the patient to maintain and obtain a healthy body weight.

In a study comparing women with breast cancer and women without breast cancer, there was no difference in resting energy expenditure between the groups.[6] Compared to the Mifflin-St. Jeor and Harris-Benedict equations for predicting daily energy needs, the quick formula of 25 kcal/kg of

Box 17.2
Endocrine, Targeted, and Maintenance Therapy for Breast Cancer Patients[4,5]

Therapeutic drug class	Mechanism of action	Length of treatment
HER2-targeted agent	Targets *ERBB2* (formerly HER2/neu) receptors to prevent further cancer growth	1 year following surgery
Aromatase inhibitor	Blocks the enzyme that converts androgens to estrogen	5 years in postmenopausal women
Osteoclast inhibitor	Prevents bone fractures, bone pain, and skeletal-related events	May continue for 3 to 10 years
Selective estrogen receptor modulator	Blocks estrogen in breast tissue	5 to 10 years

body weight was most accurate for predicting the energy needs of women with breast cancer.[3] Daily protein intakes of 1.2 to 1.5 g/kg of body weight may help prevent loss of muscle mass.[7] More information on nutrition assessment can be found in Chapter 5.

Nutrition Problems and Interventions

Fatigue

Fatigue is the most frequently reported side effect of breast cancer treatment, affecting an estimated 60% to 96% of patients.[8] Cancer-related fatigue has been associated with a body mass index (BMI) higher than 25, premenopausal status, and endocrine therapy.[9]

Regular exercise and healthy eating habits may help combat cancer-related fatigue. In a randomized, placebo-controlled, double-blind, crossover trial of multivitamin use in breast cancer patients receiving radiotherapy, multivitamin use was associated with higher rates of fatigue compared to placebo.[9] One study reported reduced rates and intensity of fatigue in those achieving 13.7 metabolic-equivalent hours of exercise per week.[8] A study of 633 patients with breast cancer concluded that those consuming higher amounts of omega-6 fatty acid than omega-3 fatty acid reported higher rates of fatigue. However, omega-3 fatty acid supplementation as an intervention to decrease fatigue in breast cancer patients has not been evaluated.[10] Soy intake has been associated with decreased fatigue in breast cancer patients consuming more than 24 g/d versus those consuming 0 g/d in a cross-sectional study of 365 patients with breast cancer.[11]

Lymphedema

Researches estimate that 20% to 42% of women with breast cancer have breast cancer–related lymphedema (BCRL). Upper-extremity lymphedema can affect full function of the arms and quality of life. Factors that increase the risk for BCRL include:

- lymph node dissection;
- adjuvant radiation to regional lymph nodes;
- BMI greater than 26[12];
- some cardiovascular conditions; and
- age.[13]

Primary BCRL treatment recommendations include the following:

- compression bandaging[14]
- manual lymphatic drainage
- exercise[15]

There is limited evidence to support specific nutrition recommendations for BCRL. One study with a 12-week weight-loss intervention reported decreased lymphedema-related arm volume in the group with a mean weight loss of 3.3 kg.[13] In a study of a similar 24-week intervention, decrease in excess arm volume was significantly correlated with weight loss (mean loss of 4 kg) in overweight participants.[16] Until more data are available, it is reasonable to assume that weight loss may help reduce BCRL.

Vasomotor Symptoms

Vasomotor symptoms (including hot flashes, intense sweating, and flushing) occur in two-thirds of postmenopausal women with breast cancer.[17] Isoflavones, a type of phytoestrogen that may exert an estrogenic or antiestrogenic effect by binding to estrogen receptors, may help control menopausal symptoms.[18] In one study, increased consumption of soy, which is naturally high in isoflavones, resulted in a 25% to 55% improvement in menopausal symptoms, including decreased frequency or intensity of hot flashes and night sweats.[19] There is no association between soy supplements and frequency of hot flashes. Vitamin E supplementation (800 IU/d) decreased the frequency of hot flashes by one less episode per day in patients with breast cancer.[20]

Aromatase Inhibitor–Induced Musculoskeletal Symptoms

Musculoskeletal symptoms have been associated with the adjuvant use of aromatase inhibitors (AIs) (eg, anastrozole, letrozole, and exemestane) in 19%

to 50% of breast cancer patients.[21] Pain can occur in various areas, including hands, knees, hips, back, shoulders, and feet, with some women reporting "every bone in the body hurts."[22] This may limit treatment adherence and result in discontinuation of AI therapy.

A randomized, placebo-controlled trial of 60 women with early breast cancer showed that supplementing with 50,000 IU of vitamin D weekly for 15 weeks and then monthly for 2 months, resulted in improved AI-induced musculoskeletal symptoms (AIMSS).[22] Conversely, in another randomized trial, women with serum 25-hydroxyvitamin D levels below 40 ng/mL who were undergoing treatment with letrozole were given 30,000 IU of vitamin D3 per week and experienced no difference in AIMSS events.[21] In the Women's Health Initiative (WHI) randomized clinical trial, there was no difference in joint pain between those receiving 1,000 mg of calcium and 400 IU of vitamin D3 compared to those taking a placebo.[23] Multiple studies have evaluated the use of omega-3 fatty acids to ameliorate AIMSS without significant improvements in pain in the supplementation groups.[24,25]

Bone Loss

Bone loss and fracture risk have been associated with AI initiation due to estrogen deficiency and increased bone resorption, ovarian failure due to surgery, chemotherapy, or use of luteinizing hormone.[26]

Increasing physical activity, doing weight-bearing exercises, and taking calcium and vitamin D supplements have been recommended for both men and women for bone health. In a systematic review evaluating bone mineral density in women with breast cancer, 500 to 1,500 mg of supplemental calcium and 200 to 1,000 IU of supplemental vitamin D did not prevent loss of bone mineral density.[27] The NCCN guidelines recommend aiming for 1,200 mg of calcium per day for bone health.[5] For those unable to meet their calcium needs through diet, the guidelines suggest using calcium carbonate taken with meals or calcium citrate for those on proton pump inhibitors. In the setting of vitamin D depletion (levels of 20 to 30 ng/mL), consider administering 1,000 IU of vitamin D2 or D3 daily for 3 months.[28] Calcium should not be taken at the same time as oral bisphosphonates but 2 hours before or after for maximum absorption.[29]

Neuropathy

Peripheral neuropathy has been associated with taxane-based chemotherapy. This condition affects 15% to 23% of breast cancer patients receiving taxane treatment, and there are no US Food and Drug Administration–approved treatment options.[30] Chemotherapy-induced peripheral neuropathy (CIPN) can lead to impaired mobility and decreased quality of life, and recovery can last months to years.[31] Certain lifestyle factors, such as obesity, limited fruit and vegetable intake, and use of some supplemental antioxidants, have been associated with CIPN.[30]

A double-blind, randomized controlled trial assessed the efficacy of oral acetyl-L-carnitine in women receiving taxane-based chemotherapy. When compared with a placebo group, the group receiving acetyl-L-carnitine supplementation experienced more severe CIPN.[32] In the Pathways Study, incidence of CIPN was two to three times greater among women who initiated antioxidant supplementation during taxane-based chemotherapy.[30] In a small, randomized, double-blind, placebo-controlled trial, women randomly assigned to the intervention arm received 640 mg of omega-3 fatty acid three times daily throughout paclitaxel chemotherapy and for 1 month after completion of therapy. Those taking the omega-3 fatty acid supplements had a significantly decreased incidence of CIPN and a nonsignificant ($P = .054$) decrease in severity of CIPN.[33]

Chemotherapy-Induced Nausea and Vomiting

Approximately 37% of breast cancer patients experience nausea and 13% experience vomiting within 24 hours of receiving chemotherapy.[34] Five days after receiving chemotherapy, up to 70% of breast cancer patients experience nausea.[34] Previous chemotherapy-induced nausea and vomiting (CINV), anxiety, and a history of motion sickness are associated with increased risk for CINV.[35] Use of aprepitant, ondansetron, and dexamethasone before chemotherapy and ongoing use of ondansetron and aprepitant for 3 days after chemotherapy resulted in decreased use of rescue medication, improved quality of life, and fewer treatment delays in women receiving adjuvant doxorubicin and cyclophosphamide.[36] However, in one study, 42% of patients with breast cancer self-reported noncompliance with antiemetic therapy while receiving anthracycline-based chemotherapy (doxorubicin or epirubicin).[37] Acupressure and acupuncture can also be considered in addition to standard care for the treatment of CINV.[38-41]

Mucositis

In a study of patients being treated for breast cancer with cyclophosphamide, epirubicin, and fluorouracil, no difference was seen in rates of mucositis between those receiving glutamine, a conditionally essential amino acid involved in cell replication for rapid cell turnover, primarily in the gastrointestinal mucosa and immune system, and those taking a placebo.[42] However, in a randomized, placebo-controlled trial of patients receiving anthracylcine-based chemotherapy for breast cancer, a statistically significant decreased incidence of moderate to severe mucositis was seen in the group receiving glutamine. The therapeutic dose used in the study was 2.5 g of glutamine administered as a swish and swallow three times per day starting the first day of chemotherapy and continuing for 14 days.[43]

Taste Changes

Taste changes are a common side effect of chemotherapy and can result in inadequate nutrient intake, weight loss, and emotional distress. Breast cancer patients receiving taxane- or anthracylcine-based adjuvant chemotherapy have more difficulty identifying monosodium glutamate as savory, sodium chloride as salty, and citric acid as sour. These changes are more likely to occur 4 to 6 days after receiving chemotherapy and improve throughout the cycle. Most taste changes resolve within 3 months after completion of treatment.[44] Breast cancer patients also are more likely to report disliking sweet tastes and having an increased aversion to chocolate and coffee.[44]

Fasting During Treatment

Fasting before and after chemotherapy has been suggested as a means to decrease chemotherapy-associated side effects.[45-47] Short-term starvation for 24 hours before and after docetaxel, doxorubicin, and cyclophosphamide infusion was well tolerated in a small study of patients with HER2-negative stage II and III breast cancer.[45] Although fasting (consuming <200 calories in 24 hours) has been associated with fatigue and headaches, it was well tolerated for up to 72 hours (48 hours before and 24 hours after chemotherapy) in a study that included patients receiving docetaxel, carboplatin, and trastuzumab for breast cancer.[46] A case series included four patients who fasted from 48 to 140 hours before undergoing chemotherapy for breast cancer and from 5 to 40 hours after therapy; commonly reported side effects during fasting included fatigue, dry mouth, weakness, and short-term memory impairment.[47] Until more data are available, those with a recent 10% or greater weight loss or a BMI below 20.5 should be discouraged from fasting during treatment.[47]

Weight Gain During Treatment

The pathophysiology of weight gain is not well understood. Ovarian failure, fatigue, and decreased physical activity among those with breast cancer may contribute to weight gain.[48] Typical weight gain of 8 to 10 kg was reported in breast cancer patients in the 1990s, with an average weight gain of 6 kg at 2 years postdiagnosis.[48,49] However, the treatments used in the 1990s are no longer the standard of care.[50] In more recent studies, a typical weight gain of 1.95 to 4.5 kg has been reported.[48,51] About 60% of breast cancer patients report gaining weight within the first year after diagnosis, and weight gain appears to plateau 2 to 3 years after diagnosis. In the Pulling Through Study of weight and weight change following breast cancer, 24% of patients experienced an average weight gain of 3.8 kg.[51] However, 15% experienced clinically significant weight loss. Weight loss may be concerning, as women who are leaner at the time of diagnosis have an increased mortality if they lose 10% or more of their body weight.[52]

Weight gain might be related to fatigue from treatment, transition to menopause, and higher energy intake during treatment.[53] Women who are younger, closer to their ideal body weight, and who receive chemotherapy are at higher risk for weight gain during breast cancer treatment.[50] Conversely, women who are aged 55 years or older at the time of diagnosis or who have higher prediagnosis weight are less likely to gain weight during treatment.[53] Chemotherapy—specifically a cyclophosphamide, methotrexate, and fluorouracil (CMF) regimen or a doxorubicin and cyclophosphamide regimen—is associated with a 65% increased risk for weight gain when compared with no chemotherapy for breast cancer treatment. Weight gain with CMF averages between 2 and 4.4 kg.[54] Contrary to popular belief, tamoxifen use is not associated with significant weight gain, according to a study comparing weight gain in those taking tamoxifen and those not taking tamoxifen.[55] Gains of more than 6 kg after diagnosis have been associated with increased risk for cancer recurrence, mortality, and sarcopenic obesity (obesity accompanied by decreased muscle mass).[48,50,54,56] Obesity can also influence treatment-related outcomes, leading to longer postsurgery recovery times, increased infection rates, increased risk for lymphedema, increased rates of fatigue, more frequent reports of AIMSS, and increased risk for vasomotor symptoms.[48]

While weight loss during active treatment may be discouraged in certain cancers, the American Society of Clinical Oncology suggests that weight-loss programs are feasible for breast cancer patients during adjuvant treatment, as long as no contraindications exist, such as nonhealing wounds or advanced disease.[57] Supporting intentional weight loss of 1 to 2 pounds (0.45 kg to 0.91 kg) per week can be encouraged at any time after diagnosis with ongoing monitoring and approval by the patient's oncologist.[48] Many women may prefer to focus on weight loss after treatment; however, those who gain weight during treatment are statistically less likely to return to prediagnostic weight.[48,53]

Survivorship

Research indicates that people with breast cancer are particularly interested in lifestyle modification programs, with one study reporting that 79% of breast cancer patients were interested in health promotion programs.[58]

Lifestyle

Data suggest that following the American Cancer Society (ACS) guidelines for survivorship can reduce the risk of breast cancer recurrence. In the WHI observational study, the effect of following the ACS Nutrition and Physical Activity Cancer Prevention Guidelines on cancer risk and mortality was evaluated in postmenopausal women. Women who had the highest adherence to the ACS guidelines had a 22% decreased risk for breast

cancer diagnosis, and women in whom breast cancer was already diagnosed and adhered to the guidelines had a 33% decreased risk of dying from breast cancer.[59] A meta-analysis of 18 studies also reported decreased breast cancer risk in those who followed a healthy eating pattern.[60]

Low-Fat Diet

A high fat intake has been associated with breast cancer incidence.[61] The nutrition cohort of the Cancer Prevention Study II evaluated postmenopausal women prior to breast cancer diagnosis. Women with the highest intake of dietary energy had a statistically significant higher risk of developing breast cancer than those in the lowest quintile for dietary energy intake.[62] Similarly, in the European Prospective Investigation into Cancer and Nutrition (EPIC) study, high intake of saturated fat was weakly associated with a higher risk for breast cancer in postmenopausal women who did not use hormone therapy at baseline.[61]

Studies have evaluated the impact of a low-fat diet on breast cancer recurrence and survival.[61] The WHI dietary modification study of postmenopausal women found a reduced incidence of ER+, PR− breast cancer in those who lost 3% of their weight, decreased their fat intake, and increased their intake of fruits, vegetables, and grains. However, the result in the initial study did not reach statistical significance.[63] In a follow-up study, postmenopausal women who ate a high-fat diet (>37% of energy from fat) before diagnosis and who had ER+, PR− breast cancer had a modest decrease in risk of death after breast cancer diagnosis in the intervention group.[64] This is consistent with a study that evaluated potential dietary risk factors and mortality risk in postmenopausal women with breast cancer. Women consuming the highest percentage of energy from fat were nearly three times more likely to die than those with the lowest fat intake. The study also found that those who ate the most vegetables and fiber before diagnosis had a 40%

to 50% reduced risk of dying after breast cancer diagnosis.[65] Data from the Women's Intervention Nutrition Study showed that lifestyle intervention can be successful in reducing fat intake, which may also support subsequent weight loss. Fat intake was significantly less in the intervention group (23% of energy from fat versus 31.2% in the control group). In an analysis performed 5 years after intervention, the risk of relapse was 24% lower in the intervention group than in the control group. Reduction of dietary fat had the largest impact on relapse-free survival in ER-negative (ER-) breast cancer. It is important to note that the women enrolled were postmenopausal and the intervention group had a statistically significant greater weight loss than the control group (change in BMI of 1 in the intervention group).[66] In the Women's Healthy Eating and Living (WHEL) study, patients with early-stage breast cancer were encouraged to increase their fruit, vegetable, and fiber intakes while decreasing fat intake. The authors concluded that a high-fiber (29 g/d), low-fat (21% of energy from fat) diet is associated with decreased levels of estradiol in women with breast cancer.[67] However, they found no difference in breast cancer–related events or mortality when compared with a control group.[68] While breast cancer incidence did not differ between the two groups, the intervention group did not decrease fat intake to the study target of 15% to 20% of total energy intake and did not lose weight.

Considering the available data, a low-fat diet may be beneficial for postmenopausal women with ER+, PR– breast cancer who may benefit from weight loss and who followed a high-fat diet before diagnosis.

Fruits, Vegetables, and Fiber

In the EPIC study, increased fiber intake from vegetable sources was inversely associated with ER–, PR– breast cancer.[69] Those in the highest quintile for total vegetable intake in the Pooling Project had statistically decreased risk for ER– breast cancer compared with those in the lowest quintile for vegetable intake.[70] In the Black Women's Health Study, decreased risk for ER– and PR– breast cancer was associated with the consumption of at least one serving of vegetables per day, compared with fewer than four servings per week. Further analysis revealed that eating more than six servings of cruciferous vegetables weekly or more than three servings of carrots weekly may decrease breast cancer risk in Black women.[71] Women with the highest vegetable intake had significantly decreased rates of breast cancer recurrence in a secondary analysis of the WHEL study.[72] Furthermore, those receiving tamoxifen showed the highest association between vegetable intake and decreased risk of new primary breast cancer. In a prospective study of patients with early-stage breast cancer, consuming at least five servings of fruits and vegetables, and being active for at least 540 metabolic equivalent minutes per week (30 minutes of walking 6 days a week) resulted in a 6% to 7% decrease in 10-year mortality risk. The survival effect was most pronounced for ER+ tumors.[73] When comparing those in the highest quartile of total fruit intake to those in the lowest quartile, a decrease in breast cancer risk was inversely associated with total fruit intake, especially for ER+ breast cancer.[74] These study results conflict with the results of a meta-analysis of 15 prospective studies that found no association between vegetable intake and breast cancer risk.[75]

A meta-analysis published in 2012 showed that women who eat more than 25 g of fiber daily had a lower risk of breast cancer. The results correlated with a 5% lower breast cancer risk for each 10-g increase in fiber per day.[76] In the EPIC study, total fiber intake in the highest quintile versus the lowest quintile was inversely associated with breast cancer risk, especially for fiber consumption from vegetables and for ER– and PR– tumors.[77] Although fruits, vegetables, and fiber appear to provide a beneficial role in reducing breast cancer risk, no difference in rate of breast cancer diagnosis was found between vegetarians and nonvegetarians.[78]

Carotenoids

Carotenoids have been shown to inhibit mammary cell proliferation, induce apoptosis, and provide antioxidant activity.[79,80] In the WHEL study, women with early-stage breast cancer and high levels of plasma carotenoids had a 43% reduction in new breast cancer events when compared with women with lower levels of plasma carotenoids.[81] A pooled analysis of eight prospective studies concluded that breast cancer risk was significantly decreased for women who had higher levels of α carotene, β carotene, and other carotenoids. The strongest association was among those with a BMI of 25 or lower and ER– tumors.[82] In a nested case-control study of 1,502 women, being in the highest versus the lowest quartile of plasma total carotenoid concentration was associated with a 43% reduction in risk for a new breast cancer diagnosis.[81] Although these studies show an inverse association between plasma carotenoids and breast cancer risk, long-term exposure to a diet high in fruit and vegetables may be more responsible for positive outcomes than a short-term intervention aimed at increasing carotenoid intake. During a 7-year follow-up of the WHEL study, breast cancer–free survival in patients with early breast cancer was associated with a higher lifetime exposure to carotenoids.[83] This is further supported by a meta-analysis that found an association between serum carotenoids and decreased breast cancer risk but no association with total dietary carotenoid intake.[84]

Lignans

Flaxseeds are rich in α-linolenic acid (a polyunsaturated fatty acid) and lignans, which are phytoestrogens. Researchers estimated that up to 50% of breast cancer patients consume flaxseed.[85] In a case-control study of flaxseed and breast cancer risk, consuming ¼ cup of flaxseed at least monthly or one slice of flax bread (equivalent to 2.5 to 5 g of flaxseed) at least weekly was associated with a 20% to 30% decreased risk for breast cancer.[86] As little as ½ tsp of flaxseed per day may be associated with a decreased risk for breast cancer.[87] Flaxseed consumption may slow tumor growth, as evidenced by a randomized, double-blind, placebo-controlled trial in postmenopausal women. When women in this study consumed one muffin containing 25 g of ground flax (about 3½ Tbsp) every day for 1 month, expression of the Ki-67 and HER2 proteins in tumors was significantly decreased and apoptosis was increased when compared with the control group.[88]

Concern about flaxseeds interacting with tamoxifen has been evaluated in preclinical studies; no interaction was found, and a possible increased efficacy of tamoxifen in mice fed a diet higher in flaxseed was noted.[89] Although observational studies have reported significantly reduced rates of mortality in postmenopausal women who have high lignan exposure, not all studies have shown lignan intake to be associated with breast cancer risk.[85,90]

Soy

Soy contains isoflavones (primarily daidzein, genistein, and glycitein) that are structurally similar to endogenous estrogens, such as 17β-estradiol. In addition to having antioxidant and anti-inflammatory properties, soy isoflavones compete for binding to estrogen receptors.[91] Data from preclinical and epidemiological studies of soy and breast cancer risk offer conflicting information. Concerns about genistein activating the estrogen receptors in breast cells and increasing proliferation of breast cancer cells have been evaluated.

Multiple cohort studies and case-control studies have suggested that consuming soy in amounts found in a typical Asian diet can be considered safe and possibly beneficial for those at risk for breast cancer and those with breast cancer. Additional studies have found that soy consumption might decrease breast cancer risk for women in Asian countries.[92] In the Shanghai Women's Health Study, high intake of soy foods during adolescence was associated with a decreased risk for premenopausal breast cancer in Chinese women.[93] In a large 2012 meta-analysis, an inverse association between high isoflavone intake and decreased breast cancer recurrence was noted.[94] In this study, breast cancer recurrence was 36% lower, and breast cancer–specific mortality was decreased by 29%, in women consuming 10 mg or more of isoflavones per day when compared with those consuming less than 4 mg per day.[95] Soy intake also has been inversely associated with recurrence of ER– breast cancer.[93] See Table 17.1 for a list of soy foods and their isoflavone content.

Preclinical studies have raised concerns about soy competing with tamoxifen.[96,97] However, postmenopausal tamoxifen users with increased intakes of glycetin had significantly decreased risk for breast cancer recurrence.[91] Increased intakes of isoflavones were associated with a decreased risk for recurrence in ER+ or PR+ breast cancers. In a meta-analysis, women taking tamoxifen who had higher intakes of soy isoflavones had a 37% decrease risk for breast cancer recurrence.[94]

Dairy

A meta-analysis of 11 prospective studies showed an inverse relationship between dietary calcium intake and breast cancer risk. For premenopausal women, an 8% decrease in breast cancer risk was associated with each increase of 300 mg/d in calcium intake.[98] A meta-analysis of 18 prospective studies found that total dairy intake may be associated with a decrease in breast cancer risk. The association was strongest for postmenopausal women consuming low-fat dairy.[99] In the Life After Cancer Epidemiology cohort, those with early-stage breast cancer who ate more than one serving of high-fat dairy per day had an increased risk for breast cancer mortality and all-cause mortality. This

Table 17.1
Isoflavone Content of Soy Foods[95]

Food	Serving size	Total isoflavones (mg)
Miso	½ c	57.0
Tempeh	3 oz	51.5
Dry roasted soybeans	1 oz	41.6
Soy milk, low-fat	1 c	6.2
Tofu yogurt	½ c	21.3
Tofu, soft	3 oz	19.2
Edamame	½ c	16.1
Meatless soy burger	1 patty	4.5
Soy cheese, cheddar	1 oz	1.9

association was not seen for those who ate low-fat dairy foods.[100] Until more research is available, breast cancer patients who enjoy consuming dairy should be encouraged to choose lower-fat dairy.

Red Meat

Mechanisms by which red-meat intake can increase cancer risk include bioavailable iron content, presence of carcinogens produced during cooking, and higher fat content. In addition, increased cholesterol intake (>370 mg/d) has been associated with increased risk for breast cancer.[101] Epidemiology reports and case-control studies have found conflicting results on the association between meat and breast cancer risk.[54] However, recent studies have identified a positive association with red-meat intake. In the Nurses' Health Study II, consuming more than three servings of red meat per week was associated with increased risk for ER+, PR+ breast cancer.[102] These results are consistent with the UK Women's Cohort Study, in which postmenopausal breast cancer was strongly associated with processed and red meat intake, while premenopausal breast cancer was associated with total meat intake. For each 50-g increment of red-meat intake, breast cancer risk increased by 12%.[103]

Omega-3 Fatty Acids

The three main omega-3 fatty acids are α-linolenic acid, which is found mainly in plants, and docosahexaenoic acid (DHA) and eicosapentaenoic acid (EPA), which are found mainly in fish and seafood. Intake of omega-3 fatty acids and its relation to breast cancer prevention and survivorship is increasingly being studied. Some studies have suggested that while omega-6 fatty acids may have a stimulatory effect on breast cancer cells, omega-3 fatty acids may inhibit the growth of these cells.[104] A 2013 meta-analysis of 16 cohort studies reported that higher intakes of omega-3 polyunsaturated fatty acids from marine sources was associated

with a 14% decrease in risk for breast cancer.[105] In a population-based, 15-year follow-up study of more than 1,400 women with newly diagnosed breast cancer, all-cause mortality decreased by 16% to 34% for those reporting the highest intakes of fish and omega-3 fatty acids.[106] Table 17.2 lists the DHA and EPA content for a variety of fish and seafood.

Weight and Breast Cancer Risk

Weight at the time of breast cancer diagnosis has been associated with increased risk for recurrence and decreased survival in premenopausal and postmenopausal women.[108] Excess weight may increase blood concentrations of estradiol, insulin, and insulin-like growth factor 1, leading to increased risk for breast cancer recurrence. In addition, hyperinsulinemia and hyperglycemia associated with obesity may be related to increased breast cancer risk, as people who have type 2 diabetes mellitus have a 13% to 27% increased risk for breast cancer.[109,110]

Weight gain in middle adulthood may increase the risk of breast cancer diagnosis before age 50 years.[111] Women with a BMI of 35 or higher have a 58% increased risk of postmenopausal breast cancer—especially ER+, PR+ cancer—compared to normal-weight women (BMI <25).[112] In the Nurses' Health Study, postmenopausal women aged 30 to 55 years who gained more than 25 kg since they were 18 years old had a statistically significant higher risk for breast cancer than those who maintained their weight. The authors concluded that 15% of breast cancer incidence in the postmenopausal study population was associated with a 2-kg weight gain in adulthood.[113]

Research has suggested that obesity negatively affects survival in women with early-stage breast cancer.[108] A 2010 meta-analysis of 43 studies concluded that women with obesity in whom breast cancer is newly diagnosed have a 33% higher risk of death when compared to nonobese patients with breast cancer.[114] A 2014 meta-analysis of 82 studies

Table 17.2
Docosahexaenoic Acid and Eicosapentaenoic Acid Content of Seafoods[107]

Type of seafood	Docosahexaenoic acid (g per 3-oz serving)	Eicosapentaenoic acid (g per 3-oz serving)
Salmon, Atlantic, farmed, cooked	1.24	0.59
Salmon, Atlantic, wild, cooked	1.22	0.35
Herring, Atlantic, cooked	0.94	0.77
Sardines, canned in tomato sauce, drained	0.74	0.45
Mackerel, Atlantic, cooked	0.59	0.43
Salmon, pink, canned, drained	0.63	0.28
Trout, rainbow, wild, cooked	0.44	0.40
Oysters, eastern, wild, cooked	0.23	0.30
Sea bass, cooked	0.47	0.18
Shrimp, cooked	0.12	0.12
Lobster, cooked	0.07	0.10
Tuna, light, canned in water, drained	0.17	0.02
Tilapia, cooked	0.11	0.09
Scallops, cooked	0.09	0.06
Cod, Pacific, cooked	0.10	0.04
Tuna, yellowfin, cooked	0.09	0.01

reported that a BMI greater than 30 at any point before diagnosis, within a year of diagnosis, or more than a year after diagnosis was associated with a 21% to 41% higher total mortality and a 25% to 68% higher breast cancer mortality compared to a healthy BMI.[115] It is important to note that being underweight (BMI <20) has also been associated with an increased risk for breast cancer recurrence and mortality.[76]

Weight-Loss Interventions

For breast cancer patients, programs that include diet, physical activity, and behavioral support offer the highest likelihood of weight-loss success.[48] However, it is unclear what approach to diet and macronutrient distribution would best support weight loss. Postmenopausal women with breast cancer who were enrolled in the CHOICE study's weight-loss program lost 12.5% of their initial weight in 6 months, and there were no statistically significant differences between the low-fat-diet group and low-carbohydrate-diet group.[116] Encouraging a Mediterranean diet resulted in improved BMI after 2 months and reduced waist circumference after 6 months in 100 patients with breast cancer.[117] The Exercise and Nutrition to Enhance Recovery and Good Health for You (ENERGY) study encouraged a reduced-calorie diet with a focus on fruits, vegetables, and whole grains along with 60 minutes of intentional exercise per day and 2 to 3 days of strengthening exercises per week.[118] Initial weight loss in the intervention group reached 5.9% at 6 months and was maintained at 1 year. However, at the end of 24 months, total weight loss was only 3.7%.[119] A randomized pilot study found that breast cancer patients with obesity who received individualized counseling while on Weight Watchers (now WW) achieved a mean weight loss of 9.4 kg in 12 months, which was significantly more than the control group, which gained a mean of 0.85 kg in the same time frame.[120]

Physical activity has been associated with decreased risk for breast cancer diagnosis; all-cause and breast cancer–related death; and progression and recurrence of breast cancer.[121] In the Nurses' Health Study, increased hours of physical activity per week was inversely associated with breast cancer–related death. This relationship was strongest for those with hormonally responsive tumors.[122,123] Patients with breast cancer who complete 3 to 5 hours of brisk walking per week have a reduced risk for breast cancer–associated death. Physical activity during adjuvant chemotherapy has also been associated with improved disease-free survival.[124] Those who are physically active before diagnosis should be encouraged to continue activity, since those with decreasing physical activity after diagnosis have an increased risk for death.[125] Leisure and recreational activity have also been associated with a 30% decreased risk for mortality.

Behavioral approaches, in addition to diet, have resulted in weight loss; however, ongoing support after 1 year might be required to avoid regaining weight. Interfacing with patients through in-person, telephone, or electronic interactions also might help prevent weight gain. Use of self-tracking for food intake and activity, use of accountability partners, and weekly weigh-ins have contributed to weight-loss success.[126]

Fasting

A National Health and Nutrition Examination Survey study showed that longer nighttime fasting was associated with decreased blood glucose levels and a non–statistically significant decrease in glycated hemoglobin (HbA1c). Diabetes has been associated with increased risk for breast cancer diagnosis, and nighttime fasting may lower breast cancer risk.[127] In a cohort of the WHEL study, patients with breast cancer who fasted more than 13 hours at night had decreased rates of breast cancer recurrence, compared with those who fasted for less than 13 hours per night.[128]

See Box 17.3 for a summary of nutrition advice for patients with breast cancer.

Dietary Supplements

An estimated 67% to 87% of those with breast cancer use at least one vitamin or mineral supplement.[138] A systematic review found that, when compared with cancer-free controls, patients with breast cancer were 11% to 20% more likely to take dietary supplements, such as multivitamins, calcium, vitamin E, and vitamin B6.[138]

Antioxidant Supplements

Antioxidants are one of the more commonly used supplements. One study reported that 81% of women diagnosed with early-stage breast cancer used at least one antioxidant supplement.[130] A case-control study of postmenopausal women with early-stage breast cancer showed that women who

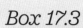

Box 17.3
Evidence for Food and Lifestyle Advice for Patients With Breast Cancer[52,56,59,64,67,73,76,85,91,94,98,101,105,128-137]

Component	Guideline
Healthy lifestyle	Follow American Cancer Society guidelines for a plant-based approach to eating.[59]
Low-fat diet	Limit fat to 15% to 20% of total energy intake, especially for postmenopausal women with estrogen receptor negative, progesterone receptor negative breast cancer; limit saturated fat; and limit cholesterol intake to <370 mg/d.[56,101]
Fruit intake	Aim for two to three servings per day.[73]
Vegetable intake	Aim for two to three servings per day; for cruciferous vegetables, aim for four to six servings per week.[129]
Carotenoid intake	Eat foods containing carotenoids three times per week; supplemental carotenoids are not recommended.[130]
Fiber intake	Aim for 30 g/d.[64,67]
Flaxseed intake	Aim for 1 to 3 Tbsp of ground flaxseed per day.[85]
Omega-3 fatty acid intake	Aim for one to two servings per week of fish high in docosahexaenoic acid (DHA) and eicosapentaenoic acid (EPA).[105,131]
Soy intake	Aim for one to two servings per day of whole soy foods (10 to 40 mg of soy isoflavones per day).[91,94,132]
Dairy intake	Aim for two to three servings per day; choose low-fat dairy products.[133]
Red-meat intake	Limit to three or fewer servings per week; limit consumption of grilled, barbecued, and smoked red meat.[134]
Green-tea intake	Limited data are available; suggested intake is more than 5 cups per day.[135]
Fasting	Aim to fast for 13 hours per night.[128]
Weight	Obtain and maintain a healthy body weight (body mass index of 18.5 to 25).[52,56]
Calcium intake	Aim for 1,200 mg/d through food; use supplements if necessary.[98]
Vitamin D intake	Consider supplements in cases of deficiency.[136]
Alcohol intake	Limit to three or four drinks per week, particularly in postmenopausal and overweight or obese women.[137]
Activity	Aim for the equivalent of walking for 30 minutes 6 days a week.[76]

reported using antioxidant supplements were less likely to have breast cancer recurrence or breast cancer–related death than those who did not report supplement use.[139] However, the results did not reach statistical significance. In a prospective study evaluating antioxidant use after breast cancer diagnosis, those who reported frequent intake of vitamin C and vitamin E had a decreased risk for breast cancer recurrence compared with those who did not report vitamin C and vitamin E supplementation.[130] A meta-analysis of vitamin C intake and supplement use in women with breast cancer suggested decreased mortality may be associated with vitamin C supplement use or with increasing vitamin C intake after diagnosis.[140] Similarly, in the After Breast Cancer Pooling Project (ABCPP), which included four large cohorts totaling more than 12,000 breast cancer patients, decreased recurrence of breast cancer was associated with use of vitamin E supplements, and decreased risk for death was associated with vitamin C use.[141] On the other hand, a two-thirds increased risk for death from breast cancer was identified in those using combination carotenoids after breast cancer diagnosis.[130]

Coenzyme Q10 (CoQ10) is a potent antioxidant. Studies have shown that women with breast cancer have low plasma levels of CoQ10. CoQ10 administration has been evaluated as a potential intervention to reduce and prevent anthracycline-induced cardiotoxicity.[142] A small study found that breast cancer patients who took CoQ10 supplements while undergoing chemotherapy with the anthracycline doxorubicin experienced fewer episodes of arrhythmias and decreased severity of echocardiogram changes.[143] Doses of 50 to 100 mg of CoQ10 were administered twice a day for 3 to 7 days before the first dose of doxorubicin and continued throughout the chemotherapy regimen.[142] The antineoplastic efficacy of doxorubicin in breast cancer cells does not appear to be affected by CoQ10 supplementation.[144]

Overall, there is limited evidence to support or to refute routine supplementation with antioxidants during treatment for breast cancer. Greenlee and colleagues[20] present a comprehensive review of antioxidant use during breast cancer treatment and urge caution when recommending antioxidants during treatment because most studies to date lack statistical power and are of insufficient duration to determine impact on recurrence and survival.

Multivitamin and Mineral Supplements
A study of the WHI cohorts found that using multivitamins over 8 years had no influence on invasive breast cancer in postmenopausal women when compared to nonusers.[145] A follow-up study found that breast cancer mortality was 30% lower in those using multivitamin and mineral (MVM) supplements than in nonusers.[146] The authors stated that no data on MVM use during treatment were obtained, and, therefore, they could not draw conclusions about the impact of MVM use during chemotherapy or radiotherapy for breast cancer. A small, randomized, placebo-controlled trial found that multivitamin supplementation during radiation resulted in increased fatigue in those taking the supplements when compared with those taking the placebo.[9]

Vitamin D Supplements
Numerous studies have evaluated the risk of breast cancer diagnosis in relation to serum 25-hydroxyvitamin D and vitamin D supplementation. An inverse association between vitamin D levels and breast cancer risk was identified in a 2010 meta-analysis. The authors concluded that a 45% decreased risk for breast cancer was seen in those in the highest quantile for serum 25-hydroxyvitamin D levels versus those in the lowest quantile. In addition, premenopausal and perimenopausal women consuming higher amounts of vitamin D had a 17% decreased risk of breast cancer.[147] A dose-response meta-analysis including only prospective studies found an inverse association between

breast cancer risk in postmenopausal women and 25-hydroxyvitamin D levels of 25 to 35 ng/mL.[141] However, not all studies show an inverse association between serum vitamin D levels or vitamin D intake and breast cancer risk. In the EPIC study, serum 25-hydroxyvitamin D levels prior to breast cancer diagnosis were not related to breast cancer risk.[148] In a large, prospective, nested case-control study, no association between plasma 25-hydroxyvitamin D levels and breast cancer risk in predominantly premenopausal women was identified.[149]

One study reported that 74% of breast cancer patients are deficient in 25-hydroxyvitamin D during adjuvant therapy.[150] Insufficient or deficient vitamin D levels during neoadjuvant chemotherapy for women with HER2-negative breast cancer enrolled in the I-SPY trial did not influence pathological tumor response to treatment or 3-year relapse-free survival.[151] Lohmann and colleagues[136] concluded that 25-hydroxyvitamin D levels did not correlate with relapse-free survival, overall survival, or breast cancer–specific survival in those receiving adjuvant chemotherapy. However, in a retrospective study of HER2-positive breast cancer patients receiving neoadjuvant trastuzumab-based chemotherapy, disease-free survival was significantly improved in those receiving a vitamin D supplement throughout their neoadjuvant treatment. Most of the patients in this study were postmenopausal, living in the southern part of the United States, and taking less than 10,000 IU of vitamin D per week.[152]

Vitamin D intake and serum 25-hydroxyvitamin D levels have been evaluated in relationship to risk of breast cancer recurrence. A 2017 meta-analysis found that circulating 25-hydroxyvitamin D levels in women with a breast cancer diagnosis had a significant dose-response linear relationship with overall survival. For each 4 ng/mL increment above 9.3 ng/mL, overall mortality rate decreased by 6%.[153] No relationship between serum 25-hydroxyvitamin D and breast cancer recurrence was seen in the WHEL study.[154] In a meta-analysis of 30 prospective studies, higher serum 25-hydroxyvitamin D was associated with improved breast cancer survival.[155] In the ABCPP study, vitamin D use was associated with a 46% decreased risk of recurrence, but only for those with ER+ breast cancer.[141]

Omega-3 Fatty Acid Supplements

In the Vitamins and Lifestyle Cohort study, postmenopausal women who were using fish oil supplements had a statistically significant lower risk for breast cancer compared to those not taking a fish oil supplement. However, the authors noted a twofold increase in the risk for breast cancer among those who were previously diagnosed with coronary artery disease and using fish oil supplements compared to those who did not use a fish oil supplement. Therefore, they concluded that until more data on timing, dosage, and mechanisms of action become available, fish oil supplements should not be routinely recommended in an effort to reduce breast cancer risk.[156] Intake of marine EPA and DHA from food (ie, fish and seafood) and from supplements was assessed in early-stage breast cancer patients. When compared to those with the lowest intakes of EPA and DHA from food (lowest tertile), those with the highest intakes had a 25% decreased risk of recurrence. There was no significant association between consuming fish oil supplements and breast cancer outcomes.[131]

Some research suggests that mammary tumors may be sensitized to chemotherapy in the presence of DHA intake. Bougnoux and colleagues[157] provided a limited number of patients with metastatic breast cancer receiving anthracycline-based chemotherapy (cyclophosphamide, fluorouracil, and epirubicin administered every 3 weeks) with 1.8 g of DHA daily throughout 5 months of chemotherapy. When comparing patients with the highest level of plasma DHA to those with the lowest level of plasma DHA, the high-DHA group had a longer time to progression (8.7 months) than the low-DHA group (3.5 months). Overall survival in the high-DHA group was also significantly greater, to a survival time of 34 months, compared with an overall survival of 18 months in the low-DHA group. The study also suggests that chemotherapy was better tolerated in the group with high DHA levels, as anemia and thrombocytopenia were less frequent.

Although omega-3 fatty acid supplementation is generally well tolerated, diarrhea, heartburn, indigestion, nausea, and abdominal bloating may occur. Fish oil supplementation might also affect bleeding risk (especially in doses >3 g/d) and may need to be discontinued for 1 to 2 weeks before surgery. In addition, hemorrhagic strokes have been associated with very high daily intake of omega-3 fatty acids (>10 g/d).[104]

Summary

Despite a large body of preclinical, population-based, observational, and interventional studies evaluating the impact of nutrition on breast cancer, results often are conflicting and lead to confusion for providers and for patients. Future research should emphasize the use of nutrition to ameliorate treatment-related side effects, targeted recommendations for patients based on menopausal status and tumor characteristics, and best practices for successfully implementing lifestyle changes.

Sample PES Statements for Breast Cancer

Intake domain: Excessive oral intake related to hormonal manipulation from breast cancer therapy, as evidenced by dietary intake >130% of estimated needs, per diet recall, and unintentional weight gain of 5% in 1 month.

Behavioral-environmental domain: Food- and nutrition-related knowledge deficit related to non–evidence-based information, as evidenced by reports of following a low-carbohydrate diet (approximately 30 g of carbohydrates per day), per diet recall.

References

1. *SEER Cancer Stat Facts: Female Breast Cancer*. National Cancer Institute. Accessed March 28, 2020. https://seer.cancer.gov /statfacts/html/breast.html

2. American Cancer Society. *Breast Cancer Facts & Figures 2019-2020*. American Cancer Society, Inc; 2019.

3. American Cancer Society Breast Cancer Early Detection and Diagnosis website. Accessed January 21, 2019. www.cancer .org/cancer/breast-cancer /screening-tests-and-early -detection.html

4. Taghian A, El-Ghamry M, Merajver S. Overview of the treatment of newly diagnosed, non-metastatic breast cancer. In: DF Hays & SR Vora (Eds), *UptoDate*. UpToDate; 2019. Accessed January 28, 2019. www.uptodate.com/contents /overview-of-the-treatment-of -newly-diagnosed-invasive -non-metastatic-breast-cancer

5. Zuconi C, Ceolin Alves A, Toulson Davisson Correia M. Energy expenditure in women with breast cancer. *Nutrition*. 2015;31:556-559.

6. National Comprehensive Cancer Network. *NCCN Clinical Practice Guidelines in Oncology (NCCN Guidelines): Breast Cancer*. Version 2.2017. National Comprehensive Cancer Network; 2017. Accessed April 10, 2019. www.nccn.org/professionals /physician_gls/pdf/breast.pdf

7. Limon-Miro A, Lopez-Teros V, Astiazaran-Garcia A. Dietary guidelines for breast cancer patients: a critical review. *Adv Nutr*. 2017;8(4):613-623.

8. Huang X, Zhang Q, Kang K, Song Y, Zhao W. Factors associated with cancer-related fatigue in breast cancer patients undergoing endocrine therapy in an urban setting: a cross-sectional study. *BMC Cancer*. 2010;10:453. doi:10.1186/1471 -2407-10-453

9. de Souza Fede A, Bensi C, Trufelli D, et al. Multivitamins do not improve radiation therapy-related fatigue: results of a double-blind randomized crossover trial. *Am J Clin Oncol*. 2007;30(4):432-436.

10. Alfano C, Imayama I, Neuhouser M, et al. Fatigue, inflammation, and omega-3 and omega-6 fatty acid intake among breast cancer survivors. *J Clin Oncol*. 2012;30(12):1280-1287. doi:10 .1200/JCO.2011.36.4109

11. Nomura S, Hwang Y, Gomez S, et al. Dietary intake of soy and cruciferous vegetables and treatment-related symptoms in Chinese-American and non-Hispanic White breast cancer survivors. *Breast Cancer Res Treat*. 2018;168(2):467-479. doi:10 .1007/s10549-017-4578-9

12. Clark B, Sitzia J, Harlow W. Incidence and risk of arm oedema following treatment for breast cancer: a three-year follow-up study. *QJ:M*. 2005;98(5):343-348.

13. Shaw C, Mortimer P, Judd P. A randomized controlled trial of weight reduction as a treatment for breast cancer -related lymphedema. *Cancer*. 2007;110:1868-1874.

14. Kligman L, Wong R, Johnston M, Laetsch N. The treatment of lymphedema related to breast cancer: a systematic review and evidence summary. *Support Care Cancer*. 2004;12(6):421-431.

15. Dawson R, Piller N. Diet and BCRL: facts and fallacies on the web. *J Lymphoedema*. 2011;6(1):36-42.

16. Shaw C, Mortimer P, Judd P. Randomized controlled trial comparing a low-fat diet with a weight-reduction diet in breast cancer-related lymphedema. *Cancer*. 2007;109(10):1949-1956.

17. Hot flashes and night sweats PDQ. National Cancer Institute. Accessed January 25, 2019. www.cancer.gov/about-cancer /treatment/side-effects/hot-flashes -hp-pdq

18. Clarkson T, Utian W, Barnes S, et al. The role of soy isoflavones in menopausal health: report of The North American Menopause Society. *Menopause*. 2011;18(7):732-753. doi:10.1097 /gme.0b013e31821fc8e0

19. Newton K, Reed S, LaCroix A, Grothaus L, Ehrlich K, Guiltinan J. Treatment of vasomotor symptoms of menopausal with black cohosh, multibotanicals, soy, hormone therapy, or placebo: a randomized trial. *Ann Intern Med*. 2006;145(12):869-879.

20. Greenlee H, Hershman D, Jacobson J. Use of antioxidant supplements during breast cancer treatment: a comprehensive review. *Breast Cancer Res Treat.* 2009;115(3):437-452. doi:10.1007/s10549-008-0193-0

21. Khan Q, Kimler B, Reddy P, et al. Randomized trial of vitamin D3 to prevent worsening of musculoskeletal symptoms in women with breast cancer receiving adjuvant letrozole. The VITAL trial. *Breast Cancer Res Treat.* 2017;166(2):491-500. doi:10.1007/s1059-017-4429-8

22. Rastelli A, Taylor M, Armamento-Villareal R, Jamalabadi-Majidi S, Napilo N, Ellis M. Vitamin D and aromatase inhibitor-induced musculoskeletal symptoms (AIMSS): a phase II, double-blind, placebo-controlled, randomized trial. *Breast Cancer Res Treat.* 2011;129(1):107-116. doi:10.1007/s10549-011-1644-6

23. Chlebowski R. Vitamin D and breast cancer incidence and outcome. *Anticancer Agents Med Chem.* 2013;13(1):98-106.

24. Lustberg M, Orchard T, Reinbolt R, et al. Randomized placebo-controlled pilot trial of omega 3 fatty acids for prevention of aromatase inhibitor-induced musculoskeletal pain. *Breast Cancer Res Treat.* 2018;167(3):709-718. doi:10.1007/s10549-017-4559

25. Hershman D, Unger J, Crew K, et al. Randomized multicenter placebo-controlled trial of omega-3 fatty acids for the control of aromatase inhibitor-induced musculoskeletal pain: SWOG S0927. *J Clin Oncol.* 2015;33(7):1910-1917. doi:10.1200/JCO.2014.59.5595

26. Michaud L. Managing cancer treatment-induced bone loss and osteoporosis in patients with breast or prostate cancer. *Am J Health Syst Pharm.* 2010;67(7 suppl 3):S20-30. doi:10.2146/ajhp100078

27. Datta M, Schwartz G. Calcium and vitamin D supplementation and loss of bone mineral density in women undergoing breast cancer therapy. *Crit Rev Oncol Hematol.* 2013;88(3):1-19. doi:10.1016/j.critrevonc.2013.07.002

28. Gralow J, Biermann J, Farooki A, et al. NCCN Task Force report: Bone health in cancer care. *J Natl Compr Canc Netw.* 2013 (suppl 3):S1-50.

29. Rosen H. The use of bisphosphonates in postmenopausal women with osteoporosis. In: Rosen CJ, Schmader KE, & Mulder JE (Eds). *UptoDate.* UpToDate. 2019. Accessed January 28, 2019. www.uptodate.com

30. Greenlee H, Hershman D, Shi Z, et al. BMI, lifestyle factors, and taxane-induced neuropathy in breast cancer patients: The Pathways Study. *J Natl Cancer Inst.* 2016;109(2):1-8.

31. Brami C, Bao T, Deng G. Natural products and complementary therapies for chemotherapy-induced peripheral neuropathy: a systematic review. *Crit Rev Oncol Hematol.* 2016;98:325-334. doi:10.1016/j.critrevonc.2015.11.014

32. Hershman D, Unger J, Minasian L, et al. Randomized double-blind placebo-controlled trial of acetyl-L-carnitine for the prevention of taxane-induced neuropathy in women undergoing adjuvant breast cancer therapy. *J Clin Oncol.* 2013;31(20):2627-2633. doi:10.1200/JCO.2012.44.8738

33. Ghoreishi Z, Esfahani A, Djazayeri A, et al. Omega-3 fatty acids are protective against paclitaxel-induced peripheral neuropathy: A randomized double-blind placebo controlled trial. *BMC Cancer.* 2012;12:355. doi:10.1186/1471-2407-12-355

34. Booth C, Clemons M, Dranitsans G, et al. Chemotherapy-induced nausea and vomiting in breast cancer patients: a prospective observational study. *J Support Oncol.* 2007;5(8):374-380.

35. Shih V, Wan H, Chan A. Clinical predictors of chemotherapy-induced nausea and vomiting in breast cancer patients receiving adjuvant doxorubicin and cyclophosphamide. *Ann Pharmacother.* 2009;43(3):444-452. doi:10.1345/aph.1L437

36. Yeo W, Mo F, Suen J, et al. A randomized study of aprepitant, ondansetron and dexamethasone for chemotherapy-induced nausea and vomiting in Chinese breast cancer patients receiving moderately emetogenic chemotherapy. *Breast Cancer Res Treat*. 2009;113(3):529-535. doi:10.1007/s10549-008-9957

37. Chan A, Low X, Yap K. Assessment of the relationship between adherence with antiemetic drug therapy and control of nausea and vomiting in breast cancer patients receiving anthracycline-based chemotherapy. *J Manag Care Pharm*. 2012;18(5):385-394.

38. Greenlee H, DuPont-Reyes M, Blaneaves L, et al. Clinical practice guidelines on the evidence-based use of integrative therapies during and after breast cancer treatment. *CA Cancer J Clin*. 2017;67(3):194-232. doi:10.3322/caac.21397

39. Dibble SL, Chapman J, Mack KA, Shih AS. Acupressure for nausea: results of a pilot study. *Oncol Nurs Forum*. 2000;27(1):41-47.

40. Dibble SL, Luce J, Cooper BA, et al. Acupressure for chemotherapy-induced nausea and vomiting: randomized clinical trial. *Oncol Nurs Forum*. 2007;24(4):813-820.

41. Lee J, Dodd M, Dibble S, Abrams D. Review of acupressure studies for chemotherapy-induced nausea and vomiting control. *J Pain Symptom Manage*. 2008;36(5):529-544.

42. Li Y, Yu Z, Liu F, Wu B, Li J. Oral glutamine ameliorates chemotherapy-induced changes of intestinal permeability and does not interfere with the antitumor effect of chemotherapy in patients with breast cancer: a prospective randomized trial. *Tumori*. 2006;92:396-401.

43. Peterson D, Jones J, Petit R. Randomized, placebo-controlled trial of Saforis for prevention and treatment of oral mucositis in breast cancer patients receiving anthracycline-based chemotherapy. *Cancer*. 2007;109(2):322-331.

44. Boltong A, Aranda S, Keast R, et al. A prospective cohort study of the effects of adjuvant breast cancer chemotherapy on taste function, food liking, appetite and associated nutritional outcomes. *PLos ONE*. 9(7):2014. doi:10.1371/jounral.pone.0103512

45. de Groot S, Vreeswijk M, Welters M, et al. The effects of short-term fasting on tolerance to (neo) adjuvant chemotherapy in HER2-negative breast cancer patients: a randomized pilot study. *BMC Cancer*. 2015;15:652-661. doi:10.1186/s12885-015-1663-5

46. Dorff T, Groshen S, Garcia A, et al. Safety and feasibility of fasting in combination with platinum-based chemotherapy. *BMC Cancer*. 2016;16:360-369. doi:10.1186/s12885-016-2370-6

47. Safdie F, Dorff T, Quinn D, et al. Fasting and cancer treatment in humans: a case series report. *Aging*. 2009;1(12):988-1007. doi:10.18632/aging.100114

48. Demark-Wahnefried W, Campbell K, Hayes S. Weight management and its role in breast cancer rehabilitation. *Cancer*. 2012;118(80):1-16. doi:10.1002/cncr.27466

49. Levine E, Raczynski J, Carpenter J. Weight gain with breast cancer adjuvant treatment. *Cancer*. 1991;67(7):1954-1959. doi:10.1002/1097-0142

50. Makari-Judson G, Braun B, Jerry D, Mertens W. Weight gain following breast cancer diagnosis: Implication and proposed mechanisms. *World J Clin Oncol*. 2014;5(3):272-282. doi:10.5306/wjco.v5.i3.272

51. Vagenas D, DiSipio T, Battistutta D, et al. Weight and weight change following breast cancer: evidence from a prospective, population-based, breast cancer cohort study. *BMC Cancer*. 2015;15(28):1-9. doi:10.1186/s12885-015-1026-2

52. Caan B, Kwan M, Shu X, et al. Weight change and survival after breast cancer in the after breast cancer pooling project. *Cancer Epidemiol Biomark Prev*. 2012;21(8):1260-1271. doi:10.1158/1055-9965

53. Saquib N, Flatt S, Natarajan L, et al. Weight gain and recovery of pre-cancer weight after breast cancer treatments: evidence from the women's healthy eating and living (WHEL) study. *Breast Cancer Res Treat*. 2007;105(2):177-186.

54. Mourouti N, Kontogianni M, Papavagelis C, Panagiotakos D. Diet and breast cancer: a systematic review. *Int J Food Sci Nutr*. 2015;66(1):1-42. doi:10.3109/09637486.2014.950207

55. Kumar NB, Allen K, Cantor A, Cox CE, Greenberg H, Shah S. Weight gain associated with adjuvant tamoxifen therapy in stage I and II breast cancer: fact or artifact? *Breast Cancer Res Treat*. 1997;44(2):135-143.

56. Playdon M, Bracken M, Sanft T, Ligibel J, Harrigan M, Irwin M. Weight gain after breast cancer diagnosis and all-cause mortality: systematic review and meta-analysis. *J Natl Cancer Inst*. 2015;107(2):1-15. doi:10.1093/jnci/djv275

57. Obesity and cancer: A guide for oncology providers. Accessed March 9, 2018. https://asco.org/sites/new-www.asco.org/files/content-files/blog-release/documents/obesity-provider-guide.pdf

58. Demark-Wahnefried W, Peterson B, McBride C, et al. Current health behaviors and readiness to pursue life-style changes among men and women diagnosed with early stage prostate and breast carcinomas. *Cancer*. 2000;88(3):674-684.

59. Thomson C, McCullough M, Wertheim B, et al. Nutrition and physical activity cancer prevention guidelines, cancer risk, and mortality in the Women's Health Initiative. *Cancer Prev Res*. 2014;7(1):42-53. doi:10.1158/1940-6207.CAPR-13-0258

60. Brennan S, Cantwell M, Cardwell C, Velentzis L, Woodside J. Dietary patterns and breast cancer risk: a systematic review and meta-analysis. *Am J Clin Nutr*. 2010;91(5):1294-1302. doi:10.3945/ajcn.2009.28796

61. Sieri S, Krogh V, Ferrari P, et al. Dietary fat and breast cancer risk in the European Prospective Investigation into Cancer and Nutrition. *Am J Clin Nutr*. 1304;2008(88):5.

62. Hartman T, Gapstur S, Gaudet M, et al. Dietary energy density and postmenopausal breast cancer incidence in the Cancer Prevention Study II nutrition cohort. *J Nutr*. 146(10):2045-2050.

63. Prentice R, Caan B, Chlebowski R, et al. Low-fat dietary pattern and risk of invasive breast cancer: the Women's Health Initiative Randomized Controlled Dietary Modification Trial. *JAMA*. 2006;295(6):629-642.

64. Chlebowski R, Aragaki A, Anderson G, et al. Low-fat dietary pattern and breast cancer mortality in the Women's Health Initiative Randomized Controlled Trial. *J Clin Oncol*. 2017;35(25):2919-2926. doi:10.1200/JCO.2016.72.0326

65. McEligot A, Largent J, Ziggas A, Peel D, Anton-Culver H. Dietary fat, fiber, vegetable, and micronutrients are associated with overall survival in postmenopausal women diagnosed with breast cancer. *Nutr Cancer*. 2006;55(2):132-140.

66. Chlebowski R, Blackburn G, Thomson C, et al. Dietary fat reduction and breast cancer outcome: interim efficacy results from the Women's Intervention Nutrition Study. *J Natl Cancer Inst*. 1767;2006(98):24.

67. Rock C, Flatt S, Thomson C, et al. Effects of a high-fiber, low-fat diet intervention on serum concentrations of reproductive steroid hormones in women with a history of breast cancer. *J Clin Oncol*. 2004;22(12):2379-2387.

68. Pierce J, Natarajan L, Caan B, et al. Influence of a diet very high in vegetables, fruit, and fiber and low in fat on prognosis following treatment for breast cancer. The Women's Healthy Eating and Living Randomized Trial. *JAMA*. 2007;298(3):289-298.

69. Ferrari P, Rinaldi S, Jenab M, et al. Dietary fiber intake and risk of hormonal receptor-defined breast cancer in the European Prospective Investigation into Cancer and Nutrition study. *Am J Clin Nutr*. 2013;97(2):344-353. doi:10.3945/ajcn.112.034025

70. Jung S, Spiegelman D, Baglietto L, et al. Fruit and vegetable intake and risk of breast cancer by hormone receptor status. *J Natl Cancer Inst*. 2013;105(3):219-236. doi:10.1093/jnci/djs635

71. Boggs D, Palmer J, Wise L, et al. Fruit and vegetable intake in relation to risk of breast cancer in the Black Women's Health Study. *Am J Epidemiol*. 2010;172(11):1268-1279. doi:10.1093/aje/kwq293

72. Thomson C, Rock C, Thompson P, et al. Vegetable intake is associated with reduced breast cancer recurrence in tamoxifen users: a secondary analysis from the Women's Healthy Eating and Living Study. *Breast Cancer Res Treat*. 2011;125(2):519-527. doi:10.1007/s10549-010-1014-9

73. Pierce J, Stefanick M, Flatt S, et al. Greater survival after breast cancer in physically active women with high vegetable-fruit intake regardless of obesity. *J Clin Oncol*. 2007;25(17):2345-2351.

74. Lissowska J, Gaudet M, Brinton L, et al. Intake of fruits, and vegetables in relation to breast cancer risk by hormone receptor status. *Breast Cancer Res Treat*. 2008;107(1):113-117.

75. Aune D, Chan D, Vieira A, et al. Fruits, vegetables and breast cancer risk: a systematic review and meta-analysis of prospective studies. *Breast Cancer Res Treat*. 2012;134(2):479-493. doi:10.1007/s10549-012-2118-1

76. Aune D, Chan D, Greenwood D, et al. Dietary fiber and breast cancer risk: a systematic review and meta-analysis of prospective studies. *Ann Oncol*. 2012;23(6):1394-1402.

77. Bradbury K, Appleby P, Key T. Fruit, vegetable, and fiber intake in relation to cancer risk: findings from the European Prospective Investigation into Cancer and Nutrition (EPIC). *Am J Clin Nutr*. 2014;100(suppl 1):394S-398S. doi:10.3945/ajcn.113.071357

78. Penniecook-Sawyers J, Jaceldo-Siegl K, Fan J, Beeson L, Knutsen S, Herring P. Vegetarian dietary patterns and the risk of breast cancer in a low-risk population. *Br J Nutr*. 2016;115(10):1790-1797. doi:10.1017/S0007114516000751

79. Pool-Zobel BL, Bub A, Liegibel UM, Treptow-van Lishaut S, Rechkemmer G. Mechanisms by which vegetable consumption reduces genetic damage in humans. *Cancer Epidemiol Biomarkers Prev*. 1998;7(10):891-899.

80. Borek C. Dietary antioxidants and human cancer. *Integr Cancer Ther*. 2004;3:333-341.

81. Rock C, Flatt S, Natarajan L, et al. Plasma carotenoids and recurrence-free survival in women with a history of breast cancer. *J Clin Oncol*. 2005;23(27):6631-6638.

82. Eliassen A, Hendrickson S, Brinton L, et al. Circulating carotenoids and risk of breast cancer: pooled analysis of eight prospective studies. *J Natl Cancer Inst*. 2012;104(24):1905-1916. doi:10.1093/jnci/djs461

83. Rock C, Natarajan L, Pu M, et al. Longitudinal biological exposure to carotenoids is associated with breast cancer-free survival in the Women's Healthy Eating and Living Study. *Cancer Epidemiol Biomark Prev*. 2009;18(2):486-494. doi:10.1158/1055-9965

84. Aune D, Chan D, Vieira A, et al. Dietary compared with blood concentrations of carotenoids and breast cancer risk: a systematic review and meta-analysis of prospective studies. *Am J Clin Nutr*. 2012;96(2):356-373. doi:10.3945/ajcn.112.034165

85. Mason J, Thompson L. Flaxseed and its lignan and oil components: can they play a role in reducing the risk of and improving the treatment of breast cancer? *Appl Physiol Nutr Metab*. 2014;39(6):663-678. doi:10.1139/apnm-2013-0420

86. Lowcock E, Cotterchio M, Boucher B. Consumption of flaxseed, a rich source of lignans, is associated with reduced breast cancer risk. *Cancer Causes Control*. 2013;24(4):813-816. doi:10.1007/s10552-013-0155-7

87. Cotterchio M, Boucher B, Kreiger N, Mills C, Thompson L. Dietary phytoestrogen intake-lignans and isoflavones-and breast cancer risk. *Cancer Causes Control*. 2008;19(3):259-272.

88. Thompson L, Chen J, Li T, Strasser-Weippl K, Goss P. Dietary flaxseed alters tumor biological markers in postmenopausal breast cancer. *Clin Cancer Res*. 2005;11(10):3828-3835.

89. Calado A, Neves P, Santos T, Ravasco P. The effect of flaxseed in breast cancer: a literature review. *Front Nutr*. 2018;5(4):4-11. doi:10.3389/fnut.2018.00004

90. Zamora-Ros R, Forouhi NG, Sharp SJ, et al. The association between dietary flavonoid and lignan intakes and incident type 2 diabetes in European populations: the EPIC-InterAct study. *Diabetes Care*. 2013;36(12):3961-3970.

91. Guha N, Kwan M, Quesenberry C, Weltzien E, Castillo A, Caan B. Soy isoflavones and risk of cancer recurrence in a cohort of breast cancer survivors: the Life After Cancer Epidemiology study. *Breast Cancer Res Treat*. 2009;118(2):395-405. doi:10.1007/s10549-009-0321-5

92. Chen M, Rao Y, Zheng Y, Wei S, Li Y, Yin P. Association between soy isoflavone intake and breast cancer risk for pre- and post-menopausal women: a meta-analysis of epidemiological studies. *PLos ONE*. 2014;9(2):1-10. doi:10.1371/journal.pone.0089288

93. Lee S, Shu X, Li H, et al. Adolescent and adult soy food intake and breast cancer risk: results from the Shanghai Women's Health Study. *Am J Clin Nutr*. 2009;89(6):1920-1926. doi:10.3945/ajcn.2008.27361

94. Nechuta S, Caan B, Chen W, Lu W, Chen Z, Kwan M. Soy food intake after diagnosis of breast cancer and survival: an in-depth analysis of combined evidence from cohort studies of US and Chinese women. *Am J Clin Nutr*. 2012;96(2):1.

95. Oregon State. Soy isoflavones. Accessed March 9, 2018. http://lpi.oregonstate.edu/mic/dietary-factors/phytochemicals/soy-isoflavones

96. Ju Y, Doerge D, Allred K, Allred C, Helferich W. Dietary genistein negates the inhibitory effect of tamoxifen on growth of estrogen-dependent human breast cancer (MCF-7) cells implanted in athymic mice. *Cancer Res*. 2002;62:2474-2477.

97. Liu B, Edgerton S, Yang X, et al. Low-dose dietary phytoestrogen abrogates tamoxifen-associated mammary tumor prevention. *Cancer Res*. 2005;65(3):879-886.

98. Hidayat K, Chen G, Zhang R, et al. Calcium intake and breast cancer risk: meta-analysis of prospective cohort studies. *Br J Nutr*. 116(1):158-166. doi:10.1017/S0007114516001768

99. Dong J, Zhang L, He K, Qin L. Dairy consumption and risk of breast cancer: a meta-analysis of prospective cohort studies. *Breast Cancer Res Treat*. 2011;127(1):23-31. doi:10.1007/s10549-011-1467-5

100. Kroenke C, Kwan M, Sweeney C, Castillo A, Caan B. High- and low-fat dairy intake, recurrence, and mortality after breast cancer diagnosis. *J Natl Cancer Inst*. 2013;105(9):616-623. doi:10.1093/jnci/djt027

101. Li C, Yang L, Zhang D, Jiang W. Systematic review and meta-analysis suggest that dietary cholesterol intake increases risk of breast cancer. *Nutr Res*. 2016;36(7):627-635. doi:10.1016/j.nutres.2016.04.009

102. Cho E, Chen W, Hunter D, et al. Red meat intake and risk of breast cancer among premenopausal women. *Arch Intern Med*. 2006;166(20):2253-2259.

103. Taylor E, Burley V, Greenwood D, Cade J. Meat consumption and risk of breast cancer in the UK Women's Cohort Study. *Br J Cancer*. 2007;96(7):1139-1146. doi:10.1038/sj.bjc.6603689

104. Janos A, Logomarsino J. Role of omega-3 fatty acids in the risk and treatment of breast cancer. *Top Clin Nutr*. 2011;26(3):246-256.

105. Zheng J, Hu X, Zhao Y, Yang J, Li D. Intake of fish and marine n-3 polyunsaturated fatty acids and risk of breast cancer: meta-analysis of data from 21 independent prospective cohort studies. *BMJ*. 213AD;346:f3706. doi:10.1136/bmj.f3706

106. Khankari N, Bradshaw P, Steck S, et al. Dietary intake of fish, polyunsaturated fatty acids, and survival after breast cancer: a population-based follow-up study on Long Island, New York. *Cancer*. 2015;121(13):2244-2252. doi:10.1002/cncr.29329

107. U.S. Department of Agriculture, Agricultural Research Service. FoodData Central, 2019. Accessed March 19, 2020. https://fdc.nal.usda.gov

108. Chlebowski R, Aiello E, McTiernan A. Weight loss in breast cancer patient management. *J Clin Oncol*. 2002;20(4):1128-1143.

109. Larsson S, Mantzoros C, Wolk A. Diabetes mellitus and risk of breast cancer: a meta-analysis. *Int J Cancer*. 2007;121:856-862.

110. Boyle P, Boniol M, Koechlin A, et al. Diabetes and breast cancer risk: a meta-analysis. *Br J Cancer*. 2012;107:1608-1617. doi:10.1038/bjc.2012.414

111. Emaus M, van Gils C, Bakker M, et al. Weight change in middle adulthood and breast cancer risk in the EPIC-PANACEA study. *Int J Cancer*. 2014;135:2887-2899.

112. Neuhouser M, Aragaki A, Prentice R, et al. Overweight, obesity and postmenopausal invasive bresat cancer risk. *JAMA Oncol*. 2015;1(5):611-621. doi:10.1001/jamaoncol.2015.1546

113. Eliassen H, Colditz G, Rosner B, Willett W, Hankinson S. Adult weight change and risk of postmenopausal breast cancer. *JAMA*. 2006;296(2):193-201.

114. Protani M, Coory M, Martin J. Effect of obesity on survival of women with breast cancer: systematic review and meta-analysis. *Breast Cancer Res Treat*. 2010;123(3):627-635. doi:10.1007/s10549-010-0990-0

115. Chan D, Vieira A, Aune D, et al. Body mass index and survival in women with breast cancer-systematic literature review and meta-analysis of 82 follow-up studies. *Ann Oncol*. 2014;25(10):1901-1914. doi:10.1093/annonc/mdu042

116. Thompson H, Sedlacek S, Playdon M, et al. Weight loss interventions for breast cancer survivors: impact of dietary pattern. *PLos ONE*. 2015;10(5):1-17. doi:10.1371/journal.pone.0127366

117. Finocchiaro C, Ossola M, Monge T, et al. Effect of specific educational program on dietary change and weight loss in breast cancer survivors. *Clin Nutr*. 2016;35:864-870. doi:10.1016/j.clnu.2015.05.018

118. Rock C, Byers T, Colditz G, et al. Reducing breast cancer recurrence with weight loss, a Vanguard Trial: The Exercise and Nutrition to Enhance Recovery and Good Health for You (ENERGY) trial. *Contemp Clin Trials*. 2013;34(2):282-295. doi:10.1016/j.cct.2012.12.003

119. Rock C, Flatt S, Byers T, et al. Results of the Exercise and Nutrition to Enhance Recovery and Good Health for You (ENERGY) trial: a behavioral weight loss intervention in overweight or obese breast cancer survivors. *J Clin Oncol*. 2015;33:1-8. doi:10.1200/jco.2015.61.1095

120. Djuric Z, DiLaura N, Jenkins I, et al. Combining weight-loss counseling with the Weight Watchers plan for obese breast cancer survivors. *Obes Res*. 10(7):657-665.

121. Dieli-Conwright C, Lee K, Kiwata J. Reducing the risk of breast cancer recurrence: an evaluation of the effects and mechanisms of diet and exercise. *Curr Breast Cancer Rep*. 2016;8(3):139-150. doi:10.1007/s12609-016-0218-3

122. Holmes M, Chen W, Feskanich D, Kroenke C, Colditz G. Physical activity and survival after breast cancer diagnosis. *JAMA*. 2005;293(20):2479-2486.

123. Ibrahim E, Al-Homaidh A. Physical activity and survival after breast cancer diagnosis: meta-analysis of published studies. *Med Oncol*. 2011;28(3):753-765. doi:10.1007/s12032-010-9536-x

124. Courneya K, Segal R, McKenzie D, et al. Effects of exercise during adjuvant chemotherapy on breast cancer outcomes. *Med Sci Sports Exerc*. 2014;46(9):1744-1751.

125. Irwin M, Smith A, McTiernan A, et al. Influence of pre- and postdiagnosis physical activity on mortality in breast cancer survivors: the health, eating, activity, and lifestyle study. *J Clin Oncol*. 2008;26(24):3958-3964. doi:10.1200/JCO.2077.15.9822

126. Harris M, Swift D, Myers V, et al. Cancer Survival Through Lifestyle Change (CASTLE): a pilot study of weight loss. *Int J Behav Med*. 2013;20:403-412. doi:10.1007/s12529-012-9234-5

127. Marinac C, Natarajan L, Sears D, et al. Prolonged nightly fasting and breast cancer risk: findings from NHANES (2009-2010). *Cancer Epidemiol Biomark Prev*. 2015;24(5):783-789. doi:10.1158/1055-9965

128. Marinac C, Nelson S, Breen C, et al. Prolonged nightly fasting and breast cancer prognosis. *JAMA Oncol*. 2016;2(8):1049-1055. doi:10.1001/jamaoncol.2016.0164

129. Emaus M, Peeters P, Bakker M, et al. Vegetable and fruit consumption and the risk of hormone receptor-defined breast cancer in the EPIC cohort. *Am J Clin Nutr*. 2016;103(1):168-177. doi:10.3945/ajcn.114.101436

130. Greenlee H, Kwan M, Kushi L, et al. Antioxidant supplement use after breast cancer diagnosis and mortality in the LACE cohort. *Cancer*. 2012;118(8):2048-2058. doi:10.1002/cncr.26526

131. Patterson R, Flatt S, Newman V, et al. Marine fatty acid intake is associated with breast cancer prognosis. *J Nutr*. 2011;141(2):201-206. doi:10.3945/jn.110.128777

132. Shu X, Zheng Y, Cai H, Gu K, Chen Z, Zheng W. Soy food intake and breast cancer survival. *JAMA*. 2009;302(22):2437-2443. doi:10.1001/jama.2009.1783

133. Zang J, Shen M, Du S, Chen T, Zou S. The association between dairy intake and breast cancer in Western and Asian populations: a systematic review and meta-analysis. *J Breast Cancer*. 2015;18(4):313-322. doi:10.4048/jbc.2015.18.1.313

134. Parada HJ, Steck S, Bradshaw P, et al. Grilled, barbecued, and smoked meat intake and survival following breast cancer. *J Natl Cancer Inst*. 2017;109(6). doi:10.1093/jnci/djw299

135. Seely D, Mills E, Wu P, Verma S, Guyatt G. The effects of green tea consumption on incidence of breast cancer and recurrence of breast cancer: a systematic review and meta-analysis. *Integr Cancer Ther*. 2005;4(2):144-155. doi:10.1177/1534735405276420

136. Lohmann A, Chapman J, Burnell M, et al. Prognostic associations of 25 hydroxy vitamin D in NCIC CTG MA.21, a phase III adjuvant randomized clinical trial of three chemotherapy regimens in high-risk breast cancer. *Breast Cancer Res Treat*. 2015;150(3):605-611. doi:10.1007/s10549-015-3355-x

137. Kwan M, Kushi L, Weltzien E, et al. Alcohol consumption and breast cancer recurrence and survival among women with early-stage breast cancer: the life after cancer epidemiology study. *J Clin Oncol*. 2010;28(29):4410-4416. doi:10.1200/JCO.2010.29.2730

138. Velicer C, Ulrich C. Vitamin and mineral supplement use among US adults after cancer diagnosis: a systematic review. *J Clin Oncol*. 2008;26(4):665-673. doi:10.1200/jco.2007.13.5905

139. Fleischauer A, Simonsen N, Arab L. Antioxidant supplements and risk of breast cancer recurrence and breast cancer-related mortality among postmenopausal women. *Nutr Cancer*. 2003;46(1):15-22.

140. Harris H, Orsini N, Wolk A. Vitamin C and survival among women with breast cancer: a meta-analysis. *Eur J Cancer*. 2014;50(7):1223-1231. doi:10.1016/j.ejca.2014.02.013

141. Bauer S, Hankinson S, Bertone-Johnson E, Ding E. Plasma vitamin D levels, menopause, and risk of breast cancer: dose-response meta-analysis of prospective studies. *Medicine (Baltimore)*. 2013;92(3):123-131. doi:10.1097/MD.0b013e3182943bc2

142. Conklin K. Coenzyme q10 for prevention of anthracycline-induced cardiotoxicity. *Integr Cancer Ther*. 2005;4(2):110-130.

143. Takimoto M, Sakurai T, Kodama K, et al. Protective effect of CoQ10 administration on cardial toxicity in FAC therapy. *Gan To Kagaku Rhoho*. 1984;11:1420-1427.

144. Greenlee H, Shaw J, Lau Y, Naini A, Maurer M. Effect of coenzyme Q10 on doxorubicin cytotoxicity in breast cancer cell cultures. *Integr Cancer Ther*. 2012;11(3):1-12. doi:10.1177/1534735412439749

145. Neuhouser M, Wassertheil-Smoller S, Thomson C, et al. Multivitamin use and risk of cancer and cardiovascular disease in the Women's Health Initiative cohorts. *Arch Intern Med*. 2009;169(3):294-304. doi:10.1001/archinternmed.2008.540

146. Wassertheil-Smoller S, McGinn A, Budrys N, et al. Multivitamin and mineral use and breast cancer mortality in older women with invasive breast cancer in the Women's Health Initiative. *Breast Cancer Res Treat*. 2013;141(3):495-505. doi:10.1007/s10549-013-2712-x

147. Chen P, Hu P, Zie D, Qin Y, Wang F, Wang H. Meta-analysis of vitamin D, calcium and the prevention of breast cancer. *Breast Cancer Res Treat*. 2010;121(2):469-477. doi:10.1007/s10549-009-0593-9

148. Kuhn T, Kaaks R, Becker S, et al. Plasma 25-hyroxyvitamin D and the risk of breast cancer in the European Prospective Investigation into Cancer and Nutrition: a nested case-control study. *Int J Cancer*. 2013;133(7):1689-1700. doi:10.1002/ijc.28172

149. Eliassen A, Warner E, Rosner B, et al. Plasma 25-hydroxyvitamin D and risk of breast cancer in women followed over 20 years. *Cancer Res*. 2016;76(18):5423-5430. doi:10.1158/0008-5472.CAN-16-0353

150. Crew K, Shane E, Cremers S, McMahon D, Irani D, Hershman D. High prevalence of vitamin D deficiency despite supplementation in premenopausal women with breast cancer undergoing adjuvant chemotherapy. *J Clin Oncol*. 2151;2009(27):13. doi:10.1200/JCO.2008.19.6162

151. Clark A, Chen J, Kapoor S, et al. Pretreatment vitamin D level and response to neoadjuvant chemotherapy in women with breast cancer on the I-SPY trial (CALGB 15007/150015/ACRIN6657). *Cancer Med*. 2014;3(3):693-701. doi:10.1002/cam4.235

152. Zeichner S, Koru-Sengul T, Shah N, et al. Improved clinical outcomes associated with vitamin D supplementation during adjuvant chemotherapy in patients with HER2+ nonmetastatic breast cancer. *Clin Breast Cancer*. 2015;15(1):e1-11. doi:10.1016/j.clbc.2014.08.001

153. Hu K, Callen D, Li J, Zheng H. Circulating vitamin D and overall survival in breast cancer patients: a dose-response meta-analysis of cohort studies. *Integr Cancer Ther*. 2017. doi:10.1177/1534735417712007

154. Jacobs E, Thomson C, Flatt S, et al. Vitamin D and breast cancer recurrence in the Women's Healthy Eating and Living (WHEL) Study. *Am J Clin Nutr*. 2011;93(1):108-117. doi:10.3945/ajcn.2010.30009

155. Kim Y, Je Y. Vitamin D intake, blood 25(OH)D levels, and breast cancer risk or mortality: a meta-analysis. *Br J Cancer*. 2014;110(11):2772-2784. doi:10.1038/bjc.2014.175

156. Brasky T, Lampe J, Potter J, Patterson R, White E. Specialty supplements and breast cancer risk in the VITamins And Lifestyle (VITAL) cohort. *Cancer Epidemiol Biomark Prev*. 2010;19(7):1696-1708. doi:10.1158/1055-9965.EPI-10-0318

157. Bougnoux P, Hajjaji N, Ferrasson M, Giraudeau B, Couet C, Le Floch O. Improving outcome of chemotherapy of metastatic breast cancer by docosahexaenoic acid: a phase II trial. *Br J Cancer*. 2009;101(12):1978-1985. doi:10.1038/sj.bjc.6605441

Chapter 18
Medical Nutrition Therapy for Esophageal and Gastric Cancers

Kacie Merchand, MS, RD, CSO, LD
Jeannine B. Mills, MS, RDN, CSO, LD

Esophageal cancer (EC) is the uncontrolled growth of cancerous cells in the esophagus, with the lining of the esophagus as the most common region for cancers to originate. EC is the eighth most common cancer worldwide and the sixth most common cause of cancer-related death.[1] Expected death rates are more than four times higher in men than in women.[2] The 5-year survival rate for esophageal cancer is about 20% in the United States,[3] approximately 10% in Europe, and lower in less developed countries.[4] The survival rate more than doubles with early diagnosis.[3,5] Discussion of gastric cancer begins on page 382.

Esophageal Cancer

Esophageal squamous cell carcinomas (ESCCs) and esophageal adenocarcinomas (EACs) account for most cases of EC. Box 18.1 on page 376 summarizes the prevalence and risk factors for these two types of ECs. ESCCs originate in the inner layers of the esophagus—arising from squamous cells—and commonly occur in the upper two-thirds of the esophagus. EACs originate in the inner layers of the esophagus and spread outward—arising from gland cells that replace squamous cells (Barrett's esophagus)—and are typically found in the lower third of the esophagus. Adenocarcinoma at the gastroesophageal junction is treated like esophageal cancer. Other rare cancers can start in the esophagus (eg, lymphomas, sarcomas, and melanomas).[6]

Diagnosis of EC typically occurs after presentation of symptoms. Symptoms of ED rarely occur when the disease is localized, and may include dysphagia, odynophagia, reflux-like pain, throat or back pain, and weight loss. Results from diagnostic tests used in staging may include barium swallow, chest or abdominal computed tomography (CT), magnetic resonance imaging (MRI), positron emission tomography (PET) scans, endoscopy, biopsies, laboratory tests, and physical examination.[7] The most common staging system is that of the American Joint Committee on Cancer (available from the American Cancer Society on its website).[8]

Treatment of Esophageal Cancer

A range of treatments for EC are available. Box 18.2 on page 376 summarizes the common treatment options and interventions for both curative and palliative intent, as well as several nutrition impact symptoms related to treatment. Multimodal treatment—incorporating chemotherapy, radiation, targeted therapy, and surgery—is often used.[9] Treatment is based on tumor resectability. If resectable, then surgery may be a part of the treatment plan; if nonresectable, then treatment may involve nonsurgical methods or palliative care. Refer to the *NCCN Clinical Practice Guidelines in Oncology (NCCN Guidelines): Esophageal and Esophagogastric Junction Cancers* for details of specific therapies.[7,9]

Surgery

Patients with EC who are eligible for surgery commonly undergo esophagectomy or esophagogastrectomy through open or minimally invasive surgery, such as laparoscopic or robotic-assisted surgery.[10] Many surgical approaches fall under the category of transthoracic or transhiatal esophagectomy. In most cases, the stomach is used to create a new esophagus; however, the colon or

Box 18.1
Esophageal Cancer Prevalence and Risk Factors[2,4,6,12-18]

	Esophageal adenocarcinoma	Esophageal squamous cell carcinoma
Prevalence[a]	In the United States, EAC is the most common type of esophageal adenocarcinoma esophageal cancer(EC) among White people. The number of EAC cases, especially among men, is expected to continue to increase rapidly (2005 through 2030) in high-income countries.	In the United States, Esophageal squamous cell carcinoma (ESCC) is the most common type of EC among African Americans. Worldwide, ESCC makes up the majority of EC cases.
Risk factors	Obesity, body fatness Gastroesophageal reflux disease and Barrett's esophagus Smoking Gender, race, genetic aspects	Smoking Alcohol Human papillomavirus infection Yerba mate consumption Gender, race, genetics Processed and red meats[b]

[a] Lower rates of esophageal cancer are found in American Indian and Alaskan native peoples, Hispanics, and Asians and Pacific Islanders.

[b] Limited or suggestive evidence.

Box 18.2
Common Esophageal Cancer Treatments and Related Nutrition Impact Symptoms[a,7,9,19,20]

Curative treatment options	Chemotherapy, radiation therapy, chemoradiation, targeted therapy, surgery (partial or total esophagectomy), endoscopic mucosal resection
Palliative care interventions	Chemotherapy, radiation therapy (including brachytherapy), targeted therapy, endoscopic treatment Diet modification, stent, dilation, feeding tube, medications for symptom management (eg, pain, nausea, reflux, anxiety)
Nutrition impact symptoms	Esophagitis (common during weeks 3 through 6 of concurrent chemoradiation therapy), nausea, vomiting, anorexia, dysphagia, odynophagia, reflux, dysgeusia, fatigue, constipation or diarrhea, xerostomia

[a] See Chapters 9 and 10 for details of treatments and their side effects.

small intestine may be used if needed.[11] See Figure 18.1 on page 378 for before and after illustrations of surgical esophagectomy.

Esophageal Stents

Several studies have demonstrated improved swallowing ability and quality of life (QOL) with stent placement in palliative care management of dysphagia, but also with neoadjuvant treatment.[21-24] Self-expanding stents allow quick return to oral intake of most foods[25]; however, complications such as stent migration are possible. A 2014 Cochrane review of palliative management of dysphagia found that self-expanding metal stents did not offer greater QOL improvement or length of survival than other techniques, such as radiotherapy or brachytherapy.[20] Box 18.3 outlines diet recommendations for patients with esophageal stents.

Nutrition Assessment in Patients With Esophageal Cancer

Criteria that should trigger a positive nutrition risk screening for patients with EC include dysphagia, weight loss, and poor oral intake. Studies demonstrating benefits to early nutrition intervention indicate that a standard nutrition pathway in patients with EC who are receiving definitive chemoradiation therapy or surgery may help reduce weight loss, treatment breaks, complications, unplanned hospital admissions, length of stay (LOS), and inpatient costs.[26-32] Energy expenditure may be elevated in men with a new EC diagnosis who are losing weight, as well as in patients undergoing esophagectomy.[33-35] See Chapter 4 for general nutrition assessment information and Chapter 5 for discussion of energy and nutrient requirements.

> ### Box 18.3
> #### Best-Practice Diet Recommendations for Patients With Esophageal Stents[25]
>
> Typically, liquids followed by moist, soft, easily chewed foods within 24 hours of stent placement (eg, crackers or breads dipped in soups, cooked or pureed vegetables, peeled or canned fruit, ground or bite-size soft or moist meats)
>
> Adequate chewing
>
> Small bites or food bolus
>
> Sitting upright during and following meals (for 30 to 60 minutes)
>
> Fluids with oral food intake, though may need to save most beverages for between meals (eg, early satiety)
>
> Sips of carbonated beverages if food does not pass through stent

Nutrition Problems and Interventions Specific to Esophageal Cancer

Nutrition Impact Symptoms

Side effects of treatment for esophageal cancer vary depending on the modality of treatment, concurrent therapy, and whether therapy is adjuvant or neoadjuvant. Treatment-related nutrition impact symptoms vary by treatment modality and can include esophagitis, nausea, vomiting, anorexia, dysphagia, odynophagia, reflux, dysgeusia, fatigue, constipation, diarrhea, early satiety, and xerostomia. See Chapters 9 and 10 for a detailed description of side effects due to chemotherapy and radiotherapy and Chapter 11 for symptom management.

Preesophagectomy

Postesophagectomy

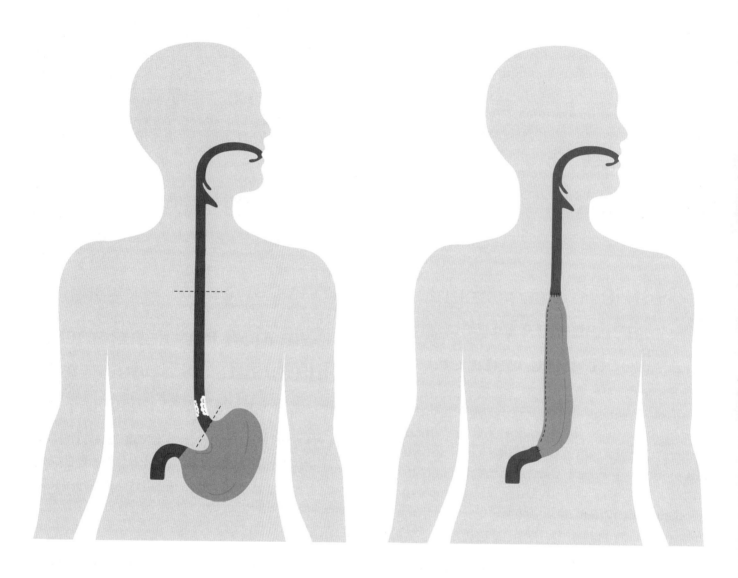

Figure 18.1
Esophagectomy

Malnutrition

Malnutrition, weight loss, cachexia, and inadequate oral intake are experienced by many patients being treated for EC[33,36-38] and may have a negative impact on overall survival.[39,40] Prevalence of malnutrition has been reported in more than 75% of patients.[36] Risk of dose-limiting toxicity has been shown to significantly increase in sarcopenic obese patients with EC.[41] Additionally, lower pretreatment hand-grip strength in patients with EC has been associated with treatment modifications.[42]

Weight Loss and Sarcopenia

Nutritional status and underweight status have been identified as risk factors for predicting postoperative complications following esophagectomy.[43,44] Studies indicate that loss of muscle mass, and specifically sarcopenia, have correlated with postoperative complications,[45] such as pulmonary complications,[46] unplanned postoperative readmissions,[47] postoperative mortality (stage III through IV),[48] and worse survival rates in esophagectomy patients.[47,49] Other studies are inconclusive, indicating that sarcopenia was not associated with increased morbidity or mortality in esophagectomy patients[50]; and in a separate study, those with more than 10% preoperative weight loss experienced decreased 5-year survival rates with no increase in postoperative complications.[51]

Dysphagia

Dysphagia is the most common symptom of EC. Symptoms caused by EC, such as difficulty swallowing, often prompt findings of the cancer.[8] Interventions may include modified diet and eating practices (eg, increased time chewing foods), feeding-tube placement, esophageal stent, dilation, chemotherapy, radiotherapy, brachytherapy, cryoablation, and surgery.[20] See Chapter 11 for details of symptom management of dysphagia.

Nutrition Support

Enteral nutrition (EN) is used as an intervention for dysphagia during treatment as a palliative measure, or following surgery. Jejunostomy feeding tubes are often preferred in surgical candidates, though gastrostomy or nasogastric tubes may also be placed.

The Oncology Guideline in the Academy of Nutrition and Dietetics Evidence Analysis Library states there are limited data showing that EN for severely dysphagic patients with EC helps maintain weight during concurrent chemoradiation therapy (CCRT).[52] EN has demonstrated favorable outcomes when compared with parenteral nutrition (PN) in EC patients receiving CCRT[53]; however, the optimal nutrition approach during CCRT for patients with resectable EC remains unclear.[21] Immunonutrition (IN) formula has been studied in EC with varying findings.[54,55] Additional research is needed before this becomes widely recommended.

Postoperative Nutrition

Many medical centers use EN postoperatively, given delays in adequate oral intake.[56] Early EN has been shown to be safe and valid for esophagectomy patients.[57,58] It has been associated with significantly shorter LOS and improved outcomes[59] and was found to be effective in meeting nutrition goals.[58] Reduced weight loss and greater hand grip strength were found in patients receiving EN for 6 weeks postprocedure compared with feeding-tube removal at the time of hospital discharge.[60] EN combined with PN was found to be superior at maintaining weight than EN alone,[61] though EN is typically favored over PN, given EN's lower rates of postoperative pneumonia[62,63] and life-threatening complications.[64]

Standard formula is typically used for EN in esophagectomy patients. Clinicians may test a patient's tolerance of an energy-dense formula (eg, 1.5 kcal/mL), which is generally well tolerated in the jejunum, to decrease feeding time. The potential benefits of IN formulas have been studied in the perioperative setting.[65-67] In one study, patients experienced reduced surgical wound infection and postoperative systemic inflammatory response syndrome on perioperative IN.[65] Reduced inflammatory response and decreased interruption or reduction of EN due to abdominal symptoms was demonstrated in esophagectomy patients using perioperative synbiotics.[66] Conversely, some randomized controlled trials using IN perioperatively in oral and enteral feeds did not establish any benefit over standard nutrition.[68,69] Additional evidence is needed before IN can be widely recommended in EC surgical patients.

Early Oral Feeding After Surgery

The European Society for Clinical Nutrition and Metabolism recommends early oral feeding for most surgical patients[70]; however, this is not currently standard practice in patients undergoing surgery for EC. Oral intake is often delayed out of concern for possible complications, such as anastomotic leaks and aspiration pneumonia, despite a lack of evidence to support increased risk for these complications with early oral feeding.[71] Recent studies found early oral intake (started postoperative day 0 to 1) to be safe and feasible for patients receiving esophagectomy[71-77] and have demonstrated favorable outcomes, such as significantly shorter LOS,[73,74] quicker return of bowel movement and improved short-term QOL,[77] lower rates of pneumonia and anastomotic leakage, and shorter stay in intensive care units.[73] The feasibility, safety, and potential benefits of early oral nutrition, with or without EN, continue to be studied in patients undergoing surgery for EC.

Postoperative Nutrition Complications

Oral diet typically progresses from liquids to soft solids, followed by the reintroduction of regular foods, as tolerated. Emphasis on well-chewed, small, frequent meals consumed slowly is advisable. Sitting upright following meals, leaving 2 to 3 hours between the final meal of the day and bedtime, and keeping the head elevated while lying down can help patients manage reflux and reduce aspiration risk.

Special consideration should be given to postoperative anatomical changes and complications that may affect the nutrition advice given to esophagectomy patients. The following should be kept in mind[78]:

- Anastomotic complications, such as leaks and strictures, may occur, and strictures can result in dysphagia.

- Removal of the lower esophageal sphincter contributes to postoperative reflux.

- Chylothorax may occur, at which time a very-low-fat EN formula or oral diet may be indicated.

- The size, shape, and position of the postoperative stomach can cause postprandial symptoms, such as delayed emptying, reflux, and dumping syndrome.

- Pylorus dysfunction, decreased gastric capacity, devascularization, and resection of the vagus nerve can result in dysmotility, which may present as early satiety, emesis, or dumping syndrome, alone or in combination. Box 18.4 discusses dumping syndrome and its management.

Postsurgical malabsorption has been highly associated with advanced tumor stage.[82] In addition to dumping syndrome, possible factors affecting absorption may be small intestinal bacterial overgrowth, exocrine pancreatic insufficiency (EPI), or

Box 18.4
Dumping Syndrome[79-81]

Definition	Rapid gastric emptying, allowing incompletely digested and hyperosmolar chyme to enter the small intestine. When fluids rush to the small intestine to normalize osmolarity, the high fluid volume, along with hormonal and vasomotor changes, may result in bloating, abdominal cramps, nausea, or diarrhea. Symptoms often diminish or resolve when medical nutrition therapy is implemented.	
Medical management	In severe cases, medications such as octreotide or acarbose may be used to manage symptoms.	
	Timing	**Symptoms**
Early dumping (75% of cases)	10 to 30 minutes postprandial	Epigastric fullness, nausea, vomiting, abdominal cramps, bloating, diarrhea, lightheadedness, diaphoresis, desire to lie down, borborygmus, pallor, palpitations
Late dumping (25% of cases)	1 to 3 hours postprandial	Hunger, perspiration, tremors, difficulty concentrating
Medical nutrition therapy for dumping syndrome	Limit foods high in concentrated sugars. Test tolerance to lactose-containing foods. Avoid fried and greasy foods, but test tolerance to small amounts of fats. Eat protein-rich foods and complex carbohydrates, specifically foods high in soluble fiber. Drink liquids 30 minutes before or after meals but not during meals. Eat five to six small meals daily and avoid large portions. Eat slowly and chew food into very small pieces or until liquefied.	

bile acid malabsorption.[82] There is some evidence that pancreatic enzyme replacement therapy may provide benefit.[82-84] See Chapter 20 for more information on the management of EPI, also known as pancreatic exocrine insufficiency (PEI).

Survivorship and Esophageal Cancer

With increasing postoperative survival rates,[85] researchers are paying attention to health-related QOL in survivorship.[82] Symptoms influencing QOL, such as early satiety, diarrhea, dumping syndrome, no appetite, nausea, and reflux, can persist for several years after esophagectomy.[86-88] In a single study, long-term nutrition, gastrointestinal (GI) function, and QOL were found to be "excellent" in survivors at 10 or more years after surgery,[89] though it may take more than 12 months for health-related QOL to return to a level similar to that of the general population.[86]

A systematic review found that patients may not take in adequate energy and protein in the early postoperative years,[88,90] which is in line with ongoing weight-loss findings[82,83] and high rates of sarcopenia.[82] There is limited evidence to support routine monitoring of micronutrients in this population.[82,90] Further research on long-term postoperative diet and micronutrient status is needed.

❧ ❧ ❧

Gastric Cancer

The wall of the stomach is made up of three layers of tissue: (from innermost to outermost) the mucosal layer, the muscularis layer, and the serosal layer. See Figure 18.2 for normal anatomy of the stomach. Gastric (stomach) cancers occur when malignant tumors form in the cells lining the stomach and can invade from the innermost layer to the outermost layer as it grows.[91]

Prevalence

Gastric cancer ranks 15th in incidence among the major types of cancer in the United States, is the 5th most common cancer in the world, and is the 3rd leading cause of cancer-related deaths worldwide, with Korea having the highest global incidence.[91,92] Over 27,000 new cases in the United States were estimated for 2020, with a projection of 11,010 deaths associated with gastric cancer; the 5-year survival rate is 32%.[91] Gastric cancer is more common in men than in women, and it is more frequently diagnosed among people aged 65 to 74 years, with the median age at the time of diagnosis being 68 years.[91]

Prognosis and Survival

The prognosis for patients with gastric cancer depends on tumor extent, nodal involvement, and direct tumor extension beyond the gastric wall. Tumor grade is also considered.[93]

More than 50% of patients in whom localized distal gastric cancer is diagnosed can be cured. Unfortunately, early-stage disease is only discovered in 10% to 20% of all cases diagnosed in the United States, while the remaining patients present with metastatic disease in either regional or distant sites with overall 5-year survival rates. Advanced gastric cancers account for about 40% of those diagnosed.[94] For those patients with metastatic disease, survival rates range from nearly no survival to no more than 50% survival for patients with localized and resectable distal gastric cancers. The 5-year survival rate for patients with proximal gastric cancer with localized disease is only 10% to 15%.[93]

Gastronitestinal stromal tumors (GISTs) occur most commonly in the stomach but are not covered in this chapter. See the National Cancer Institute's PDQ summary on treatment of GISTs for more information.[93]

Types of Gastric Cancer

Adenocarcinoma accounts for 90% to 95% of all gastric malignancies, and the rest are lymphomas, sarcomas, and carcinoid tumors. There are two types of gastric cancer: intestinal and diffuse.[93]

Intestinal adenocarcinomas, often described as tubular, papillary, or mucinous, are well differentiated with the cells often configured into tubular or glandular structures. Diffuse adenocarcinomas are undifferentiated or poorly differentiated, and no gland formation is present. Infiltration of the gastric wall by diffuse adenocarcinomas can cause a condition known as linitis plastica. Tumors can have mixed features of both types of adenocarcinoma.[93]

Risk factors for gastric cancer are listed in Box 18.5 on page 384.

Diagnosis of Gastric Cancer

The number of annual new gastric cancer cases has been declining over the past 10 years, and from 2007 to 2016, the death rates for gastric cancer decreased by 2.1% each year. The incidence of early gastric cancer has been increasing compared to that

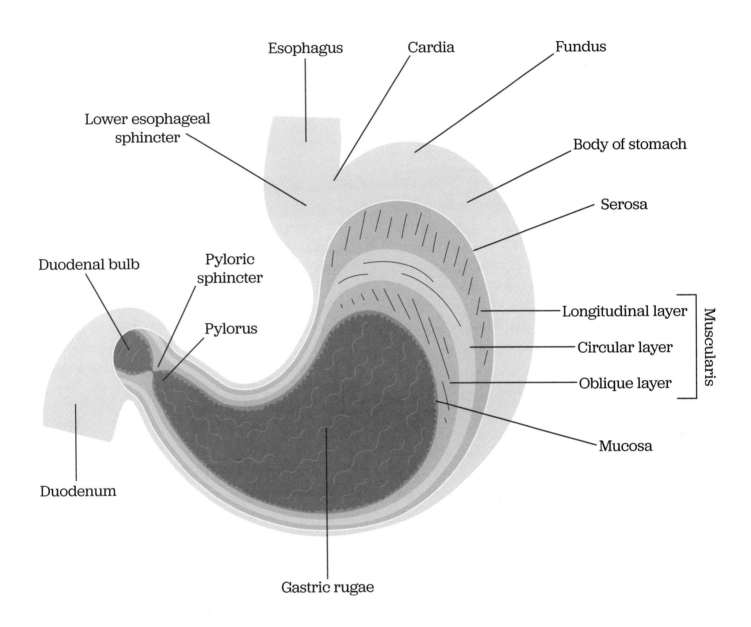

Esophagus   Cardia   Fundus

Lower esophageal
sphincter

Body of stomach

Serosa

Duodenal bulb   Pyloric
sphincter

Pylorus

Longitudinal layer
Circular layer   Muscularis
Oblique layer

Mucosa

Duodenum

Gastric rugae

Figure 18.2
Normal anatomy of the stomach

Helicobacter pylori gastric infection

Advanced age

Male sex

Diet low in fruits and vegetables

Diet high in salted, smoked, or preserved foods

Chronic atrophic gastritis

Intestinal metaplasia

Pernicious anemia

Gastric adenomatous polyps

Family history of gastric cancer

Cigarette smoking

Ménétrier disease

Epstein-Barr virus

Familial sydromes including familial adenomatous polyposis

of advanced gastric cancer due to increased efforts to screen and the use of advanced diagnostic instruments. Gastric cancers are diagnosed by upper GI endoscopy and biopsy, and possibly via upper endoscopic ultrasound. Staging of gastric cancer may use results from the following: endoscopic ultrasound, computed tomography scan, positron emission tomography scan, magnetic resonance imaging, and laparoscopy.[93]

Symptoms

Symptoms that present at the early stages of gastric cancer may include indigestion, postprandial bloating, nausea, decreased appetite, and reflux. As cancer progresses, and in more advanced stages of gastric cancer, patients may be more symptomatic, presenting with heme-positive stools, vomiting, stomach pain, jaundice, ascites, and dysphagia.[93]

Malnutrition can occur in up to 80% of patients with advanced stages of gastric cancer. Weight loss of more than 10% in 6 months is evident in 15% of patients with gastroesophageal cancers.[95]

Treatment of Gastric Cancer

Gastric cancer is often treated using a multimodal approach. Treatment is based on tumor resectability,

according to the *NCCN Clinical Practice Guidelines in Oncology (NCCN Guidelines): Gastric Cancer*.[96] Patients with potentially resectable tumors may require perioperative chemotherapy or preoperative chemoradiation therapy followed by adjuvant chemotherapy after surgical resection. Patients with unresectable disease may elect to have chemoradiation, systemic therapy, or palliative management. Nonsurgical candidates may have chemoradiation or palliative management. Refer to the NCCN guidelines for details of specific therapies.[96]

Surgery

Figure 18.3 illustrates several types of reconstruction following gastrectomy. Standard treatment options for stage I, II, and III include any one of the following surgeries[93]:

- distal subtotal gastrectomy (if the lesion is not in the fundus or at the cardioesophageal junction)

- proximal subtotal gastrectomy or total gastrectomy (if the lesion involves the cardia)

- total gastrectomy (if the tumor involves the stomach diffusely or arises in the body of the stomach and extends to within 6 cm of the cardia)

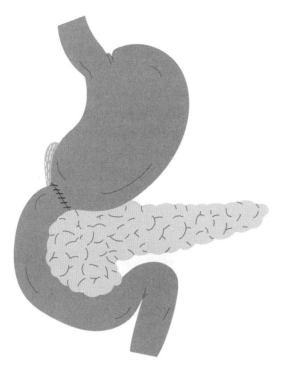

Partial gastrectomy (Billroth I) involves a gastroduodenostomy, with anastomosis between the distal gastric segment and the proximal duodenum.

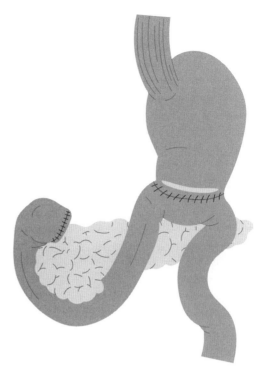

Partial gastrectomy (Billroth II) involves gastrojejunostomy, with anastomosis between the distal gastric segment and the proximal jejunum. A blind loop of duodenum is created to maintain flow of bile salts and pancreatic enzymes.

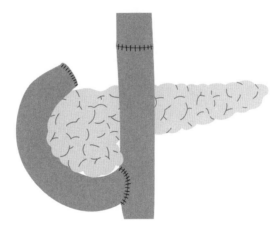

Total gastrectomy involves removal of the stomach with Roux-en-Y reconstruction (ie, the jejunum is pulled up and anastomosed to the esophagus). The duodenum is connected to the small bowel so bile salts and pancreatic enzymes can continue to flow into the intestine.

Figure 18.3
Types of reconstruction after gastrectomy

A partial gastrectomy with reconstruction may be performed as a Billroth I or Billroth II procedure. In a study comparing outcomes in patients who received Billroth I vs Billroth II gastrectomy, nutritional indexes and body weight were similar when compared in the short and the long term.[97] Size of remnant stomach after distal gastrectomy was associated with benefits, such as reduced reflux esophagitis, more stable body weight, and better food intake in the Billroth I group. In patients with cancers in the lower third of the stomach, a larger remnant stomach can improve nutritional status and reduce symptoms.[98]

Nutrition Problems and Interventions Specific to Gastric Cancer

Nutrition Impact Symptoms

Side effects of the treatment for gastric cancer vary depending on the modality of treatment, concurrent therapy, and whether therapy is adjuvant or neoadjuvant. Disease-related issues that affect nutritional status in this population include anorexia-cachexia, dysphagia, early satiety, nausea, and vomiting.[95] Treatment-related nutrition impact symptoms vary by treatment modality and can include nausea, vomiting, constipation, diarrhea, reflux, early and prolonged satiety, anorexia, and mouth sores. See Chapters 9 and 10 for a detailed description of side effects due to chemotherapy and radiation and Chapter 11 for symptom management.

Perioperative Medical Nutrition Therapy

Consensus guidelines for enhanced recovery after gastrectomy were published by the ERAS Study Group in 2014.[99] The procedure-specific guidelines consist of eight elements: preoperative nutrition, preoperative oral pharmaconutrition, access, wound catheters and transversus abdominis plane block, nasogastric or nasojejunal decompression, perianastomotic drains, early postoperative diet and artificial nutrition, and audit. The ERAS Study Group protocol for gastric cancer surgery has helped to reduce costs and shorten hospital LOS and has not increased surgical complication rates.[99,100]

The evidence was graded for each summary and recommendation. Despite very low evidence to support routine use of preoperative artificial nutrition, there is a strong recommendation that this is not warranted unless the patient is significantly malnourished.[99] Moderate evidence supports early postoperative diet, with the recommendation that patients undergoing total gastrectomy be offered food and drink at will from postoperative day one. This recommendation is based on the fact that no study to date has reported an adverse effect as a result of early oral feeding.[101-103] Patients who are unable to meet 60% of their energy intake needs by postoperative day 6 should be considered individually for nutrition support.[99]

There is no clear evidence of improved clinical outcomes with the use of enteral IN in patients undergoing gastrectomy.[99]

Sarcopenia

The incidence of sarcopenia in this population is reported to be 21.2%. When preoperative energy and protein intakes were compared, they were found to be significantly lower in sarcopenic vs nonsarcopenic patients. Sarcopenia also has been identified as an independent risk factor for postoperative severe complications. One study examined a preoperative nutrition and exercise program for elderly patients with gastric cancer who had sarcopenia and were undergoing gastrectomy. Although this was a pilot study with small sample size, it was the first to look at an organized preoperative program for patients with gastric cancer. Measures of handgrip strength, gait speed, and skeletal muscle mass index increased as a result of the program with the potential to improve sarcopenia.[104]

Nutrition Support

Patients with gastric cancer may require nutrition support if there are obstructive symptoms that impede their ability to maintain adequate nutrition. Patients generally undergo placement of a jejunostomy feeding tube, which can be performed open, laparoscopically, or percutaneously. PN may be reserved for short-term instances to include advancement to EN support or during recovery

from complications or surgery in specific situations.[105] Box 18.6 reviews the available evidence regarding the role of nutrition support in gastric cancer.

Common Postgastrectomy Complications

Malnutrition is among the more common postoperative complications of subtotal or total gastrectomy. Preoperative risk factors for severe postoperative malnutrition include age of more than 60 years, preoperative weight loss, gastric cancer, and open surgical procedure.[112] The most common nutrition-related postoperative complications include weight

---

Box 18.6
Evidence Regarding the Role of Nutrition Support in Gastric Cancer[106-112]

Type of support	Evidence
Preoperative	Preoperative nutritional status directly affects postoperative, disease-specific, and overall survival.[106]
Perioperative	Perioperative nutrition support for patients who are moderately or severely malnourished may reduce overall complications and hospital length of stay (LOS).[107]
	Perioperative and postoperative parenteral nutrition (PN) may reduce mortality and morbidity[106] in patients who are malnourished.[108]
	Perioperative nutritional parameters, such as body mass index, total lymphocyte count, and prognostic nutritional index, are independent prognostic factors.[109]
Postoperative	Early enteral nutrition (EN) improves early and long-term postoperative nutritional status.[106]
	Early postoperative enteral immunonutrition is superior to isocaloric formula, as it reduces hospital LOS, postoperative infections, and anastomotic leaks, and improves cellular immunity.[110]
	Enriched enteral formulas do not improve long-term survival but may affect survival within the first 6 months postoperatively.[111]
In advanced gastric cancer	Stage IV patients treated with chemotherapy and receiving medical nutrition therapy (MNT) have improved nutrition risk scores, indicating improved prognosis.[112]
	Short-term PN may improve quality of life and functional status in malnourished patients. PN may be considered in patients who are unable to take oral nutrition or EN.[106]

---

loss, gastric stasis, dumping syndrome, fat malabsorption, and nutrient deficiencies. Reportedly, patients who have undergone distal gastrectomy can experience up to 13% weight loss within 6 months, and patients who have undergone a total gastrectomy can experience up to 17% weight loss in 6 months.[113]

Malnutrition following surgery can have an impact on postoperative recovery and survival. One study examined the nutritional status in postoperative patients using the nutritional risk index (NRI) and nutritional risk screening (NRS). Malnourished patients (NRI < 97.5) showed a greater incidence of wound complications than nonmalnourished patients (NRI ≥ 97.5). Patients at high risk for malnutrition (NRS ≥ 3) with advanced gastric cancer showed significantly lower survival rates than those at low risk (NRS < 3) (median survival: 25.7 months vs 31.9 months, $P < .001$). Surgical patients who participated in a multidisciplinary program (eg, nutrition support) had shorter hospital length of stay than those receiving conventional treatment (mean length of stay 11.29 days vs 14.04 days, $P = .023$).[101] There are few studies examining postoperative nutritional status in patients, and most consider only short-term nutritional outcomes.[114]

Postgastrectomy syndromes result from altered form and function of the stomach. Early recognition and treatment of these symptoms and treatment of vitamin and mineral deficiencies to reduce chronic complications involves a team approach in risk assessment, patient education, and postoperative management to promote optimal care.[115] Box 18.7 on pages 390 to 393 discusses common postgastrectomy syndromes including incidence, mechanism, symptoms, evaluation, and management.

Nutritional deficiencies are most pronounced after gastrectomy. Given that gastric cancer is asymptomatic or minimally symptomatic for an extended period before diagnosis, preoperative nutritional deficiencies and weight loss can develop insidiously.[115] Box 18.8 on pages 394 to 395 outlines nutrient deficiencies associated with gastrectomy surgery.

Vitamin and mineral deficiencies should be monitored and replenished and peripheral blood levels should be monitored to guide therapy. Some programs recommend a multivitamin supplement that includes vitamin B12, vitamin D, calcium, and iron. At 1, 3, 6, 9, and 12 months after surgery, patients should be weighed and evaluated by a registered dietitian nutritionist (RDN); serum levels for thiamine, red blood cell folate, iron, vitamin B12, methylmalonic acid, zinc, 25-hydroxyvitamin D, prealbumin, and C-reactive protein should be checked; and a complete blood count and basic metabolic panel should be obtained.[115]

Palliative Nutrition Management of Gastric Cancer

In patients with advanced gastric cancer who are not surgical candidates and who may be undergoing palliative treatment, often symptom management is the priority and should involve a multidisciplinary team. Symptoms can include dysphagia and gastric outlet obstruction, pending degree of tumor burden in the lumen of the stomach. Symptoms can be quantified using the Dysphagia Grading Score or the Gastric Outlet Obstruction Grading Score. Palliation of obstruction or dysphagia may include gastric dilation using endoscopy. This may provide instant but not often durable relief. Gastric stenting performed via endoscopy, which more often provides long-lasting relief from obstruction by a tumor, can also be considered. Gastroduodenal stent placement has been found to be feasible, effective, and safe in the management of gastric outlet obstruction. It can provide immediate relief of symptoms but is not without risk; risks include perforation, a sense of pressure experienced by patient, and stent migration, or it can lead to obstruction with tumor progression. Other therapies that may be used in conjunction with dilation or stenting include endoluminal brachytherapy, photodynamic therapy, laser therapy, endoscopic alcohol injection, endoscopic injection of chemotherapy, argon plasma coagulation, and cryoablation. Surgical palliation of obstruction or dysphagia, which may involve bypass procedures (such as gastrojejunostomy) or palliative resection, can also be considered. Retrospective studies indicate that the median symptom-free duration was longer in patients who received surgical palliative procedures, with the longest overall survival in the palliative resection group.[105]

Survivorship and Gastric Cancer

Postoperative nutrition surveillance of patients undergoing total gastrectomy is imperative. Adjuvant therapy for 6 months or more has been identified as the single independent risk factor for significant postoperative loss of skeletal muscle mass.[116]

There are few studies investigating long-term postoperative medical nutrition therapy for patients with gastric cancer. Future studies may need to include additional ways to improve the quality of long-term intervention in these patients.[101] Patients who undergo total or distal gastrectomy with Roux-en-Y anastomosis or adjuvant therapy should be monitored for malnutrition for the first postoperative year. Patients who undergo total gastrectomy should be monitored for both malnutrition and anemia for 5 years. Patients who have received adjuvant chemotherapy also should be monitored for anemia for 1 year after surgery.[92]

Summary

RDNs are an integral part of the multidisciplinary team in the management of patients with EC. Routine nutrition screening and assessment are indicated at the time of diagnosis, throughout the course of treatment, and during recovery. Standardized postoperative nutrition pathways are lacking, and the pursuit of early EN and early oral feeding warrants further research.

In newly diagnosed gastric cancer, the incidence of malnutrition ranges from 65% to 85%. Research demonstrates that weight loss at presentation may be an independent prognostic variable of outcome in patients with gastric cancer.[112]

Early and intensive medical nutrition therapy may reduce complications, malnutrition, morbidity, and mortality in patients with gastric cancer. Preoperative nutritional deficiencies are common in this population. Nutritional assessment and preoperative management with a focus on preventive treatment are likely to decrease the incidence of severe complications. Care of patients after gastrectomy is enhanced through an integrated team approach to preoperative assessment, patient education, and effective management of postoperative symptoms and expected nutritional deficiencies.[115] Palliative supportive care is critical in managing obstruction and dysphagia in patients with metastatic disease to assure adequate nutrition in an effort to best support quality of life.

Box 18.7
Postgastrectomy Syndromes[115,117]

Small gastric remnant or early satiety syndrome

Incidence	Symptoms occur most often when more than 80% of the stomach is removed.
Mechanism	Loss of gastric capacity through resection or vagotomy resulting in loss of receptive relaxation and accommodation
Symptoms	Early satiety Epigastric pain soon after eating Vomiting
Management	Diet modifications: ■ Small-volume, frequent meals ■ Liquids consumed separate from solids at meals

Gastric stasis or Roux stasis syndrome

Incidence	0.4% to 30%
Mechanism	Hypomotility of remnant stomach Motor disturbances in jejunal limb Vagotomy and transection of the proximal small bowel during Roux creation. Vagotomy results in delayed gastric emptying, whereas small bowel transection disrupts coordination of small bowel contractions.
Symptoms	Nausea Pain Gas, bloating Postprandial fullness Symptoms relieved by vomiting

(continued)

Box 18.7

Postgastrectomy Syndromes[115,117] *(continued)*

Gastric stasis or Roux stasis syndrome (continued)

Evaluation	Gastric emptying may be evaluated by scintigraphy.
	Syndrome is diagnosed as early (occurring < 90 days postoperatively) or late.
	In the early syndrome, rule out small bowel obstruction.
	In the late syndrome, rule out internal hernia, adhesive bowel obstruction, malignant recurrence, and possible anastomotic stricture.
	Order endoscopy and fluoroscopic upper gastrointestinal (GI) studies to rule out other disorders because this syndrome is a diagnosis of exclusion. Most useful is scintigraphic imaging, which can measure gastric emptying and Roux limb transit.
	Treatment depends on severity of symptoms.
	Increased risk for small intestinal bacterial overgrowth (similar symptoms)
Management	Consider use of prokinetic or antiemetic medications.
	Consider diet modifications.
	Possible diet modifications for nausea and vomiting after meals:
	▪ Small-volume, frequent meals
	▪ Liquids rather than solid foods, as they are better tolerated
	▪ Liquid calories and pureed foods for easier emptying
	For persistent symptoms despite medications and diet modifications:
	▪ Initiate low-fat, low-fiber diet. Consumption of moderate- to high-fat liquids is usually tolerated.
	Surgical treatment: Consists of resection of the remnant stomach with Roux-en-Y esophagojejunostomy. If patient had a total gastrectomy or if the Roux limb is contributing to this syndrome, the only surgical management consists of placing a jejunostomy tube to maintain adequate nutrition.

Dumping syndrome

Incidence	20% to 50%
Mechanism	Decreased gastric reservoir and loss of pyloric sphincter
	Rapid influx of hyperosmolar contents into small bowel resulting in fluid shift from the intravascular space into the bowel lumen and release of hormones, including vasoactive inhibitory peptide, gastric inhibitory peptide, neurotensin, and serotonin, which affects GI secretion, motility, and splanchnic blood flow.
	Creation of intravascular hypovolemia lends to the release of epinephrine, resulting in the classic vasomotor symptoms of the syndrome.
	Luminal carbohydrate also increases release of enteroglucagon, resulting in hyperinsulinism and hypoglycemia, contributing to vasomotor symptoms and adrenaline response in late dumping.

(continued)

Box 18.7
Postgastrectomy Syndromes[115,117] *(continued)*

Dumping syndrome (continued)

Symptoms	Symptoms vary depending on timing of dumping (early vs late).[a]
Evaluation	Symptom evaluation Oral glucose tolerance test Diagnostic tests: ■ Technetium-labeled meal to assess gastric emptying ■ Clinical scoring system developed by Sigstad ■ Oral glucose challenge—highly sensitive and specific for dumping ■ Quality of life (QOL) questionnaires to assess GI symptoms ■ Endoscopy and contrast-enhanced fluoroscopic imaging of the upper GI tract
Management	In severe cases, medications such as octreotide or acarbose may be used to manage symptoms. Diet modifications may include: ■ Limit foods high in concentrated sugars. ■ Test tolerance to lactose-containing foods. ■ Avoid fried and greasy foods, but test tolerance to small amounts of fats. ■ Eat protein-rich foods and complex carbohydrates, specifically foods high in soluble fiber. ■ Drink liquids 30 minutes before or after meals but not during meals. ■ Eat five to six small meals daily and avoid large portions. ■ Eat slowly and chew food into very small pieces or until liquefied.

Postvagotomy diarrhea

Incidence	Occurs in any type of gastrectomy but more commonly with vagotomy
Mechanism	Multifactorial mechanisms; can include alterations in the rate of flow of enteric contents, including gastric emptying of liquids, small bowel and biliary vagal denervation, and malabsorption related to altered anatomy and transit
Symptoms	Episodic, explosive diarrhea unrelated to oral intake
Evaluation	Diagnosis can be challenging; all sources of diarrhea should be considered.

(continued)

[a] See Box 18.4 on page 381.

Box 18.7
Postgastrectomy Syndromes[115,117] (continued)

Postvagotomy diarrhea (continued)

Management	Watchful waiting, as symptoms may improve after several months
	Diet modifications
	Avoidance of instigating foods
	Fiber supplementation (may be effective)
	Addition of antidiarrheal agents (eg, loperamide) and cholestyramine

Bile reflux gastritis

Incidence	Most frequently found after Billroth II gastrectomy; decreased incidence after Billroth I gastrectomy and pyloroplasty
Mechanism	Bile reflux gastritis as a result of chronic exposure of the gastric remnant to biliopancreatic secretions caused by loss of the pylorus
Symptoms	Burning epigastric pain
	Nausea with vomiting that does not relieve the pain, and pain is only partially associated with meals
	Vomitus containing bile mixed with food
	Possible weight loss and anemia
Evaluation	Evaluate for pain, nausea, and bilious vomiting associated with endoscopic findings of bile and inflammation in the distal stomach.
	Hepatobiliary iminodiacetic acid scan may indicate pooling of bile in the stomach.
	Scintigraphy may reveal lack of gastric emptying.
	Endoscopy can assess the anastomosis and the gastric remnant. Biopsy may be required.
Management	Medical treatment has been found to be ineffective or does not lead to consistent symptom relief.
	Cholestyramine has been used.
	Ursodeoxycholic acid and sucralfate have shown minimal effect.
	Other options are antacids, promotility agents, histamine receptor blockers, proton pump inhibitors, and anticholinergics.
	Surgical therapy is the mainstay of treatment, which includes Roux-en-Y gastrojejunostomy to persuade biliopancreatic contents away from the gastric remnant.

Box 18.8
Nutrient Deficiencies and Related Conditions After Partial or Total Gastrectomy[115,117]

Vitamin B12 deficiency

Mechanism and incidence rates

Loss in gastric acid and intrinsic factor; may occur in presence of small intestinal bacterial overgrowth (SIBO)

Common after gastrectomy and often develops in less than 1 year

Recommendation

1,000 mcg of vitamin B12 intramuscularly once monthly, or 1,000 to 2,000 mcg/d orally

Folate deficiency

Mechanism and incidence rates

Secondary to malabsorption

Recommendation

Use red blood cell folate to measure serum levels

5 mg of folate daily to replete deficiency

Iron deficiency

Mechanism and incidence rates

Bypass of the duodenum after Roux-en-Y anastomosis, and less gastric acid and intrinsic factor are produced after a total gastrectomy.

Iron deficiency anemia in 50% of patients. Primary cause is lack of absorption from decreased gastric acid secretion, decreased intrinsic factor production, and bypass of the duodenum. Patients have a higher degree of anemia after total gastrectomy versus partial gastrectomy, and after Roux-en-Y gastrojejunostomy versus Billroth I reconstruction.

Recommendation

200 mg of ferrous sulfate three times daily (provides 67 mg of elemental iron per 200-mg tablet)

Bone disease

Mechanism and incidence rates

Incidence and mechanism are not definitive.

Decreased intake of calcium and vitamin D

Malabsorption of calcium—secondary to reconstruction of duodenum or rapid transit

Vitamin D loss results in calcium deficiency, which may lead to early-onset osteoporosis. Osteoporosis and fracture risk also are related to calcium malabsorption caused by decreased gastric acid production.

Recommendation

Check total calcium, ionized calcium, and parathyroid hormone levels to evaluate calcium deficiencies.

Monitor bone mineral density.

Increase consumption of calcium-rich foods.

Increase calcium intake (1,500 mg/d) if bone disease is confirmed.

Monitor serum 25-hydroxyvitamin D levels.

(continued)

Box 18.8
Nutrient Deficiencies and Related Conditions After Partial or Total Gastrectomy[115,117] (continued)

Fat malabsorption

Mechanism and incidence rates	Recommendation
Occurs in about 10% of patients	Evaluation can include 72-hour fecal fat test and fecal elastase concentration.[b]
More common when the duodenum is bypassed	Consider empirically treating SIBO.
Alterations in gastric lipase secretions, exocrine pancreatic insufficiency, altered cholecystokinin release, pancreaticobiliary asynchrony, SIBO	If no improvement is noted, consider pancreatic enzymes.[c]
Symptoms include steatorrhea, cramping, abdominal pain, and oily or foul-smelling diarrhea.	

[b] See Chapter 20 for more information.

[c] See Chapter 11 for more on symptom management.

Sample PES Statements for Esophageal and Gastric Cancers

Clinical domain: Unintended weight loss related to inadequate oral intake, as evidenced by ≥5% weight loss within 30 days.

Intake domain: Inadequate oral intake related to radiation-induced dysphagia, as evidenced by weight loss of 5 lbs in 1 week.

Clinical domain: Moderate, chronic disease- or condition-related malnutrition related to change in GI structure and function following esophageal surgery, as evidenced by dumping syndrome, a weight loss of 5% in past month, and observed mild muscle wasting of quadriceps.

References

1. Ferlay J, Soerjomataram I, Dikshit R, et al. Cancer incidence and mortality worldwide: sources, methods and major patterns in GLOBOCAN 2012. *Int J Cancer.* 2015;136(5):359-386. doi:10.1002/ijc.29210

2. American Cancer Society. Key statistics for esophageal cancer. American Cancer Society. Updated March 20, 2020. Accessed November 4, 2020. https://cancer.org/cancer/esophagus-cancer/about/key-statistics.html

3. Surveillance Epidemiology and End Results Program. Cancer stat facts: esophageal cancer. National Cancer Institute. Accessed November 4, 2020. https://seer.cancer.gov/statfacts/html/esoph.html

4. World Cancer Research Fund International/American Institute for Cancer Research. Continuous update project report: diet, nutrition, physical activity and oesophageal cancer. Published 2016. Accessed December 6, 2017. http://aicr.org/continuous-update-project/reports/oesophageal-cancer-cup-report.pdf

5. Rubenstein JH, Shaheen NJ. Epidemiology, diagnosis, and management of esophageal adenocarcinoma. *Gastroenterology.* 2015;149(2):302-317. doi:10.1053/j.gastro.2015.04.053

6. American Cancer Society. Esophagus cancer. American Cancer Society. Accessed November 4, 2020. https://cancer.org/cancer/esophagus-cancer.html

7. National Comprehensive Cancer Network. *NCCN Clinical Guidelines for Patients: Esophageal Cancer.* National Comprehensive Cancer Network; Accessed April 28, 2019. https://nccn.org/patients/guidelines/content/PDF/esophageal.pdf

8. Esophagus cancer: early detection, diagnosis, and staging. American Cancer Society website. Updated June 14, 2017. Accessed April 28, 2019. www.cancer.org/cancer/esophagus-cancer/detection-diagnosis-staging.html

9. National Comprehensive Cancer Network. *NCCN Clinical Practice Guidelines in Oncology: Esophageal and Esophagogastric Junction Cancers.* Version 1.2021. National Comprehensive Cancer Network; 2021. Accessed March 1, 2021. http://isesnet.org/wp-content/uploads/2013/02/NCCN-esophagus-2012.pdf

10. Straughan DM, Azoury SC, Bennett RD, Pimiento JM, Fontaine JP, Toloza EM. Robotic-assisted esophageal surgery. *Cancer Control.* 2015;22(3):335-339. doi:10.1177/107327481502200312

11. Barreto JC, Posner MC. Transhiatal versus transthoracic esophagectomy for esophageal cancer. *World J Gastroenterol.* 2010;16(30):3804-3810. doi:10.3748/wjg.v16.i30.3804

12. Arnold M, Laversanne M, Brown LM, Devesa SS, Bray F. Predicting the future burden of esophageal cancer by histological subtype: international trends in incidence up to 2030. *Am J Gastroenterol.* 2017;112(8):1247-1255. doi:10.1038/ajg.2017.155

13. Arnal MJD, Arenas ÁF, Arbeloa ÁL. Esophageal cancer: risk factors, screening and endoscopic treatment in western and eastern countries. *World J Gastroenterol.* 2015;21(26):7933-7943. doi:10.3748/wjg.v21.i26.7933

14. Lauby-Secretan B, Scoccianti C, Loomis D, Grosse Y, Bianchini F, Straif K. Body fatness and cancer—viewpoint of the IARC working group. *N Engl J Med.* 2016;375:794-798. doi:10.1056/NEJMsr1606602

15. Vingeliene S, Chan DSM, Vieira AR, et al. An update of the WCRF/AICR systematic literature review and meta-analysis on dietary and anthropometric factors and esophageal cancer risk. *Ann Oncol.* 2017;28(7):2409-2419. doi:10.1007/s10552-016-0755-0

16. American Cancer Society. *Cancer Facts & Figures 2020.* American Cancer Society; 2020. www.cancer.org/research/cancer-facts-statistics/all-cancer-facts-figures/cancer-facts-figures-2020.html

17. Katada C, Yokoyama T, Yano T, et al. Alcohol consumption and multiple dysplastic lesions increase risk of squamous cell carcinoma in the esophagus, head, and neck. *Gastroenterology*. 2016;151(5):860-869. doi:10.1053/j.gastro.2016.07.040

18. Moore SC, Lee IM, Weiderpass E, et al. Association of leisure-time physical activity with risk of 26 types of cancer in 1.44 million adults. *JAMA Intern Med*. 2016;176(6):816-825. doi:10.1001/jamainternmed.2016.1548

19. National Cancer Institute. Esophageal cancer treatment (PDQ)–health professional version. Updated 2017. Accessed January 3, 2018. https://cancer.gov/types/esophageal/hp/esophageal-treatment-pdq

20. Dai Y, Li C, Xie Y, et al. Interventions for dysphagia in oesophageal cancer. *Cochrane Database Syst Rev*. 2014;(10). doi:10.1002/14651858.CD005048.pub4

21. Huddy JR, Huddy FMS, Markar SR, Tucker O. Nutritional optimization during neoadjuvant therapy prior to surgical resection of esophageal cancer—a narrative review. *Dis Esophagus*. 2017;31(1):1-11. doi:10.1093/dote/dox110

22. Martin RC, Cannon RM, Brown, RE, et al. Evaluation of quality of life following placement of self-expanding plastic stents as a bridge to surgery in patients receiving neoadjuvant therapy for esophageal cancer. *Oncologist*. 2014;19(3):259-265. doi:10.1634/theoncologist.2013-0344

23. Smith ZL, Gonzaga JE, Haasler GB, Gore EM, Dua KS. Self-expanding metal stents improve swallowing and maintain nutrition during neoadjuvant therapy for esophageal cancer. *Dig Dis Sci*. 2017;62(6):1647-1656. doi:10.1007/s10620-017-4562-6

24. So H, Ahn JY, Han S, et al. Efficacy and safety of fully covered self-expanding metal stents for malignant esophageal obstruction. *Dig Dis Sci*. 2018;63(1):234-241. doi:10.1007/s10620-017-4839-9

25. Bower M, Jones W, Vessels B, Scoggins C, Martin R. Role of esophageal stents in the nutrition support of patients with esophageal malignancy. *Nutr Clin Pract*. 2010;25(3):244-249. doi:10.1177/0884533610368871024

26. Academy of Nutrition and Dietetics Evidence Analysis Library. ONC chemotherapy: protein, intervention, by a dietitian and chemoradiation therapy: esophogeal cancer. Accessed December 6, 2017. www.andeal.org/topic.cfm?cat=2959&evidence_summary id=250546&highlight=esophogeal&home=1

27. Thompson KL, Elliott L, Fuchs-Tarlovsky V, Levin RM, Voss AC, Piemonte T. Oncology evidence-based nutrition practice guideline for adults. *J Acad Nutr Diet*. 2017;117(2):297-310. doi:10.1016/j.jand.2016.05.010

28. Xu Y-J, Cheng JC-H, Lee J-M, Huang P-M, et al. A walk-and-eat intervention improves outcomes for patients with esophageal cancer undergoing neoadjuvant chemoradiotherapy. *Oncologist*. 2015;20:1216-1222. doi:10.1634/theoncologist.2015-0178

29. Silvers MA, Savva J, Huggins CE, Truby H, Haines T. Potential benefits of early nutritional intervention in adults with upper gastrointestinal cancer: a pilot randomised trial. *Support Care Cancer*. 2014;22:3035-3044. doi:10.1007/s00520-014-2311-3

30. Cong M-H, Li S-L, Cheng G-W, et al. An interdisciplinary nutrition support team improves clinical and hospitalized outcomes of esophageal cancer patients with concurrent chemoradiotherapy. *Chin Med J*. 2015;128(22):3003-3007. doi:10.4103/0366-6999.168963

31. Odelli C, Burgess D, Bateman L, et al. Nutrition support improves patient outcomes, treatment tolerance and admission characteristics in oesophageal cancer. *Clin Oncol (R Coll Radiol)*. 2005;17(8):639-645.

32. Wang JY, Hong X, Chen GH, Li QC, Liu ZM. Clinical application of the fast track surgery model based on preoperative nutritional risk screening in patients with esophageal cancer. *Asia Pac J Clin Nutr*. 2015;24(2):206-211. doi:10.6133/apjcn.2015.24.2.18

33. Wu J, Huang C, Xiao H, Tang Q, Cai W. Weight loss and resting energy expenditure in male patients with newly diagnosed esophageal cancer. *Nutrition*. 2013;29:1310-1314. doi:10.1016/j.nut.2013.04.010

34. Ceolin Alves AL, Zuconi CP, Correia MI. Energy expenditure in patients with esophageal, gastric, and colorectal cancer. *J Parenter Enter Nutr*. 2016;40(4):499-506. doi:10.1177/0148607114567336

35. Okamoto H, Saki M, Johtatsu T, et al. Resting energy expenditure and nutritional status in patients undergoing transthoracic esophagectomy for esophageal cancer. *J Clin Biochem Nutr*. 2011;49(3):169-173. doi:10.3164/jcbn.11-13

36. Larrea J, Vega S, Martínez T, Torrent JM, Vega V, Nunez V. The nutritional status and immunological situation of cancer patients. *Nutr Hosp*. 1992;7(3):178-184.

37. Quyen TC, Angkatavanich J, Van Thuan T, Van Xuan V, Tuyen LD, Tu DA. Nutrition assessment and its relationship with performance and Glasgow prognostic scores in Vietnamese patients with esophageal cancer. *Asia Pac J Clin Nutr*. 2017;26(1):49-58. doi:10.6133/apjcn.122015.02

38. Grace EM, Shaw C, Lalji A, Mohammed K, Andreyev HJN, Whelan K. Nutritional status, the development and persistence of malnutrition and dietary intake in oesophago-gastric cancer: a longitudinal cohort study. *J Hum Nutr Diet*. 2018;31:785-792. doi:10.1111/jhn.12588

39. Cox S, Powell C, Carter B, Hurt C, Mukherjee S, Crosby TDL. Role of nutritional status and intervention in oesophageal cancer treated with definitive chemoradiotherapy: outcomes from SCOPE1. *Br J Cancer*. 2016;115:172-177. doi:10.1038/bjc.2016.129

40. Martin L, Birdsell L, MacDonald N, et al. Cancer cachexia in the age of obesity: skeletal muscle depletion is a powerful prognostic factor, independent of body mass index. *J Clin Oncol*. 2013;31(12):1539-1547. doi:10.1200/JCO.2012.45.2722

41. Anandavadivelan P, Brismar TB, Nilsson M, Johar AM, Martin L. Sarcopenic obesity: a probable risk factor for dose limiting toxicity during neo-adjuvant chemotherapy in oesophageal cancer patients. *Clin Nutr*. 2016;35(3):724-730. doi:10.1016/j.clnu.2015.05.011

42. Lakenman P, Ottens-Oussoren K, Witvliet-van Nierop J, van der Peet D, de van der Schueren M. Handgrip strength is associated with treatment modifications during neoadjuvant chemoradiation in patients with esophageal cancer. *Nutr Clin Pract*. 2017;32(5):652-657. doi:10.1177/0884533617700862

43. Filip B, Scarpa M, Cavallin F, et al. Postoperative outcome after oesophagectomy for cancer: nutritional status is the missing ring in the current prognostic scores. *Eur J Surg Oncol*. 2015;41(6):787-794. doi:10.1016/j.ejso.2015.02.014

44. Sunpaweravong S, Ruangsin S, Laohawiriyakamol S, Mahattanobon S, Geater A. Prediction of major postoperative complications and survival for locally advanced esophageal carcinoma patients. *Asian J Surg*. 2012;35:104-109. doi:10.1016/j.asjsur.2012.04.029

45. Elliott JA, Doyle SL, Murphy CF, et al. Sarcopenia: prevalence, and impact on operative and oncologic outcomes in the multimodal management of locally advanced esophageal cancer. *Ann Surg.* 2017;266(5):822–830. doi:10.1097/SLA.0000000000002398

46. Ida S, Watanabe M, Yoshida N, et al. Sarcopenia is a predictor of postoperative respiratory complications in patients with esophageal cancer. *Ann Surg Oncol.* 2015;22:4432-4437. doi:10.1245/s10434-015-4559-3

47. Makiura D, Ono R, Inoue J, et al. Impact of sarcopenia on unplanned readmission and survival after esophagectomy in patients with esophageal cancer. *Ann Surg Oncol.* 2018;25:456-464. doi:10.1245/s10434-017-6294-4

48. Reisinger KW, Bosmans JWAM, Uittenbogaart M, et al. Loss of skeletal muscle mass during neoadjuvant chemoradiotherapy predicts postoperative mortality in esophageal cancer surgery. *Ann Surg Oncol.* 2015;22(13):4445–4452. doi:10.1245/s10434-015-4558-4

49. Järvinen T, Ilonen I, Kauppi J, Salo J, Räsänen J. Loss of skeletal muscle mass during neoadjuvant treatments correlates with worse prognosis in esophageal cancer: a retrospective cohort study. *World J Surg Oncol.* 2018;16:27. doi:10.1186/s12957-018-1327-4

50. Siegal SR, Dolan JP, Dewey EN, et al. Sarcopenia is not associated with morbidity, mortality, or recurrence after esophagectomy for cancer. *Am J Surg.* 2017;1-5. doi:10.1016/j.amjsurg.2017.12.017

51. van der Schaaf MK, Tilanus HW, van Lanschot JJB, et al. The influence of preoperative weight loss on the postoperative course after esophageal cancer resection. *J Thorac Cardiovasc Surg.* 2014;147(1):490-495. doi:10.1016/j.jtcvs.2013.07.072

52. Academy of Nutrition and Dietetics Evidence Analysis Library. Esophageal Cancer (2007). Is there a relationship between enteral nutrition to enhance nutritional intake (protein, kcals) to improve tolerance and support recovery from chemoradiation therapy for esophageal cancer patients, and the reduction of complications associated with treatment? Accessed October 29, 2020. www.andeal.org/topic.cfm?menu=5291&pcat=1058&cat=3239

53. Miyata H, Yano M, Yasuda T, et al. Randomized study of clinical effect of enteral nutrition support during neoadjuvant chemotherapy on chemotherapy-related toxicity in patients with esophageal cancer. *Clin Nutr.* 2012;31(3):330-336. doi:10.1016/j.clnu.2011.11.002

54. Sunpaweravong S, Puttawibul P, Ruangsin S. Randomized study of antiinflammatory and immune-modulatory effects of enteral immunonutrition during concurrent chemoradiotherapy for esophageal cancer. *Nutr Cancer.* 2014;66(1):1-5. doi:10.1080/01635581.2014.847473

55. Miyata H, Yano M, Yasuda T, et al. Randomized study of the clinical effects of ω-3 fatty acid–containing enteral nutrition support during neoadjuvant chemotherapy on chemotherapy-related toxicity in patients with esophageal cancer. *Nutrition.* 2017;33:204-210. doi:10.1016/j.nut.2016.07.004

56. Gupta V. Benefits versus risks: a prospective audit. Feeding jejunostomy during esophagectomy. *World J Surg.* 2009;33(7):1432-1538.

57. Wang G, Chen H, Liu J, Ma Y, Jia H. A comparison of postoperative early enteral nutrition with delayed enteral nutrition in patients with esophageal cancer. *Nutrients.* 2015;7(6):4308-4317. doi:10.3390/nu7064308

58. Wani ML, Ahangar AG, Lone GN, et al. Feeding jejunostomy: does the benefit overweight the risk (a retrospective study from a single centre). *Int J Surg.* 2010;8(5):387-390. doi:10.1016/j.ijsu.2010.05.009

59. Barlow R, Price P, Reid TD, et al. Prospective multicentre randomised controlled trial of early enteral nutrition for patients undergoing major upper gastrointestinal surgical resection. *Clin Nutr*. 2011;30(5):560-566. doi:10.1016/j.clnu.2011.02.006

60. Bowrey DJ, Baker M, Halliday V, et al. A randomised controlled trial of six weeks of home enteral nutrition versus standard care after oesophagectomy or total gastrectomy for cancer: report on a pilot and feasibility study. *Trials*. 2015;16(531). doi:10.1186/s13063-015-1053-y

61. Wu W, Zhong M, Zhu D, et al. Effect of early full-calorie nutrition support following esophagectomy. *JPEN J Parenter Enter Nutr*. 2017;41(7):1146-1154. doi:10.1177/0148607116651509

62. Takesue T, Takeuchi H, Ogura M, et al. A prospective randomized trial of enteral nutrition after thoracoscopic esophagectomy for esophageal cancer. *Ann Surg Oncol*. 2015;22:802-809. doi:10.1245/s10434-015-4767-x

63. Yu HM, Tang CW, Feng WM, Chen QQ, Xu YQ, Bao Y. Early enteral nutrition versus parenteral nutrition after resection of esophageal cancer: a retrospective analysis. *Indian J Surg*. 2017;79(1):13-18. doi:10.1007/s12262-015-1420-7

64. Fujita T, Daiko H, Nishimura M. Early enteral nutrition reduces the rate of life-threatening complications after thoracic esophagectomy in patients with esophageal cancer. *Eur Surg Res*. 2012;48(2):79-84. doi:10.1159/000336574

65. Takeuchi H, Ikeuchi S, Kawaguchi Y, et al. Clinical significance of perioperative immunonutrition for patients with esophageal cancer. *World J Surg*. 2007;31(11):2160-2167. doi:10.1007/s00268-007-9219-8

66. Tanaka K, Yano M, Motoori M, Kishi K, et al. Impact of perioperative administration of synbiotics in patients with esophageal cancer undergoing esophagectomy: a prospective randomized controlled trial. *Surgery*. 2012;152(5):832-842. doi:10.1016/j.surg.2012.02.021

67. Matsuda Y, Habu D, Lee S, Kishida S, Osugi H. Enteral diet enriched with omega-3 fatty acid improves oxygenation after thoracic esophagectomy for cancer: A randomized controlled trial. *World J Surg*. 2018;41:1584. doi:10.1007/s00268-017-3893-y

68. Healy LA, Ryan A, Doyle SL, et al. Does prolonged enteral feeding with supplemental omega-3 fatty acids impact on recovery post-esophagectomy: results of a double blind randomized trial. *Ann* Surg. 2017;266(5):720-728. doi:10.1097/SLA.0000000000002390

69. Mudge LA, Watson DI, Smithers BM, Isenring EA, Smith L and Jamieson GG. Multicentre factorial randomized clinical trial of perioperative immunonutrition versus standard nutrition for patients undergoing surgical resection of oesophageal cancer. *BJS*. 2018;105:1262-72. doi:10.1002/bjs.10923

70. Weimann A, Braga M, Carli F, et al. ESPEN guideline: clinical nutrition in surgery. *Clin Nutr*. 2017;36:623-650. doi:10.1016/j.clnu.2017.02.013

71. Sun H, Liu X, Zhang R, et al. Early oral feeding following thoracolaparoscopic oesophagectomy for oesophageal cancer. *Eur J Cardiothorac Surg*. 2015;47(2):227-233. doi:10.1093/ejcts/ezu168

72. Giacopuzzi S, Weindelmayer J, Treppiedi E, et al. Enhanced recovery after surgery protocol in patients undergoing esophagectomy for cancer: a single center experience. *Dis Esophagus*. 2017;30(4):1-6. doi:10.1093/dote/dow024

73. Weijs TJ, Nieuwenhuijzen GA, Dolmans AC, et al. Immediate postoperative oral nutrition following esophagectomy: a multicenter clinical trial. *Ann Thorac Surg*. 2016;102(4):1141-1148. doi:10.1016/j.athoracsur.2016.04.067

74. Mahmoodzadeh H, Shoar S, Sirati F, Khorgami Z. Early initiation of oral feeding following upper gastrointestinal tumor surgery: a randomized controlled trial. *Surg Today*. 2015;45(2):203-208. doi:10.1007/s00595-014-0937-x

75. Lopes LP, Menezes TM, Toledo DO, De-Oliveira ATT, Longatto-Filho A, Nascimento JEA. Early oral feeding post-upper gastrointestinal tract resection and primary anastomosis in oncology. *ABCD Arq Bras Cir Dig*. 2018;31(1): e1359. doi:10.1590/0102-672020180001e1359

76. Zhu Z, Li Y, Zheng Y, et al. Chewing 50 times per bite could help to resume oral feeding on the first postoperative day following minimally invasive oesophagectomy. *Eur J Cardiothorac Surg*. 2018;53:325-30. doi:10.1093/ejcts/ezx291

77. Sun HB, Li Y, Liu XB, et al. Early oral feeding following McKeown minimally invasive esophagectomy an open-label, randomized, controlled, noninferiority trial. *Ann Surg*. 2018;267(3):435-442. doi:10.1097/SLA.0000000000002304

78. Chen KN. Managing complications I: leaks, strictures, emptying, reflux, chylothorax. *J Thorac Dis*. 2014;6(suppl 3):355-363. doi:10.3978/j.issn.2072-1439.2014.03.36

79. Tack J, Arts J, Caenepeel P, De Wulf D, Bisschops R. Pathophysiology, diagnosis and management of postoperative dumping syndrome. *Nat Rev Gastroenterol Hepatol*. 2009.6(10):583-590. doi:10.1038/nrgastro.2009.148

80. Ukleja A. Dumping syndrome. *Pract Gastroenterol*. 2006;35:32-46.

81. van Beek AP, Emous M, Laville M, Tack J. Dumping syndrome after esophageal, gastric or bariatric surgery: pathophysiology, diagnosis, and management. *Obes Rev*. 2017;18(1):68-85. doi:10.1111/obr.12467

82. Heneghan HM, Zaborowski A, Fanning M, et al. Prospective study of malabsorption and malnutrition after esophageal and gastric cancer surgery. *Ann Surg*. 2015;262(5):803-808. doi:10.1097/SLA.0000000000001445

83. Kiefer T, Krahl D, Osthoff K, et al. Importance of pancreatic enzyme replacement therapy after surgery of cancer of the esophagus or the esophagogastric junction. *Nutr Cancer*. 2018;70(1):69-72. doi:10.1080/01635581.2017.1374419

84. Huddy JR, Macharg FM, Lawn AM, Preston SR. Exocrine pancreatic insufficiency following esophagectomy. *Dis Esophagus*. 2013;26(6):594–597. doi:10.1111/dote.12004

85. Reynolds JV, Donohoe CL, McGillycuddy E, et al. Evolving progress in oncologic and operative outcomes for esophageal and junctional cancer: lessons from the experience of a high-volume center. *J Thorac Cardiovasc Surg*. 2012;143(5):1130-1137. doi:10.1016/j.jtcvs.2011.12.003

86. Sorianoa TT, Eslick GD, Vanniasinkam T. Long-term nutritional outcome and health related quality of life of patients following esophageal cancer surgery: a meta-analysis. *Nutr Cancer*. 2018;70(2);192-203. doi:10.1080/01635581.2018.1412471

87. Haverkort EB, Binnekade JM, Busch ORC, van Berge Henegouwen MI, de Haan RJ, Gouma DJ. Presence and persistence of nutrition-related symptoms during the first year following esophagectomy with gastric tube reconstruction in clinically disease-free patients. *World J Surg*. 2010;34(12):2844-2852. doi:10.1007/s00268-010-0786-8

88. Baker M, Halliday V, Williams RN, Bowrey DJ. A systematic review of the nutritional consequences of esophagectomy. *Clin Nutr*. 2016;35(5):987-994. doi:10.1016/j.clnu.2015.08.010

89. Greene CL, DeMeester SR, Worrell SG, Oh DS, Hagen JA, DeMeester TR. Alimentary satisfaction, gastrointestinal symptoms, and quality of life 10 or more years after esophagectomy with gastric pull-up. *J Thorac Cardiovasc Surg*. 2014;147(3):909-914. doi:10.1016/j.jtcvs.2013.11.004

90. Haverkort EB, Binnekade JM, de Haan RJ, Busch OR, van Berge Henegouwen MI, Gouma DJ. Suboptimal intake of nutrients after esophagectomy with gastric tube reconstruction. *J Acad Nutr Diet*. 2012;112(7):1080-1087. doi:10.1016/j.jand.2012.03.032

91. Surveillance Epidemiology and End Results Program. Cancer stat facts: stomach cancer. National Cancer Institute. Accessed October 29, 2020. https://seer.cancer.gov/statfacts/html/stomach.html

92. Kim KH, Park DJ, Park YS, Ahn SH, Park DJ, Kim HH. Actual 5-year nutritional outcomes of patients with gastric cancer. *J Gastric Cancer*. 2017;17(2):99-109. doi:10.5230/jgc.2017.17.e12

93. National Cancer Institute. Gastric cancer treatment (PDQ)–health professional version. Accessed May 19, 2019. www.cancer.gov/types/stomach/hp/stomach-treatment-pdq

94. Kim DW. Actual compliance to adjuvant chemotherapy in gastric cancer. *Ann of Surg Treatment and Research*. 2019;96(4):185-190. doi:10.4174/astr.2019.96.4.185

95. Rosania R, Chiapponi C, Malfertheiner P, Venerito M. Nutrition in patients with gastric cancer: an update. *Gastrointest Tumors*. 2016;2:178-187. doi:10.1159/000445188

96. National Comprehensive Cancer Network. *NCCN Clinical Practice Guidelines in Oncology: Gastric Cancer*. Version 1.2021. National Comprehensive Cancer Network; 2012. Accessed March 1, 2021. www.isesnet.org/wp-content/uploads/2013/02/NCCN-gastric-2012.pdf

97. Inokuchi M, Kojima K, Yamada H, et al. Long-term outcomes of Roux-en-Y and Billroth-I reconstruction after laparoscopic distal gastrectomy. *Gastric Cancer*. 2013;16(1):67-73. doi:10.1007/s10120-012-0154-5

98. Nomura E, Lee SW, Bouras G, Tokuhara T, Hayashi M H, M et al. Functional outcomes according to the size of the gastric remnant and type of reconstruction following laparoscopic distal gastrectomy for gastric cancer. *Gastric Cancer*. 2011;14:279-284. doi:10.1007/s10120-011-0046-0

99. Yamagata y. Yoshikawa T, et al. Current status of the "enhanced recovery after surgery" program in gastric cancer surgery. *Ang Gastroenteral Surg*. 2019;3:231-238. doi:10.1002/ags3.12232

100. Willcutts KF, Chung MC, Erenberg C, et al. Early oral feeding as compared with traditional timing of oral feeding after upper gastrointestinal surgery: a systematic review with meta-analysis. *Ann of Surg*. 2016;264:54-63. doi:10.1097/SLA.0000000000001644

101. Choi WJ, Kim J. Nutritional care of gastric cancer patients with clinical outcomes and complications: a review. *Clin Nutr Res*. 2016;(2):65-78. doi:10.7762/cnr.2016.5.2.65

102. Yamada T, Hayashi T, Cho H, et al. Usefulness of enhanced recovery after surgery protocol as compared with conventional perioperative care in gastric surgery. *Gastric Cancer*. 2012;15(1):34-41. doi:10.1007/s10120-011-0057-x

103. Jo DH, Jeong O, Sun JW, Jeong MR, Ryu SY, Park YK. Feasibility study of early oral intake after gastrectomy for gastric carcinoma. *J Gastric Cancer*. 2011;11(2):101-108. doi:10.5230/jgc.2011.11.2.101

104. Yamamoto K, Nagatsuma Y, Fukuda Y, et al. Effectiveness of a preoperative exercise and nutritional support program for elderly sarcopenic patients with gastric cancer. *Gastric Cancer*. 2017;20(5):913-918. doi:10.1007/s10120-016-0683-4

105. Halpern AL, McCarter MD. Palliative management of gastric and esophageal cancer. *Surg Clin North Am*. 2019;99(3):555-569. doi:10.1016/j.suc.2019.02.007

106. Rosania R, Chiapponi C, Malfertheiner P, Venerito M. Nutrition in patients with gastric cancer: an update. *Gastrointest Tumors*. 2016;2(4):178-187. doi:10.1159/000445188

107. Wu GH, Liu ZH, Wu ZH, Wu ZG. Perioperative artificial nutrition in malnourished gastrointestinal cancer patients. *World J Gastroenterol*. 2006;12(15):2441-2444. doi:10.3748/wjg.v12.i15.2441

108. Wu MH, Lin MT, Chen WJ. Effect of perioperative parenteral nutritional support for gastric cancer patients undergoing gastrectomy. *Hepatogastroenterology*. 2008;55(82-83):799-802.

109. Oh SE, Choi MG, Seo JM, et al. Prognostic significance of perioperative nutritional parameters in patients with gastric cancer. *Clin Nutr*. 2019;38(2):870-876. doi:10.1016/j.clnu.2018.02.015

110. Marano L, Porfidia R, Pezzella M, et al. Clinical and immunological impact of early postoperative enteral immunonutrition after total gastrectomy in gastric cancer patients: a prospective randomized study. *Ann Surg Oncol*. 2013;20(12):3912-3918. doi:10.1245/s10434-013-3088-1

111. Klek S, Scislo L, Walewska E, Choruz R, Galas A. Enriched enteral nutrition may improve short-term survival in stage IV gastric cancer patients: A randomized, controlled trial. *Nutrition*. 2017;36:46-53. doi:10.1016/j.nut.2016.03.016

112. Shim H. Perioperative Nutritional status changes in gastrointestinal cancer patients. *Yonsei Med J*. 2013;54(6):1370-1376. doi:10.3349/ymj.2013.54.6.1370

113. Qiu M, YX Z, Jin Y, et al. Nutrition support can bring survival benefit to high nutrition risk gastric cancer patients who received chemotherapy. *Support Care Cancer*. 2015;23(7):1933-1939. doi:10.1007/s00520-014-2523-6

114. Zheng HL. Effects of preoperative malnutrition on short- and long-term outcomes of patients with gastric cancer: can we do better? *Ann Surg Oncol*. 2017;24(11):3376-3385. doi:10.1245/s10434-017-5998-9

115. Davis JL, Ripley RT. Postgastrectomy syndromes and nutritional considerations following gastric surgery. *Surg Clin N Am*. 2017;97:277-293. doi:10.1016/j.suc.2016.11.005

116. Rogers C. Postgastrectomy Nutrition. *Nutr Clin Pract*. 2011;26(2):126-136. doi:10.1177/0884533611400070

117. Yamaoka Y, Fujitani K, Tsujinaka T, Yamamoto K, Hirao M, Sekimoto M. Skeletal muscle loss after total gastrectomy, exacerbated by adjuvant chemotherapy. *Gastric Cancer*. 2014:382-389. doi:10.1007/s10120-014-0365-z

Chapter 19

Medical Nutrition Therapy for Cancers of the Liver, Bile Duct, Gallbladder, Small Bowel, Colon, Rectum, and Anus

Colleen Gill, MS, RDN, CSO

The hollow organs that make up the gastrointestinal (GI) tract have multiple roles. Digestion begins in the mouth through the secretion of amylase and the mastication and lubrication of food, which is then delivered to the stomach via the esophagus. Gastric contractions break down food and mix in fluid to create a chyme that passes into the small bowel over 1 to 2 hours. The transit time is influenced by meal composition. Food exiting the stomach triggers hormone signals that stimulate the release of bile from the gallbladder (to emulsify fat) and enzymes from the pancreas (to further break down food).

Macronutrients (carbohydrates, fats, and proteins) and most fluids are absorbed into circulation during the 1- to 4-hour transit through the approximately 20 feet of small bowel. Referred to as the second brain, the small bowel also functions as an essential component of the immune system, as 70% to 80% of the body's immune cells are located there. Gut-associated lymphoid tissue determines what is allowed to pass through the GI mucosa and into the bloodstream.[1] Any drugs ingested and some nutrients are then sent to the liver for further processing or storage or both. Residual fluid and electrolytes are absorbed during the much slower transit through the colon, leaving waste for excretion via the rectum and anus.

A thorough understanding of GI tract function and the changes that can result from cancer and its treatment is essential for optimizing medical nutrition therapy, quality of life (QOL), and treatment outcomes. Early symptoms are often nonspecific but may compromise nutritional status even before diagnosis.[2] Managing disease and treatment-related symptoms to improve nutritional intake is critical throughout the continuum of care, and estimated needs in GI cancers are similar to needs in other cancer diagnoses.[3]

Types of Gastrointestinal Cancers

The six types of GI cancer discussed in this chapter, in anatomical order, are as follows: hepatocellular carcinoma (HCC), cholangiocarcinoma (CCA), gallbladder carcinoma (GBC), neuroendocrine tumor of the small bowel (GI NET), colorectal cancer (CRC), and anal carcinoma (AC). Esophageal and gastric cancers are discussed in Chapter 18 and pancreatic cancer in Chapter 20. Important characteristics of the cancers discussed in this chapter are summarized in Figure 19.1 on page 406 and detailed information on each specific disease is found in the sections that follow. Statistical data compiled by the American Cancer Society regarding the incidence of the six cancers are listed in Table 19.1 on page 407. Risk factors are summarized in Table 19.2 on page 408.

Treatment of Gastrointestinal Cancers

For all GI cancers, oncologists base their treatment decisions on evidence-based guidelines outlined in the National Comprehensive Cancer Network (NCCN) Clinical Practice Guidelines in Oncology.[25] More information can be found in the

Hepatocellular Carcinoma

- Associated with cirrhosis of the liver due to chronic hepatitis C, alcohol abuse, or nonalcoholic fatty liver disease
- Signs and symptoms: nausea, vomiting, enlarged liver, abdominal pain or swelling, itching, jaundice, worsening of existing cirrhosis or hepatitis, loss of appetite, early satiety, fatigue, unintended weight loss
- Some hepatocellular carcinoma tumors secrete hormones and can cause hypercalcemia, hypoglycemia, gynecomastia, increased cholesterol levels, and erythrocytosis (ie, facial redness and flushing).

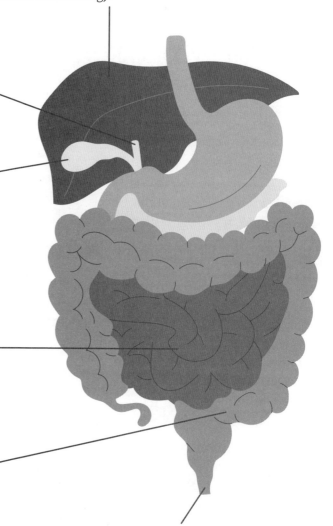

Cholangiocarcinoma

- Subtypes: intrahepatic, perihilar, and distal
- Signs and symptoms: jaundice, itching, fatigue, abdominal pain, weight loss, acholic stools

Gallbladder Carcinoma

- Initial symptoms are vague, and disease is often advanced at diagnosis.
- Signs and symptoms: nonspecific abdominal pain, nausea, vomiting, fever, taste change, anorexia, jaundice due to bile duct compression

Neuroendocrine Tumor of the Small Bowel

- Small, slow-growing tumor in the neuroendocrine cells of the gastrointestinal tract
- Signs and symptoms: nonfunctional bloating, pain, diarrhea

Colorectal Cancer

- Subtypes: adenocarcinoma (85%–90% of cases), mucinous adenocarcinoma (10%–15% of cases), and signet ring cell carcinoma (1%)
- Signs and symptoms: change in bowel habits (eg, diarrhea, constipation, or narrowing of the stool); unexplained anemia; visible blood in stool; abdominal pain, nausea, and vomiting; unintended weight loss; fatigue

Anal Carcinoma

- Signs and symptoms: itching or pain, change in stool diameter, abnormal anal discharge, swollen lymph nodes in the groin
- Most patients experience bleeding, which can be falsely attributed to hemorrhoids and delay diagnosis.

Figure 19.1
Cancers of the liver, bile duct, gallbladder, small bowel, colon, rectum, and anus[4-10]

Table 19.1
Gastrointestinal Cancer Statistics, United States

Type	New cases per year	Deaths per year	5-year relative survival rate
Hepatocellular carcinoma[4,11,12]	42,810	30,160	2.4%-18.4%
Gallbladder carcinoma[5-12]	11,980	4,090	2%-62%
Cholangiocarcinoma[6,12]	8,000	Not available	8%-24%
Neuroendocrine tumor of the small bowel[7,12]	12,000	Not available	67%-97%
Colorectal cancer[8,12]	104,610 (colon) 43,340 (rectal)	53,200 (colon and rectal combined)	63% (colorectal) 90% (localized)
Anal carcinoma[9,12]	8,590	1,350	82% (stage I–II) 32% (stage IV)

Chapter 19 *Medical Nutrition Therapy for Cancers of the Liver, Bile Duct, Gallbladder, Small Bowel, Colon, Rectum, and Anus*

407

Table 19.2
Risk Factors for Different Types of Gastrointestinal Cancers[13-24]

	Increased Risk				
Type of Cancer	Gender	Obesity	Smoking	Alcohol consumption	Ethnicity and race
Hepatocellular carcinoma	2-6 times greater risk in males than females	30% increased risk per 5 body mass index (BMI) units	Highest increase in risk with concurrent hepatitis or alcohol intake	More than 45 g of alcohol per day	--
Gallbladder carcinoma	2-6 times greater risk in females than males	25% increased risk per 5 BMI units	Implicated	Significant intake	Highest in Mexicans and Native Americans
Cholangio-carcinoma	1.5 times greater risk in males than females	Implicated	Implicated	Implicated	--

Chronic conditions	Diet and environmental exposure	Oral contraceptive use	Other	Decreased Risk
Type 2 diabetes mellitus Hemochromatosis α1-antitrypsin deficiency Primary sclerosing cholangitis Hepatitis B and hepatitis C infection Cirrhosis	Drinking water contaminated with arsenic Chewing betel nuts Aflatoxins	Long-term use	Markers of inflammation associated with increased hepatocellular carcinoma	Coffee consumption (14% decrease in risk per cup per day) Fish consumption Physical activity
Primary sclerosing cholangitis Biliary abnormalities Gallstones Insulin resistance and diabetes Salmonella or *Helicobacter pylori* infection	Industrial and environmental chemicals Sweetened beverages (doubles risk) Capsicum and other pepper	--	--	--
Chronic inflammation Cholestasis of biliary tract Parasitic infections Hepatitis C Cirrhosis Bile duct cysts Hepatolithiasis Cholelithiasis Primary sclerosing cholangitis Lynch syndrome Metabolic syndrome	Thorotrast contrast exposure Parasitic infection from liver flukes in undercooked fish	--	--	High intake of vegetables and fruits

(continued)

Chapter 19 *Medical Nutrition Therapy for Cancers of the Liver, Bile Duct, Gallbladder, Small Bowel, Colon, Rectum, and Anus*

409

Table 19.2
Risk Factors for Different Types of Gastrointestinal Cancers [9-29] (continued)

Increased Risk					
Type of Cancer	Gender	Obesity	Smoking	Alcohol consumption	Ethnicity and race
Neuroendocrine tumor of the small bowel	Risk greater in females than males	--	Implicated	--	--
Colorectal cancer	More proximal cancers in females; males have higher risk of recurrence	Implicated	40% increased risk	7% increased risk per 10 g of alcohol per day	Black males Multifactorial ethnic disparities, influenced by access to care
Anal cancer	Risk greater in females than males	--	Implicated	Implicated	--

Chronic conditions	Diet and environmental exposure	Oral contraceptive use	Other	Decreased Risk
Multiple endocrine neoplasia type 1 Family history of cancer	--	--	--	--
Lynch syndrome Peutz-Jeghers syndrome Other inherited syndromes Inflammatory bowel disease Ulcerative colitis Crohn disease Primary sclerosing cholangitis Type 2 diabetes Insulin resistance Cholecystectomy	Age 50+ years Family history of colorectal cancer (first-degree relative doubles risk) High intake of red and processed meats Low serum vitamin D Low calcium intake Physical inactivity Androgen deprivation therapy	--	Colon's direct contact with food and carcinogens accounts for strong association with nutrition and lifestyle factors	Nonsteroidal anti-inflammatory drug use Calcium (preferably dietary) Normal serum 25-hydroxyvitamin D protective Coffee
Human papillomavirus 16 and 18 associated with 90% of anal cancers Immune suppression and HIV Organ transplant Sexually transmitted disease (herpes, genital warts, chlamydia, gonorrhea) Other cancers Cervical dysplasia	--	--	--	Human papillomavirus vaccine in adolescence

Chapter 19 *Medical Nutrition Therapy for Cancers of the Liver, Bile Duct, Gallbladder, Small Bowel, Colon, Rectum, and Anus*

411

National Cancer Institute's Physician Data Query Summaries[26] or on the UpToDate website (www.uptodate.com).

Multimodal therapies—combinations of surgery, systemic therapies, radiation, and liver-directed therapies—are the standard of care in neoadjuvant, adjuvant, salvage, and palliative interventions. Surgical resection can be curative or palliative, potentially altering the anatomy of the GI tract and affecting its function. Systemic therapies, including chemotherapy, targeted therapy, and immunotherapies, are used in combination, either sequenced with site-specific radiation therapies or paired in chemoradiation. Targeting the tumor from multiple pathways is effective but often toxic to the rapidly dividing cells of the GI tract. Mucositis,

changes in bowel movements, nausea, vomiting, fatigue, and early satiety can lead to loss of weight, loss of muscle mass, and diminished QOL, which can affect optimal treatment delivery as described in the NCCN guidelines.[25] Clinical experience suggests that anything that alters surface area, or the messaging and secretions orchestrating the timing of GI transit, can significantly affect GI function and status.

Common treatment-related issues and recommended interventions related to the various cancers of the GI tract discussed in this chapter are detailed in Box 19.1, and specific issues and interventions are discussed in the cancer-specific sections that follow.

Box 19.1
Common Treatment-Related Nutrition Issues in Gastrointestinal Cancers and Recommended Interventions[27,28,30,31-38]

General surgery-related issues, including ileus, gastroparesis, infection, wound or anastomosis dehisence, dehydration, gas pains

Interventions

Enhanced recovery after surgery (ERAS), also known as fast-track surgery:

- ERAS is becoming a standard of care.
- It minimizes fasting and bowel preparation and includes carbohydrate loading.
- It prescribes early enteral nutrition (EN) and mobilization.
- It limits risk of postoperative ileus with oral magnesium, helps avoid necessity of nasogastric tube, encourages chewing gum, and utilizes alvimopan as needed.

Preoperative nutrition

- Preoperative nutrition replenishes nutritional status in malnourished patients prior to anticipated surgery, reducing length of stay, morbidity, and mortality.
- Parenteral nutrition (PN) is an option where EN is not feasible.
- Oral immune-enhanced formulas perioperatively decrease infectious complications in malnourished gastrointestinal (GI) patients.
- Standard oral nutritional supplements limit postoperative complications in patients with a history of weight loss.

Postoperative nutrition

- Postoperative follow-up over approximately 6 weeks of recovery can maximize nutritional status in preparation for adjuvant chemotherapy.
- Gastroparesis and ileus are common postoperative issues, and dehydration is a major cause of readmission.
- Gas pains improve with walking, chewing gum, and use of heating pads.
- Clarify duration of diet restrictions postoperatively.

(continued)

Box 19.1

Common Treatment-Related Nutrition Issues in Gastrointestinal Cancers and Recommended Interventions *(continued)*

Issues related to small-bowel resections, including diarrhea, insufficient nutrient absorption, small intestinal bacterial overgrowth, dehydration

Interventions

Although <150 cm of small bowel remaining is the technical definition of short bowel, any side effect of therapy that affects the functional surface area of the bowel can make advancing to a normal diet challenging and involve weeks to months. Some patients require long-term supplemental EN or parenteral nutrition (PN) to maintain nutritional status, and management goals often change over time.

Fluid and electrolytes should be provided frequently in small amounts. Consider oral rehydration solutions and intravenous (IV) fluids when fluid losses routinely exceed intake.

With terminal ileum resection:

- Question bile acid malabsorption with any perianal burning, and recommend bile acid sequestrants such as colesevelam.
- Monitor vitamin B12 levels and supplement as needed.
- Keep serum vitamin D level >30 mg/dL; supplement calcium for a total intake of 1,500 mg/d if >100 cm of the ileum is resected.

Consider probiotics to limit the risk of small intestinal bacterial overgrowth (SIBO).

Enterocutaneous fistulas

Interventions

Replenish fluid and electrolyte losses.

Adjust macronutrient and micronutrient needs to promote wound healing.

Consider PN if oral diet increases protein and output losses.

Consider support with EN below the fistula or PN for bowel rest as needed to support closure.

The following treatment algorithm is used for high-output fistula and enterostomy:

- High-dose acid-suppressive therapy with proton pump inhibitor (PPIs) opting for IV forms over oral forms. Substitute histamine H2-receptor antagonist if hypomagnesemia is present.
- Antidiarrheal, eg, loperamide (Imodium AD), up to 32 mg/d. Add codeine if diarrhea persists.

Changes in bowel movements

Interventions

Ask the patient specific questions about the frequency and consistency of bowel movements to help define the patient's "normal." The Bristol Scale offers a common, descriptive language.

Encourage the patient to titrate rather than hold medications (such as loperamide [Imodium AD] and senna) to avoid recurrence of diarrhea or overcorrection leading to extreme swings in bowel movements.

Consider the impact of any change in narcotic use.

Malabsorptive symptoms may reflect exocrine pancreatic insufficiency, rapid transit issues, SIBO, or different etiologies that must be identified and addressed. Supplement with fat-soluble vitamins (A, D, E, K) and calcium, zinc, and magnesium as needed.

Vitamin B12 deficiency (serum B12 level <300 pg/mL)

Interventions

Risk is present with the loss of more than 20 cm of ileum, short bowel, radiation enteritis, neuroendocrine tumor, cirrhosis, achlorhydria (from aging or chronic PPI use), and metformin use.

Liver disease limits vitamin B12 reserves. Check methylmalonic acid levels because serum levels may be elevated with liver destruction.

Supplement orally with 1,000 mcg/d for 4 weeks, followed by 500 mcg/d for maintenance of synthetic vitamin B12 (effective for most patients).

Recommend intramuscular dosing of vitamin B12 for severe short bowel, ileal resection, and noncompliance with oral supplementation.

Nutrition Assessment for Gastrointestinal Cancers

See Chapter 5 for details on assessing nutrition needs for patients with cancer. Nutrition assessment guidelines that may be specific to GI cancers are discussed in the sections that follow.

Hepatocellular Carcinoma

The liver is the largest organ in the body and the only one that regenerates. It is essential to survival through its roles in waste removal, production of cholesterol and proteins (such as albumin and clotting factors), and processing and storing of nutrients (including glycogen). All blood circulating from the stomach and bowel flows through the liver, where carcinogens and drugs are detoxified. Waste products are secreted into bile and excreted in stool or secreted into the blood and excreted in urine. Bile also plays a role in fat digestion.

HCC is the second leading cause of cancer-related deaths worldwide. Most cases (83%) occur in developing countries, including Asian countries, and are linked to perinatally acquired hepatitis B virus (HBV), which confers a 100-times-higher lifetime risk for HCC. Incidence is low in North America. Although increased HBV detection and new antiviral therapies are expected to decrease overall HCC incidence, the opioid epidemic has resulted in a doubling of incidence in people aged 20 to 39 years. Early diagnosis is key, and at-risk patients with cirrhosis or HBV should be monitored routinely.[39]

Treatment

Due to the essential functions of the liver, underlying and progressive liver disease have a major impact on viable treatment options for HCC and long-term survival. Treatment options include surgical resection, liver transplantation, systemic therapies (including chemotherapy, targeted therapies, and immunotherapy), radiation, and liver-directed therapies. Refer to the *NCCN Clinical Practice Guidelines in Oncology (NCCN Guidelines): Hepatobiliary Cancers* regarding details of specific therapies.[40]

Surgical Resection and Liver Transplantation

Surgical resection and liver transplantation are the only curative interventions for HCC, and they improve the survival rate to 50%.[41] However, most tumors are inoperable or occur in patients who are not surgical candidates.[40] Similarly, few qualify for liver transplantation, which offers a long-term survival rate of 60% to 79%. Feasibility depends on baseline liver function, tumor burden, and tumor location. Preoperative prealbumin serum level is a predictive factor for postoperative liver insufficiency in patients with liver function of Child-Pugh class A who are undergoing hepatectomy.[42] Side effects of liver surgery include bleeding, blood clots, infection, diarrhea, pain, fatigue, and damage to the remaining liver or rejection of the transplanted organ.

Liver-Directed Therapies

Liver-directed therapies include ablation and embolization. Types of ablation include radiofrequency, cryoablation, percutaneous ethanol, and microwave. Types of embolization include bland embolization, transarterial chemoembolization (TACE), and radioembolization. TACE is avoided before planned surgical resection. Weight loss is common after liver-directed therapies due to side effects, which include abdominal pain, nausea, vomiting, liver infection and inflammation, fever, and fatigue.

Systemic Therapies

Targeted therapy and immunotherapy are commonly used in the treatment of HCC. Chemotherapy is often poorly tolerated due to liver dysfunction, and data regarding its effectiveness in the treatment of HCC are limited.[40,41] Side effects commonly associated with specific systemic therapies are listed in Chapter 9.

Disease-Specific Nutrition Problems and Interventions

Nutritional needs and concerns in patients with HCC and recommended interventions are summarized in Box 19.2 on page 416. See Chapters 9 and 10 for a detailed description of side effects of systemic and radiation therapy and Chapter 11 for symptom management.

Cholangiocarcinoma

CCA is cancer that forms in the bile ducts—the tubes that carry bile from the liver to the gallbladder to the small intestine. The three main types of bile ducts are the intrahepatic (within the liver), the perihilar (just outside the liver), and the distal (nearest the small intestine). The types of CCA are defined accordingly, depending on the tumor location within the bile duct or biliary, system (see Figure 19.2 on page 417). More than 90% of these tumors are adenocarcinomas, and they make up 10% to 20% of hepatobiliary cancers. Biology and management vary depending on the location of the tumor.[43]

Treatment

Tumor location influences the chosen treatment modalities for CCA. Chemotherapy, radiation therapy, liver-directed therapies, and surgery are used in the treatment of CCA, either alone or often in combination.[43,44] Immunotherapy may be used in microsatellite instability–high (MSI-H) tumors. Microsatellite instability (MSI) is the disruption or mutation of caretaker genes that maintain genetic stability. Refer to the NCCN guidelines for hepatobiliary cancers regarding details of specific therapies.[40]

Surgery

Resection is the sole curative intervention, although many cases are determined to be unresectable upon exploratory laparotomy. Pancreaticoduodenectomy, or Whipple resection, is the surgical intervention for distal CCA and perihilar CCA. See Chapter 20 for surgery details for these procedures. Surgical bypass may be performed for palliation of bile duct obstruction and often as part of a failed resection attempt. Orthotic liver transplantation may be used in carefully selected patients or as part of a clinic trial. Acute surgical complications may include intra-abdominal abscess and bile duct leak.

Palliative Interventions

CCA may obstruct the bile duct. Bile duct stenting and external biliary drain placement may be used to treat a biliary obstruction. Stenting involves the placement of a plastic or metal stent in the bile duct. Biliary stenting may increase survival, especially when combined with photodynamic therapy. Plastic stents have a greater risk of reocclusion than metal stents and, therefore, require replacement every 3 to 6 months or placement of a metal stent in replacement of a plastic stent, or both. Procedural side effects include nausea and anorexia.[44]

External biliary drains or biliary obstruction distal to the common bile duct with decompression above the obstruction will reduce the bile salt pool that typically recycles via the terminal ileum. In the setting of malabsorption due to this, reinfusion of biliary secretions of 100 to 200 mL every 4 to 6 hours via the Y-port to coincide with enteral feedings or use of a semielemental enteral formula may need to be considered.[45]

Disease-Specific Nutrition Problems and Interventions

Disease-specific nutrition problems associated with CCA are influenced by disease location and treatment modalities used. Nutrition problems of GI cancers and interventions are summarized in Box 19.1.

Box 19.2
Estimated Nutritional Needs and Concerns in Patients With Hepatic Compromise and Recommended Interventions[46-53]

Energy intake

Interventions[46-47]

Ensure intake of 25 to 40 kcal/kg/d—based on the patient's dry (euvolemic) weight—for patients with stable cirrhosis, varying with degree of disease.

Ensure 15 to 20 kcal/kg/d to start, if there is refeeding risk.

Protein intake

Interventions[46-49]

Ensure 1.0 to 1.5 g/kg/d; intake should be liberal as tolerated. Note that protein needs increase with decompensated liver disease, and inadequate support risks more loss of muscle.

With acute encephalopathy, ensure a daily intake of 1 g/kg/d. Avoid glutamine supplementation due to metabolism to glutamate and ammonia.

Data are mixed regarding benefits from branched-chain amino acids.

Vitamin and mineral intake

Interventions[50-51]

With cirrhosis, ensure a thiamin intake of 1 to 2 mg/d.

Use a multivitamin and mineral supplement to limit deficiency related to poor intake.

Note that low selenium levels are linked to increased risk of hepatocellular carcinoma (HCC).

Because of the elevated osteoporosis risk with cirrhosis, promote a daily intake of vitamin D3 of 2,000 IU and a daily calcium intake of 1,200 to 1,500 mg.

Maximization of nutritional status

Interventions[50,52]

Given lower glycogen reserves in this population, minimize time without nutrition support and consider dextrose-containing intravenous (IV) hydration when the patient is nothing by mouth (npo).

Recommend six small meals with a carbohydrate-rich snack at bedtime.

Be aware that patients with HCC commonly require the use of oral nutrition supplements.

Sarcopenia and muscle wasting due to metabolic mediators, limited appetite associated with cirrhosis, and losses with ascites

Interventions[50,53]

Assess temporal, clavicle, and scapular regions, which are less affected by fluid overload.

Note that handgrip strength best predicts malnutrition and related complications in patients with cirrhosis.

(continued)

Box 19.2
Estimated Nutritional Needs and Concerns in Patients With Hepatic Compromise and Recommended Interventions[46-53] *(continued)*

Ascites, fluid overload, edema

Interventions[46,47]

Estimate the patient's dry weight by subtracting average weight of ascitic fluid from the patient's actual body weight. Average ascitic-fluid weights are as follows:

- In mild ascites: 3 to 5 kg
- In moderate ascites: 7 to 9 kg
- In severe ascites: 14 to 15 kg

Early satiety will worsen between paracenteses.

Liberalize the patient's diet to avoid limiting intake, but apply a sodium diet restriction of 2 to 3 g/d as needed.

Encourage liquid protein sources to replace protein losses.

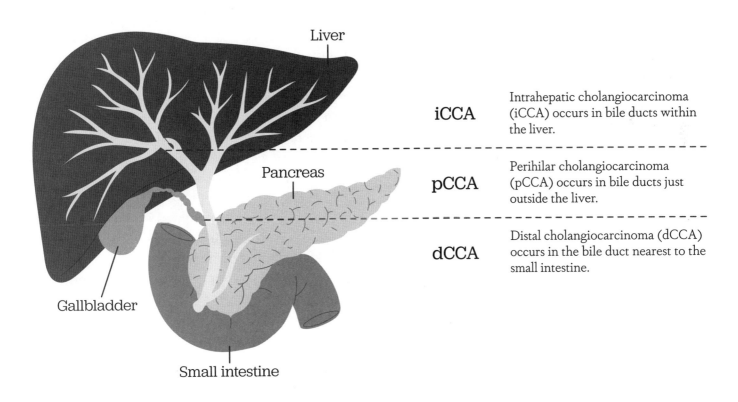

Figure 19.2
The biliary system and types of cholangiocarcinoma

Chapter 19 *Medical Nutrition Therapy for Cancers of the Liver, Bile Duct, Gallbladder, Small Bowel, Colon, Rectum, and Anus*

417

See Chapters 9 and 10 for a detailed description of side effects due to systemic and radiation therapy and Chapter 11 for symptom management.

Gallbladder Carcinoma

The gallbladder is a small, pear-shaped organ that collects and stores the bile that flows from the liver via the bile ducts. When food enters the duodenum, secretion of cholecystokinin precipitates gallbladder contractions that release alkaline bile into the duodenum via the common bile duct. The alkaline bile helps neutralize acid from the stomach and emulsifies fats, thereby assisting pancreatic enzymes to break down fat for absorption.

GBC is the most common of biliary tract tumors. Though uncommon in the United States (one to two cases per 100,000 people), it is a leading cause of cancer mortality in Mexican and Southwest Native Americans and in geographical areas including Chile, North India, and East Asia.[5] It is linked to a genetic susceptibility, exacerbated by prolonged irritation and inflammation due to gallstones or chronic infection.[15] Poor prognosis for GBC is related to both anatomical issues (ie, a gallbladder wall <3 mm thick and close adjacent structures) and to lymph nodes' contributing to metastatic spread. Better prognosis occurs with early identification, usually occurring during 1% to 2% of cholecystectomies.[5]

Treatment

Surgery, chemotherapy, and radiation therapy are used in the treatment of GBC, either alone or in combination.[54] Immunotherapy may be used in MSI-H tumors. Refer to the NCCN Clinical guidelines for hepatobiliary cancers regarding details of specific therapies.[40] Palliative measures include bile duct stenting and biliary bypass to reduce jaundice and allow bile to drain. Anorexia and nausea can occur acutely after bile duct stenting.

Disease-Specific Nutrition Problems and Interventions

Disease-specific nutrition problems associated with GBC are influenced by disease location and treatment modalities used. Nutrition problems and interventions of GI cancers are summarized in Box 19.1 on pages 412 and 413. See Chapters 9 and 10 for a detailed description of side effects due to systemic and radiation therapy and Chapter 11 for symptom management.

Neuroendocrine Tumors of the Small Bowel

Neuroendocrine tumors of the small bowel (GI NETs; also abbreviated NETSBs) account for 70% of all neuroendocrine tumors.[55] The tumors are small (<1 cm), slow growing, and can be non-functional or functional (ie, secreting bioactive hormones, amines, and peptides). Functional GI NETs produce an excess of serotonin, in addition to other hormones. Most remain clinically silent until there is mass effect or symptoms develop after liver metastases circumvent hepatic metabolism and increase circulating hormone levels. Because the initial symptoms are vague, diagnosis often is delayed by more than 4 years.[56]

Diagnostic testing and monitoring for GI NETs are unique compared to that for other cancers of the GI tract. Testing includes measuring hormone levels, including urinary and serum levels of 5-hydroxyindoleacetic acid (5-HIAA), a primary metabolite of serotonin. Blood 5-HIAA level may be affected by renal impairment and is useful in diagnosis but less helpful in monitoring.[57,58] Chromogranin A is used as a tumor marker for GI NETs and is elevated in 90% of patients with the disease, independent of hormone secretion; it is a biomarker of tumor burden but is also elevated with use of proton pump inhibitors and with renal or hepatic insufficiency. Positron emission tomography (PET) scans using somatostatin analogues, such as the single-photon emission computed tomography octreotide scan and Ga-68 dotatate PET/CT scan, are used to identify tumors expressing somatostatin receptors.[59]

Treatment

Surgery, somatostatin analogues, and radiopharmaceuticals are common treatment modalities for GI NETs and may be used alone or in combination.[60] Systemic therapies are limited for GI NETs.[61] Liver-directed therapies may be used for the treatment of hepatic metastases. Refer to the *NCCN Clinical Practice Guidelines in Oncology (NCCN Guidelines): Neuroendocrine Tumors* regarding details of specific therapies.[62]

Surgery

Surgery for GI NETs includes small-bowel resection. Location of the tumor influences the area and amount of small bowel resected. Side effects of surgery can include small intestinal bacterial overgrowth and exocrine pancreatic insufficiency. Carcinoid crisis can be triggered by anesthesia; therefore, somatostatin analogues are used preventatively during surgery.

Somatostatin Analogue Therapy

A somatostatin analogue (SSA) is a drug that is similar to the hormone somatostatin. Somatostatin is responsible for the release of certain other hormones in the body. SSAs reduce the amount of hormones secreted from functional tumors and help stabilize tumor growth. SSAs include octreotide, lanreotide, and pasireotide, which are given via depot injection, commonly every 4 weeks. SSAs improve diarrhea and flushing. Side effects of SSAs include malabsorption, due to the drug's limiting of pancreatic and gallbladder function and secretions; hyperglycemia, especially with pasireotide; and hypothyroidism.[63,64]

Radiopharmaceuticals

Peptide receptor radionuclide therapy (PRRT) uses a radiolabeled somatostatin analogue to deliver a cytotoxic radiolabeled compound directly to the tumor and has demonstrated improved survival times. Common side effects of radiopharmaceuticals include fatigue, nausea, vomiting, and risk of kidney damage.[65]

Additional Therapies

Telotristat ethyl is a tryptophan hydroxylase inhibitor that blocks serotonin synthesis peripherally.[66] This may be combined with an SSA for the management of refractory diarrhea and to limit progression of carcinoid heart disease.

Disease-Specific Nutrition Problems and Interventions

Among patients with a GI NET, malnutrition occurs in 14% of patients in the outpatient setting and 25% of patients in the inpatient setting.[67,68] Patients with a symptomatic GI NET benefit from nutrition interventions. They present unique issues that require management not only of the side effects of treatment but also of the side effects of excess hormone secretion. Nutrition problems and interventions of GI cancers are summarized in Box 19.1. See Chapters 9 and 10 for a detailed description of side effects due to systemic and radiation therapy and Chapter 11 for symptom management.

Carcinoid Syndrome

Carcinoid syndrome develops due to vasoactive substances, including serotonin, secreted by the tumor. GI NETs are involved in 72% of carcinoid-syndrome cases. Symptoms include cutaneous flushing, abdominal cramps, and diarrhea, as well as right-sided valvular heart disease. Carcinoid syndrome is more common in patients with a metastatic GI NET and occurs more frequently in women.[69]

Food sources of tyramine and dopamine increase catecholamine production, which stimulates tumor secretion of excess serotonin, leading to carcinoid symptoms of diarrhea and flushing.[68] Significant dietary sources of tyramine include aged cheeses, alcohol, smoked and salted animal proteins, yeast extracts, fava beans, soybeans, and fermented foods. Moderate dietary sources of tyramine include chocolate, peanuts, coconut, Brazil nuts, raspberries, avocados, bananas, and caffeine-containing beverages. Dietary sources of dopamine include dairy products; unprocessed meats, such as beef, chicken, and turkey; omega-3-containing fish, such as salmon, herring, and mackerel; eggs; nuts, such as almonds and walnuts; fruits and vegetables but especially bananas; and dark chocolate. For patients experiencing carcinoid syndrome, limiting foods high in tyramine and dopamine can assist with managing symptoms.[60,68]

Dry flushing of the upper body without perspiration occurs as a symptom of carcinoid syndrome. Flushing is exacerbated by the "five Es": eating, epinephrine, emotion, ethanol, and exercise. Nutrition interventions include avoiding large meals and alcohol. Foods that may trigger symptoms include alcohol (especially wine), spicy food, and foods high in tyramine or dopamine. Large meals—especially those with beef, spicy foods, or sources of sodium nitrates and sulfites—may worsen symptoms.

Secretory Diarrhea

Secretory diarrhea is a differentiating feature of serotonin-secreting tumors. The diarrhea is due to extremely rapid GI transit time through the small bowel and colon that does not slow nocturnally or with fasting and has only a limited response to antidiarrheal medications. Ondansetron is a serotonin receptor antagonist that may assist in the management of secretory diarrhea.[70] A study of Enterade, a proprietary beverage containing amino acids and electrolytes, demonstrated benefit,[71] but further research is needed to fully support its benefit and wider usage in cases of secretory diarrhea.

Niacin Deficiency

Niacin deficiency can occur when niacin synthesis is limited by tryptophan diversion to serotonin production. Low serum levels were identified in 45% of patients with neuroendocrine tumors in one study but were normalized with supplementation.[72] Scaly brown patches on the arms and legs may be observed, although overt pellagra is rare. Nutrition interventions include a high-protein diet (1.5 g of protein per kg of body weight daily) and supplementation with a daily multivitamin and niacin. Niacin supplementation can be given as niacinamide, 20 to 50 mg twice daily, or niacin combined with half a baby aspirin, to counter prostacyclin that causes flushing.[69,72]

Colorectal Cancer

The colon is a muscular tube stretching approximately 5 feet from the ileum to the rectum, helping maintain hydration and conserve electrolytes by reabsorbing fluid and salts. Transit through the small bowel occurs over 1 to 4 hours, but passage through the colon may take 10 times as long and varies with diet. The walls of the colon contract via peristalsis, which can be slowed significantly by narcotics. Stool remains in the sigmoid colon until evacuation into the rectum, typically one to two times a day. The rectum is an 8-inch reservoir with a sphincter that relaxes when signaled by the nervous system, followed by contractions that expel stool.

According to the American Cancer Society, colorectal cancer (CRC) is the third most common cancer in the United States, with a 4% lifetime risk.[12] The 10-fold global variations reflect environmental influences, with increased rates where a Western lifestyle is adopted.[73] Incidence has declined 3% annually due to improved colonoscopy rates, despite underutilization (<60%) by eligible patients and an increase in incidence of early onset CRC.[74]

The majority of CRC develops over a multi-year transition of adenomatous polyps, involving cumulative changes that are described as adenoma-carcinoma sequence.[74] Chromosomal instability involves disruption or mutation of gatekeeper or growth regulatory genes (eg, *APC*, *TP53*, *PI3K*, *KRAS*, and *BRAF*), which accounts for more than 80% of CRC cases. Another 15% of cases result from mutation or disruption of caretaker genes that maintain genetic stability; this is termed microsatellite instability (MSI) and can be deemed "high" or "low." These variants are used by oncologists in determining appropriate therapy.[75]

The colon is home to healthy bacteria (probiotics) that have a symbiotic relationship when intestinal flora use fiber (prebiotics) as fuel to produce the short-chain fatty acids that support colon health. The colon also can be infected with harmful types of bacteria, such as *Clostridium difficile* and pathogenic strains of *Escherichia coli*. *Bacteroides fragilis* produces a toxin that causes inflammation and triggers oncogenic pathways.[76] Infections and antibiotic use can disrupt the microbiome balance, and probiotic therapies have shown potential benefit in maintaining and restoring that balance.[75,77]

Treatment

Treatment modalities for CRC include surgery, chemotherapy, radiation, targeted therapy, and immunotherapy. Except in early stage CRC, multiple treatment modalities are often used. Multimodal therapy can result in anorexia, mucositis, diarrhea, nausea, vomiting, fatigue, and unintended weight loss. Refer to the *NCCN Clinical Practice Guidelines in Oncology for Colon and Rectal Cancers* regarding details of specific therapies.[78,79]

Surgery

Surgery can be curative or palliative to relieve obstruction. Typical complications can include hernias, adhesions, and leaks. Several surgeries are illustrated in Figure 19.3 on page 422. Colon surgeries include endoscopic polypectomy, local excision, and colectomy. Rectal surgeries include transanal excision (used to remove rectal tumors and polyps), low anterior resection, abdominal perineal resection with colostomy, and proctectomy with coloanal anastomosis (the rectum is removed then the colon is connected to the anus). Resection of isolated metastases is used when CRC recurs and for metastatic disease. When CRC recurs, it is typically within 3 years and most often in the liver or lung. Resection of isolated metastases may still be curative.

Cytoreductive Surgery and Hyperthermic Intraperitoneal Chemotherapy

Cytoreductive surgery (CRS) and hyperthermic intraperitoneal chemotherapy (HIPEC) are used in patients with metastatic CRC with peritoneal carcinomatosis.[80] Peritoneal carcinomatosis occurs most frequently in patients with mucinous and signet ring cell carcinomas. Peritoneal carcinomatosis can result in impaired peritoneal blood supply, making traditional systemic therapy of limited benefit.[81]

CRS and HIPEC can be curative in small percentages, but defining which patients will benefit remains controversial. Because 90% of chemotherapy stays in the abdomen, acting locally, this may potentially minimize systemic side effects. Nutrition impact symptoms are often influenced by the extent of surgical resection. Additionally, development of abscesses and postoperative delayed gastric emptying can affect nutritional status and interventions. Clinical experience shows that GI recovery can also require 2 weeks of enteral nutrition or parenteral nutrition.

Disease-Specific Nutrition Problems and Interventions

Nutrition problems and interventions for GI cancers are summarized in Box 19.1 on pages 412 and 413. See Chapters 9 and 10 for a detailed description of side effects due to systemic and

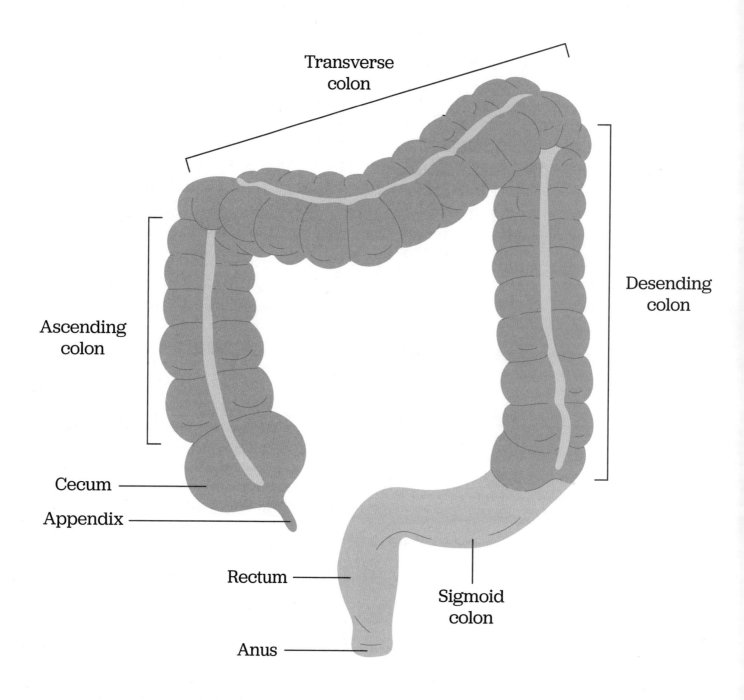

Transverse
colon

Desending
colon

Ascending
colon

Cecum

Appendix

Rectum

Sigmoid
colon

Anus

Figure 19.3
Selected surgeries for colorectal cancer

Adapted with permission from Christine Eberle Barron.

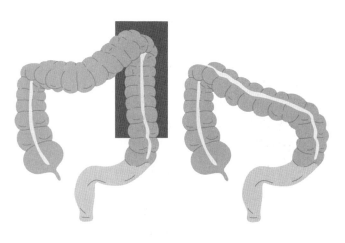

Left colectomy

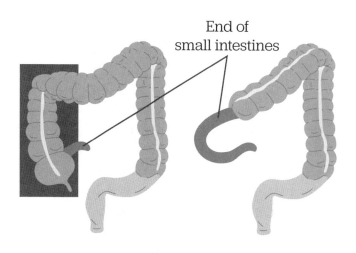

End of
small intestines

Right colectomy

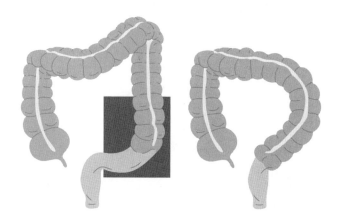

Sigmoid colectomy

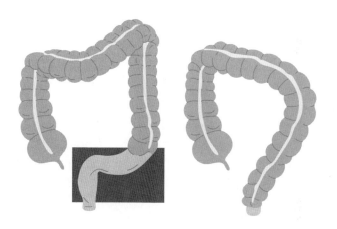

Low anterior resection

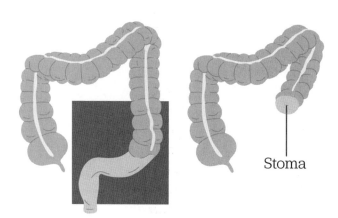

Stoma

Abdominal perineal resection

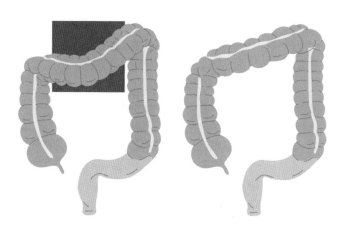

Segmental resection

radiation therapy and Chapter 11 for symptom management.

Bowel Management

Following surgery, while the body adapts to its new anatomy, dietary modifications and medications can help slow food transit through the GI tract, improving absorption. Most patients will ultimately tolerate a variety of foods. Management of loose stools is necessary in rectal resections and with colon anastomosis. A firmer, formed stool decreases urgency, and leaking and allows more complete elimination. The optimal goal is fewer than four bowel movements per day.

Nutrition interventions for bowel management may include the following:

- Start the patient on 1 teaspoon of psyllium, with little or no additional water, twice daily with morning and evening meals. The psyllium is best mixed with oatmeal, pudding, yogurt, mashed potatoes, applesauce, or peanut butter, with no additional fluid for 1 hour before or after meals. This will assist with absorbing excess fluid and slowing transit. Increase by 1 teaspoon every 3 to 5 days to a maximum of 1 tablespoon twice daily.

- Advise the patient to avoid hot beverages.

- Recommend foods to thicken stools, including marshmallows.

- Adjust doses of medications to slow transit. See Chapter 11 for additional details on bowel management.

Ostomy Management

Ostomies are more common with rectal surgeries and may be temporary (with plans for reversal) or permanent. After the adaptation period, normal ileostomy output is 500 to 1,000 mL/d, and 200 to 600 mL/d for a colostomy.[36] Patients can benefit from referral to a wound care and ostomy nurse for education and evaluation of problems. Extensive resources and links to support groups can be found on the United Ostomy Associations of America website (www.ostomy.org).

Nutrition interventions for ostomy management may include the following:

- Use appropriate dietary strategies based on stool consistency and odor.

- Integrate fiber slowly, titrating to volume and consistency of output. Note that different functional fibers in the gut play specific roles.[82]

- Monitor for fluid and electrolyte losses, which are especially problematic with ileostomy. Replace fluid and electrolytes as follows:

    - Aim for a daily intake goal of 1 L more than output.

    - Use oral rehydration solutions, sports drinks, broth, and vegetable juices to address losses of fluid, sodium, and potassium.

Low Anterior Resection Syndrome

Low rectal anastomosis avoids an abdominal perineal resection with colostomy, but more than 80% of patients who undergo low anterior resection remain symptomatic due to changes in anal sphincter function, sensation, and the rectoanal inhibitory reflex.[83] Symptoms of low anterior resection syndrome include increased frequency and clustering of bowel movements, urgency, and incontinence or constipation with feelings of incomplete emptying.[84] A history of radiation therapy may exacerbate outcomes. Changes are considered permanent at 2 years postsurgery. Repeat ostomy is an option for improved symptom control.

Nutrition interventions for lower anterior resection syndrome may include the following[84,85]:

- Recommend a soft, low-fiber diet for 2 weeks postoperatively.

- Recommend consumption of larger meals earlier in the day.

- Use psyllium fiber to jell stools.

- If stool frequency slows after 6 weeks with extensive and consistent use of antidiarrheal medications, advise taking one to two tablets of loperamide (Imodium AD) 30 minutes before meals and bedtime. Adjust dosing as needed. Consider prescription options, if needed.

- Consider the use of type 3 serotonin receptor antagonists or the bile acid sequestrant colesevelam to reduce urgency and frequency.

- Note that neither the proprietary probiotic preparation VSL#3 (VSL Pharmaceuticals)[86] nor steroids offer any benefit.

- If incomplete rectal emptying and clustered stools persist despite interventions through the recovery period, the surgeon may allow deliberate evacuation with a tap-water enema, instilled and held for 30 seconds.

- Sacral nerve stimulation may be considered after 1 year.[87] Biofeedback and pelvic floor rehabilitation significantly improve symptoms, with tolerance of rectal volumes improving over 6 to 12 months.[88]

Neorectal Reservoirs

Neorectal reservoirs are surgical procedures creating an internal reservoir using the distal 20 to 30 cm of ileum, either in a one-step or two-step process that includes a temporary ileostomy that is reversed at 8 to 12 weeks to reestablish continuity. Neorectal reservoirs include colonic J-pouch anal anastomosis, side-to-end anal anastomosis (a one-step process), and transverse coloplasty pouch. Five to seven loose bowel movements a day with urgency despite optimizing medications to slow transit is considered normal for up to 6 weeks after surgery.[89]

Bowel movements become less frequent and thicken as the pouch stretches over 6 months after surgery. Long-term complications include inflammation of the reservoir, known as pouchitis, causing diarrhea, cramps, and bloating; stricturing at the connection of the reservoir and anus, making it difficult to empty the reservoir; incontinence; and diarrhea or ongoing frequent bowel movements. Pouchitis can occur in one-third of patients, and antibiotic therapy may worsen diarrhea. Antidiarrheal medication may be used to manage symptoms and should be taken before meals to be most effective.

Vitamin and Mineral Malabsorption

Vitamin and mineral malabsorption is common following surgeries that result in rapid transit through the digestive tract.

Nutrition interventions for vitamin and mineral malabsorption may include the following:

- Monitor serum vitamin D levels and provide appropriate supplementation to achieve normal serum levels.

- Recommend a calcium-rich diet with supplementation as needed to meet total needs.

- Monitor vitamin B12 levels after ileocecal resections and begin supplementation as needed.

- Be aware that a multivitamin supplement may be indicated with perceived or actual diet restrictions.

Anal Carcinoma

A 1.5-inch anal canal connects the rectum to the anus. The anal sphincter is a muscular sphincter at the distal end of the rectum that surrounds the anus and helps maintain stool continence. The point at which the anal canal meets the skin is called the anal verge, and the area beyond the anal verge is described as perianal. Stool is stored in the rectum before it passes through the anal canal and anus, at which time the anal sphincter relaxes, allowing a bowel movement.

Anal carcinoma (AC) accounts for less than 3% of all GI cancers in the United States.[9,12] The majority of ACs are squamous cell carcinomas arising from the squamous cells that line most of the anal canal. Adenocarcinomas are rare, developing in cells that line the upper anal canal adjacent to the rectum, and respond best to rectal cancer treatments. Infrequently, malignant melanomas and sarcomas can involve the anal canal.

Treatment

Treatment modalities for AC include surgery, chemotherapy, and radiation. Multimodal treatments are often used. Concurrent chemoradiation is first-line therapy for AC and often results in significant side effects that can alter QOL.[90] Chemotherapy-related nutrition impact symptoms include mucositis, nausea, vomiting, diarrhea, and decreased appetite. Radiation therapy–related nutrition impact symptoms include skin changes; anal irritation and pain; nausea; vomiting; diarrhea; discomfort with bowel movements; and fatigue. Refer to the *NCCN Clinical Practice Guidelines in Oncology (NCCN Guidelines): Anal Carcinoma* regarding details of specific therapies.[91]

Surgery

Surgical intervention is reserved for persistent disease, which is evaluated at 12 to 26 weeks after chemoradiation. Salvage surgeries include abdominal perineal resection with complete removal of the anus, anal sphincter, surrounding tissue, and lymph nodes, which then results in a colostomy. This surgery offers a 5-year disease-free survival of 30% to 45%.[92]

Disease-Specific Nutrition Problems and Interventions

The majority of disease-specific nutrition problems among patients with AC are related to treatment, especially chemotherapy and radiation. Nutrition problems and interventions for GI cancers are summarized in Box 19.1 on pages 412 and 413. See Chapters 9 and 10 for a detailed description of side effects due to systemic and radiation therapy and Chapter 11 for symptom management.

Summary

GI cancers pose multiple challenges to patients, caregivers, and clinicians. The management of these challenges can benefit from the specialized knowledge of an oncology registered dietitian nutritionist as part of the multidisciplinary team. Evidence-based medical nutrition therapy is essential for improving the functional status and QOL of patients with these cancers.

Sample PES Statements for Cancers of the Gastrointestinal Tract

Intake domain: Inadequate fluid intake related to ileostomy, as evidenced by dehydration and altered laboratory values, specifically elevated blood urea nitrogen (BUN) and sodium.

Clinical domain: Moderate, chronic disease- or condition-related malnutrition related to malabsorptive diarrhea, as evidenced by a weight loss of >5% in the past month and a medical diagnosis of malnutrition.

Chapter 19 *Medical Nutrition Therapy for Cancers of the Liver, Bile Duct, Gallbladder, Small Bowel, Colon, Rectum, and Anus*

427

References

1. Ahluwalia B, Magnusson MK, Ohman L. Mucosal immune system of the gastrointestinal tract: maintaining balance between the good and the bad. *Scand J Gastroenterol.* 2017;52(11):1185-1193.

2. Andreyev HJ, Norman AR, Oates J, Cunningham D. Why do patients with weight loss have a worse outcome when undergoing chemotherapy for gastrointestinal malignancies? *Eur J Cancer.* 1998;34(4):503-509.

3. Ceolin Alves AL, Zuconi CP, Correia MI. Energy expenditure in patients with esophageal, gastric, and colorectal cancer. *JPEN J Parenter Enter Nutr.* 2016;40(4):499-506.

4. American Cancer Society. About liver cancer. Accessed June 11, 2020. www.cancer.org/cancer /liver-cancer/about/what-is-key -statistics.html

5. American Cancer Society. Key statistics about gall bladder cancer. 2020. Accessed June 11, 2020. www.cancer.org/cancer /gallbladder-cancer/about/key -statistics.html

6. American Cancer Society. Key statistics about bile duct cancer. Accessed June 11, 2020. www .cancer.org/cancer/bile-duct -cancer/about/key-statistics.html

7. American Cancer Society. Survival rates for gastrointestinal carcinoid tumors. Accessed July 20, 2019. https://cancer.org /cancer/gastrointestinal-carcinoid -tumor/detection-diagnosis -staging/survival-rates.html

8. American Cancer Society. Survival rates for colorectal cancer. Accessed June 11, 2020. https://www.cancer.org/cancer /colon-rectal-cancer/detertion -diagnosis-staging/survival -rates.html

9. American Cancer Society. Key Statistics for anal cancer. Accessed June 11, 2020. https:// www.cancer.org/cancer/anal -cancer/about/what-is-key -statistics.html

10. American Cancer Society. Liver cancer risk factors. Accessed June 11, 2020. www.cancer.org /cancer/liver-cancer/causes-risks -prevention/risk-factors.html

11. Cicalese L. What is the prognosis for hepatocellular carcinoma? Medscape. Updated June 5, 2020. Accessed June 11, 2020. www .medscape.com/answers/197319 -39201/what-is-the-prognosis-for -hepatocellular-carcinoma-hcc

12. Siegel RL, Miller KD, Jemal A. Cancer statistics, 2020. CA: *Cancer J Clin.* 2020;70(1):7-30.

13. World Cancer Research Fund International/American Institute for Cancer Research. Continuous Update Project Expert Report 2018. *Diet, Nutrition, Physical Activity and Cancer: A Global Perspective.* Accessed May 18, 2020. http://www.aicr.org/assets /docs/pdf/reports/cup-report-liver -cancer.pdf

14. Aleksandrova K, Boeing H, Nothlings U, et al. Inflammatory and metabolic biomarkers and risk of liver and biliary tract cancer. *Hepatology.* 2014;60(3):858-871.

15. Campbell PT, Newton CC, Kitahara CM, et al. Body size indicators and risk of gallbladder cancer: pooled analysis of individual-level data from 19 prospective cohort studies. *Cancer Epidemiol Biomarkers Prev.* 2017;26(4):597-606.

16. Bagnardi V, Rota M, Botteri E, et al. Alcohol consumption and site-specific cancer risk: a comprehensive dose-response meta-analysis. *Br J Cancer.* 2015;112(3):580-593.

17. Shafqet M, Sharzehi K. Diabetes and the pancreatobiliary diseases. *Curr Treat Options Gastroenterol.* 2017;15(4):508-519.

18. Cen L, Pan J, Zhou B, et al. Helicobacter Pylori infection of the gallbladder and the risk of chronic cholecystitis and cholelithiasis: a systematic review and meta-analysis. *Helicobacter.* 2018;23(1). doi:10.1111/hel.12457

19. Larsson SC, Giovannucci EL, Wolk A. Sweetened beverage consumption and risk of biliary tract and gallbladder cancer in a prospective study. *J Natl Cancer Inst*. 2016;108(10). doi:10.1093/jnci/djw125

20. Makiuchi T, Sobue T, Kitamura T, et al. The relationship between vegetable/fruit consumption and gallbladder/bile duct cancer: A population-based cohort study in Japan. *Int J Cancer*. 2017;140(5):1009-1019.

21. National Comprehensive Cancer Network. *NCCN Clinical Practice Guidelines (NCCN Guidelines): Genetic/Familial High-Risk Assessment: Colorectal*. Version 1.2020. National Comprehensive Cancer Network; 2020. Accessed February 24, 2021. www.nccn.org/professionals/physician_gls/pdf/genetics_colon.pdf

22. Komaki Y, Komaki F, Micic D, Ido A, Sakuraba A. Risk of colorectal cancer in chronic liver diseases: a systematic review and meta-analysis. *Gastrointest Endosc*. 2017;86(1):93-104.

23. Kreimer AR, Brennan P, Lang Kuhs KA, et al. Human papillomavirus antibodies and future risk of anogenital cancer: a nested case-control study in the European prospective investigation into cancer and nutrition study. *J Clin Oncol*. 2015;33(8):877-884.

24. Palefsky J. Human papillomavirus infections: epidemiology and disease associations. Uptodate.com. Accessed February 24, 2021. www.uptodate.com/contents/human-papillomavirus-infections-epidemiology-and-disease-associations

25. National Comprehensive Cancer Network. NCCN Guidelines and Clinical Resources. National Comprehensive Cancer Network. website. Accessed February 24, 2021. www.nccn.org/professionals/physician_gls/default.aspx#site

26. National Cancer Institute. Gastrointestinal carcinoid tumors treatment (Adult) (PDQ)–health professional version. Accessed June 11, 2020. www.cancer.gov/types/gi-carcinoid-tumors/hp/gi-carcinoid-treatment-pdq

27. Nanavati AJ, Prabhakar S. Enhanced recovery after surgery: if you are not implementing it, why not? Nutrition Issues in Gastroenterology 2016. Accessed June 11, 2020. https://med.virginia.edu/ginutrition/wp-content/uploads/sites/199/2014/06/Parrish-April-2016.pdf

28. Gustafsson UO, Scott MJ, Schwenk W, et al. Guidelines for perioperative care in elective colonic surgery: Enhanced Recovery After Surgery (ERAS(R)) Society recommendations. *Clin Nutr*. 2012;31(6):783-800.

29. Moya, P, Soriano-Irigaray L, Ramirez JM, et al. Perioperative standard oral nutrition supplements verses immunonutrition in patients undergoing colorectal resection in an Enhanced Recvovery (ERAS) Protocol: a multi center randomized clinical trial (SONVI Study). *Medicine*. 2016;95(21):e3704.

30. Kabata P, Jastrzebski T, Kakol M, et al. Preoperative nutritional support in cancer patients with no clinical signs of malnutrition-prospective randomized controlled trial. *Support Care Cancer*. 2015;23(2):365-370.

31. Parrish CR, DiBaise JK. Short bowel syndrome in adults-part 2: nutrition therapy for short bowel syndrome in the adult patient. *Nutr Issues in Gastroenterol* 2014. https://med.virginia.edu/ginutrition/wp-content/uploads/sites/199/2014/06/Parrish-October-14.pdf

32. Islam RS, DiBaise JK. Bile acids: an underrecongnized and underappreciated cause of chronic diarrhea. *Pract Gastroenterol*. 2012;36(10):32-44. Accessed February 24, 2021. https://med.virginia.edu/ginutrition/wp-content/uploads/sites/199/2014/06/Parrish_Oct_12.pdf

Chapter 19 *Medical Nutrition Therapy for Cancers of the Liver, Bile Duct, Gallbladder, Small Bowel, Colon, Rectum, and Anus*

429

33. Han Z, Margulies S, Kurlan,D, Elliott M. Vitamin D deficiencies in patients with disorder of the digestive system: current knowledge and practical considerations. *Pract Gastroenterol*. 2016;40:36-43. Accessed February 24, 2021. https://med.virginia.edu/ginutrition/wp-content/uploads/sites/199/2014/06/Parrish-July-16.pdf

34. Liang S, Xu L, Zhang D, Wu Z. Effect of probiotics on small intestinal bacterial overgrowth in patients with gastric and colorectal cancer. *Turk J Gastroenterol*. 2016;27(3):227-232.

35. Adike A, DiBaise JK. Small intestinal bacterial overgrowth: nutritional implications, diagnosis, and management. *Gastroenterol Clin North Am*. 2018;47(1):193-208. doi: 10.1016/j.gtc.2017.09.008

36. de Vries FEE, Reeskamp LF, van Ruler O, et al. Systematic review: pharmacotherapy for high-output enterostomies or enteral fistulas. *Aliment Pharmacol Ther*. 2017;46(3):266-273.

37. Lewis S, Heaton K. Stool form scale as a useful guide to intestinal transit time. *Scand J Gastroenterol*. 1997;32(9):920–924.

38. Lind A, Wangberg B, Ellegard L. Vitamin D and vitamin B12 deficiencies are common in patients with midgut carcinoid (SI-NET). *Eur J Clin Nutr*. 2016;70(9):990-99.

39. American Cancer Society. Can liver cancer be found early? Accessed June 11, 2020. https://cancer.org/cancer/liver-cancer/detection-diagnosis-staging/detection.html.

40. National Comprehensive Cancer Network. *NCCN Clinical Practice Guidelines (NCCN Guidelines): Hepatobilary Cancers*. Version 5.2020. National Comprehensive Cancer Network; 2020. Accessed March 26, 2020. https://www.nccn.org/professionals/physician_gls/pdf/hepatobiliary.pdf

41. Curley SA BC, Abdalla EK, Singai AG. Management of potentially resectable hepatocellular carcinoma: prognosis, role of neoadjuvant and adjuvant therapy, and posttreatment surveillance. Uptodate.com. Accessed June 10, 2020. www.uptodate.com/contents/management-of-potentially-resectable-hepatocellular-carcinoma-prognosis-role-of-neoadjuvant-and-adjuvant-therapy-and-posttreatment-surveillance

42. Huang L, Li J, Yan JJ, Liu CF, Wu MC, Yan YQ. Prealbumin is predictive for postoperative liver insufficiency in patients undergoing liver resection. *World J Gastroenterol*. 2012;18(47):7021-7025.

43. Blechacz B. Cholangiocarcinoma: current knowledge and new developments. *Gut Liver*. 2017;11(1):13-26.

44. Anderson CD, Stuart KE, Palta M. Treatment of locally advanced, unresectable, but nonmetastatic cholangiocarcinoma. UpToDat.com. Accessed June 10, 2020. www.uptodate.com/contents/treatment-options-for-locally-advanced-unresectable-but-nonmetastatic-cholangiocarcinoma

45. Parrish CR, Quattra B. Reinfusion of intestinal secretions: a valuable option for select patients. *Pract Gastrenterol*. 2010;34:28-40. Accessed February 24, 2021. https://med.virginia.edu/ginutrition/wp-content/uploads/sites/199/2014/06/ParrishArticle_4-10.pdf

46. Johnson TM, Overgard EB, Cohen AE, DiBaise JK. Nutrition assessment and management in advanced liver disease. *Nutr Clin Pract*. 2013;28(1):15-29.

47. Krenitsky J. Nutrition update in hepatic failure. Nutrition Issues in Gastroenterology. 2014. Accessed June 11, 2020. https://med.virginia.edu/ginutrition/wp-content/uploads/sites/199/2014/06/Parrish-April-14.pdf

48. Cordoba J, Lopez-Hellin J, Planas M, et al. Normal protein diet for episodic hepatic encephalopathy: results of a randomized study. *J Hepatol*. 2004;41(1):38-43.

49. Gluud LL, Dam G, Les I, et al. Branched-chain amino acids for people with hepatic encephalopathy. *Cochrane Database Syst Rev*. 2015;(2):Cd001939.

50. Bemeur C, Desjardins P, Butterworth RF. Role of nutrition in the management of hepatic encephalopathy in end-stage liver failure. *J Nutr Metab*. 2010;2010:489823. doi:10.1155/2010/48982

51. Hughes DJ, Duarte-Salles T, Hybsier S, et al. Prediagnostic selenium status and hepatobiliary cancer risk in the European Prospective Investigation into Cancer and Nutrition cohort. *Amer J Clin Nutr*. 2016;104(2):406-414.

52. Kerwin AJ, Nussbaum MS. Adjuvant nutrition management of patients with liver failure, including transplant. *Surg Clin North Am*. 2011;91(3):565-578.

53. Huisman EJ, Trip EJ, Siersema PD, van Hoek B, van Erpecum KJ. Protein energy malnutrition predicts complications in liver cirrhosis. *Eur J Gastroenterol Hepatol*. 2011;23(11):982-989.

54. Mehrotra B, Bekaii-Saab T. Adjuvant treatment for localized, resected gallbladder cancer. UpToDate.com. Accessed January 1, 2018. https://uptodate.com/contents/adjuvant-treatment-for-localized-resected-gallbladder-cancer

55. Klimstra DS. Pathologic classification of neuroendocrine neoplasms. *Hematol Oncol Clin North Am*. 2016;30(1):1-19.

56. Basuroy R, Bouvier C, Ramage J, Sissons M, Srirajaskanthan R. Delays and routes to diagnosis of neuroendocrine tumours. *BMC Cancer*. 2018;18(1):1122. doi:10.1186/s12885-01

57. Al-Efraij K, Aljama MA, Kennecke HF. Association of dose escalation of octreotide long-acting release on clinical symptoms and tumor markers and response among patients with neuroendocrine tumors. *Cancer Med*. 2015;4(6):864-870.

58. Adaway JE, Dobson R, Walsh J, et al. Serum and plasma 5-hydroxyindoleacetic acid as an alternative to 24-h urine 5-hydroxyindoleacetic acid measurement. *Ann Clin Biochem*. 2016;53(pt 5):554-560.

59. Mojtahedi A, Thamake S, Tworowska I, Ranganathan D, Delpassand ES. The value of (68)Ga-DOTATATE PET/CT in diagnosis and management of neuroendocrine tumors compared to current FDA approved imaging modalities: a review of literature. *Am J Nucl Med Mol Imaging*. 2014;4(5):426-434.

60. Ito T, Lee L, Jensen RT. Carcinoid-syndrome: recent advances, current status and controversies. *Curr Opin Endocrinol Diabetes Obes*. 2018; 25(1):22-25.

61. Caplin ME, Pavel M, Cwikla JB, et al. Anti-tumour effects of lanreotide for pancreatic and intestinal neuroendocrine tumours: the CLARINET open-label extension study. *Endocr Relat Cancer*. 2016;23(3):191-199.

62. National Comprehensive Cancer Network. *NCCN Clinical Practice Guidelines (NCCN Guidelines): Neuroendocrine and Adrenal Tumors*. Version 2. 2020. National Comprehensive Cancer Network; 2020. Accessed July 26, 2020. www.nccn.org/professionals/physician_gls/pdf/neuroendocrine.pdf

63. Saif MW LH, Kaley K, Shaib W. Chronic octreotide therapy can induce pancreatic insufficiency: a common but under-recognized adverse effect. *Expert Opin Drug Saf 2010*; Accessed December 31, 2017. doi:10.1517/14740338.2010.510130

64. Henry RR, Ciaraldi TP, Armstrong D, Burke P, Ligueros-Saylan M, Mudaliar S. Hyperglycemia associated with pasireotide: results from a mechanistic study in healthy volunteers. *J Clin Endocrinol Met*. 2013;98(8):3446-3453.

Chapter 19 *Medical Nutrition Therapy for Cancers of the Liver, Bile Duct, Gallbladder, Small Bowel, Colon, Rectum, and Anus*

431

65. Sharma N, Naraev BG, Engelman EG, et al. Peptide receptor radionuclide therapy outcomes in a north american cohort with metastatic well-differentiated neuroendocrine tumors. *Pancreas*. 2017;46(2):151-156.

66. Kulke MH, Horsch D, Caplin ME, et al. Telotristat Ethyl, a tryptophan hydroxylase inhibitor for the treatment of carcinoid syndrome. *J Clin Oncol*. 2017;35(1):14-23.

67. Qureshi SA, Burch N, Druce M, et al. Screening for malnutrition in patients with gastro-entero-pancreatic neuroendocrine tumours: a cross-sectional study. *BMJ Open*. 2016;6(5):e010765.

68. Warner M. Nutritional concerns for the carcinoid patient: developing nutrition guidelines for persons with carcinoid disesase. 2009; Accessed February 24, 2021. https://carcinoid.org/for-patients/general-information/nutrition/nutritional-concerns-for-the-carcinoid-patient-developing-nutrition-guidelines-for-persons-with-carcinoid-disease

69. Ducreux M. Carcinoid syndrome in neuroendocrine tumors: a prognostic effect? *Lancet Oncol*. 2017;18(4):426-428.

70. Kiesewetter B, Raderer M. Ondansetron for diarrhea associated with neuroendocrine tumors. *N Engl J Med*. 2013;368(20):1947-1948.

71. Chauhan A, Miller RC, Yu Q, Aslam B, Weiss H. The antidiarrheal efficacy of a proprietary amino acid mixture in gastroenteropancreatic neuroendocrine patients. *J Clin Oncol*. 2018;36(supple 4S):Abstract 509.

72. Bouma G, van Faassen M, Kats-Ugurlu G, de Vries EG, Kema IP, Walenkamp AM. Niacin (vitamin B3) supplementation in patients with serotonin-producing neuroendocrine tumor. *Neuroendocrinology*. 2016;103(5):489-494.

73. Brenner H, Kloor M, Pox C. Colorectal cancer. *Lancet*. 2014;383(9927):1490-1502. doi:10.1016/S0140-6736(13)61649-9

74. Bibbins-Domingo K, Grossman DC, Curry SJ, et al. Screening for colorectal cancer: US preventive services task force recommendation statement. *JAMA*. 2016;315(23):2564-2575.

75. Marmol I, Sanchez-de-Diego C, Pradilla Dieste A, Cerrada E, Rodriguez Yoldi MJ. Colorectal carcinoma: a general overview and future perspectives in colorectal cancer. *Int J Mol Sci. 2017*;18(1). doi:10.3390/ijms18010197

76. Chung L, Thiele Orberg E, Geis AL, et al. Bacteroides fragilis toxin coordinates a pro-carcinogenic inflammatory cascade via targeting of colonic epithelial cells. *Cell Host Microbe*. 2018;23(2):203-214.e205.

77. Dasari S, Kathera C, Janardhan A, Praveen Kumar A, Viswanath B. Surfacing role of probiotics in cancer prophylaxis and therapy: a systematic review. *Clin Nutr*. 2017;36(6):1465-1472.

78. National Comprehensive Cancer Network. *NCCN Clinical Practice Guidelines (NCCN Guidelines): Genetic/Familial High-Risk Assessment: Colorectal*. Version 2. 2021. National Comprehensive Cancer Network; 2021. Accessed February 24, 2021. www.nccn.org/professionals/physician_gls/pdf/colon.pdf

79. National Comprehensive Cancer Network. *NCCN Clinical Practice Guidelines (NCCN Guidelines): Rectal Cancer*. Version 1.2021. National Comprehensive Cancer Network; 2021. Accessed February 24, 2021. www.nccn.org/professionals/physician_gls/pdf/rectal.pdf

80. Simkens GA, Rovers KP, Nienhuijs SW, de Hingh IH. Patient selection for cytoreductive surgery and HIPEC for the treatment of peritoneal metastases from colorectal cancer. *Cancer Manag Res*. 2017;9:259-266.

81. Esquivel J. Cytoreductive surgery and hyperthermic intraperitoneal chemotherapy for colorectal cancer: survival outcomes and patient selection. *J Gastrointest Oncol*. 2016;7(1):72-78.

82. McRorie JW, Jr., McKeown NM. Understanding the physics of functional fibers in the gastrointestinal tract: an evidence-based approach to resolving enduring misconceptions about insoluble and soluble fiber. *J Acad Nutr Diet*. 2017;117(2):251-264.

83. Dulskas A, Smolskas E, Kildusiene I, Samalavicius NE. Treatment possibilities for low anterior resection syndrome: a review of the literature. *Int J Colorectal Dis*. 2018;33(3):251-260.

84. Ridolfi TJ, Berger N, Ludwig KA. Low anterior resection syndrome: current management and future directions. *Clin Colon Rectal Surg*. 2016;29(3):239-245.

85. Martellucci J. Low anterior resection syndrome: a treatment algorithm. *Dis Colon Rectum*. 2016;59(1):79-82.

86. Stephens JH, Hewett PJ. Clinical trial assessing VSL#3 for the treatment of anterior resection syndrome. *ANZ J Surg*. 2012;82(6):420-427.

87. Eftaiha SM, Balachandran B, Marecik SJ, et al. Sacral nerve stimulation can be an effective treatment for low anterior resection syndrome. *Colorectal Dis*. 2017;19(10):927-933.

88. Visser WS, te Riele WW, Boerma D, van Ramshorst B, van Westreenen HL. Pelvic floor rehabilitation to improve functional outcome after a low anterior resection: a systematic review. *Ann Colorproctol*. 2015;30(3):109-114. doi:10.3393/ac.2014.30.3.109

89. Hallbook O. Neorectal reservoirs and their revision. In: Zbar A., Madoff R., Wexner S. eds. *Reconstructive Surgery of the Rectum, Anus and Perineum*. Springer; 2013:105-112.

90. Ryan DP, Willett CG. Clinical features, staging and treatment of anal cancers. UptoDate.com. Accessed February 24, 2021. www.uptodate.com/contents/clinical-features-staging-and-treatment-of-anal-cancer

91. National Comprehensive Cancer Network. *NCCN Clinical Practice Guidelines (NCCN Guidelines): Anal Carcinoma*. Version 1.2021. National Comprehensive Cancer Network; 2021. Accessed February 21, 2021. www.www.nccn.org/professionals/physician_gls/pdf/anal.pdf

92. Gilshtein H, Khoury W. Surgical management of anal cancer. *Minerva Chir*. 2015;70(2):141-145.

Chapter 20
Medical Nutrition Therapy for Pancreatic Cancer

Maria Q. B. Petzel, RD, CSO, LD, CNSC, FAND

The pancreas is located in the abdomen behind the stomach. It functions as part of the endocrine and exocrine systems and consists of a head, body, and tail (see Figure 20.1). Endocrine cells in the pancreas produce hormones (eg, insulin and glucagon) that are released directly into the blood to regulate blood glucose. Exocrine cells produce pancreatic secretions containing bicarbonate and the digestive enzymes lipase, amylase, and proteases (including trypsin and chymotrypsin); these secretions help neutralize stomach acid and digest fats, carbohydrate, and proteins from food.

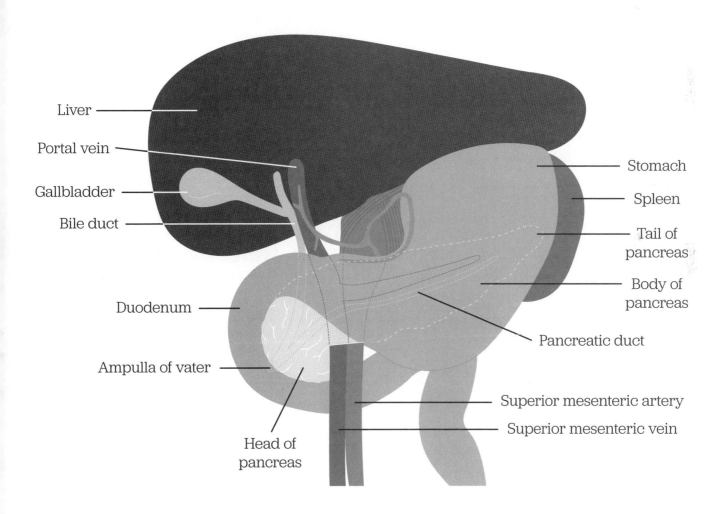

Figure 20.1
Normal anatomy of the abdominal region and pancreas

Types of Pancreatic Cancer

Pancreatic tumors arise from exocrine or endocrine cells. Exocrine tumors account for 93% of pancreatic cancer (PC) cases, while 7% of cases are endocrine tumors.[1] Although exocrine tumors are more common than endocrine tumors, survival rates are poorer for patients with exocrine tumors. The most common type of PC is adenocarcinoma, a cancer of the exocrine cells. Pancreatic adenocarcinoma is also known as ductal cell carcinoma or ductal adenocarcinoma.[2] Ninety-five percent of all exocrine tumors are pancreatic adenocarcinomas.[3] Other, less common types of exocrine tumors include acinar cell carcinoma, adenosquamous carcinoma, cystadenocarcinoma, squamous cell carcinoma, and giant cell carcinoma.

Types of endocrine (neuroendocrine or islet cell) tumors include the following[4]:

- carcinoid tumor
- insulinoma
- glucagonoma
- gastrinoma
- somatostatinoma
- VIPoma

Other regional tumors (periampullary) include ampullary, distal common bile duct (cholangiocarcinoma), and duodenal tumors. Premalignant or nonmalignant tumors (cysts) include solid pseudopapillary neoplasm, intraductal papillary mucinous neoplasm, mucinous cystic neoplasm, and serous cystadenoma.[5] Although these arise from different cells, side effects and surgeries are similar for these types of cancer or premalignant conditions due to their anatomic location.

Treatments and responses to treatment vary greatly among tumor types. Because nonexocrine tumors of the pancreas are rare, the remainder of this chapter focuses on pancreatic exocrine tumors (adenocarcinoma), unless otherwise specified.

Statistics on estimated new cases, deaths and 5-year relative survival rates for pancreatic adenocarcinoma and pancreatic neuroendocrine tumors in the United States are shown in Box 20.1.

Pancreatic secretions are released into side ducts, which merge to form the main pancreatic duct. Bile, which promotes digestion and absorption of dietary fat, passes from the liver and gallbladder to the small intestine via the common bile duct. The common bile duct merges with the main pancreatic duct, emptying secretions into the small

Box 20.1
Pancreatic Cancer Statistics, United States [3,4]

Pancreatic adenocarcinoma

Estimated new cases in 2020: 57,600

Estimated deaths in 2020: 47,050

Five-year relative survival rate:
- Overall: 9%
  - Localized (resectable) at diagnosis: 34%
  - Regional at diagnosis: 12%
  - Metastatic (unresectable) at diagnosis: 3%

Pancreatic neuroendocrine tumor

Estimated new cases in 2020: 4,030

Five-year relative survival rate:
- Overall: 54%
  - Localized (resectable) at diagnosis: 94%
  - Regional at diagnosis: 76%
  - Metastatic (unresectable) at diagnosis: 27%

intestine (duodenum) at the ampulla of Vater. The superior mesenteric artery and superior mesenteric vein cross behind the pancreas; tumor involvement with these vessels may determine if the tumor is resectable or not.

Risk factors for pancreatic adenocarcinoma include[3,6,7]:

- family history;

- cigarette smoking;

- obesity and abdominal adiposity;

- chronic pancreatitis;

- diabetes mellitus;

- heavy drinking, defined as more than three drinks per day (evidence is limited but suggestive); and

- a diet high in total fat, saturated fat, red meat, processed meat, or foods and beverages containing fructose (evidence is limited but suggestive).

Diagnosis

There is no tumor-specific marker for pancreatic exocrine tumors, but carbohydrate antigen 19-9 (CA 19-9) is elevated in most patients with PC and may be followed during or after treatment as a potential indicator of tumor response.[2,8]

There are two main staging methods for PC[9,10]:

- Resectability staging is based on imaging, CA19-9 level, and patient performance status. Tumors are divided into three groups: resectable (potentially curable), borderline resectable, and unresectable (locally advanced or metastatic).

- The American Joint Committee on Cancer staging method requires surgery to determine disease stage.

Because most patients with PC do not undergo surgery, resectability staging is used most often.[10] The American Society of Clinical Oncology and the National Comprehensive Cancer Network (NCCN) generally outline treatment plans based on resectability staging.

Treatment

Systemic therapy is used for all stages of PC. Sequence and duration of treatment varies depending on disease stage and treatment modality.[10] Refer to the *NCCN Clinical Practice Guidelines in Oncology (NCCN Guidelines): Pancreatic Cancer* for details of specific therapies.[10]

For unresectable PC, treatment is generally limited to systemic treatment only, and it is largely palliative.[11-14] A combination of surgery and systemic treatment is recommended for resectable PC; chemoradiation may or may not be included. The sequence of treatment for resectable disease may be influenced by general institutional beliefs or dictated by clinical trial protocols. Treatment for borderline resectable PC begins with systemic treatment; subsequent treatment may or may not include radiation therapy, surgery, or both.[10,15-17]

Systemic Therapy

Systemic chemotherapy has been shown to extend survival and improve quality of life (QOL) in patients with unresectable PC.[11-14] It generally is given as a combination of two or more drugs, but single agents may be given in cases of poor performance status. Chemotherapy is often given at the same time as radiation therapy to enhance radiosensitization of the tumor.[18] Box 20.2 lists the drugs and drug combinations commonly used to treat PC and associated nutrition impact symptoms (NIS). See also Chapter 9 for a comprehensive list of chemotherapeutic agents and strategies to manage NIS.

Box 20.2
Systemic Treatment Agents for Pancreatic Adenocarcinoma and Corresponding Nutrition Impact Symptoms[10,13,14,16,19-22]

Treatments	Anorexia	Taste Changes	Mucositis, Stomatitis	Nausea, Vomiting	Diarrhea	Other
Chemotherapy						
Capecitabine (Xeloda)			✓	✓	✓	
Cisplatin (Platinol-AQ)	✓	✓		✓	✓	Sodium wasting; magnesium wasting
Docetaxel (Taxotere)	✓		✓	✓	✓	
Fluorouracil		✓	✓	✓	✓	
Gemcitabine (Gemzar)	✓			✓		
Irinotecan (Camptosar) Liposomal irinotecan (Onivyde)	✓		✓	✓	✓	
Oxaliplatin (Eloxatin)		✓		✓	✓	Cold sensitivity (dysesthesia)
Paclitaxel (Taxol, Abraxane)			✓	✓	✓	
Targeted therapy						
Erlotinib (Tarceva)	✓			✓	✓	
Immunotherapy						
Pembrolizumab (Keytruda)	✓			✓	✓	Constipation

Drug combinations

First- or second-line therapy for patients with good performance status

FOLFIRINOX	Fluorouracil, leucovorin, oxaliplatin, and irinotecan
GA	Gemcitabine and albumin-bound paclitaxel, also known as nab-paclitaxel (Abraxane)

First-line therapy for patients with poorer performance status

GX	Gemcitabine and capecitabine (Xeloda)
GEM-E	Gemcitabine and erlotinib (Tarceva)

Less common, per guidelines

CapeOx or XELOX	Capecitabine (Xeloda) and oxaliplatin
FOLFIRI	Fluorouracil, leucovorin, and irinotecan (or liposomal irinotecan)
FOLFOX	Fluorouracil, leucovorin, and oxaliplatin
GemCis	Gemcitabine and cisplatin
GTX	Gemcitabine, docetaxel (Taxotere), and capecitabine (Xeloda)

Treatment duration and sequence depend on disease stage and response to therapy:

- For unresectable disease, treatment may be ongoing from initiation until treatment options are exhausted or until last days of life. Patients who have good response to treatment may be able to take a treatment holiday. Next-line treatment is initiated only after evidence of disease progression.[10,12,14]

- For borderline resectable tumors, chemotherapy or chemoradiation (or a combination of both) is given before resection, to improve the chances of getting clean margins.[10,15-17]

- For resectable and resected tumors, systemic treatment is recommended, although the appropriate sequence remains debated. It is recommended that any adjuvant (ie, postsurgery) systemic treatment commence within 8 to 12 weeks postoperatively. A total of 6 months (neoadjuvant or adjuvant, or both) of systemic treatment is recommended.[15-17]

Radiotherapy

The goal of radiotherapy depends on the clinical scenario. It may be given in the neoadjuvant setting to improve the chances of having clean surgical margins, as adjuvant treatment to help sterilize positive margins, or in those with positive lymph nodes to help reduce the chance of local recurrence. Radiotherapy may be part of a definitive treatment plan for locally advanced or unresectable tumors to prevent or delay progression of local disease. Treatment also may be given for palliation of symptoms, such as pain or bleeding; to relieve obstructive symptoms; or as palliative treatment for patients with poor performance status, advanced age, or comorbidities that prevent other definitive treatment strategies.[10]

Special nutrition considerations for individuals receiving radiotherapy to the pancreas may include adjustments to timing of meals, adjustments to food intake, and management of side effects caused by exposing the pancreas as well as surrounding organs to radiation. Patients receiving radiotherapy for tumors in the pancreatic body or tail may be asked to come to treatment on an empty stomach and then drink a specific volume of fluid to aid with mimicking simulation anatomy.[10]

Common side effects include anorexia, diarrhea, fatigue, nausea, vomiting, and weight loss.[23] Tolerance and side effects of treatment generally are affected by the type of concurrent therapy, planned total volume, the exposure of surrounding organs to the radiation, and the type of radiotherapy (conventional vs three-dimensional, intensity-modulated, or stereotactic body). See Chapter 10 for more about radiotherapy in general. Concurrent chemotherapy generally includes capecitabine, fluorouracil, or gemcitabine.[10,19] Exocrine pancreatic insufficiency (EPI), also referred to as pancreatic exocrine insufficiency (PEI), may develop or worsen following radiotherapy.[24]

Radiotherapy regimens typically are given in 10 or 28 treatments. Use of stereotactic body radiation therapy given over 3 to 5 treatments is emerging as a regimen for locally advanced disease, and its use for borderline disease is being examined in clinical trials. The sequence of radiotherapy vs chemotherapy can vary. In the case of resectable and borderline resectable disease, radiotherapy may be given after neoadjuvant induction chemotherapy or as first-line treatment. When given neoadjuvantly, surgery generally follows 4 to 8 weeks later to allow optimal downstaging and sterilization of the margin before significant formation of radiation-induced fibrosis.[10]

Surgery

Surgical types and techniques are determined by anatomic location of the cancer, rather than by pathologic type. In general, surgical considerations and side effects can be similarly managed based on anatomical location. See Chapter 19 for more information about nonsurgical treatment for neuroendocrine tumors of the pancreas or common bile duct. Box 20.3 and Figures 20.2 through 20.5 on pages 442 to 445 show more detailed information about the nutrition and anatomical impact of the most common pancreatic and periampullary surgeries

Two surgeries may typically be performed to resect pancreatic and periampullary tumors: pancreaticoduodenectomy (PD) or distal pancreatectomy. Figures 20.2 and 20.3 on pages 442 and 443 show the anatomical changes as a result of PD surgery. The two types of PD are standard and pylorus-preserving (PPPD). Figure 20.4 on page 444 shows the anatomical changes as a result of PPPD surgery and 20.5 on page 445 shows the anatomical changes as a result of distal pancreatectomy. Less common surgical procedures include total pancreatectomy, central pancreatectomy, and enucleation. PD and total pancreatectomy have greater nutritional implications than distal pancreatectomy. The mortality rate is 2% when surgery is performed at a high-volume center, and morbidity is reported at 30% to 60% for infectious (pneumonia, abscess, cholangitis, wound, and urinary tract infection) and noninfectious (bile leak, pancreatic fistula or leak) complications.[25-29] Regardless of the type of surgery, patients who are malnourished at the time of surgery have an increased risk for morbidity and mortality.[27]

Nutrition Assessment

Regardless of disease stage, nutrition plays a role in a patient's QOL. Patients with PC have an especially high risk for nutrition problems due to the anatomic location of the cancer and its potential effects on exocrine, endocrine, and biliary function.[33] Weight loss and malnutrition (one or both) occur in 50% to 90% of patients and are correlated with shorter progression-free survival, decreased chemotherapy response, decreased QOL and performance status, and greater surgical morbidity and mortality.[34-36] Weight stabilization is associated with improved survival, improved QOL, and better surgical outcomes,[37-39] but 70% to 80% of patients with pancreatic adenocarcinoma experience cachexia by the time of death.[36]

Studies to determine energy expenditure in patients with PC (vs healthy controls) show mixed results for resting energy expenditure (REE). Some studies suggest patients with PC are hypermetabolic,[40,41] while others suggest normometabolism or hypometabolism.[42,43] There are also variable results suggesting that tumor burden may or may not have a significant effect on REE.[40,42] The variation in findings is likely due to the heterogeneity in analysis of the data. There is also an absence of literature evaluating or reporting protein needs in patients with PC. Ultimately, the variation in study findings demonstrates the importance of an individualized nutrition assessment.

PC and its treatments may require modifications to usual nutrition interventions for NIS. Patients with PC may not tolerate typical recommendations for nutrition buildup, such as high-fat food or calorie-dense oral nutrition supplement drinks. For patients with precachexia and cachexia, there are no special interventions for PC, but practitioners should pay careful attention to optimal management of the side effects unique to PC. Strategies for these are discussed in the sections that follow. See Chapter 11 for strategies to manage common NIS.

Box 20.3
Common Surgeries for Pancreatic and Periampullary Tumors, Resulting Anatomic Changes, and Associated Nutrition Impact Symptoms[30-32]

Surgical procedure	Anatomic changes	Nutrition Impact Symptoms				
		Pancreatic exocrine insufficiency	Dumping syndrome	Delayed gastric emptying	Lactose intolerance	Diabetes mellitus
Pancreatico-duodenectomy (PD) (also known as a Whipple procedure)	Anatomy resected: head of pancreas, duodenum, gallbladder,* distal stomach, and part of common bile duct Reconstruction: hepaticojejunostomy,* pancreaticojejunostomy,** and gastrojejunostomy	✓	✓	✓	✓	✓
Pylorus-preserving pancreatico-duodenectomy (PPPD) (also known as a pylorus-preserving Whipple procedure)	Anatomy resected: head of pancreas, duodenum, gallbladder,* and part of common bile duct Reconstruction: hepaticojejunostomy,* pancreaticojejunostomy,** and duodenojejunostomy	✓		✓	✓	✓
Total pancreatectomy	Anatomy resected: same as PD or PPPD except entire pancreas is removed Spleen may be removed Reconstruction: same as PD or PPPD without pancreatojejunostomy or pancreaticogastrostomy	‡	✓	✓	✓	‡
Distal pancreatectomy	Anatomy resected: tail of pancreas or tail and body of pancreas Spleen may be removed Reconstruction: N/A	✓				✓

✓ = possible occurrence

‡ = definite occurrence

* Variation of resection and reconstruction may include leaving the gallbladder intact and reconstruction with choledocojejunostomy (jejunum to common bile duct) or cholecystojejunostomy (jejunum to gallbladder).

** Variation of reconstruction may include pancreaticogastrostomy (connecting remnant pancreas to stomach) instead of jejunum; may be performed more often in minimally invasive operations for technical reasons.

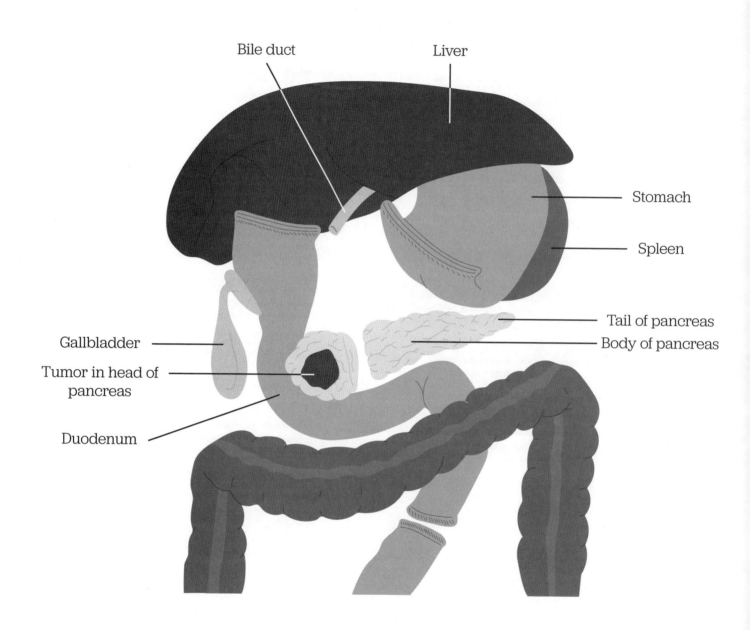

Figure 20.2
Pancreaticoduodenectomy (resected anatomy)

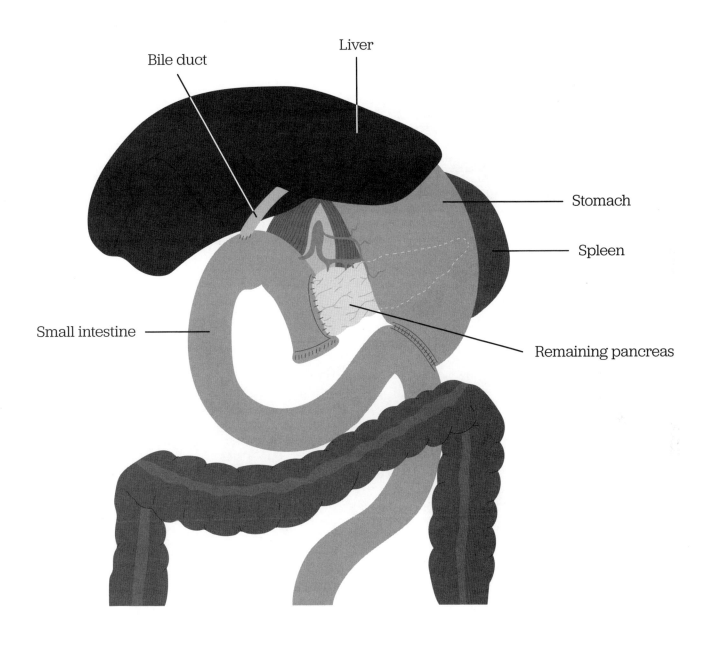

Bile duct

Liver

Stomach

Spleen

Small intestine

Remaining pancreas

Figure 20.3
Pancreaticoduodenectomy (anatomical reconstruction)

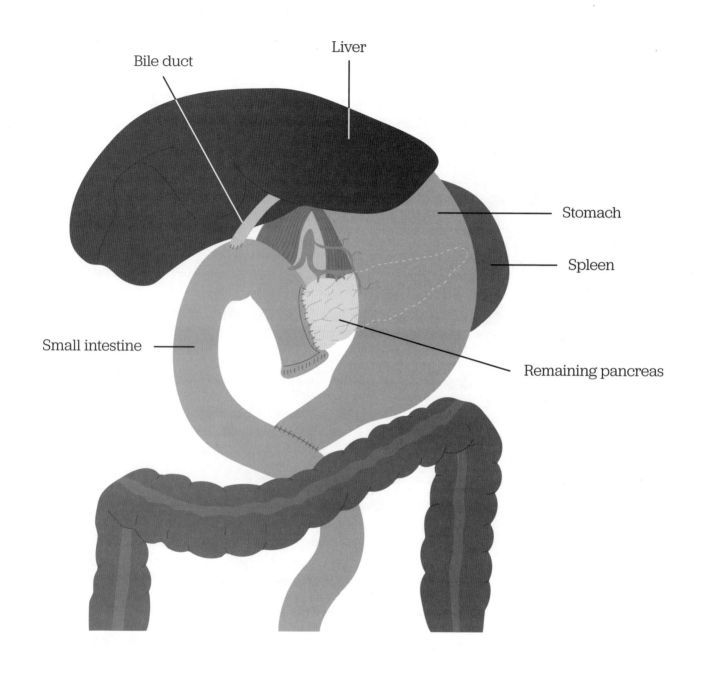

Figure 20.4
Pylorus-preserving pancreaticoduodenectomy (anatomical reconstruction)

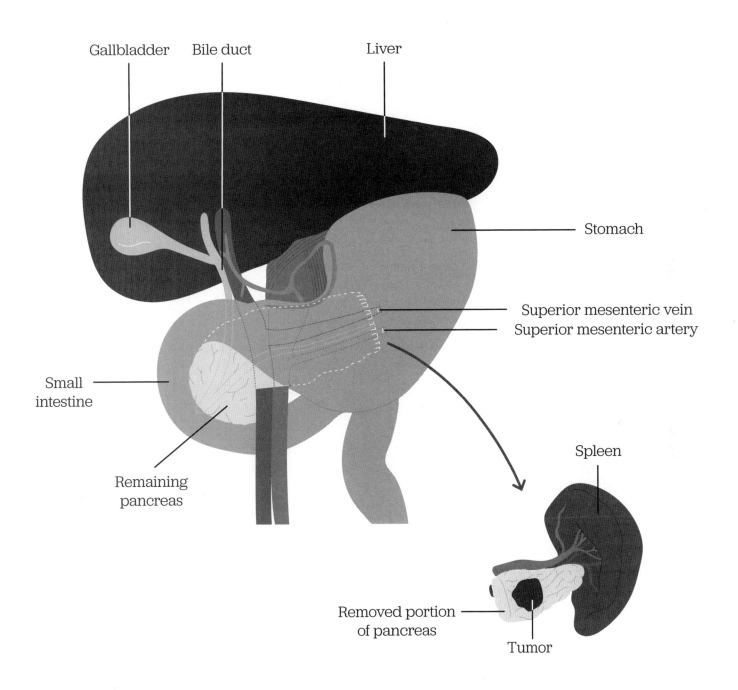

Figure 20.5
Distal pancreatectomy

Nutrition Problems and Interventions

The location and type of tumor and the stage of disease may affect symptoms that trigger the need for a diagnostic workup for PC. Box 20.4 lists NIS common at the time of diagnosis and their prevalence. Symptoms are more common in patients with advanced-stage disease. Some may present without NIS but develop symptoms associated with disease progression or resulting from treatment.[44-48] Depending on etiology, some NIS may be reversible (eg, loss of appetite and weight due to bile duct blockage and malabsorption) vs irreversible weight loss related to cancer cachexia.[49-51]

Malabsorption and Pancreatic Exocrine Insufficiency

Malabsorption may be attributed to insufficient digestion or absorption of food. PEI may be caused by loss of pancreatic parenchyma, obstructed pancreatic or common bile duct, changes in gastrointestinal (GI) tract synchrony, or reduced pancreatic secretions,[56,57] resulting in inadequate food digestion. Malabsorption may be observed in patients at the time of diagnosis, during nonsurgical treatment, following surgery, or with disease progression.[33,58] Symptoms of malabsorption can also be attributed to inadequate bile salts in the GI tract,[59] leading to inadequate fat absorption; therefore, biliary obstruction can lead to weight loss even if exocrine activity is sufficient.[55,60,61] However, studies indicate that 50% to 94% of patients with PC may have PEI and malabsorption,[56,58,62-64] and they may develop at any point during the disease.[58]

PEI often is associated with the hallmark characteristics of frequent or loose bowel movements. However, because narcotic pain medications also slow gut motility, the typically characteristic loose or frequent bowel movements may not be present. Other signs and symptoms are listed in Box 20.5 on page 448.

Tests to diagnose PEI can be cumbersome, difficult to conduct in clinical practice, and expensive; therefore, it is often diagnosed clinically and through response to empiric treatment.[65] Diagnostic tests[57,66,67] include the following:

- coefficient of fat absorption
- fecal chymotrypsin level
- fecal elastase (fecal elastase 1)
- fecal fat excretion
- urinary paraaminobenzoid acid excretion rate
- carbon 13–labeled mixed triglyceride breath test

Unfortunately, clinical diagnosis is less sensitive than functional testing and may lead to underdiagnosis and undertreatment; therefore, recent publications[56-58,66,67] suggest initiating treatment with pancreatic enzyme replacement therapy if a patient has clinical symptoms of PEI. In the absence of clinical symptoms, functional testing (most commonly fecal elastase) should be performed.[28,57,58,68] Screening for PEI should be repeated throughout the continuum of care.[58]

Box 20.4
Common Symptoms at the Time of Diagnosis of Pancreatic or Periampullary Tumors [5,23,28,44,48,52-55]

Symptom	Prevalence (% of patients)	Possible etiology
Jaundice Light-colored ("clay-colored") stools, dark urine, yellow skin, itchy skin	51% to 72%	Blocked bile duct
Pain	72% to 80%	Tumor involving or invading nerves Blocked digestive tract Pancreatic exocrine insufficiency
Weight loss	70% to 80%	Cancer cachexia Malabsorption
Decreased appetite	28% to 48%	Cancer cachexia Jaundice
Malabsorption	50% to 94%	Blocked pancreatic duct Reduced pancreatic enzyme production Blocked bile duct
Delayed gastric emptying or gastric outlet obstruction	2% to 38% (gastric outlet obstruction)	Partial or full blockage of the duodenum
Diabetes mellitus	50% to 80%	Reduced insulin production
Ascites Occurring within 0 to 2 months of diagnosis	22%	Cancer spread to peritoneum Portal vein hypertension Hepatic insufficiency Blockage of lymph system

Medical Nutrition Therapy for Malabsorption and Pancreatic Exocrine Insufficiency

Pancreatic Enzymes The primary strategy for management of malabsorption is pancreatic enzyme replacement therapy (PERT), which involves a prescription of pancreatic enzymes (pancrelipase). PERT is demonstrated to have a positive effect on body weight, stool frequency, total calorie intake, and total protein intake, even in the absence of symptomatic improvement.[72] Table 20.1 lists pancrelipase products currently approved by the US Food and Drug Administration (FDA), and Table 20.2 describes approved dosing regimens.

The most common practice is meal-based dosing. Enzyme dose should be divided throughout the meal.[65] Taking enzymes with the first bite of food, throughout the meal, and at the end of the meal ensures that enzymes are delivered with the food.[68,73] Supplemental pancreatic enzyme doses should not exceed 10,000 lipase units per kg of body weight per day, or 2,500 lipase units per kg of

body weight per meal up to four times a day.[68] The wide range of dosing reflects diet variation—some patients may present having already self-restricted the fat content of their diet or meal sizes and, therefore, need lower doses of PERT, whereas those who are still eating regular-size meals or large amounts of fat may need higher doses. It is often more prudent to begin at the low end of the range for meal-based dosing[32] and titrate up every few days as needed, while considering the characteristics of stools, clinical symptoms, and nutrition intake.[68,74] See Figure 20.8 on page 450 for guidance regarding initiation, titrating dose, and troubleshooting problems. Achieving optimal management of PEI often requires paying close attention to detail that gives registered dietitian nutritionists (RDNs) an opportunity to be the expert member of the health care team and an integral part of the patient's team.[68,75]

A physiologically basic environment is required both for enzyme function and bile acids to transport fatty acids into the bloodstream.[69,73] When pancreatic exocrine function is compromised, it is suggested that a histamine H2-receptor antagonist (eg, ranitidine or famotidine) or a proton pump inhibitor (eg, pantoprazole or omeprazole) be used because bicarbonate production and transport to the small intestine could be impaired.[65]

Because the clinical symptoms are not specific only to PEI and can be indicative of other physiologic or disease-related issues, it is important to understand that PERT may not completely resolve symptoms. If possible, complete PERT optimization during treatment breaks in order to eliminate the variable that anticancer treatment may be contributing to GI symptoms. While it may be impossible to eliminate steatorrhea completely, treatment can reduce symptoms by 60% to 70%.[69,73]

The cost of enzymes can be burdensome, and patients may seek to use an over-the-counter (OTC) preparation. OTC enzyme preparations may include bromelain, papain, trypsin, and chymotrypsin, or may be a combination product.[76]

Table 20.1
Pancreatic Enzyme Replacement Products (Pancrelipase) Approved by the Food and Drug Administration[74,77-80]

Brand	Available strengths (lipase USP units)		Dosage form	Manufacturer
Creon	3,000 6,000 12,000	24,000 36,000	Delayed-release capsule; enteric-coated spheres, beads, or microtablets	AbbVie
Pancreaze	2,600 4,200 10,500	16,800 21,000	Delayed-release capsule; enteric-coated spheres, beads, or microtablets	Vivus
Pertzye	4,000 8,000	16,000 24,000	Delayed-release capsule; bicarbonate-buffered enteric-coated spheres, beads, or microtablets	Digestive Care
Viokace	10,440	20,880	Tablet, no enteric coating	Allergan
Zenpep	3,000 5,000 10,000 15,000	20,000 25,000 40,000	Delayed-release capsule; enteric-coated spheres, beads, or microtablets	Allergan

Table 20.2
Pancreatic Enzyme Replacement Dosing Regimens [33,56,57,60,67,68,70,73,74,79,81-84]

Dosing method	Starting dose (lipase USP units)	Maximum dose (lipase USP units)
Per meal or snack	20,000-75,000 per meal 5,000-50,000 per snack	2,500 per kg of body weight per meal or 10,000 per kg of body weight per day
By body weight	500 per kg of body weight per meal 250 per kg of body weight per snack	2,500 per kg of body weight per meal or 10,000 per kg of body weight per day
Per fat content of meal or snack	500-1,000 per g of fat ingested	4,000 per g of fat ingested

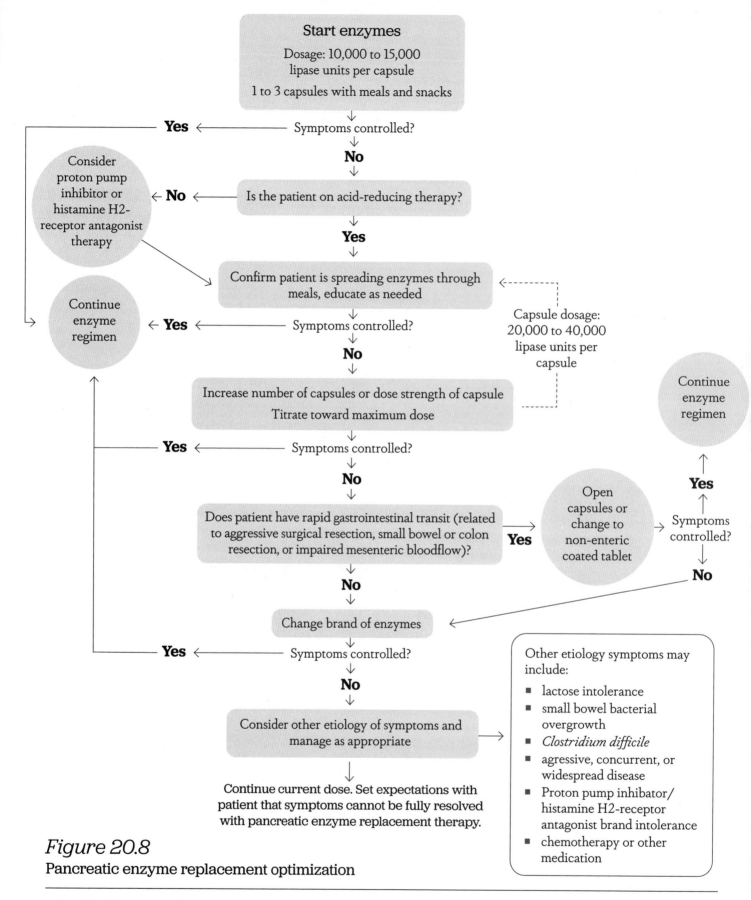

Figure 20.8
Pancreatic enzyme replacement optimization

Adapted with permission from EDP Consulting, LLC, Houston, Texas.

Oncology Nutrition *for* Clinical Practice

There is a lack of strong data to support the use of these supplements and, as with all OTC supplements, individuals should be counseled regarding concerns with the nonregulated industry and potential for nonstandardized or appropriately concentrated products. Efforts should be made to keep patients on FDA-approved products. They should be advised of FDA-approved products and encouraged to review their insurance formulary for the best option covered by their insurance. See Box 20.6 for possible financial resources for prescription enzymes.

Enteral Nutrition Regardless of the indication, for those patients with known or suspected PEI, the use of a semielemental enteral nutrition (EN) formula high in medium-chain triglycerides (MCTs) is recommended to limit the need for supplemental pancreatic enzymes during tube feeding.[85,86] For patients with severe PEI or when semielemental formula is cost prohibitive, administration of PERT still may be necessary.

If supplemental pancreatic enzymes are required with enteral feeding, enzymes should be administered about every 3 hours during continuous feedings. If feedings are given intermittently via gravity or bolus feeding, enzymes may be delivered with each feeding. If the patient has a large-bore gastrostomy tube (G-tube), the enzyme microspheres may be delivered in a thickened liquid. If the tube is small-bore or a jejunostomy tube (J-tube), enzymes should be crushed or dissolved with bicarbonate (or both) before administration.[85] Refer to Ferrie and colleagues[85] for methods of enzyme delivery via feeding tube, and to Berry[87] for recommendations for taking enzymes by mouth in tandem with EN infusion.

Though data are limited at this time, studies in humans with cystic fibrosis demonstrate that lipid absorption from EN is enhanced with the use of an in-line digestive cartridge, such as Relizorb (Alcresta Therapeutics).[88,89] These findings suggest potential benefit in patients with other etiologies of PEI.

Box 20.6
Resources for Financial Assistance for Pancreatic Enzyme Products

General resources	Brand-specific programs
CancerCare www.cancercare.org/financial_assistance	AbbVie patient assistance (for Creon) www.abbviepaf.org
NeedyMeds www.needymeds.org	Vivus patient assistance (for Pancreaze): https://pancreaze.com/patient-support
Medicine Assistance Tool www.medicine assistancetool.org	Chiesi CareDirect patient support (for Pertzye): www.pertzyecf.com/savings-support
	Allergan patient assistance (for Zenpep) www.allergan.com/responsibility/patient-resources/patient-assistance-programs

Diet Modification Patients with PEI or who have had pancreatic surgery are at risk for several micronutrient deficiencies. It is important for PERT to be adequate in order to maximize absorption of dietary sources of vitamins. With adequate PERT, patients may not need to restrict dietary fat.[33,48,69] However, fat restriction to less than 75 g/d may benefit some patients with severe steatorrhea.[73]

For patients having trouble consuming adequate calories due to limited fat tolerance, MCT oil may be substituted for other fats because MCTs do not require enzymatic action or bile salts for digestion or absorption.[73,90] MCT oil should not be used as a patient's only source of fat because it can lead to essential fatty acid deficiency.[73] Side effects can include diarrhea, vomiting, nausea, stomach discomfort, and intestinal gas. Compliance may be an issue because liquid MCT is not very palatable; however, recipes are available from some manufacturers. Though MCT oil is available in pill form, dosage per pill is very low and requires a significant number of pills to equate to 1 tablespoon of liquid. Although coconut oil does not provide MCTs exclusively, it is very high in MCTs and may be substituted for other fat sources in the regular diet. Malabsorption related to biliary obstruction may be reduced by following a low-fat diet until the obstruction is corrected.[55]

Diabetes Mellitus and Hyperglycemia

Diabetes mellitus (DM) may be a symptom of or a risk factor for PC.[28,91] Approximately 50% of all patients have DM at the time of their PC diagnosis[28]; and in about 50% to 75% of these patients, DM had been diagnosed within the 24 months prior to the PC diagnosis.[28,91] DM and hyperglycemia are newly reported in 17% to 24% of patients following pancreatic resection,[28,92] in 15% to 41% of patients following PD or PPPD, and in 8% to 54% of patients following distal pancreatectomy.[28] Preexisting DM has been shown to improve, worsen, or remain stable following surgery.[28,92] One study reported that preexisting DM worsened in about 50% of patients following PD and in 25% following distal pancreatectomy.[92] Other studies report an improvement in DM in 20% to 57% of patients following PD and in 13% following distal pancreatectomy.[28] Patients with preoperative chronic pancreatitis, long-standing DM, insulin use, previous glucose intolerance, and malignancy are less likely to have resolution.[28]

Medical Nutrition Therapy for Diabetes Mellitus and Hyperglycemia

The role of nutrition in management of DM varies depending on the side effects or symptoms a patient is experiencing and his or her stage of disease. It is appropriate to be more liberal with the diet and to use more aggressive medication or insulin management due to PC side effects or symptoms that reduce or limit oral intake.[73,93] Diet and blood glucose targets should be liberalized—to a hemoglobin A1c (HbA1c) level of less than 8%—for patients with progressive disease and older age.[93,94] In general, advise patients to minimize the use of refined carbohydrates, consume meals and snacks at regular intervals, and include a mix of protein, complex carbohydrates, and fat (as tolerated) in meals and snacks.

In patients with no evidence of PC and who have completed treatment, carbohydrate counting is appropriate to improve glycemic control,[73,95,96] with a goal HbA1c level of less than 7% (fasting blood glucose level, 70 to 130 mg/dL) without episodes of hypoglycemia.[95,97] Research shows that better postoperative glucose control following a total pancreatectomy (fasting blood glucose level <155 mg/dL and HbA1c level <7%) was associated with better recurrence-free survival and better overall survival.[98] As with all patients, dietary education is a key component of treatment: At least one study has shown improved outcomes (fewer hospitalizations, decreased health care expenditures, and fewer emergency visits) for patients with

Gastric Outlet Obstruction and Small Bowel Obstruction

Gastric outlet obstruction, also known as duodenal obstruction, is typically a late-onset side effect PC.[100-104] Small bowel obstruction, a malignant obstruction in the intestine beyond the ligament of Treitz, may occur as a result of peritoneal disease metastasis in advanced stages.[105] Symptoms of obstruction are the same for both types of obstruction and include nausea, vomiting (often containing retained, undigested food), abdominal distention, or pain. These symptoms can lead to dehydration, electrolyte imbalances, weight loss, and poor QOL.

Treatment for gastric outlet obstruction may be surgical[106] or endoscopic. Surgery typically involves gastrojejunostomy (gastric bypass), in which a loop of jejunum is connected to a new opening in the stomach, allowing food to pass from the stomach and bypass the blocked portion of the small bowel. Even with gastric bypass, delayed gastric emptying may endure in 30% to 50% of patients.[102] If endoscopic treatment is chosen, a metallic stent is placed into the duodenum to hold open the obstructed area.[100] The choice of surgery or stenting may be guided by life expectancy. NCCN guideline recommendations favor surgery for patients who are fit and have a life expectancy of more than 3 to 6 months.[10] Sometimes, stenting or gastric bypass is not possible; in these cases, a G-tube is inserted for drainage.[102] Placement of a feeding J-tube may also be inserted at the time of gastric bypass or G-tube placement.[10]

Medical Nutrition Therapy for Gastric Outlet Obstruction and Small Bowel Obstruction

Little information is published on appropriate diet after duodenal stent or drainage G-tube. Practice may vary, but for both circumstances the diet is generally the same. Literature suggests that after a duodenal stent is placed, patients should first establish tolerance of liquids before transitioning to a soft, low-fiber diet, as tolerated, a few days later. Patients should be instructed to chew all foods well and to drink plenty of liquids with meals.[107-109] Kobayashi and colleagues[101] advanced their patients' diet from liquids-only on day 1 to soft solids on day 2, and finally to a regular diet on day 3. It is recommended that patients with drainage G-tubes follow the same parameters as patients with duodenal stents; however, at some institutions these patients may be instructed to consume blended foods before progressing to a diet of soft solids.[110,111] Others may be allowed to progress to a regular diet as tolerated.[111-113] Episodes of blockage may often be managed by flushing the tube and avoiding the specific food that caused the blockage in the future.[113]

Patients with advanced PC are at risk of developing small bowel obstruction; risk factors for development include abdominal carcinomatosis, enlarged retroperitoneal nodes, or pelvic masses. McCallum and colleagues[114] suggest that all patients at high risk for bowel obstruction should be educated about appropriate diet (soft foods low in fiber and chewed thoroughly) and the use of laxatives to prevent obstruction.

Ascites

Ascites may be present at diagnosis in advanced disease or may develop later in the disease course (median 8.8 months after diagnosis of PC). Medical management includes diuretics or therapeutic paracentesis.[54] Poor appetite and early satiety may accompany ascites.

Medical Nutrition Therapy for Ascites
Helpful dietary strategies are similar to those for delayed gastric emptying (see Changes in Gastrointestinal Transit Time later in the chapter). There is no evidence regarding the effectiveness of sodium restriction in cancer-associated ascites;

however, research has suggested restricting sodium in practice[115] and is found to be beneficial for patients who have a high (≥1 g/dL) serum-ascites albumin gradient (SAAG).[116-118] In patients who are not already limiting sodium consumption through decreased volume of food intake, it is reasonable to consider a no-added-salt diet (a sodium intake of approximately 2 g/d) for those with a high SAAG.

Perioperative Nutrition Considerations

NIS associated with surgery (see Table 20.2 on page 449) may be either transient or enduring. Some symptoms influence the patient's ability to take in and absorb adequate nutrition, while others require specific nutrition interventions to promote resolution. Common postoperative problems reported by patients include struggling with weight loss and feeling pressured to eat. At least one study has reported that patients perceive they are given insufficient detailed information about diet following pancreatic surgery.[119] Patients expressed a desire for more information about what to eat and how often, about the use of PERT, and about long-term issues and survivorship.[119]

Energy Requirements

As with general macronutrient needs, the literature on postoperative energy needs is limited. A study by Sasaki and colleagues[43] sought to determine the effect of PD on REE. Much like in other metabolic studies, Sasaki and colleagues' patient population consisted only of nonobese patients. REE of study participants was measured using indirect calorimetry during a preoperative visit and at 7 and 14 days after surgery. REE at both postoperative time points was about 115% of preoperative REE. Based on their data, the authors recommended that individual energy needs be estimated at 25 kcal per kg of body weight per day preoperatively, and at 30 kcal per kg of body weight per day in the postoperative recovery weeks. Alternatively, a stress factor of 1.2 to 1.3 can be used if daily needs are calculated using REE predictive equations.[43]

Perioperative Medical Nutrition Therapy

Nutrition optimization for surgery should be considered a continuum. In the preoperative setting, it is important to manage side effects and to recover from neoadjuvant treatment, if received. The use of immunonutrition products containing arginine, omega-3 fatty acids, and nucleotides for 5 days before surgery is likely beneficial. Studies demonstrate reduced postoperative morbidity, surgical complications, and length of stay in both well-nourished and malnourished individuals undergoing major surgery, including pancreatic resection.[28,120-125]

The use of nutrition support in the perioperative setting continues to be debated. For patients at severe nutritional risk, the European Society for Clinical Nutrition and Metabolism recommends nutrition support for 7 to 14 days preoperatively, even if it causes the operation to be delayed.[126] Use of EN is generally favored over PN[127-129]; however, there are concerns that the placement of a feeding tube itself is associated with increased complications, leading to a delay in resuming a regular diet. Tube-specific complications, reported to occur in 5% to 20% of patients, include site infection, pneumatosis intestinalis, diarrhea, and tube malfunction.[28,130] Use of nasojejunal tubes seems to show no difference in complications, infections, or length of stay over directly placed feeding tubes.[131] Much of the use of nutrition support is left to the individual surgeon. If EN is used, initiating feeding with an immunonutrition formula may reduce the risk of postoperative complications and infections, and may be associated with decreased length of stay.[28] A study by Worsh and colleagues[132] found that patients with delayed gastric emptying (DGE) and other postoperative complications (eg, surgical site infection or postoperative pancreatic fistula) were most likely to need and benefit from PN administration for more than 3 days. A systematic review by Gerritsen and colleagues[133] found no evidence to support the routine use of nutrition support following PD or PPPD and that oral diet is preferred.

Early Postoperative Oral Diet

In the era of "enhanced recovery after surgery" protocols, many programs are now starting oral diet earlier.[134] Early oral feeding following PD has been associated with decreased length of stay and no differences in complications, DGE, hemorrhage, and mortality when compared to early enteral feeding via nasojejunal tube.[133]

In the short-term postoperative period after PD, PPPD, or total pancreatectomy, diet is often started as clear liquids and transitioned to soft solids. Research suggests that patients may be safely transitioned to a "regular diet" shortly after surgery; however, this diet is generally not outlined, and many of these studies take place outside the United States, where the health care and food service model may be different. For example, the regular solid-food diet outlined by Fujii and colleagues[135] in their study of postoperative pancreatic fistula is considered low-fat (45 g of fat per day) in the United States.

Therefore, it is the practice of the University of Texas MD Anderson to start patients on a diet that is very low in insoluble fiber, low in fat, and low in refined carbohydrates, generally on postoperative day 4, and transition to a less restrictive yet still low-fiber, low-fat diet 1 to 2 weeks following surgery. After 4 to 8 weeks, in the absence of enduring side effects or surgical complications, the patient is transitioned to a regular diet. For many patients, symptoms may best be managed by avoiding high-fat foods (eg, fried foods, cream sauces, and full-fat dairy products) over the long term and limiting fat intake to 75 g/d.[73]

PEI and Malabsorption PEI and malabsorption are reported in 50% to 100% of patients after PD and in 0% to 42% after distal pancreatectomy.[32] Variations in reported incidence generally are due to variation in diagnostic method and timing of evaluation. PEI may be transient after surgery, in patients with normal pancreatic function before surgery (measured by fecal elastase level). One study found that normal amounts of elastase were present in stool in most patients within 24 months after extended distal pancreatectomy,[136] and in 50% of patients 24 months after PD or PPPD.[137] It is important to note that these results represent only patients with a reduction in pancreatic exocrine enzyme production as measured by fecal elastase level. Even patients with normal fecal elastase levels may experience long-term malabsorption after PD or PPPD, because the anatomic changes resulting from the procedure can lead to GI asynchrony and consequent malabsorption (because endogenous enzymes do not digest food at the appropriate point in the digestive system).[57,66] Surgical reconstruction (such as pancreaticogastrostomy) may also influence effectiveness of endogenous pancreatic enzymes and lead to increased need for supplemental enzymes, since direct exposure of pancreatic secretions to gastric acid inactivates endogenous pancreatic enzymes.[138,139]

Changes in Gastrointestinal Transit Time

Changes in GI transit time may result in DGE, gastroparesis, or an increase in transit due to dumping syndrome or denervation of the mesentery. The effects on transit time have been compared in patients who have undergone PD vs PPPD. Studies suggest that PPPD may result in less dumping and diarrhea, better weight recovery, better QOL, and improved postoperative nutrition parameters[140-145]; however, a recent Cochrane review does not support any significant advantages of PPPD over

PD[145] and found that DGE may be more prevalent in PPPD. Conclusions are difficult to draw due to the heterogeneity of studies and definitions of DGE. Using the 2007 International Study Group of Pancreatic Surgery (ISGPS) consensus definition,[146] DGE is reported to occur in 15% to 45% of patients after surgery (including distal pancreatectomy).[147-152] Regardless of the type of resection, risk factors for DGE are male sex, advanced age, presence of pancreatic fistula, and postoperative intra-abdominal abscess.[147-151] DGE is reported to last a median of 9 to 10 days in less severe cases and 15 to 31 days in more severe cases (individual reports ranged from 3 to 356 days).[147,148,152,153]

Although concern for dumping syndrome is a suggested reason for using PPPD over PD, it is not commonly observed.[145,154] In patients who do experience dumping syndrome, however, the symptoms and nutrition consequences can be significant (see Chapter 18 for signs, symptoms, and management of dumping syndrome).

Aggressive resection to free tumors from the superior mesenteric artery may be necessary in PD and PPPD and may lead to rapid intestinal transit. To access the superior mesenteric artery, the surgeon may dissect the nerve plexus around the artery, interrupting the normal dampening effect of the sympathetic nerves, resulting in severe diarrhea.[28,155,156] The duration of rapid intestinal transit is not well documented; however, one study reported diarrhea in patients up to 4 months postoperatively.[156]

Medical Nutrition Therapy for Delayed Gastric Emptying

Instructions for patients with DGE may include following a low-fiber and low-fat diet, drinking fluids with meals, and eating small meals six to eight times per day. For practitioners working with these patients, the following special guidelines should also be followed:

- Make it a goal to achieve glycemic control if the patient has DM, as hyperglycemia can contribute to DGE.

- If gastroparesis is or is anticipated to be prolonged (more than 7 to 14 days),[153,157] nutrition support may be initiated (enteral feeding on a cyclic schedule).[153,158]

- Semisolid and liquid meals or nutritional supplements may be better tolerated than solid foods.[159]

- Prokinetic medications (metoclopramide, erythromycin) may be prescribed by the medical team.[153]

Medical Nutrition Therapy for Diarrhea and Rapid Intestinal Transit

In addition to diet modifications (see Chapter 11), the following special interventions for diarrhea are recommended:

- Consider prescription of medications to slow transit (see Table 20.3).

- Consider use of absorptive fiber, one to four times per day after meals,[160-162] according to the following guidelines:

  - One dose is 3.4 g of psyllium powder or 1 tsp of methylcellulose powder blended with 2 oz of water; or two psyllium fiber wafers.

  - Fiber should be taken once a day after a meal, and patients should avoid drinking fluid for 1 hour after.

  - Start once a day and gradually increase as needed up to four times per day.

- Consider these other factors and interventions:

  - Metformin may contribute to GI side effects, including diarrhea; therefore, gradual dose escalation is advised and

Table 20.3
Intestinal Transit–Inhibiting Medications [23,162]

Medication	Common dosing	Maximum dose
Loperamide (Imodium AD) May be used with diphenoxylate-atropine, each taken every 6 hours; alternating use resulting in individual taking one or the other every 3 hours	4 mg orally once, then 2 mg after each bowel movement 2-4 mg four times a day (every 6 hours)	16 mg/d
Diphenoxylate-atropine (Lomotil)	1-2 tablets orally three to four times a day	8 tablets/d
Deodorized tincture of opium	0.3-1 mL orally four times a day	6 mL/d
Codeine Used less commonly due to sedation and nausea	15-30 mg orally three or four times a day	

possible use of extended-release preparation if appropriate.[95]

■ A common method of pain control is regional neurolysis using a celiac plexus block, which may result in diarrhea[23]; though this may be a transient side effect, a diet strategy may be helpful.

■ For patients suspected of having bile acid–related diarrhea, a bile acid sequestrant (cholestyramine or colestipol) may be prescribed.[162]

Postoperative Pancreatic Fistula

Postoperative pancreatic fistula (POPF) is reported to occur in 13% to 41% of patients following pancreatectomy and leads to leakage of pancreatic fluid into the abdomen.[163] POPF is diagnosed by a drain amylase concentration of more than three times the upper limit of normal serum value (other factors are used to determine severity).[164] Obesity, malnutrition, and sarcopenia are risk factors for development of POPF.[163,165] Some surgeons prefer to attach the pancreatic remnant to the stomach (pancreaticogastrostomy) instead of the small

intestine as a proposed method for reducing pancreatic fistula[166,167]; however, this does not appear to reduce incidence.[138,139,163] Development of POPF is a risk factor for development of DGE.[147,163]

Medical Nutrition Therapy for Postoperative Pancreatic Fistula

Although there is a theoretical concern that food intake will exacerbate POPF or inhibit healing because it increases the secretion of digestive juices, this is not supported by current research.[135,168] To resume oral diet as usual in patients with pancreaticojejunostomy or no anastomosis (distal pancreatectomy) and in pancreaticogastrostomy, Research recommends to first rule out a mechanical anastomotic leak.[163] Although oral diet appears to be safe, if the patient requires nutrition support, EN is superior to parenteral nutrition (PN)—that is, EN leads to increased rates of spontaneous fistula closure compared to PN.[169]

Chyle Leak

Chyle leak may occur in up to 10% of patients following all types of pancreatic resection and 12.5% of patients following PD.[170] It is defined by the

International Study Group for Pancreatic Surgery as an "output of milky-colored fluid from drain, drain site, or wound," on or after postoperative day 3, with a triglyceride content of 110 mg/dL or higher (1.2 mmol/L or higher)[170] and is generally recognized at a median of 5 to 6 days after surgery. Duration of abdominal drainage has been shown to last a median of 14 days (range: 7 to 41 days) following pancreatic resection.[171] Initial and maximum drainage are predictive of time to resolution.[170]

Medical Nutrition Therapy for Chyle Leak

Interventions suggested for chyle leak include a fat-free diet (generally acknowledged as limiting fat intake to less than 0.5 g per serving); a low-fat diet; a diet supplemented with MCTs; a low-fat, high-MCT EN formula; nothing by mouth or a clear liquid diet with PN; or a combination thereof.[170,172] There is a lack of data to conclude that one intervention is better than another.[173] As is the goal in general, patients should ideally be maintained on oral diet. If that is not possible, then EN is preferred over PN. Lipids administered intravenously will not contribute to chyle volume—they may be used as part of PN or administered three times per week to avoid essential fatty acid deficiency in a patient otherwise maintained on a fat-free diet. Sriram and colleagues[172] recommend that patients be maintained on the intervention of choice for 7 to 10 days and that diet be advanced as chyle drainage volume decreases.

Survivorship

Studies of long-term survivors of PC are limited, and recommendations for nutrition evaluation are largely based on small series or case studies of patients presenting with micronutrient deficiency (see Box 20.7). Because of the limited literature, the incidence of deficiency in this population remains unknown. Deficiency may be due to inadequate dietary intake, loss of absorptive site, altered physiology and synchrony of the GI tract, and altered chemistry (including changes in production of intrinsic factor and pH).[32] In addition to vitamin and mineral deficiencies, and chronic conditions such as DM, long-term survivors are at risk for developing nonalcoholic fatty liver disease and early bone-density loss.

Deficiency Replacement

Micronutrient replacement should be individualized (see Box 20.8 on pages 460 to 461). When deciding on a plan for replacement, RDNs should consider whether a single nutrient or multiple nutrients are deficient. Most reports of patients with nutrient deficiency following surgery demonstrated poorly managed EPI symptoms.[32] In addition to nutrient replacement, therefore, it is important to make sure that PERT is also optimized and maintained. Historically, practice-based recommendations for replacement have suggested the use of water-miscible forms of fat-soluble vitamins; however, most reports suggest that replacement may be achieved with adequate PERT and high doses of standard vitamins. Water-miscible forms of fat-soluble vitamins should be considered if replacement with standard preparations fails.

Although its etiology is poorly understood, nonalcoholic fatty liver disease (NAFLD), or hepatic steatosis, is reported to occur in 7% to 40% of patients after pancreatectomy.[32] PERT has been suggested and is being studied as a possible treatment for NAFLD. Current studies are compelling and suggest the importance of adequate PEI control, even in the absence of nutritional deficiency.[32]

Decreased Bone Density

Because the duodenum, the primary site of calcium absorption, is removed as part of PD and many patients are on acid-suppressive therapy that changes the solubility of calcium salts, it is also important to monitor bone density. Although supporting literature is sparse, literature evaluating

Box 20.7
Recommendations for Micronutrient Evaluation in Survivors of Pancreatic Cancer[32]

Bone mineral density

Baseline evaluation	After completion of surgical recovery and any adjuvant treatment, within 2 years following surgery
Follow-up	*Normal*: every 5 years
	Abnormal: reevaluate; refer to primary care team or bone health clinic for management

Bloodwork

Complete blood count	Iron	Serum retinol
Vitamin B12	Copper	α-Tocopherol (vitamin E)
Methylmalonic acid	Zinc	25-hydroxyvitamin D
Folate	Selenium	Hemoglobin A1C
Ferritin	Retinol binding protein (vitamin A)	Magnesium
Total iron binding capacity		

Baseline evaluation	Within 1 year after surgical resection or sooner if individual has signs and symptoms of malabsorption
Follow-up	*Normal*: annually
	Abnormal: attempt repletion and recheck in 3 months

patients with PEI, Roux-en-Y gastric bypass, and total-pancreatectomy suggests that an increased risk of osteopenia or osteoporosis is not reflective of natural disease. Therefore, it is recommended that adequate calcium intake, adequate serum 25-hydroxyvitamin D, and adherence to weight-bearing activities are ensured.

Summary

It is important for the oncology registered dietitian nutritionist to help patients with PC cope with nutrition issues throughout the course of their treatment and survivorship. Though disease prognosis is poor, medical nutrition therapy can improve treatment outcomes and empower patients to play an active role in their own care and for families to play an active role as well. For long-term survivors, the nutrition implications of the disease and its treatments are likely to endure for the rest of their lives, and continued nutrition intervention may be necessary.

Box 20.8

Recommendations for Micronutrient Replacement in Survivors of Pancreatic Cancer [32,174-179]

Vitamin A [174]

Rebuild	30,000 IU of retinol palmitate orally once daily for 4 weeks
Maintain	Dietary Reference Intake (DRI)
Problem solving	Parenteral administration may be necessary if unable to normalize serum level.

Vitamin B12 [175]

Rebuild	1,000 mcg of cyanocobalamin by intramuscular (IM) injection once monthly
Maintain	1,000 mcg of cyanocobalamin by IM injection once monthly, or 1,000 mcg of vitamin B12 orally once daily
Problem solving	If unable to maintain with oral dosage, change to monthly intramuscular injection.

Vitamin D [176]

Rebuild	50,000 IU of cholecalciferol or ergocalciferol, nothing by mouth, once weekly for 8 weeks 6,000 IU of cholecalciferol or ergocalciferol once daily for 8 weeks
Maintain	1,500 to 2,000 IU of cholecalciferol orally once daily, or 50,000 IU of cholecalciferol or ergocalciferol, nothing by mouth, once every other week 1,500 to 2,000 IU of cholecalciferol orally once daily
Problem solving	Patients who are obese or have malabsorption may require two to three times the stated dose. (See below for vitamin D obese or malabsorbing.) Patients who are obese or have malabsorption may require two to three times the stated dose. (See below for vitamin D obese or malabsorbing)

Vitamin D for obese or malabsorbing patient [174,176]

Rebuild	50,000 IU of cholecalciferol or ergocalciferol, nothing by mouth, three times weekly for 4 to 8 weeks 6,000 to 20,000 IU of cholecalciferol or ergocalciferol, nothing by mouth, once daily for 8 weeks
Maintain	3,000 to 6,000 IU of cholecalciferol orally once daily

(continued)

Box 20.8
Recommendations for Micronutrient Replacement in Survivors of Pancreatic Cancer [32,174-179] (continued)

Vitamin E [174]

Rebuild	400 IU of vitamin E orally once daily for 2 weeks
Maintain	DRI

Copper [177]

Rebuild	3 to 8 mg of elemental copper orally daily until levels normalize
Maintain	DRI
Problem solving	Ensure that the patient is not taking excessive amounts of zinc.

Iron [32,178]

Rebuild	150 to 200 mcg of elemental iron orally daily or every other day in two or three divided doses
Maintain	DRI
Problem solving	Intravenous administration may be necessary if unable to normalize serum level.

Selenium [177]

Rebuild	100 mcg of selenium orally once daily until levels normalize
Maintain	DRI

Zinc [177,179]

Rebuild	50 to 60 mg of elemental zinc orally once or twice daily for 3 months
Maintain	DRI

Sample PES Statements for Pancreatic and Bile Duct Cancers

Intake domain: Inadequate oral intake related to decreased ability to consume sufficient energy due to side effects of cancer therapy, as evidenced by nausea, weight loss of ≥3% in the last week, and a dietary intake of 50% to 75% of estimated needs.

Clinical domain: Impaired nutrient utilization related to pancreatic exocrine insufficiency, as evidenced by steatorrhea.

References

1. The Pancreatic Cancer Action Network. Types of pancreatic cancer. 2020. Accessed April 20, 2020. www.pancan.org /facing-pancreatic-cancer/about -pancreatic-cancer/types-of -pancreatic-cancer

2. National Cancer Institute. Pancreatic cancer treatment (adult) (PDQ)–health professional version. Accessed April 20, 2020. https://cancer.gov/types /pancreatic/hp/pancreatic -treatment-pdq

3. American Cancer Society. American Cancer Society: Cancer Facts and Figures 2020. https://www.cancer.org/content /dam/cancer-org/research /cancer-facts-and-statistics /annual-cancer-facts-and-figures /2020/cancer-facts-and-figures -2020.pdf

4. American Cancer Society. Pancreatic neuroendocrine tumor (NET). 2020. Accessed May 19, 2020. www.cancer .org/cancer/pancreatic -neuroendocrine-tumor/about /what-is-pnet.html

5. Nassour I, Choti MA. Types of Pancreatic Cysts. *JAMA*. 2016;316(11):1226.

6. World Cancer Research Fund/ American Institute for Cancer Research. Continuous update project expert report. *Diet, Nutrition, Physical Activity and Pancreatic Cancer: A Global Perspective*. Revised 2018. Accessed May 19, 2020. www.wcrf.org/dietandcancer /pancreatic-cancer

7. Weisbeck A, Jansen RJ. Nutrients and the pancreas: an epigenetic perspective. *Nutrients*. 2017;9(3).

8. American Cancer Society. Treating pancreatic cancer. Accessed May 19, 2020. https:// cancer.org/content/dam/CRC/PDF /Public/8781.00.pdf

9. Isaji S, Mizuno S, Windsor JA, et al. International consensus on definition and criteria of borderline resectable pancreatic ductal adenocarcinoma 2017. *Pancreatology*. Jan 2018;18(1): 2-11.

10. National Comprehensive Cancer Network. *NCCN Clinical Practice Guidelines in Oncology (NCCN Guidelines): Pancreatic Adenocarcinoma* Version 1.2020. National Comprehensive Cancer Network; 2020. Accessed May 12, 2020. https://nccn.org /professionals/physician_gls/PDF /pancreatic.pdf

11. Sohal DP, Mangu PB, Laheru D. Metastatic pancreatic cancer: American Society of Clinical Oncology Clinical Practice Guideline Summary. *J Oncol Pract*. 2017;13(4):261-264.

12. Balaban EP, Mangu PB, Yee NS. Locally advanced unresectable pancreatic cancer: American Society of Clinical Oncology Clinical Practice Guideline Summary. *J Oncol Pract*. 2017;13(4):265-269.

13. Sohal DP, Mangu PB, Khorana AA, et al. Metastatic pancreatic cancer: American Society of Clinical Oncology Clinical Practice Guideline. *J Clin Oncol*. 2016;34(23):2784-2796.

14. Balaban EP, Mangu PB, Khorana AA, et al. Locally advanced, unresectable pancreatic cancer: American Society of Clinical Oncology Clinical Practice Guideline. *J Clin Oncol*. 2016;34(22):2654-2668.

15. Khorana AA, Mangu PB, Katz MHG. Potentially curable pancreatic cancer: American Society of Clinical Oncology Clinical Practice Guideline Update Summary. *J Oncol Pract*. 2017;13(6):388-391.

16. Khorana AA, Mangu PB, Berlin J, et al. Potentially curable pancreatic cancer: American Society of Clinical Oncology Clinical Practice Guideline Update. *J Clin Oncol*. 2017;35(20):2324-2328.

17. Khorana AA, Mangu PB, Berlin J, et al. Potentially curable pancreatic cancer: American Society of Clinical Oncology Clinical Practice Guideline. *J Clin Oncol*. 2016;34(21):2541-2556.

18. American Society of Clinical Oncology. Pancreatic cancer. 2012. Accessed May 19, 2020. http://cancer .net/patient/Cancer+Types /Pancreatic+Cancer?sectionTitle =Treatment

19. Polovich M, Olsen M, LeFebvre K. *Chemotherapy and Biotherapy Guidelines and Recommendations for Practice*. 4th ed. Oncology Nursing Society; 2014.

20. Eloxatin. Package insert. Sanofi-Aventis LLC; 2015.

21. Tarceva Package insert. OSI Pharmaceuticals, LLC; 2016.

22. Keytruda Package insert. Merck & Co, Inc; 2017.

23. Rabow MW, Petzel MQB, Adkins SH. Symptom management and palliative care in pancreatic cancer. *Cancer J.* 2017;23(6): 362-373.

24. Horst E, Seidel M, Micke O, et al. Accelerated radiochemotherapy in pancreatic cancer is not necessarily related to a pathologic pancreatic function decline in the early period. *Int J Radiat Oncol Biol Phys.* 2002;52(2):304-309.

25. Ji HB, Zhu WT, Wei Q, Wang XX, Wang HB, Chen QP. Impact of enhanced recovery after surgery programs on pancreatic surgery: A meta-analysis. *World J Gastroenterol.* 2018;24(15): 1666-1678.

26. De Pastena M, Paiella S, Marchegiani G, et al. Postoperative infections represent a major determinant of outcome after pancreaticoduodenectomy: Results from a high-volume center. *Surgery.* Oct 2017;162(4):792-801.

27. Pappas S, Krzywda E, McDowell N. Nutrition and pancreaticoduodenectomy. *Nutr Clin Pract.* 2010;25(3):234-243.

28. Gilliland TM, Villafane-Ferriol N, Shah KP, et al. Nutritional and metabolic derangements in pancreatic cancer and pancreatic resection. *Nutrients.* 2017;9(3).

29. Watanabe J, Otani S, Sakamoto T, et al. Prognostic indicators based on inflammatory and nutritional factors after pancreaticoduodenectomy for pancreatic cancer. *Surg Today.* 2016;46(11):1258-1267.

30. American Cancer Society. Surgery for pancreatic cancer. Accessed May 20, 2020. https://cancer.org/cancer/pancreatic-cancer/treating/surgery.html

31. Pancreatic Cancer Action Network. Surgery. 2017. Accessed May 20, 2020. www.pancan.org/facing-pancreatic-cancer/treatment/treatment-types/surgery

32. Petzel MQB, Hoffman L. Nutrition implications for long-term survivors of pancreatic cancer surgery. *Nutr Clin Pract.* 2017;32(5):588-598.

33. Ottery F. Supportive nutritional management of the patient with pancreatic cancer. *Oncology (Williston Park).* 1996;10(9 suppl):26-32.

34. Bruera E. ABC of palliative care. Anorexia, cachexia, and nutrition. *BMJ.* 1997;315(7117):1219-1222.

35. Vashi P, Popiel B, Lammersfeld C, Gupta D. Outcomes of systematic nutritional assessment and medical nutrition therapy in pancreatic cancer. *Pancreas.* 2015;44(5):750-755.

36. Mueller TC, Burmeister MA, Bachmann J, Martignoni ME. Cachexia and pancreatic cancer: are there treatment options? *World J Gastroenterol.* 2014;20(28):9361-9373.

37. Davidson W, Ash S, Capra S, Bauer J. Weight stabilisation is associated with improved survival duration and quality of life in unresectable pancreatic cancer. *Clin Nutr.* 2004;23(2): 239-247.

38. Richter E, Denecke A, Klapdor S, Klapdor R. Parenteral nutrition support for patients with pancreatic cancer—improvement of the nutritional status and the therapeutic outcome. *Anticancer Res.* 2012;32(5):2111-2118.

39. Bauer J, Capra S, Battistutta D, Davidson W, Ash S. Compliance with nutrition prescription improves outcomes in patients with unresectable pancreatic cancer. *Clin Nutr.* 2005;24(6): 998-1004.

40. Cao DX, Wu GH, Zhang B, et al. Resting energy expenditure and body composition in patients with newly detected cancer. *Clin Nutr.* 2010;29(1):72-77.

41. Falconer JS, Fearon KC, Plester CE, Ross JA, Carter DC. Cytokines, the acute-phase response, and resting energy expenditure in cachectic patients with pancreatic cancer. *Ann Surg.* 1994;219(4):325-331.

42. Vaisman N, Lusthaus M, Niv E, et al. Effect of tumor load on energy expenditure in patients with pancreatic cancer. *Pancreas.* 2012;41(2):230-232.

43. Sasaki M, Okamoto H, Johtatsu T, et al. Resting energy expenditure in patients undergoing pylorus preserving pancreatoduodenectomies for bile duct cancer or pancreatic tumors. *J Clin Biochem Nutr.* 2011;48(3):183-186.

44. American Cancer Society. Pancreatic cancer detailed guide. Accessed May 20, 2020. http://cancer.org/Cancer/PancreaticCancer/DetailedGuide/index

45. National Cancer Institute. Bile duct cancer (cholangiocarcinoma) treatment (PDQ)–health professional version. Accessed May 20, 2020. www.cancer.gov/types/liver/hp/bile-duct-treatment-pdq

46. National Cancer Institute. If you have pancreatic cancer. Accessed May 20, 2020. www.cancer.org/cancer/pancreatic-cancer/if-you-have-pancreatic-cancer.html

47. Pancreatic Cancer Action Network. Learn about pancreatic cancer. Accessed May 20, 2020. www.pancan.org/facing-pancreatic-cancer/learn

48. DiMagno EP, Reber HA, Tempero MA. AGA technical review on the epidemiology, diagnosis, and treatment of pancreatic ductal adenocarcinoma. American Gastroenterological Association. *Gastroenterology.* 1999;117(6):1464-1484.

49. Ballinger AB, McHugh M, Catnach SM, Alstead EM, Clark ML. Symptom relief and quality of life after stenting for malignant bile duct obstruction. *Gut.* 1994;35(4):467-470.

50. Barkay O, Mosler P, Schmitt CM, et al. Effect of endoscopic stenting of malignant bile duct obstruction on quality of life. *J Clin Gastroenterol.* 2013;47(6):526-531.

51. Fearon K, Strasser F, Anker SD, et al. Definition and classification of cancer cachexia: an international consensus. *Lancet Oncol.* 2011;12(5):489-495.

52. Pancreatic Cancer Action Network. Facing pancreatic cancer. Accessed May 20, 2020. https://pancan.org/facing-pancreatic-cancer

53. Walter FM, Mills K, Mendonca SC, et al. Symptoms and patient factors associated with diagnostic intervals for pancreatic cancer (SYMPTOM pancreatic study): a prospective cohort study. *Lancet Gastroenterol Hepatol.* 2016;1(4):298-306.

54. Hicks AM, Chou J, Capanu M, Lowery MA, Yu KH, O'Reilly EM. Pancreas adenocarcinoma: ascites, clinical manifestations, and management implications. *Clin Colorectal Cancer.* 2016;15(4):360-368.

55. Rege RV. Adverse effects of biliary obstruction: implications for treatment of patients with obstructive jaundice. *AJR Am J Roentgenol.* 1995;164(2):287-293.

56. Phillips ME. Pancreatic exocrine insufficiency following pancreatic resection. *Pancreatology.* 2015;15(5):449-455.

57. Sabater L, Ausania F, Bakker OJ, et al. Evidence-based guidelines for the management of exocrine pancreatic insufficiency after pancreatic surgery. *Ann Surg.* 2016;264(6):949-958.

58. Sikkens EC, Cahen DL, de Wit J, Looman CW, van Eijck C, Bruno MJ. A prospective assessment of the natural course of the exocrine pancreatic function in patients with a pancreatic head tumor. *J Clin Gastroenterol.* 2014;48(5):e43-46.

59. Tokumo H, Ishida K, Komatsu H, Machino H, Morinaka K. External biliary jejunal drainage through a percutaneous endoscopic gastrostomy for tube-fed patients with obstructive jaundice. *J Clin Gastroenterol.* 1997;24(2):103-105.

60. Layer P, Keller J, Lankisch PG. Pancreatic enzyme replacement therapy. *Curr Gastroenterol Rep.* 2001;3(2):101-108.

61. Heedman PA, Astradsson E, Blomquist K, Sjodahl R. Palliation of malignant biliary obstruction: adverse events are common after percutaneous transhepatic biliary drainage. *Scand J Surg.* 2018;107(1):48-53.

62. Imrie CW, Connett G, Hall RI, Charnley RM. Review article: enzyme supplementation in cystic fibrosis, chronic pancreatitis, pancreatic and periampullary cancer. *Aliment Pharmacol Ther.* 2010;32 (suppl 1):1-25.

63. Wakasugi H, Hara Y, Abe M. A study of malabsorption in pancreatic cancer. *J Gastroenterol.* 1996;31(1):81-85.

64. Landers A, Muircroft W, Brown H. Pancreatic enzyme replacement therapy (PERT) for malabsorption in patients with metastatic pancreatic cancer. *BMJ Support Palliat Care*. 2016;6(1):75-79.

65. Struyvenberg MR, Martin CR, Freedman SD. Practical guide to exocrine pancreatic insufficiency—breaking the myths. *BMC Med*. 2017;15(1):29.

66. Lindkvist B, Phillips ME, Dominguez-Munoz JE. Clinical, anthropometric and laboratory nutritional markers of pancreatic exocrine insufficiency: prevalence and diagnostic use. *Pancreatology*. 2015;15(6):589-597.

67. Bartel MJ, Asbun H, Stauffer J, Raimondo M. Pancreatic exocrine insufficiency in pancreatic cancer: a review of the literature. *Dig Liver Dis*. 2015;47(12):1013-1020.

68. Hendifar AE, Petzel MQB, Zimmers TA, et al. Pancreas cancer-associated weight loss. *Oncologist*. 2018 doi:10.1634/theoncologist.2018-0266

69. Dominguez-Munoz JE. Pancreatic exocrine insufficiency: diagnosis and treatment. *J Gastroenterol Hepatol*. 2011;26 Suppl 2:12-16.

70. Dominguez-Munoz JE. Pancreatic enzyme therapy for pancreatic exocrine insufficiency. *Gastroenterol Hepatol*. 2011;7(6):401-403.

71. Fieker A, Philpott J, Armand M. Enzyme replacement therapy for pancreatic insufficiency: present and future. *Clin Exp Gastroenterol*. 2011;4:55-73.

72. Bruno MJ, Haverkort EB, Tijssen GP, Tytgat GN, van Leeuwen DJ. Placebo controlled trial of enteric coated pancreatin microsphere treatment in patients with unresectable cancer of the pancreatic head region. *Gut*. 1998;42(1):92-96.

73. Sarner M. Treatment of pancreatic exocrine deficiency. *World J Surg*. 2003;27(11):1192-1195.

74. Creon Package insert. AbbVie Inc; 2015.

75. Toouli J, Biankin AV, Oliver MR, et al. Management of pancreatic exocrine insufficiency: Australasian Pancreatic Club recommendations. *Med J Aust*. 2010;193(8):461-467.

76. Edakkanambeth VJ, Bauer BA, Hurt RT. Over-the-counter enzyme supplements: what a clinician needs to know. *Mayo Clin Proc*. Sep 2014;89(9):1307-1312.

77. PERTZYE (R) Package insert. Digestive Care, Inc; 2017.

78. Viokace(TM) Package insert. Aptalis Pharma US, Inc; 2012.

79. Zenpep(R) Package insert. Allergan; 2017.

80. Pancreaze Package insert. Vivus, Inc.; 2016.

81. Ellison NM, Chevlen E, Still CD, Dubagunta S. Supportive care for patients with pancreatic adenocarcinoma: symptom control and nutrition. *Hemat Oncol Clin North Am*. 2002;16(1):105-121.

82. Borowitz DS, Grand RJ, Durie PR, Consensus Committee. Use of pancreatic enzyme supplements for patients with cystic fibrosis in the context of fibrosing colonopathy. *J Pediatr*. 1995;127(5):681-684.

83. Schwarzenberg SJ. Cystic fibrosis foundation pancreatic enzymes clinical care guidelines: executive summary. 2018. Accessed May 20, 2020. www.cff.org/Care/Clinician-Resources/Network-News/January-2018/Executive-Summaries-of-Clinical-Care-Guidelines

84. Gan KH, Heijerman HG, Geus WP, Bakker W, Lamers CB. Comparison of a high lipase pancreatic enzyme extract with a regular pancreatin preparation in adult cystic fibrosis patients. *Aliment Pharmacol Ther*. 1994;8(6):603-607.

85. Ferrie S, Graham C, Hoyle M. Pancreatic enzyme supplementation for patients receiving enteral feeds. *Nutr Clin Pract*. 2011;26(3):349-351.

86. Alexander DD, Bylsma LC, Elkayam L, Nguyen DL. Nutritional and health benefits of semi-elemental diets: a comprehensive summary of the literature. *World J Gastrointest Pharmacol Ther*. 2016;7(2):306-319.

87. Berry AJ. Pancreatic enzyme replacement therapy during pancreatic insufficiency. *Nutr Clin Pract*. 2014;29(3):312-321.

88. Freedman SD. Options for addressing exocrine pancreatic insufficiency in patients receiving enteral nutrition supplementation. *Am J Manag Care*. 2017;23(12 suppl):S220-S228.

89. Freedman S, Orenstein D, Black P, et al. Increased fat absorption from enteral formula through an in-line digestive cartridge in patients with cystic fibrosis. *J Pediatr Gastroenterol Nutr*. 2017;65(1):97-101.

90. Babayan VK. Medium chain triglycerides and structured lipids. *Lipids*. 1987;22(6):417-420.

91. Andersen DK, Korc M, Petersen GM, et al. Diabetes, pancreatogenic diabetes, and pancreatic cancer. *Diabetes*. 2017;66(5):1103-1110.

92. Burkhart RA, Gerber SM, Tholey RM, et al. Incidence and severity of pancreatogenic diabetes after pancreatic resection. *J Gastrointest Surg*. 2015;19(2):217-225.

93. Poulson J. The management of diabetes in patients with advanced cancer. *J Pain Symptom Manage*. 1997;13(6):339-346.

94. American Diabetes Association. Older adults: standards of medical care in diabetes-2018. *Diabetes Care*. 2018;41(suppl 1):S119-S125.

95. Cui Y, Andersen DK. Pancreatogenic diabetes: special considerations for management. *Pancreatology*. 2011;11(3):279-294.

96. Maeda H, Hanazaki K. Pancreatogenic diabetes after pancreatic resection. *Pancreatology*. 2011;11(2):268-276.

97. American Diabetes Association. Glycemic targets: standards of medical care in diabetes-2018. *Diabetes Care*. 2018;41(suppl 1):S55-S64.

98. Shi HJ, Jin C, Fu DL. Impact of postoperative glycemic control and nutritional status on clinical outcomes after total pancreatectomy. *World J Gastroenterol*. 2017;23(2):265-274.

99. Irizarry L, Li QE, Duncan I, et al. Effects of cancer comorbidity on disease management: making the case for diabetes education (a report from the SOAR program). *Popul Health Manag*. 2013;16(1):53-57.

100. Gaidos JK, Draganov PV. Treatment of malignant gastric outlet obstruction with endoscopically placed self-expandable metal stents. *World J Gastroenterol*. 2009;15(35):4365-4371.

101. Kobayashi S, Ueno M, Kameda R, et al. Duodenal stenting followed by systemic chemotherapy for patients with pancreatic cancer and gastric outlet obstruction. *Pancreatology*. 2016;16(6):1085-1091.

102. Perone JA, Riall TS, Olino K. Palliative care for pancreatic and periampullary cancer. *Surg Clin North Am*. 2016;96(6):1415-1430.

103. Oh SY, Edwards A, Mandelson M, et al. Survival and clinical outcome after endoscopic duodenal stent placement for malignant gastric outlet obstruction: comparison of pancreatic cancer and nonpancreatic cancer. *Gastrointest Endosc*. 2015;82(3):460-468 e462.

104. Shah A, Fehmi A, Savides TJ. Increased rates of duodenal obstruction in pancreatic cancer patients receiving modern medical management. *Dig Dis Sci*. 2014;59(9):2294-2298.

105. Laval G, Marcelin-Benazech B, Guirimand F, et al. Recommendations for bowel obstruction with peritoneal carcinomatosis. *J Pain Symptom Manage*. 2014;48(1):75-91.

106. Poruk KE, Wolfgang CL. Palliative management of unresectable pancreas cancer. *Surg Oncol Clin N Am*. 2016;25(2):327-337.

107. Adler DG, Baron TH. Endoscopic palliation of malignant gastric outlet obstruction using self-expanding metal stents: experience in 36 patients. *Amer J Gastroentol*. 2002;97(1):72-78.

108. Dormann A, Meisner S, Verin N, Wenk Lang A. Self-expanding metal stents for gastroduodenal malignancies: systematic review of their clinical effectiveness. *Endoscopy*. 2004;36(6):543-550.

109. Ly J, O'Grady G, Mittal A, Plank L, Windsor JA. A systematic review of methods to palliate malignant gastric outlet obstruction. *Surgical Endosc.* 2009;24(2):290-297.

110. Meyer L, Pothuri B. Decompressive percutaneous gastrostomy tube use in gynecologic malignancies. *Curr Treat Options Oncol.* 2006;7(2):111-120.

111. Pothuri B, Montemarano M, Gerardi M, et al. Percutaneous endoscopic gastrostomy tube placement in patients with malignant bowel obstruction due to ovarian carcinoma. *Gynecol Oncol.* 2005;96(2):330-334.

112. Teriaky A, Gregor J, Chande N. Percutaneous endoscopic gastrostomy tube placement for end-stage palliation of malignant gastrointestinal obstructions. *Saudi J Gastroenterol.* 2012;18(2):95-98.

113. Brooksbank MA, Game PA, Ashby MA. Palliative venting gastrostomy in malignant intestinal obstruction. *Palliat Med.* 2002;16(6):520-526.

114. McCallum P, Walsh D, Nelson KA. Can a soft diet prevent bowel obstruction in advanced pancreatic cancer? *Support Care Cancer.* 2002;10(2):174-175.

115. Saif MW, Siddiqui IA, Sohail MA. Management of ascites due to gastrointestinal malignancy. *Ann Saudi Med.* 2009;29(5):369-377.

116. White A. Outpatient interventions for hepatology patients with fluid retention: a review and synthesis of the literature. *Gastroenterol Nurs.* 2014;37(3):236-244.

117. Moore KP, Aithal GP. Guidelines on the management of ascites in cirrhosis. *Gut.* 2006;55 (suppl 6):vi1-12.

118. Yu AS, Hu KQ. Management of ascites. *Clin Liver Dis.* 2001;5(2):541-568.

119. Cooper C, Burden ST, Molassiotis A. An explorative study of the views and experiences of food and weight loss in patients with operable pancreatic cancer perioperatively and following surgical intervention. *Support Care Cancer.* 2015;23(4):1025-1033.

120. Burden S, Todd C, Hill J, Lal S. Pre-operative nutrition support in patients undergoing gastrointestinal surgery. *Cochrane Database Syst Rev.* Nov 14 2012;11:CD008879.

121. Martin RC, Agle S, Schlegel M, et al. Efficacy of preoperative immunonutrition in locally advanced pancreatic cancer undergoing irreversible electroporation (IRE). *Eur J Surg Oncol.* 2017;43(4):772-779.

122. Silvestri S, Franchello A, Deiro G, et al. Preoperative oral immunonutrition versus standard preoperative oral diet in well nourished patients undergoing pancreaticoduodenectomy. *Int J Surg.* 2016;31:93-99.

123. Gade J, Levring T, Hillingso J, Hansen CP, Andersen JR. The effect of preoperative oral immunonutrition on complications and length of hospital stay after elective surgery for pancreatic cancer—a randomized controlled trial. *Nutr Cancer.* 2016;68(2):225-233.

124. Shirakawa H, Kinoshita T, Gotohda N, Takahashi S, Nakagohri T, Konishi M. Compliance with and effects of preoperative immunonutrition in patients undergoing pancreaticoduodenectomy. *J Hepatobiliary Pancreat Sci.* May 2012;19(3):249-258.

125. Suzuki D, Furukawa K, Kimura F, et al. Effects of perioperative immunonutrition on cell-mediated immunity, T helper type 1 (Th1)/Th2 differentiation, and Th17 response after pancreaticoduodenectomy. *Surgery.* Sep 2010;148(3):573-581.

126. Weimann A, Braga M, Carli F, et al. ESPEN guideline: clinical nutrition in surgery. *Clin Nutr.* 2017;36(3):623-650.

127. Gianotti L, Braga M, Gentilini O, Balzano G, Zerbi A, Di Carlo V. Artificial nutrition after pancreaticoduodenectomy. *Pancreas.* 2000;21(4):344-351.

128. Liu C, Du Z, Lou C, et al. Enteral nutrition is superior to total parenteral nutrition for pancreatic cancer patients who underwent pancreaticoduodenectomy. *Asia Pac J Clin Nutr.* 2011;20(2):154-160.

129. Zhu XH, Wu YF, Qiu YD, Jiang CP, Ding YT. Effect of early enteral combined with parenteral nutrition in patients undergoing pancreaticoduodenectomy. *World J Gastroenterol*. 2013;19(35):5889-5896.

130. Nussbaum DP, Zani S, Penne K, et al. Feeding jejunostomy tube placement in patients undergoing pancreaticoduodenectomy: an ongoing dilemma. *J Gastrointest Surg*. 2014;18(10):1752-1759.

131. Perinel J, Mariette C, Dousset B, et al. Early enteral versus total parenteral nutrition in patients undergoing pancreaticoduodenectomy: a randomized multicenter controlled trial (Nutri-DPC). *Ann Surg*. 2016;264(5):731-737.

132. Worsh CE, Tatarian T, Singh A, et al. Total parenteral nutrition in patients following pancreaticoduodenectomy: lessons from 1184 patients. *J Surg Res*. 2017;218:156-161.

133. Gerritsen A, Wennink RA, Besselink MG, et al. Early oral feeding after pancreatoduodenectomy enhances recovery without increasing morbidity. *HPB (Oxford)*. 2014;16(7):656-664.

134. Lassen K, Coolsen MM, Slim K, et al. Guidelines for perioperative care for pancreaticoduodenectomy: Enhanced Recovery After Surgery (ERAS) Society recommendations. *Clin Nutr*. 2012;31(6):817-830.

135. Fujii T, Nakao A, Murotani K, et al. Influence of food intake on the healing process of postoperative pancreatic fistula after pancreatoduodenectomy: a multi-institutional randomized controlled trial. *Ann Surg Oncol*. 2015;22(12):3905-3912.

136. Speicher JE, Traverso LW. Pancreatic exocrine function is preserved after distal pancreatectomy. *J Gastrointest Surg*. 2010;14(6):1006-1011.

137. Matsumoto J, Traverso LW. Exocrine function following the Whipple operation as assessed by stool elastase. *J Gastrointest Surg*. 2006;10(9):1225-1229.

138. Ma JP, Peng L, Qin T, et al. Meta-analysis of pancreaticoduodenectomy prospective controlled trials: pancreaticogastrostomy versus pancreaticojejunostomy reconstruction. *Chin Med J (Engl)*. 2012;125(21):3891-3897.

139. Makni A, Bedioui H, Jouini M, et al. Pancreaticojejunostomy vs pancreaticogastrostomy following pancreaticoduodenectomy: results of comparative study. *Minerva Chir*. 2011;66(4): 295-302.

140. Takada T, Yasuda H, Amano H, Yoshida M, Ando H. Results of a pylorus-preserving pancreatoduodenectomy for pancreatic cancer: a comparison with results of the Whipple procedure. *Hepatogastroenterology*. 1997;44(18):1536-1540.

141. Schniewind B, Bestmann B, Henne-Bruns D, Faendrich F, Kremer B, Kuechler T. Quality of life after pancreaticoduodenectomy for ductal adenocarcinoma of the pancreatic head. *Br J Surg*. 2006;93(9):1099-1107.

142. Di Carlo V, Zerbi A, Balzano G, Corso V. Pylorus-preserving pancreaticoduodenectomy versus conventional Whipple operation. *World J Surg*. 1999;23(9):920-925.

143. Diener MK, Fitzmaurice C, Schwarzer G, et al. Pylorus-preserving pancreaticoduodenectomy (pp Whipple) versus pancreaticoduodenectomy (classic Whipple) for surgical treatment of periampullary and pancreatic carcinoma. *Cochrane Database Syst Rev*. 2011(5):CD006053.

144. Ohtsuka T, Yamaguchi K, Ohuchida J, et al. Comparison of quality of life after pylorus-preserving pancreatoduodenectomy and Whipple resection. *Hepatogastroenterology*. 2003;50(51):846-850.

145. Huttner FJ, Fitzmaurice C, Schwarzer G, et al. Pylorus-preserving pancreaticoduodenectomy (pp Whipple) versus pancreaticoduodenectomy (classic Whipple) for surgical treatment of periampullary and pancreatic carcinoma. *Cochrane Database Syst Rev*. Feb 16 2016;2:CD006053.

146. Wente MN, Bassi C, Dervenis C, et al. Delayed gastric emptying (DGE) after pancreatic surgery: a suggested definition by the International Study Group of Pancreatic Surgery (ISGPS). *Surgery*. 2007;142(5):761-768.

147. Mohammed S, Van Buren Ii G, McElhany A, Silberfein EJ, Fisher WE. Delayed gastric emptying following pancreaticoduodenectomy: incidence, risk factors, and healthcare utilization. *World J Gastrointest Surg*. 2017;9(3):73-81.

148. Park JS, Hwang HK, Kim JK, et al. Clinical validation and risk factors for delayed gastric emptying based on the International Study Group of Pancreatic Surgery (ISGPS) Classification. *Surgery*. 2009;146(5):882-887.

149. Welsch T, Borm M, Degrate L, Hinz U, Buchler MW, Wente MN. Evaluation of the International Study Group of Pancreatic Surgery definition of delayed gastric emptying after pancreatoduodenectomy in a high-volume centre. *Br J Surg*. 2010;97(7):1043-1050.

150. Noorani A, Rangelova E, Del Chiaro M, Lundell LR, Ansorge C. Delayed gastric emptying after pancreatic surgery: analysis of factors determinant for the short-term outcome. *Front Surg*. 2016;3:25.

151. Courvoisier T, Donatini G, Faure JP, Danion J, Carretier M, Richer JP. Primary versus secondary delayed gastric emptying (DGE) grades B and C of the International Study Group of Pancreatic Surgery after pancreatoduodenectomy: a retrospective analysis on a group of 132 patients. *Updates Surg*. 2015;67(3):305-309.

152. Eisenberg JD, Rosato EL, Lavu H, Yeo CJ, Winter JM. Delayed gastric emptying after pancreaticoduodenectomy: an analysis of risk factors and cost. *J Gastrointest Surg*. 2015;19(9):1572-1580.

153. Beane JD, House MG, Miller A, et al. Optimal management of delayed gastric emptying after pancreatectomy: an analysis of 1,089 patients. *Surgery*. 2014;156(4):939-946.

154. Jimenez RE, Fernandez-del Castillo C, Rattner DW, Chang Y, Warshaw AL. Outcome of pancreaticoduodenectomy with pylorus preservation or with antrectomy in the treatment of chronic pancreatitis. *Ann Surg*. 2000;231(3):293-300.

155. Thorsen Y, Stimec B, Andersen SN, et al. Bowel function and quality of life after superior mesenteric nerve plexus transection in right colectomy with D3 extended mesenterectomy. *Tech Coloproctol*. 2016;20(7):445-453.

156. Orci LA, Meyer J, Combescure C, et al. A meta-analysis of extended versus standard lymphadenectomy in patients undergoing pancreatoduodenectomy for pancreatic adenocarcinoma. *HPB (Oxford)*. 2015;17(7):565-572.

157. August DA, Huhmann MB. A.S.P.E.N. clinical guidelines: nutrition support therapy during adult anticancer treatment and in hematopoietic cell transplantation. *JPEN J Parenter Enteral Nutr*. 2009;33(5):472-500.

158. van Berge Henegouwen MI, Akkermans LM, van Gulik TM, et al. Prospective, randomized trial on the effect of cyclic versus continuous enteral nutrition on postoperative gastric function after pylorus-preserving pancreatoduodenectomy. *Ann Surg*. 1997;226(6):677-685.

159. Academy of Nutrition and Dietetics. Gastroparesis nutrition therapy. *Nutrition Care Manual*. Accessed May 20, 2020. www.nutritioncaremanual.org/client_ed.cfm?ncm_client_ed_id=168

160. Murphy J, Stacey D, Crook J, Thompson B, Panetta D. Testing control of radiation-induced diarrhea with a psyllium bulking agent: a pilot study. *Can Oncol Nurs J*. 2000;10(3):96-100.

161. Singh B. Psyllium as therapeutic and drug delivery agent. *Int J Pharm*. 2007;334(1-2):1-14.

162. Bisanz A, Tucker AM, Amin DM, et al. Summary of the causative and treatment factors of diarrhea and the use of a diarrhea assessment and treatment tool to improve patient outcomes. *Gastroenterol Nurs.* 2010;33(4):268-281.

163. Nahm CB, Connor SJ, Samra JS, Mittal A. Postoperative pancreatic fistula: a review of traditional and emerging concepts. *Clin Exp Gastroenterol.* 2018;11:105-118.

164. Bassi C, Marchegiani G, Dervenis C, et al. The 2016 update of the International Study Group (ISGPS) definition and grading of postoperative pancreatic fistula: 11 years after. *Surgery.* 2017;161(3):584-591.

165. Ecker BL, McMillan MT, Allegrini V, et al. Risk factors and mitigation strategies for pancreatic fistula after distal pancreatectomy: analysis of 2026 resections from the International, Multi-institutional Distal Pancreatectomy Study Group. *Ann Surg.* 2017;269(1):143-149.

166. Wray CJ, Ahmad SA, Matthews JB, Lowy AM. Surgery for pancreatic cancer: recent controversies and current practice. *Gastroenterology.* 2005;128(6):1626-1641.

167. Morera-Ocon FJ, Sabater-Orti L, Munoz-Forner E, Perez-Griera J, Ortega-Serrano J. Considerations on pancreatic exocrine function after pancreaticoduodenectomy. *World J Gastrointest Oncol.* 2014;6(9):325-329.

168. Fujii T, Yamada S, Murotani K, et al. Oral food intake versus fasting on postoperative pancreatic fistula after distal pancreatectomy: a multi-institutional randomized controlled trial. *Medicine (Baltimore).* 2015;94(52):e2398.

169. Klek S, Sierzega M, Turczynowski L, Szybinski P, Szczepanek K, Kulig J. Enteral and parenteral nutrition in the conservative treatment of pancreatic fistula: a randomized clinical trial. *Gastroenterology.* 2011;141(1):157-163.

170. Besselink MG, van Rijssen LB, Bassi C, et al. Definition and classification of chyle leak after pancreatic operation: a consensus statement by the International Study Group on Pancreatic Surgery. *Surgery.* 2017;161(2):365-372.

171. Abu Hilal M, Layfield DM, Di Fabio F, et al. Postoperative chyle leak after major pancreatic resections in patients who receive enteral feed: risk factors and management options. *World J Surg.* 2013;37(12):2918-2926.

172. Sriram K, Meguid RA, Meguid MM. Nutritional support in adults with chyle leaks. *Nutrition.* 2016;32(2):281-286.

173. Steven BR, Carey S. Nutritional management in patients with chyle leakage: a systematic review. *Eur J Clin Nutr.* 2015;69(7):776-780.

174. Dutta SK, Bustin MP, Russell RM, Costa BS. Deficiency of fat-soluble vitamins in treated patients with pancreatic insufficiency. *Ann Intern Med.* 1982;97(4):549-552.

175. Carmel R. How I treat cobalamin (vitamin B12) deficiency. *Blood.* 2008;112(6):2214-2221.

176. Holick MF, Binkley NC, Bischoff-Ferrari HA, et al. Evaluation, treatment, and prevention of vitamin D deficiency: an Endocrine Society clinical practice guideline. *J Clin Endocrinol Metab.* 2011;96(7):1911-1930.

177. Kushner RF, Cummings S, Herron DM. Bariatric surgery: postoperative nutritional management. In: Jones D, ed. *UpToDate*; 2019.

178. Schrier SL, Auerbach M. Treatment of iron deficiency anemia in adults. In: Mentzer WC, ed. *UpToDate*; 2019.

179. Yazbeck N, Muwakkit S, Abboud M, Saab R. Zinc and biotin deficiencies after pancreaticoduodenectomy. *Acta Gastroenterol Belg.* 2010;73(2):283-286.

Chapter 21
Medical Nutrition Therapy for Head and Neck Cancers

Audrey Caspar-Clark, MA, RDN, LDN

Head and neck cancers (HNCs) are malignant tumors that develop in and around the oral cavity (mouth), pharynx (throat), larynx, nose, and sinuses. Many of the tumors originate in the tissues lining the head and neck, often the flat squamous cells. Tumor cells may grow in the mucosa or invade further into the epithelial layer. Although HNCs are rare in the United States, accounting for approximately 4% of all cancers, they present significant challenges for patients throughout the continuum of care.[1]

The role of nutrition and the involvement of the registered dietitian nutritionist (RDN) are essential to the care of these patients during and after surgery, chemotherapy, and radiation, as well as in survivorship. Box 21.1 discusses statistics regarding oral cavity and pharynx cancers.

In older adults, both tobacco use and alcohol use have long been strongly associated with HNC, but more recently human papillomavirus (HPV) infections have been linked to HNC in younger patients who do not have a history of tobacco use. Ancestry, including Chinese ancestry (which presents an increased risk for nasopharyngeal cancer), and cultural customs (such as betel-quid chewing in people from Southeast Asia) also can increase the risk for HNC.[3] Box 21.2 presents the common risk factors for HNCs.

Types of Head and Neck Cancers

HNCs are categorized by the area of the head or neck in which they originate. See Figure 21.1 on page 475 for an illustration of the normal anatomy of this region. Cancers of the oral cavity can affect the lips, the front two-thirds of the tongue, the gums, the lining inside the cheeks and lips, the floor (bottom) of the mouth under the tongue, the hard palate (bony top of the mouth), and the small area of the gums behind the third molar teeth ("wisdom teeth").

Box 21.1
Statistics for Oral Cavity and Pharynx Cancers, United States[2]

Estimated new cases in 2020: 53,260

Estimated deaths in 2020: 10,750

Lifetime risk: 1.2%

Five-year relative survival rate (overall): 66.2%

Box 21.2
Risk Factors for Head and Neck Cancers[3]

Tobacco, alcohol, marijuana use

Prolonged sun exposure

Human papillomavirus infection

Epstein-Barr virus infection

Sex: more than twice as common among males

Age: diagnosed more often in people over age 50 years

Poor oral and dental hygiene

Environmental and occupational inhalants

Poor nutrition

Weakened immune system

Gastroesophageal reflux disease

Laryngopharyngeal reflux disease

Cancers of the pharynx can occur in the upper part of the pharynx behind the nose (nasopharynx); the middle part of the pharynx (oropharynx), including the soft palate; the base of the tongue and the tonsils; and the lower part of the pharynx (hypopharynx). HNC can occur in the larynx, also known as the voice box. The larynx is made up of cartilage, located just below the pharynx in the neck, and contains the vocal cords and epiglottis. HNC can also occur in the paranasal sinuses and nasal cavity as well as in the salivary glands.[4]

HPV-related cancers can take years to develop after an HPV infection. It is unclear if having HPV alone is enough to cause oropharyngeal (ie, mouth and throat) cancers, or if other factors, such as smoking or chewing tobacco, interact with HPV to cause these cancers. More research is needed to understand the factors leading to oropharyngeal cancers. Oral HPV is about three times more common in men than in women. About 10% of men and 3.6% of women in the United States have oral HPV, and HPV is thought to cause 70% of oropharyngeal cancers.[5]

Diagnosis

Diagnosis of HNC requires a physical examination, a complete medical history, and various diagnostic tests. A biopsy of the suspected malignant tumor is necessary for diagnosing HNCs. Additional testing is required to stage the cancer and to ascertain if it has spread.[4]

Box 21.3 lists possible symptoms that patients may present with prior to diagnosis.

Treatment

Treatments for HNCs often involve a combination of several modalities, including surgical resection, radiotherapy, chemotherapy, targeted therapy and immunotherapy.[7,8] The treatment plan is individualized based on exact location of the tumor, cancer stage, and a patient's age and general health.

Box 21.3
Symptoms of Head and Neck Cancers[6]

Sore throat that does not improve

Difficulty swallowing

Hoarseness or a change in the voice that does not go away

Swelling or a sore that does not heal (the most common symptom)

Red or white patch in the mouth

Lump, bump, or mass in the head or neck area, with or without pain

Foul mouth odor not explained by hygiene

Nasal obstruction or persistent nasal congestion

Frequent nose bleeds or unusual nasal discharge

Difficulty breathing

Double vision

Numbness or weakness of a body part in the head and neck region

Pain or difficulty chewing, swallowing, or moving the jaw or tongue

Jaw pain

Blood in the saliva or phlegm, which is mucus discharged into the mouth from respiratory passages

Loosening of teeth

Dentures that no longer fit

Unexplained weight loss

Fatigue

Ear pain or infection

Interventions, such as immune-enhancing nutrients or anticytokine pharmaceutical agents, may also be effective as adjuvant therapies, but more research is needed to quantify their clinical effect.[9] Refer to the *NCCN Clinical Practice Guidelines in Oncology (NCCN Guidelines): Head and Neck Cancers* for details of specific therapies.[8]

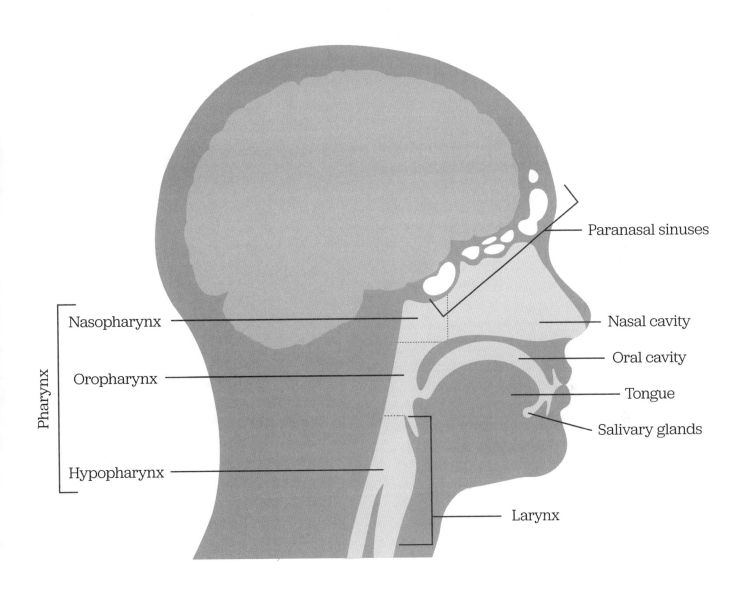

Figure 21.1
Normal anatomy of the head and neck region

Box 21.4 lists common nutrition impact symptoms (NIS) associated with HNC treatment. See Chapters 9 and 10 for detailed information on the nutritional impacts of various cancer treatments and Chapter 11 for how to manage NIS.

Nutrition and speech and swallow evaluations and respective therapies are recommended for all patients with HNC, with ongoing nutrition evaluation and rehabilitation recommended until the patient is nutritionally stable. Patients should receive regular follow-up to assess for symptoms and possible tumor recurrence and to monitor for multiple issues, including nutrition issues, as part of a comprehensive evaluation throughout treatment. Nutrition is a key component of all aspects of care, and RDNs provide appropriate nutrition interventions to help manage NIS.[10] As an integral part of the multidisciplinary team, an RDN ensures that treatment-related nutritional side effects are adequately controlled.

Box 21.4
Treatments for Head and Neck Cancers and Associated Nutrition Impact Symptoms[11]

Modality	Nutrition impact symptoms	
Radiotherapy (photons and protons)	Dysgeusia, ageusia	Thrush
	Xerostomia	Increased secretions, thick secretions
	Mucositis	Nausea
	Odynophagia	Anorexia
	Dysphagia	Anosmia
Chemotherapy	Dysgeusia, ageusia	Diarrhea
	Mucositis	Constipation, hyperglycemia, hypoglycemia
	Nausea	
	Vomiting	Anorexia
Radiotherapy and chemotherapy combined	All of the above; may also increase metabolic needs (in cases of high-dose cisplatin given concurrently with radiotherapy)	
Immunotherapy	Diarrhea	Anorexia
	Nausea	Hyperglycemia
	Mucositis	
Surgery	Dysphagia	Trismus (limited mouth opening)
	Odynophagia	Anosmia
	Xerostomia	Nasal regurgitation
	Dysgeusia, ageusia	Jaw pain, pain with chewing
	Increased secretions, thick secretions	

Oncology Nutrition *for* Clinical Practice

Radiotherapy

The effects of radiotherapy are cumulative. During radiotherapy treatment, NIS are likely to develop around the third week if the patient is receiving intensity-modulated radiation therapy (IMRT) for 30 to 35 treatments (fractions). However, patients may develop treatment-related NIS sooner or may have preexisting conditions, such as xerostomia, thrush, dysphagia, or trismus, that may increase their risk for inadequate nutrient intake. Patients treated with proton beam radiation (as opposed to IMRT) may have fewer side effects and more delayed side effects that may decrease their need for enteral feeding.[12] Patients who receive concurrent chemoradiation may develop NIS relative to chemotherapy treatment times, in addition to NIS associated with radiotherapy. Box 21.5 discusses the RDN's role in caring for patients undergoing radiation therapy and collaborating with the comprehensive care team.

Box 21.5
Comprehensive Care for Head and Neck Cancers: Collaboration With the Radiation Oncology Team[8]

Refer to the National Comprehensive Cancer Network guidelines for head and neck cancers for details on the role of the registered dietitian nutritionist (RDN) in the comprehensive care team.

The following are the key measures to be taken by the RDN:

- Discuss the treatment plan with the comprehensive care team before initiation of treatment to identify the need for prophylactic feeding tube placement.
- Ask the radiation oncologist about the size of the treatment field and if treatment will involve bilateral neck radiation.
- Identify significant or severe weight loss that has occurred before the patient's start of radiation.
- With regard to feeding tube placement and enteral nutrition:
  - If possible, meet with the patient before treatment starts to assess for weight loss, dysphagia, and other issues that may predispose the patient to inadequate oral intake.
  - Consider any comorbidities and the age of the patient.
  - If the patient might benefit from a feeding tube, determine whether the patient's insurance will cover the cost of placement and enteral supplies. Recognize that Medicare has stringent requirements for the coverage of enteral formula and supplies.
  - Determine whether the patient can self-administer tube feedings.
  - Review the current research on the use of an algorithm for determining the need for a feeding tube.
  - If the patient already has a feeding tube, assess the patient's weight, tolerance of tube feeding, condition of the tube, and any other factors that may affect his or her nutritional status.
- During radiation, monitor the patient's weight and nutrition impact symptoms weekly, if possible. If it is not possible to follow the patient closely during and after treatment, enlist the cooperation of the nursing staff to help identify whether the patient is at risk for malnutrition.

Surgery

The goal of surgery is to remove the cancerous tumor and some of the surrounding healthy tissue. Depending on the location, stage, and type of cancer, some patients may require more than one surgery. It may not be possible to completely remove all of the cancer; in such cases, additional treatments such as radiation or chemotherapy (alone or in combination) may be indicated.

Types of surgery for HNCs include laser surgery, excision, lymph node (neck) dissection, and transoral robotic surgery (TORS).

- Laser surgery is used to treat early-stage tumors, particularly tumors of the larynx.

- Excision removes the cancerous tumor and some surrounding healthy tissue (known as a margin).

- Lymph node dissection, or neck dissection, removes neck lymph nodes if the cancer has spread to that area. This may be done at the same time as excision.

- TORS uses a surgical robot to remove a tumor from the mouth or throat. In TORS, the arms of the robot are strategically placed inside the patient's mouth.[7]

- Box 21.6 discusses the RDN's role in caring for patients undergoing surgery and interfacing with the comprehensive care team.

Systemic Therapies

Chemotherapy, immunotherapy, and targeted therapy are systemic options used to treat HNCs. Chemotherapy may be used in several ways. It may be:

- combined with radiation therapy;

- given before radiation or surgery to shrink larger cancers;

- given after surgery to kill any remaining small deposits of cancer cells; or

Box 21.6

Comprehensive Care for Head and Neck Cancers: Collaboration With the Surgical Team[8,13]

The following are the key measures to be taken by the registered dietitian nutritionist when interfacing with the surgical team as part of the comprehensive care team:

- Offer a presurgical nutrition assessment to identify any risk of malnutrition that may be improved with nutrition intervention before surgery.

- Discuss the importance of minimizing postsurgery weight loss for patients who may require adjuvant therapy. Demonstrate the benefit of nutrition counseling in enhancing patients' quality of life.

- Before surgery, discuss the use of enhanced recovery after surgery protocols for optimization of nutritional status with an enhanced immunonutrition supplement and postsurgical use of short-term tube feedings via nasogastric feeding tube using immunoenhanced enteral formula.

- Recommend that patients have a postsurgery nutrition assessment to ensure nutritional needs are met to support healing.

- used to treat cancers that have spread too far to be removed by surgery.

Immunotherapy and targeted therapy have applications in the treatment of recurrent or metastatic HNCs, and their role is the subject of ongoing research and investigation.[7]

Nutrition Assessment

According to a 2013 Cochrane review, 75% to 80% of patients with HNC have significant weight loss, and 35% to 60% are malnourished at the time of diagnosis, due to obstructed dietary intake, tumor burden, anorexia, and cachexia.[14] It is essential that the RDN be included in all phases of the patient's care, as the risk for malnutrition or inadequate nutrition can occur during any phase (see Box 21.7 on page 481).

Evaluation of nutritional status by the RDN is a strong and imperative recommendation of the Academy of Nutrition and Dietetics Oncology Evidence-Based Nutrition Practice Guideline for Adults and the Cancer Council of Australia.[10] The NCCN guidelines for HNC treatment include nutrition assessment, evaluation by a speech-language pathologist, enteral nutrition support (as needed), and care by a multidisciplinary team that includes an RDN. The guidelines specifically address the need to monitor nutritional status closely, with particular emphasis on[14]:

- monitoring for weight loss (significant weight loss of 5% or more over the past month or 10% or more over the past 6 months);

- monitoring for swallowing difficulty associated with pain or location of tumor;

- nutrition counseling; and

- interventions such as nasogastric or percutaneous endoscopic gastrostomy tubes or intravenous nutrition if enteral nutrition is not feasible.

Pretreatment and posttreatment functional evaluation should include an assessment of nutritional status (particularly for patients undergoing radiotherapy) and should employ subjective and objective assessment tools.

Patients with HNC are encouraged to see an RDN before starting cancer treatments, particularly if they are having difficulty swallowing or chewing, are losing weight, or are receiving radiation therapy. The RDN can provide a nutrition care plan and monitor for the potential need for a feeding tube.[14]

Calculating Energy Needs

Calculating the nutritional needs for patients with HNC can be challenging. Weight loss during treatment may be highly correlated with a body mass index (BMI) greater than 25; a pharyngeal, oral-cavity, or supraglottic tumor site; stage III and IV cancers; and multimodality treatment regimen. Considering these predictors of weight loss may help determine whether a patient will benefit from the placement of a feeding tube.[15] Patients with HNC may have higher estimated energy and protein needs, as influenced by inflammation, tumor type, or treatment that may alter normal metabolic function and increase energy and protein needs.[16-19] Critical weight loss during radiotherapy or chemoradiation may be associated with impaired immune function and nutritional deficiencies; therefore, it is essential to determine nutritional status at the start of treatment, monitor weight loss closely during treatment and in the posttreatment recovery period, and adjust nutritional goals accordingly to stabilize weight and prevent nutritional deficiencies. Careful assessment of underweight patients with HNC is necessary to establish if a history of chronic weight loss exists. In some cases, changes in body composition may be associated with poor prognosis.[20]

The goals are weight maintenance and minimal weight loss for overweight and obese patients during radiotherapy or chemoradiation. However, the RDN needs to monitor weight and reassess frequently to determine if the patient requires more calories, protein, and fluid, as some patients may require as much as 35 to 40 kcal per kg of body weight daily after completing radiotherapy and high-dose cisplatin chemotherapy.[17,18] See Chapter 5 for general guidelines for determining the nutritional needs of cancer patients.

Nutrition Problems and Interventions

Nutrition interventions for patients with HNC should begin before treatment starts. Box 21.7 outlines the appropriate nutrition interventions throughout the care continuum. Box 21.8 discusses counseling to be provided by the RDN to patients and caregivers.

Mucositis and Thrush

Patients with HNC are at risk for mucositis and thrush (candidiasis) due to radiation-induced xerostomia, chemotherapy, and steroid use, which can contribute to pain and taste changes.[11,21] Specific interventions include:

- a thorough oral-cavity examination to identify mucositis and thrush;

- the use of medications, if needed, to alleviate the pain and oral tenderness caused by mucositis in order to help the patient tolerate adequate oral intake or to treat thrush;

- diet alterations, such as including more foods and liquids that are low in acid, smooth-textured, and very moist; and

- thorough oral care and frequent oral rinses with a solution of salt water and baking soda to help relieve minor oral discomfort.

Taste Changes

Patients may experience diminished taste (ageusia) or altered taste (dysgeusia) during and after treatment, making it challenging to find foods and fluids that are palatable. Taste changes may be due in part to surgical resection, radiotherapy, or chemotherapy and may take 3 weeks to 2 months to resolve after completion of treatment.[11,22] Patients with nasopharyngeal cancer may experience more significant taste changes and anosomia associated with the location of the tumor and the area in the radiation treatment field. It can be helpful to suggest neutral-tasting, high-calorie, high-protein foods to these patients. Chapter 11 further discusses interventions for taste changes.

Dysphagia

Dysphagia can result from the tumor, surgery, and deconditioning. Evaluation and treatment by a speech-language pathologist is necessary in combination with RDN interventions for dysphagia. Chapter 11 further discusses interventions for dysphagia.

In some cases, patients may be at risk for aspiration of oral secretions. It is critical that patients with symptoms of aspiration receive timely evaluation by a speech-language pathologist. Signs of aspiration risk include coughing during oral intake, "froggy" voice, and fever.

Oral Nutrition Interventions

All of these NIS—mucositis, thrush, taste changes, and dysphagia—can lead to poor oral intake and consequent weight loss. Interventions include the following:

- Focus on providing nutrition recommendations for high-calorie, high-protein, and easy-to-swallow soft foods and liquids.

- Recommend that patients use a blender to make milkshakes, smoothies, and pureed foods. For patients who do not have a blender or who are too fatigued to prepare meals, provide recipes and suggestions for using pureed baby foods, canned soups, frozen meals, mashed potatoes, and hot cereals (oatmeal, cream of wheat, cream of rice, grits). Enhancing these foods with extra butter, cream, or other high-fat additions can help patients and their caregivers prepare tolerable foods.

- Recommend commercial oral nutrition supplements, as well as homemade smoothies and shakes, to help patients maximize their nutrient intake, despite these NIS.

- Consult the Oncology Nutrition dietetic practice group website (www.oncologynutrition.org) for a variety of recipes, books, and online resources for patients with HNC.

Box 21.7
Nutrition Interventions for Patients With Head and Neck Cancers[8,11,13,16]

Before treatment	Assess the patient to identify significant or severe weight loss and issues impacting oral intake.
	Consider early interventions, such as feeding-tube placement, in patients at high risk for malnutrition.
	Counsel the patient on a 5 to 6 small meals a day plan, including oral nutrition supplements, as needed, that meets energy, protein, and fluid needs.
During treatment	Maintain the patient's nutritional status.
	Minimize weight loss to improve outcomes.
	Reassess the patient's oral diet tolerance, enteral nutrition tolerance, weight, hydration status, and nutrition impact symptoms (NIS).
	Adjust the nutrition care plan for increased energy needs following surgery or as needed throughout systemic treatment and radiation based on weight status.
	Revise nutrition interventions based on the patient's status. Interventions may include diet modification, enteral nutrition initiation or modification, and hydration support.
	Provide education to the patient regarding management of nutrition impact symptoms.
After treatment	Reassess for weight loss.
	Conduct a posttreatment nutrition assessment.
	Continue diet modifications for as long as needed as treatment side effects are improving (may take weeks to months).
	If a feeding tube in place, evaluate ability to chew and swallow, and implement a plan to wean enteral nutrition as NIS improve.

Box 21.8
Counseling for Patients With Head and Neck Cancers and Their Caregivers

Emphasize the importance of adequate fluid and nutrient intake to maintain or improve nutritional status along the entire continuum of care.

Remind patients and caregivers that nutritional needs may change with the phases of treatment; there may be an increased need for calories and protein after surgery, during chemoradiation, and after treatment. Therefore, continual reassessment and evaluation of adequacy of nutrients is essential.

Discuss the use of a feeding tube as a supportive measure to help meet nutritional needs versus long-term use or dependence on tube feeding as the sole source of nutrition.

Provide patients and caregivers with suggestions and recipes for soft high-calorie, high-protein foods, as well as shakes and smoothies, and tips on how to deal with nutrition impact symptoms.

Suggest participation in head and neck cancer support groups.

Enteral or Parenteral Nutrition Support

The role of feeding-tube placement in patients with HNC is often controversial. Some institutions practice prophylactic placement in all HNC patients who will be receiving radiotherapy, whereas other institutions prescribe feeding tubes on a case-by-case basis. A study comparing nutritional and clinical outcomes in patients undergoing chemoradiotherapy for HNC who had prophylactically placed feeding tubes versus reactively placed feeding tubes showed a slight statistically significant difference between the two groups. Although those with prophylactically placed tubes showed improved nutritional outcomes and fewer unplanned nutrition-related hospital admissions, the study was not large enough to demonstrate a distinct benefit.[23] These findings showed that the following factors must be considered when determining which patients may benefit from a prophylactic feeding tube[16,24]:

- tumor type and stage
- radiotherapy treatment field
- weight loss before starting treatment
- dysphagia
- significant comorbidities
- risk for aspiration
- anorexia
- pain interfering with oral intake
- dehydration

Survivorship

NCCN guidelines recommend integrating nutrition into patients' survivorship care plan.[8] Continued monitoring and intervention for NIS secondary to treatment is necessary, as many challenges can be chronic for patients with HNC (see Box 21.9).

> **Box 21.9**
> ### Chronic Challenges for Head and Neck Cancer Survivors
>
> Xerostomia
>
> Dysphagia
>
> Oral thrush
>
> Dysgeusia
>
> Ageusia
>
> Strictures
>
> Dental issues
>
> Anorexia

Using a needs assessment tool that focuses on physical, emotional, and social challenges experienced by survivors of HNC can help inform the entire multidisciplinary care team about posttreatment challenges.[23,25,26]

Specific issues to monitor after treatment include the following:

- Appropriateness and adequacy of enteral nutrition: In patients dependent on enteral nutrition, reassess their current nutritional status to determine if the enteral formula is appropriate and meeting nutritional needs.

- Swallowing and functional status: Assess to determine whether posttreatment rehabilitation with a speech-language pathologist (for swallowing therapy) and a physical therapist (to improve functional status) is indicated.

- Laboratory findings: Collaborate with the care team to monitor laboratory values and implement appropriate interventions (eg, thyroid function, complete blood count, and other values, depending on the type of treatment).

- Diet and lifestyle: Counsel survivors on diet and lifestyle to help reduce their risk for a second new cancer, cardiovascular disease, type 2 diabetes, and kidney disease.[27] The 2016 American Cancer Society guidelines for HNC survivors recommend encouraging healthy lifestyle behaviors, such as maintaining a healthy body weight and consuming a diet rich in fruits, vegetables, and whole grains, and low in saturated fats.[28] Interventions for tobacco cessation and to reduce or stop alcohol consumption are needed.[27-29]

Summary

HNCs and their treatment present a wide array of complex nutritional challenges. Undernutrition in patients with HNC is associated with poor treatment outcomes, infections, cancer recurrence, mortality and poor quality of life.[30] The role of the RDN within the multidisciplinary team and from diagnosis through survivorship is imperative to the management of the tenuous nutritional status of these patients.

Sample PES Statements for Head and Neck Cancers

Intake domain: Inadequate enteral nutrition infusion related to intolerance of enteral nutrition, as evidenced by nausea and the patient only being able to meet 50% of estimated needs via gastrostomy tube feedings.

Clinical domain: Severe, acute disease- or injury-related malnutrition related to mucositis, as evidenced by a weight loss of 4% in past week and an oral intake of less than 50% of estimated needs in the past week.

References

1. Head and neck cancer: introduction. Cancer.net website. Accessed April 25, 2020. www.cancer.net/cancer-types/head-and-neck-cancer/introduction

2. Cancer stat facts: oral cavity and pharynx cancer. National Cancer Institute Surveillance, Epidemiology, and End Results Program website. Accessed April 25, 2020. https://seer.cancer.gov/statfacts/html/oralcav.html

3. Head and neck cancer: risk factors and prevention. Cancer.net website. Accessed April 25, 2020. https://cancer.net/cancer-types/head-and-neck-cancer/risk-factors-and-prevention

4. Head and neck cancers. National Cancer Institute website. Accessed April 25, 2020. www.cancer.gov/types/head-and-neck

5. HPV and oropharyngeal cancer. Centers for Disease Control and Prevention website. Accessed April 25, 2020. https://cdc.gov/cancer/hpv/basic_info/hpv_oropharyngeal.htm

6. Head and neck cancer: signs and symptoms. Cancer.net website. Accessed April 25, 2020. https://cancer.net/cancer-types/head-and-neck-cancer/symptoms-and-signs

7. Head and neck cancer: types of treatments. Cancer.net website. Accessed April 29, 2020. www.cancer.net/cancer-types/head-and-neck-cancer/types-treatment

8. National Comprehensive Cancer Network. *NCCN Clinical Practice Guidelines in Oncology (NCCN Guidelines): Head And Neck Cancers.* Version 1.2019. National Comprehensive Cancer Network; 2019. Accessed April 26, 2019. https://nccn.org/professionals/physician_gls/pdf/head-and-neck.pdf

9. Alshadwi A, Nadershaw M, Carlson ER, et al. Nutritional considerations for head and neck cancer patients: a review of the literature. *J Oral Maxillofac Surg.* 2013 Nov;71(11):1853-60. Epub 2013 Jul 9. doi:1016/j.joms.2013.04.028

10. Thompson KL, Elliott L, Fuchs-Talovsky V, et al. Oncology evidence-based nutrition practice guideline for adults. *J Acad Nutr Diet.* 2017;117(2):297-310.

11. Kubrak C, Olson K, Baraco V. The head and neck symptom checklist: an instrument to evaluate nutrition impact symptoms effect on energy intake and weight loss. *Support Care Cancer.* 2013;21(11):3127-3136.

12. Blanchard P, Garden AS, Gunn GB, et al. Intensity modulated proton beam therapy (IMPT) versus intensity modulated photon therapy (IMRT) for oropharynx cancer patients—a case matched analysis. *Radiother Oncol.* 2016;120:(1):48-55.

13. Palma-Milla S, Lopez-Plaza B, Santamaria B, et al. New, immunomodulatory, oral nutrition formula for use prior to surgery in patients with head and neck cancer: an exploratory study. *JPEN J Parenter Enteral Nutr.* 2018;42(2):371-379.

14. Nugent B, Lewis S, O'Sullivan JM. Enteral feeding methods for nutritional management in patients with head and neck cancer being treated with radiotherapy and/or chemotherapy. *Cochrane Database Syst Rev.*2013;2013(1):CD007904. Published 2013 Jan 31. doi:10.1002/14651858.CD007904.pub3.

15. Lonbro S, Petersen, GB, Andersen, JR, Johansen J. Prediction of critical weight loss during radiation treatment in head and neck cancer patients is dependent on BMI. *Support Care Cancer.* 2016;24(5):2101-2109.

16. Head and Neck Guideline Steering Committee. Evidence-based practice guidelines for the nutritional management of adult patients with head and neck cancer. Sydney: Cancer Council Australia. Accessed May 2, 2020. https://wiki.cancer.org.au/australia/COSA:Head_and_neck_cancer_nutrition_guidelines

17. Talwar B, Donnelly R, Skelly, R, Donaldson M. Nutritional management in head and neck cancer: United Kingdom National Multidisciplinary Guidelines. *J Laryngol Otol.* 2016;130 (suppl. S2): S32-S40.

18. Ardilio, S. Calculating nutrition needs for a patient with head and neck cancer. *Clin J Oncol Nurs.* 2011;15(5):457-459.

19. Müller-Richter U, Betz C, Hartmann S, Brands R.C. Nutrition management for head and neck cancer patients improves clinical outcome and survival. *Nutr Res.* 2017;48:1-8.

20. Langius JA et al. Critical weight loss is a major prognostic indicator for disease-specific survival in patients with head and neck cancer receiving radiotherapy. *Br J Cancer*. 2013;109:1093-1099.

21. Kauffman, CA. Treatment of oropharyngeal and esophageal candidiasis. UpToDate website. Accessed April 25, 2020. www.uptodate.com/contents /treatment-of-oropharyngeal-and -esophageal-candidiasis

22. Taste changes. Cancer.net website. Accessed April 25, 2020. www.cancer.net/navigating -cancer-care/side-effects/taste -changes

23. Schoeff SS, Barrett DM, DeLassus Gress C, Jameson MJ. Nutritional management for head and neck cancer patients. Nutrition issues in gastroenterology, series #121. *Prac Gastroenterol*. 2013;43-51.

24. Brown TE, Banks MD, Huges BGM, et al. Comparison of nutritional and clinical outcomes in patients with head and neck cancer undergoing chemoradiotherapy utilizing prophylactic versus reactive nutrition support approaches. *J Acad Nutr Diet*. 2018;118(4) 627-636.

25. Sterba KR, Zapka J, LaPelle N, et al. Development of a survivorship needs assessment planning tool for head and neck cancer survivors and their caregivers: a preliminary study. *J Cancer Surviv*. 2017;11(6):822-832.

26. Ringash J, Bernstein LJ, Devins J, et al. Head and neck cancer survivorship: learning the needs, meeting the needs. *Semin Radiat Oncol*. 2017;28(1):64-74.

27. World Cancer Research Fund/ American Institute for Cancer Research. Continuous update project expert report 2018. Diet, nutrition, physical activity and cancers of the mouth, pharynx and larynx. Accessed May 2, 2020. www.aicr.org/wp-content /uploads/2020/01/mouth-pharynx -larynx-cancer.pdf

28. Cohen EEW, LaMonte SJ, Erb NL, et al. (2016), American Cancer Society Head and Neck Cancer Survivorship Care Guideline. *CA Cancer J Clin*. 2016;66:203-239.

29. Duray A, Lacremans D, Demoulin S, Delvenne P, Saussez S. Prognosis of HPV-positive head and neck cancers: implication of smoking and immunosuppression. *Advances in Cellular and Molecular Otolaryngology*. 2014;2(1):1-9.

30. Locher JL, Bonner JA, Carroll WR, et al. Prophylactic percutaneous endoscopic gastrostomy tube placement in treatment of head and neck cancer: a comprehensive review and call for evidence-based medicine. *JPEN J Parenter Enteral Nutr*. 2011;35(3):365-374. doi: 10.1177 /0148607110377097

Chapter 22
Medical Nutrition Therapy for Lung Cancer

Nicole Kiss, BSc, PhD, MNutDiet
Liz Isenring, PhD, AdvAPD

Lung cancer is the most common cancer worldwide, with an estimated global incidence in 2018 of 2.1 million new cases representing 11% of all new cancers. Global mortality from lung cancer was 9.6 million in 2018, making it the deadliest form of cancer.[1] In the United States, the National Cancer Institute (NCI) estimated more than 228,820 new cases of lung and bronchus cancer for 2020 and 135,720 estimated deaths, representing nearly one-quarter of all deaths from cancer.[2]

The incidence of lung cancer has been declining steadily over the past 20 years, most likely due to declining rates of smoking. There has been a small but steady increase in the 5-year survival rate, from 13.4% in 1990 to 20.5% estimated for 2020.[2] However, this is much lower than the 5-year survival rates of 89.9% for breast cancer, 64.4% for colorectal cancers, and 97.7% for prostate cancer over the same time period.[3]

Risk Factors

Smoking is the leading cause of lung cancer, with 80% of lung cancers attributable to smoking.[3,4] Other factors known to increase the risk for lung cancer include the following[5]:

- exposure to secondhand smoke
- exposure to asbestos
- exposure to radon (by way of radioactive gas from the breakdown of uranium in soil and rocks)
- exposure to inhaled cancer-causing chemicals in the workplace
- air pollution
- previous radiotherapy to the thoracic region
- personal or family history of lung cancer
- HIV

According to the World Cancer Research Fund and the American Institute for Cancer Research, there is probable evidence for "a decreased risk of lung cancer associated with dietary intake of fruit and foods containing carotenoids" and convincing evidence of "an increased risk of lung cancer with β-carotene supplement use."[6] Key recommendations for preventing lung cancer are to avoid smoking and environmental exposure to secondhand smoke. There is some evidence that a traditional Mediterranean diet, which is high in whole grains, fruits, and vegetables, may lower the risk for lung cancer in heavy smokers.[5]

Types of Lung Cancer

The four histologic subtypes of lung cancer are as follows[7]:

- squamous cell carcinoma
- adenocarcinoma
- large cell carcinoma
- small cell carcinoma

Squamous cell carcinoma, adenocarcinoma, and large cell carcinoma are collectively referred to as non–small cell lung cancer (NSCLC), and they account for 80% to 85% of all lung cancers. Small cell lung cancer (SCLC) accounts for 10% to 15% of lung cancers.[7] Lung cancer occurs in different areas of the lungs depending on the histological subtype. See Figure 22.1 on page 488.

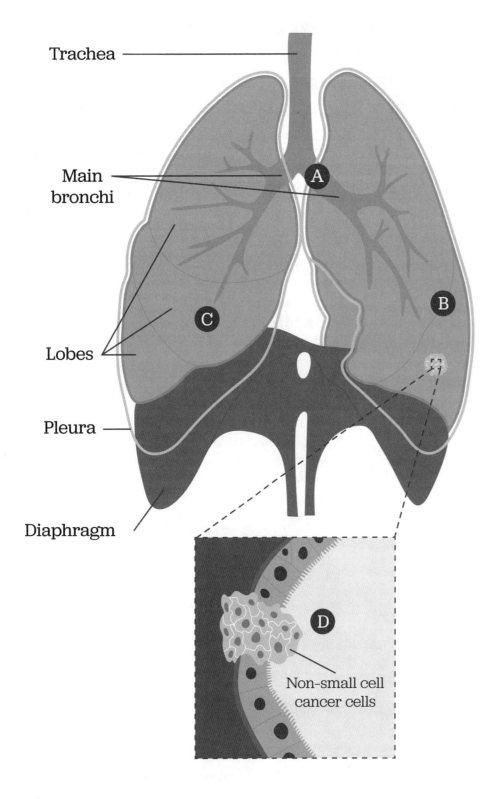

Trachea

Main bronchi

Lobes

Pleura

Diaphragm

Non-small cell cancer cells

 A

Squamous cell carcinoma begins in the squamous cells of the bronchi (in the central part of the lungs). Of all the subtypes, it appears to be the most highly related to smoking, and it tends to cause early symptoms.

 B

Small cell carcinoma can occur in multiple parts of the lung and is often asymptomatic in the early stages, but it metastasizes rapidly and, therefore, is associated with a poor prognosis.

 C

Large cell carcinoma occurs in any part of the lungs and has a tendency to metastasize rapidly. It tends to cause late symptoms.

 D

Adenocarcinoma occurs in the in mucin-producing cells in the peripheral part of the lungs. It is slower growing than other lung cancers and is associated with an improved prognosis.

Figure 22.1
The four subtypes of lung cancer

Diagnosis

Several diagnostic tests are used to determine the presence and stage of lung cancer. The following imaging tests are used to assess the size of the primary lung tumor and to determine if the tumor has metastasized to other areas of the body:

■ computed tomography (CT)

■ positron emission tomography (PET)

■ magnetic resonance imaging (MRI)

This information is then used to assign a stage to the lung cancer (see Chapter 1 for details on staging). Disease staging enables the medical team to determine the most appropriate course of treatment. NSCLC is staged using the tumor, (lymph) node, metastasis (TNM) staging system.[8] SCLC is typically staged using a two-stage system in which the disease is classified as "limited stage" or "extensive stage" disease. Limited-stage SCLC is confined to a small area and usually affects only one lung. Extensive-stage disease is more widespread across the lungs, surrounding lymph nodes, and other parts of the body.[9]

Treatment

Lung cancer can be treated with surgery, chemotherapy, targeted therapies, radiotherapy, or a combination of these modalities. The choice of treatment is guided by the disease stage, prognostic indicators (such as weight loss and performance status), and other factors, such as age and medical comorbidities. For comprehensive recommendations and details of specific therapies, refer to the National Comprehensive Cancer Network (NCCN) practice guidelines in oncology for small cell lung cancer[10] and for non–small cell lung cancer.[11]

Surgery

Surgery is often the preferred treatment for early-stage NSCLC that is localized and has not metastasized to other areas of the body.[11] However, it rarely is used to treat SCLC, as many patients with SCLC present with disease that has already spread at the time of diagnosis.[10] The nutritional consequences of surgery for lung cancer are relatively minimal, as the surgery itself does not affect the gastrointestinal tract. However, malnutrition has been associated with a higher complication rate,[12-14] and patients who present malnourished before surgery require preoperative and postoperative nutrition intervention.

Chemotherapy and Targeted Therapies

Chemotherapy might be used in any of the following ways to treat NSCLC:

■ as neoadjuvant therapy, to reduce the tumor size before surgery;

■ as adjuvant treatment, to minimize disease recurrence after surgical resection; and

■ as treatment for advanced stage disease in patients who are not suitable for curative-intent treatment with surgery or radiotherapy.[8]

For SCLC, chemotherapy is the primary treatment for extensive-stage disease.[9] The following agents are commonly used:

■ cisplatin (Platinol, Platinol-AQ)

■ carboplatin (Paraplatin)

■ paclitaxel (Taxol)

■ docetaxel (Taxotere)

■ gemcitabine (Gemzar)

■ etoposide (Etopophos)

■ vinorelbine (Navelbine)

■ pemetrexed (Alimta)

Targeted therapies are generally used to treat advanced NSCLC and may be used in combination with chemotherapy. Targeted therapies block specific physiologic processes and include:

- angiogenesis inhibitors (eg, bevacizumab and ramucirumab),

- epidermal growth factor receptor inhibitors (eg, erlotinib, gefitinib, and afatinib),

- anaplastic lymphoma kinase inhibitors (eg, crizotinib, ceritinib, alectinib, and brigatinib), and

- BRAF inhibitors (eg, dabrafenib and trametinib).[8]

The chemotherapy agents and targeted therapies used to treat lung cancer have numerous side effects, such as anorexia, mucositis, diarrhea, nausea, vomiting, and fatigue, all of which can affect dietary intake.[15] See Chapter 11 for detailed guidance on managing these symptoms.

Radiotherapy

Radiotherapy, with or without chemotherapy, is used to treat inoperable stage I and stage II NSCLC, and concurrent chemoradiation is the preferred form of treatment for stage III NSCLC. In patients with NSCLC who have poor performance status or advanced-stage disease, palliative radiotherapy may be used.[10,16] Concurrent chemoradiation is the preferred treatment for patients with limited-stage SCLC. In patients with extensive-stage SCLC who are not suitable for concurrent chemoradiation, palliative radiotherapy may be used to control symptoms.[11,17]

Radiotherapy to the thoracic region is associated with several side effects, including oesophagitis, fatigue, anorexia, and nausea, all of which can affect dietary intake.[12,18] Concurrent chemoradiation is associated with a higher incidence of severe acute esophagitis. Research indicates that this occurs in 34% of patients treated with concurrent chemoradiation, compared with 1.3% of patients treated with sequential chemoradiation.[19] See Chapter 11 for guidance on managing these symptoms.

Immunotherapy

Monoclonal antibodies, such as nivolumab (Opdivo), pembrolizumab (Keytruda), and atezolizumab (Tecentriq), may be used to treat stage IV NSCLC.[17] Monoclonal antibodies act by blocking proteins on cancer cells that prevent the immune system from recognizing them as cancerous. Through this action, the immune system can mount an attack on the cancerous cells.[20] A 2017 study showed a survival benefit with 12 months of consolidation immunotherapy treatment following completion of chemoradiation.[21] Associated side effects that can affect nutritional status include fatigue, nausea, anorexia, and diarrhea. See Chapter 11 for guidance on managing these symptoms.

Nutrition Assessment

Patients who have lung cancer are at high risk for decreased nutritional status, including malnutrition, sarcopenia, weight loss, and muscle loss before, during, and after treatment.[22,23] These conditions require early identification and treatment in order to prevent associated poor outcomes. Validated screening and assessment tools should be used from diagnosis through treatment to conduct thorough nutrition assessments and identify patients at risk for malnutrition.

Nutrient Requirements

There are no specific nutrition requirements for patients with lung cancer, and recommendations for practice are taken from general nutrition guidelines for patients with cancer (see Chapter 5).

Because indirect calorimetry often is not feasible in practice, a valid energy equation can be used to estimate resting energy expenditure. Total Energy

Expenditure (TEE) can be estimated by adding a percentage for physical activity and other factors (eg, fever or weight gain). The ratio method—for example, at least 25 to 30 kcal/kg/d—can be used as a rough indicator to calculate TEE. When using this method, ideal body weight is often used for patients with a body mass index (BMI) exceeding 30.[24] Closely monitor dietary intake and body weight (and body composition, if possible), and adjust the estimated energy requirement as needed. General nutrient requirements are as follows[24]:

■ **Protein intake** should be more than 1 g/kg/d and, if possible, up to 1.5 g/kg/d. There is general consensus that most patients with cancer requiring nutritional support for several weeks do not need any specifically formulated amino acid mixture and that high-quality protein from animal, fish, dairy, and plant sources is adequate. Future studies are required to determine if any particular amino acids help stimulate muscle anabolism.

■ **Macronutrient intake** should be similar to that for healthy persons. If hyperglycemia occurs, then a higher fat intake may be considered while reducing the carbohydrate contribution to total energy intake.

■ **Micronutrient intake** should follow recommendations from Dietary Reference Intakes, the World Health Organization, and the Food and Agriculture Organization of the United Nations, as well as from national and international nutrition societies.

■ **Omega-3 fatty acid** supplementation in patients being treated for lung cancer may help maintain body weight and fat-free mass and might improve global quality of life.[25,26] Guidelines state that the use of omega-3 fatty acids may benefit patients with advanced cancer who are undergoing chemotherapy,[24] but the overall evidence is limited.

Nutrition Problems and Interventions

Patients with lung cancer may lose weight and in particular muscle due to a combination of reduced dietary intake and various metabolic derangements, such as elevated resting metabolic rate, insulin resistance, lipolysis, and proteolysis, which may be host- or tumor-derived.[24] Many patients with lung cancer experience unintentional weight loss and may experience swallowing problems caused by the presence of the tumor itself or the impact of anticancer treatment.[27] Weight stabilization for patients with lung cancers is associated with improved survival.[2] Generally, the goals of nutrition interventions for these patients are to maintain body weight (or at least minimize unintentional weight loss) and maintain muscle mass.

Nutrition counseling plays an important role in helping patients meet their nutrition requirements, modify the impact of symptoms and side effects on their nutritional status, and make required dietary modifications.[28] Interventions may include:

■ advising the patient to eat meals and snacks rich in energy and protein;

■ counseling the patient to maintain a varied diet to meet vitamin and mineral needs;

■ instructing the patient on how to fortify food;

■ recommending small, frequent meals and snacks;

■ providing a texture-modified diet for patients with swallowing problems resulting from treatment, such as dysphagia or odynophagia;

■ artificial nutrition, such as tube feeding, if the patient is unable to eat adequately (ie, no food for more than 1 week or less than 60% of requirement for more than 2 weeks) or is malnourished with poor oral intake[24]; and

- parenteral nutrition if the patient's gastrointestinal tract is not functioning, not accessible, or unsafe to access (because of obstructions or a fistula between the trachea and esophagus, for example).

Malnutrition and Weight Loss

The prevalence of malnutrition in patients with lung cancer ranges from 45% to 69%, depending on treatment modality and disease stage.[29,30] However, the prevalence in patients with metastatic or advanced disease is generally higher.[31,32] Malnutrition in patients with lung cancer is associated with reduced survival, poorer lung function, decreased likelihood of completing treatment, and poor quality of life.[23,33-36]

Compared to other tumor types, lung cancer has been associated with a higher risk of malnutrition (odds ratio of 4.59 with a 95% confidence interval of 3.18 to 6.63; $P < .001$).[32] It is common for patients to present with clinically significant weight loss, even before starting treatment, with 35% to 75% of patients reporting unintentional weight loss in the 3 months prior to lung cancer diagnosis.[37] As many as one-third of patients experience a weight loss of 5% or more during or following radiotherapy, and, in the majority of patients, this weight loss occurs after treatment completion. This highlights the importance of posttreatment nutrition follow-up.[22] Factors associated with an increased likelihood for clinically significant weight loss during radiotherapy include:

- treatment with concurrent chemoradiation;

- disease at stage III or higher; and

- a large proportion of the esophagus receiving a dose of more than 40 Gy of radiotherapy.[22,38]

Ideally, patients with these characteristics should receive automatic nutrition referrals. A 2016 study of 151 patients with lung cancer who were treated with chemoradiation found that patients who lost more than 5% of their weight within the first 3 weeks of treatment had significantly decreased overall survival (13 months vs 23 months, $P = .017$). This indicates the importance of preventing weight loss in the first weeks of treatment.[39]

Sarcopenia and Muscle Loss

The importance of identifying patients with sarcopenia (low- and poor-quality skeletal muscle mass) and the occurrence of muscle loss during active cancer treatment have been increasingly recognized. Like malnutrition, sarcopenia is prevalent among cancer patients. Studies show that 47% of patients with lung cancer have sarcopenia before starting chemotherapy, and as many as 61% have sarcopenia before beginning chemoradiation therapy.[40,41] As with malnutrition, sarcopenia is associated with severe consequences, including reduced survival and increased likelihood of experiencing dose-limiting chemotherapy toxicities.[42-44]

Few studies have investigated muscle loss in patients with lung cancer during active treatment. However, a clinically significant muscle loss of 6 cm^2 or more, at a level associated with decreased muscle strength, has been reported in 39% of patients receiving chemotherapy for lung cancer and in 50% of patients receiving chemoradiation when assessed on CT images at the third lumbar vertebrae.[41,45] Sarcopenia occurs in patients in all BMI categories[40,45] and may not be immediately apparent from a standard nutrition assessment. To accurately identify patients with depleted muscle mass, it is important to incorporate either muscle mass or strength measurements, or both, into the nutrition assessment (see Box 22.1). Although less practical in a clinical setting, tools such as CT, dual x-ray absorptiometry, and air displacement plethysmography are ideal for measuring body composition, if they are not contraindicated. Bioelectrical impedance analysis and bioelectrical impedance spectroscopy are also feasible and useful measures, but they have some limitations.[46]

Sarcopenic Obesity

Within the context of a high prevalence of malnutrition and sarcopenia in patients with lung cancer, an increasing number of patients are also presenting as overweight or obese. Recent studies across a variety of treatment modalities consistently show that approximately 20% of patients are presenting as obese and approximately 30% to 40% are presenting as overweight.[43,47,48] Sarcopenic obesity is a known, independent predictor of survival[43,49]; however, some studies of patients with lung cancer show an independent association of obesity or a higher BMI with improved survival.[48,50] The underlying mechanism for the potential protective effect of obesity is unknown. Regardless, identifying malnutrition and sarcopenia in this patient group is of vital importance, particularly because the studies showing a protective effect of obesity have not taken into account underlying muscle mass.[51]

Box 22.1
Identifying Patients With Lung Cancer Who Are at High Nutritional Risk

Treatment stage	Steps
Before treatment	Screen for malnutrition on presentation. Automatically refer patients at high nutritional risk to a registered dietitian nutritionist for nutrition assessment and intervention. Criteria for high nutritional risk include the following: ■ combined chemoradiation ■ stage III or higher disease ■ esophagus in the radiation treatment field Incorporate a measure to assess muscle mass or strength into the nutrition assessment (eg, objective measures such as skinfold measurements, bioimpedance analysis, or handgrip strength; subjective assessments such as subjective global assessment and patient-generated subjective global assessment).
During treatment	Screen for malnutrition at regular intervals. Prevent weight loss of more than 5% during the initial weeks of treatment. Incorporate a measure to assess muscle mass or strength into the nutrition assessment (as described above).
After treatment	Screen for malnutrition at regular intervals. (Regular intervals may mean weekly as an inpatient, monthly or during outpatient visits, or when the patient reports a weight change.) Closely monitor the nutritional status of patients who have completed radiotherapy or concurrent chemoradiotherapy. Incorporate a measure to assess muscle mass or strength into the nutritional assessment (as described above).

Survivorship

Although the number of studies investigating the consequences of weight loss on health outcomes in older patients with cancer is limited, Fiorelli and colleagues[13] found that a weight loss of more than 5% before lung cancer resection was an independent risk factor for 1-year mortality in older patients (70 years and older).

Cachexia, a cancer-associated metabolic syndrome, is characterized by severe weight loss as a consequence of muscle wasting with or without loss of fat mass, anorexia, early satiety, fatigue, and systemic inflammation, all of which lead to disease-associated malnutrition.[52] The prevalence of cachexia is estimated to be as high as 80% in all patients with cancer, varying with the cancer type and stage.[53] Refractory cachexia often is identified in its late stages, when the patient has experienced severe weight loss and muscle tissue wastage, which is almost always irreversible via nutritional support.[54]

The focus of palliative care should be on symptom management (see Chapter 26), improving quality of life, and ensuring that the patient's physical, practical, emotional, and spiritual needs are addressed.[55] Hydration requirements should be considered; if the patient can only manage limited fluids orally, intravenous hydration can be considered, in discussion with the patient and the care team.

Summary

New developments and specialized treatments for lung cancer mean more patients are being treated with potentially curative therapies. However, the impacts of these anticancer treatments—namely unintentional weight loss, pain, changes in appetite, and breathlessness—contribute to a decline in the nutritional status of these patients.[19,20] The individualized nutrition interventions of medical nutrition therapy, such as dietary counseling to help maximize energy intake and manage nutrition impact symptoms, can help stabilize patients' weight and nutritional status and improve their quality of life.

Sample PES Statements for Lung Cancer

Intake domain: Inadequate oral intake related to decreased ability to consume sufficient energy due to side effects of cancer therapy evidenced by anorexia and weight loss of 4 lb (1.8 kg) in the past week.

Clinical domain: Moderate, chronic disease–related or condition-related malnutrition related to decreased ability to consume sufficient energy due to side effects of cancer therapy, as evidenced by dysgeusia, early satiety, unintentional weight loss of 7% in the past month, and a dietary intake of less than 75% of estimated needs in the past month.

References

1. World Health Organization. Cancer key facts. 2018. Accessed December 7, 2020. www.who.int /news-room/fact-sheets/detail /cancer

2. National Cancer Institute. Cancer Stat Facts: Lung and Bronchus Cancer. Accessed December 7, 2020. https://seer.cancer.gov /statfacts/html/lungb.html

3. National Cancer Institute. SEER Cancer statistics review 1975-2016. Accessed December 7, 2020. https://seer.cancer.gov/csr /1975_2016/results_merged/topic _survival.pdf

4. American Cancer Society. Lung cancer risk factors. Accessed April 8, 2020. www.cancer.org /cancer/lung-cancer/causes-risks -prevention/risk-factors.html

5. Maisonneuve P, Shivappa N, Hebert JR, et al. Dietary inflammatory index and risk of lung cancer and other respiratory conditions among heavy smokers in the COSMOS screening study. *Eur J Nutr.* 2016; 55(3):1069-1079.

6. World Cancer Research Fund/ American Institute for Cancer Research. *Food, Nutrition and Physical Activity: A Global Perspective.* WCRF/AICR; 2018. Accessed April 8, 2020. www.wcrf.org/dietandcancer /lung-cancer

7. American Cancer Society. What is lung cancer? 2020. Accessed April 8, 2020. www.cancer.org /cancer/lung-cancer/about/what -is.html

8. American Cancer Society. Non-small cell lung cancer stages. Accessed April 8, 2020. www .cancer.org/cancer/lung-cancer /detection-diagnosis-staging /staging-nsclc.html

9. American Cancer Society. Small cell lung cancer stages. Accessed April 8, 2020. www.cancer.org /cancer/lung-cancer/detection -diagnosis-staging/staging -sclc.html

10. National Comprehensive Cancer Network. *NCCN Clinical Practice Guidelines in Oncology (NCCN Guidelines): Small Cell Lung Cancer.* Version3.2020. National Comprehensive Cancer Network; 2020. Accessed April 8, 2020. www.nccn.org/professionals /physician_gls/pdf/sclc.pdf

11. National Comprehensive Cancer Network. *NCCN Clinical Practice Guidelines in Oncology (NCCN Guidelines): Non-Small Cell Lung Cancer.* Version 3.2020. National Comprehensive Cancer Network; 2020. Accessed April 9, 2020. www.nccn.org/professionals /physician_gls/pdf/nsclc.pdf

12. Zhang L, Wang C, Sha SY, et al. Mini-nutrition assessment, malnutrition, and postoperative complications in elderly Chinese patients with lung cancer. *J BUON.* 2012;17(2):323-6.

13. Fiorelli A, Vicidomini G, Mazzella A, et al. The influence of body mass index and weight loss on outcome of elderly patients undergoing lung cancer resection. *Thorac Cardiovasc Surg.* 2014;62(7):578-87.

14. Thomas PA, Berbis J, Falcoz PE, et al. National perioperative outcomes of pulmonary lobectomy for cancer: the influence of nutritional status. *Eur J Cardiothorac Surg.* 2014;45(4):652-659.

15. Cooley ME. Symptoms in adults with lung cancer: a systematic research review. *J Pain Symptom Manage.* 2000;19(2):137-153.

16. American Cancer Society. Radiation therapy for non-small cell lung cancer. Accessed April 9, 2020. www.cancer.org/cancer /lung-cancer/treating-non-small -cell/radiation-therapy.html

17. American Cancer Society. Radiation therapy for small cell lung cancer. Accessed April 9, 2020. www.cancer.org/cancer /lung-cancer/treating-small-cell /radiation-therapy.html

18. Everitt S, Krishnasamy M, Duffy M, Briffa S. Utilising evidence to inform acute toxicity scoring for patients receiving radiation therapy for lung cancer. *Aus J Cancer Nurs.* 2011;12(1):4-9.

19. Byhardt RW, Scott C, Sause WT, et al. Response, toxicity, failure patterns, and survival in five Radiation Therapy Oncology Group (RTOG) trials of sequential and/or concurrent chemotherapy and radiotherapy for locally advanced non–small-cell carcinoma of the lung. *Int J Radiat Oncol Biol Phys.* 1998;42(3):469-478.

20. National Cancer Institute. Non-small cell lung cancer treatment: treatment option overview. 2018. Accessed April 9, 2020. https://cancer.gov/types/lung/patient/non-small-cell-lung-treatment-pdq#section/_164

21. Antonia SJ, Villegas A, Daniel D, et al. Durvalumab after chemoradiotherapy in stage III non–small-cell lung cancer. *N Engl J Med.* 2017; 377(20): 1919-1929.

22. Kiss N, Isenring E, Gough K, Krishnasamy M. The prevalence of weight loss during (chemo) radiotherapy treatment for lung cancer and associated patient- and treatment-related factors. *Clin Nutr.* 2014;33(6):1074-1080.

23. van der Meij BS, Phernambucq EC, Fieten GM, et al. Nutrition during trimodality treatment in stage III non-small cell lung cancer: not only important for underweight patients. *J Thorac Oncol.* 2011;6(9):1563-1568.

24. Arends J, Bachmann P, Baracos V, et al. ESPEN guidelines on nutrition in cancer patients. *Clin Nutr.* 2017; 36(1):11-48.

25. van der Meij BS, Langius JA, Smit EF et al. Oral nutritional supplements containing (n-3) polyunsaturated fatty acids affect the nutritional status of patients with stage III non-small cell lung cancer during multimodality treatment. *J Nutr.* 2010;140(10):1774-1780.

26. van der Meij BS, Langius JA, Spreeuwenberg MD, et al. Oral nutritional supplements containing n-3 polyunsaturated fatty acids affect quality of life and functional status in lung cancer patients during multimodality treatment: an RCT. *Eur J Clin Nutr.* 2012;66(3):399-404.

27. Ashby C, Baldock E, Donald M, et al. A practical guide for lung cancer nutritional care. Accessed April 19, 2019. http://lungcancernutrition.com

28. Kiss N, Isenring I, Gough K, et al. Early and intensive dietary counseling in lung cancer patients receiving (chemo)radiotherapy—a pilot randomized controlled trial. *Nutr Cancer.* 2016;68(6):958-967.

29. Hébuterne X, Lemarie E, Michallet M, de Montreuil CB, Schneider SM, Goldwasser F. Prevalence of malnutrition and current use of nutrition support in patients with cancer. *JPEN.* 2014;38(2):196-204.

30. Read JA, Choy STB, Beale P, Clarke SJ. An evaluation of the prevalence of malnutrition in cancer patients attending the outpatient oncology clinic. *Asia Pac J Clin Oncol.* 2006;2(2): 80-86. doi:10.1111/j.1743-7563.2006.00048.x

31. Lemarie E, Goldwasser F, Michallet M, Beauvallain De Montreuil C, Hebuterne X. Prevalence of malnutrition in lung cancer patients: a one-day survey. *J Thorac Oncol.* 2007;2(Supplement 4):P1-257 [abstract].

32. Segura A, Pardo J, Jara C, et al. An epidemiological evaluation of the prevalence of malnutrition in Spanish patients with locally advanced or metastatic cancer. *Clin Nutr.* 2005;24(5):801-814.

33. Jagoe RT, Goodship TH, Gibson GJ. The influence of nutritional status on complications after operations for lung cancer. *Ann Thorac Surg.* 2001;71(3):936-943.

34. Ovesen L, Hannibal J, Mortensen EL. The interrelationship of weight loss, dietary intake, and quality of life in ambulatory patients with cancer of the lung, breast, and ovary. *Nutr Cancer.* 1993;19(2):159-167.

35. Ross PJ, Ashley S, Norton A, et al. Do patients with weight loss have a worse outcome when undergoing chemotherapy for lung cancers? *Brit J Cancer.* 2004;90(10):1905-1911.

36. Topkan E, Parlak C, Selek U. Impact of weight change during the course of concurrent chemoradiation therapy on outcomes in stage IIIB non-small cell lung cancer patients: retrospective analysis of 425 patients. *Int J Radiat Oncol Biol Phys.* 2013;87(4):697-704.

37. Morel H, Raynard B, d'Arlhac M, et al. Prediagnosis weight loss, a stronger factor than BMI, to predict survival in patients with lung cancer. *Lung Cancer.* 2018;126:55–63.

38. Kiss N, Krishnasamy M, Everitt S, et al. Dosimetric factors associated with weight loss during (chemo)radiotherapy treatment for lung cancer. *Eur J Clin Nutr*. 2014;68(12)1309-1314.

39. Sanders KJC, Hendriks LE, Troost EG, et al. Early weight loss during chemoradiotherapy has a detrimental impact on outcome in NSCLC. *J Thorac Oncol*. 2016;11(6):873-879.

40. Baracos V, Reiman T, Mourtzakis M, Gioulbasanis I, Antoun S. Body composition in patients with non-small cell lung cancer: a contemporary view of cancer cachexia with the use of computed tomography image analysis. *Amer J Clin Nutr*. 2010;91(suppl):1133S-1137S.

41. Kiss N, Beraldo J, Everitt S. Early skeletal muscle loss in non-small cell lung cancer patients receiving chemoradiation and relationship to survival. *Support Care in Cancer*. 2019;27(7):2657-2664. doi:10.1007/s00520-018-4563-9

42. Antoun S, Baracos VE, Birdsell L, et al. Low body mass index and sarcopenia associated with dose-limiting toxicity of sorafenib in patients with renal cell carcinoma. *Ann Oncol*. 2010;21(8):1594-1598.

43. Martin L, Birdsell L, Macdonald N, et al. Cancer cachexia in the age of obesity: skeletal muscle depletion is a powerful prognostic factor, independent of body mass index. *J Clin Oncol*. 2013;31(12):1539-1547.

44. Prado CM, Baracos VE, McCargar LJ, et al. Sarcopenia as a determinant of chemotherapy toxicity and time to tumor progression in metastatic breast cancer patients receiving capecitabine treatment. *Clin Cancer Res*. 2009;15(8):2920-2926.

45. Prado CM, Sawyer MB, Ghosh S, et al. Central tenet of cancer cachexia therapy: do patients with advanced cancer have exploitable anabolic potential? *Amer J Clin Nutr*. 2013;98(4):1012-1019.

46. Grundmann O, Yoon SL, Williams JJ. The value of bioelectrical impedance analysis and phase angle in the evaluation of malnutrition and quality of life in cancer patients—a comprehensive review. *Eur J Clin Nutr*. 2015;69:1290-1297.

47. Atlan P, Bayar MA, Lanoy E, et al. Factors which modulate the rates of skeletal muscle mass loss in non-small cell lung cancer patients: a pilot study. *Supportive Care Cancer*. 2017;25(11):3365-3373.

48. Lam VK, Bentzen SM, Mohindra P, et al. Obesity is associated with long-term improved survival in definitively treated locally advanced non-small cell lung cancer (NSCLC). *Lung Cancer*. 2017;104(suppl C):52-57.

49. Prado CM, Lieffers JR, McCargar LJ, et al. Prevalence and clinical implications of sarcopenic obesity in patients with solid tumours of the respiratory and gastrointestinal tracts: a population-based study. *Lancet Oncol*. 2008;9(7):629-635.

50. Wang J, Xu H, Zhou S, et al. Body mass index and mortality in lung cancer patients: a systematic review and meta-analysis. *Eur J Clin Nutr*. 2017;72(1):4-17.

51. Stenholm S, Harris TB, Rantanen T, et al. Sarcopenic obesity: definition, cause and consequences. *Curr Opin Clin Nutri Metab Care*. 2008;11(6):693-700.

52. Marshall S and Agarwal E. Comparing characteristics of malnutrition, starvation, sarcopenia and cachexia in older adults. In: Preedy V and Patel VB, eds. *Handbook of Famine, Starvation, and Nutrient Deprivation: From Biology to Policy*. Springer Link: 2017:1-23.

53. Huhmann MB and August DA. Review of American Society for Parenteral and Enteral Nutrition (ASPEN) clinical guidelines for nutrition support in cancer patients: nutrition screening and assessment. *Nutr Clin Pract*. 2008;23(2):182-188.

54. Fearon K, Strasser F, Anker SD, et al. Definition and classification of cancer cachexia: an international consensus. *Lance Oncol*.2011;12(5):489-495.

55. Isenring EA and Teleni L. Nutritional counseling and nutritional supplements: a cornerstone of multidisciplinary cancer care for cachectic patients. *Curr Opin Support Palliat Care*. 2013;7(4):390-395.

Chapter 23
Medical Nutrition Therapy for Gynecologic Cancers

Gretchen B. Gruender, MS, RDN, CSO, CD
Shayne Robinson, RD, CSO, CDN

Gynecologic cancers include cervical cancer, fallopian tube cancer, gestational trophoblastic tumor, ovarian cancer, primary peritoneal cancer, uterine cancer (endometrial cancer and uterine sarcoma), vaginal cancer, and vulvar cancer. This chapter covers primarily cervical, uterine (endometrial), and ovarian cancers. Worldwide, these three cancers, respectively, are the fourth, sixth, and eighth most commonly occurring cancers in women.[1]

With the introduction of the human papillomavirus vaccine in the 1990s, the incidence of cervical cancer has been declining in the United States. However, in many parts of the world, it remains a significant threat to women's health.[1] It is most often diagnosed in women aged 35 to 44 years; the median age at the time of diagnosis is 49 years. Nearly one-half (45.7%) of gynecologic cancers are diagnosed at an early stage and, consequently, the survival rate is 91.5%.[2]

Endometrial cancer is the fourth most common cancer among women in the United States, with a 5-year survival rate of more than 80%.[3] Recent trends indicate that cancers of the uterus, originating primarily in the endometrium, are increasing over time and with successive generations, especially in countries with improving socioeconomic status.[4]

Ovarian cancer is the leading cause of gynecologic cancer deaths in the United States, with a lifetime risk of 1 in 79.[5] It is the fifth leading cause of death from cancer in women and is the most lethal of all gynecologic cancers.[6,7] Epithelial cancers originating in the ovaries, fallopian tubes, and peritoneum exhibit similar clinical characteristics and behavior; therefore, they are often combined and defined as epithelial ovarian cancer in clinical trials and in clinical practice.[8] Unlike endometrial cancer, this condition has few symptoms, and early detection is often difficult. Overall survival is poor, due to diagnosis at advanced stages.[9] The 5-year survival rate is approximately 92.4% for localized ovarian cancer, 75.2% for regional cancer, 29.2% for distant, and 24% for unknown.[5] Successful surgery is important, because complete resection is associated with a 5-year increased survival when compared with postoperative presence of residual tumor.[10]

Table 23.1 presents prevalence data for new cases and deaths in the United States for several gynecologic cancers.

Table 23.1

Statistics for Gynecologic Cancers, United States, 2020[3,11]

Cancer type	Estimated new cases	Estimated deaths
Cervical	13,800	4,290
Uterine (all types)	65,620	12,590
Ovarian	21,750	13,940
Vulvar	6,120	1,350

Risk Factors

Evidence exists that endometrial cancer can be influenced by diet and body composition. A case-control study found decreased risk with a high intake of vegetables, particularly nonstarchy vegetables, and a possible protective effect with high fruit intake. Protective benefits may be due to modulation of steroid hormones and metabolism; activation of antioxidant mechanisms; modulation of detoxification enzymes; and immune system stimulation. Following a Mediterranean diet and the diet inflammation index also showed significantly decreased risk.[12]

Another study analyzing risk estimates for individual components of metabolic syndrome found that obesity and larger waist circumference were stronger predictors for endometrial cancer than any other component of metabolic syndrome. Observed components increasing risk for endometrial cancer included hyperglycemia, hypertension, and high triglycerides.[13]

By contrast, a case-control study examining ovarian cancer risk and adherence to the US Dietary Guidelines for Americans found that neither individual food groups nor dietary quality have been associated with ovarian cancer risk.[14]

Calcium and Ovarian Cancer

Overall, studies show conflicting data regarding ovarian cancer and dairy intake. Two case-control studies conducted in 2012 found conflicting associations for individual dairy products.[15,16] A 2002 case-control study showed a decreased risk for epithelial ovarian cancer in women who consumed lactose-containing foods and dietary calcium.[17] This same study was included in a more recent meta-analysis of 15 studies showing dietary calcium and dairy calcium may reduce the risk for ovarian cancer; however, calcium supplements plus dietary calcium did not show the same results. Subgroups of these studies conducted in North America and Europe found a significant inverse relationship between dietary calcium intake and ovarian cancer risk. Additional studies are warranted.[18]

Risk factors and protective factors for gynecologic cancers are summarized in Box 23.1.

Types of Gynecologic Cancers

The most common gynecologic cancers—uterine cancer (specifically endometrial cancer), cervical cancer, and ovarian cancer—are the focus of this chapter. See Figure 23.1 for additional details on the common types of gynecologic cancers.

Endometrial and Uterine Cancer

The uterus is a muscular organ where a fetus develops before birth. It consists of the myometrium (muscle and tissue that form the walls of the uterus) and the endometrium (the epithelial membrane that lines the uterus). The endometrium is sensitive to hormones, such as estrogen and progesterone, especially during the menstrual cycle. Endometrial cancer (also called endometrial adenocarcinoma) originates in the endometrium; it is the most common form of uterine cancer—accounting for approximately 80% of all cancers of the uterus—and, consequently, the terms *endometrial cancer* and *uterine cancer* are often used interchangeably. Uterine sarcoma, the other main type of uterine cancer, develops in the myometrium and is rare.[19]

Ovarian Cancer

The ovaries, two almond-shaped reproductive organs located on each side of the pelvis, secrete estrogen and progesterone, and in women of reproductive age they release monthly ova. After menopause, the ovaries stop releasing ova and secrete smaller volumes of hormones. While the majority of women present with ovarian epithelial cancer, less common types include ovarian low malignant potential tumors and ovarian germ cell tumors.[5]

Cervical Cancer

The cervix is the lower, narrow end of the uterus, leading from the uterus to the vagina (birth canal). The main types of cervical cancers are squamous cell carcinoma and adenocarcinoma.[2]

Box 23.1
Gynecologic Cancers: Risk Factors and Protective Factors[12,13,20-28]

Uterine—endometrial[12,13,20-23]

Factors that increase risk	*Hormones:* birth control pills, total number of menstrual cycles, obesity, pregnancy, polycystic ovarian syndrome, ovarian tumors, tamoxifen use *Age:* increased risk with advancing age *Diet and exercise:* increased risk with body fat increase; probable increase with increased glycemic load *Family history:* hereditary nonpolyosis colon cancer or Lynch syndrome *Medical history:* metabolic syndrome, diabetes mellitus, hyperglycemia, hypertension, high triglycerides, prior pelvic radiation, endometrial hyperplasia, breast or ovarian cancer
Factors that decrease risk	*Diet and exercise:* coffee consumption; vegetable consumption, particularly nonstarchy vegetables; high fruit consumption; following a Mediterranean die; physical activity (probable decrease)

Uterine sarcoma[24]

Factors that increase risk	*Medical history:* radiotherapy to the pelvis *Family history:* history of retinoblastoma due to an abnormal copy of the *RB* gene *Race:* In Black women, it is more than twice as common as in White or Asian women.

Ovarian[22,24,25-27]

Factors that increase risk	*Age:* increased risk with advancing age (half of all cases are diagnosed in women over age 63 years) *Height and body mass index (BMI):* greater linear growth (marked by adult-attained height) and BMI >30 *Family history:* history of ovarian cancer (5% to 15% of cases are genetically determined) *Genetic mutations:* BRCA1, BRCA2, and RAD51C mutations for high-grade serous ovarian cancers
Factors that decrease risk	*Reproductive history:* giving birth, taking oral contraceptives for more than 5 years, breastfeeding, tubal ligation *Body composition:* increasing hip circumference (postmenopausal women) *Medical history:* prophylactic bilateral salpingo-oophorectomy (may reduce risk by 80% in carriers of genetic mutations)

Cervical[28]

Factors that increase risk	*Medical history:* long-term infection with certain types of human papillomavirus (HPV) (causes almost all cases of cervical cancer); in utero exposure to diethylstilbestrol; immunosuppression from medication or HIV (increases risk for HPV and, thereby, for cervical cancer)
Factors that decrease risk	*Medical history:* vaccines against HPV

Diagnosis

Endometrial Cancer

Symptoms of early-stage disease include unusual vaginal bleeding or abnormal discharge, pelvic pain, and unintentional weight loss. The average age of women with endometrial cancer is 61 years; therefore, women are encouraged to be alert to early symptoms after menopause.[3]

Ovarian Cancer

Symptoms of early-stage (stage I and II) disease are vague and often ignored by women. Consequently, approximately 75% of cases are diagnosed at an advanced stage.[9] Symptoms of advanced ovarian cancer include pelvic and abdominal pain, swelling or pressure, early satiety, and gastrointestinal (GI) problems, such as gas, bloating, or constipation.[8-10]

Cervical Cancer

There usually are no signs or symptoms of early cervical cancer, but it can be detected early with regular examinations. Later signs and symptoms include vaginal bleeding and pelvic pain, unusual vaginal discharge, and pain during sexual intercourse.[28]

Treatment

Gynecologic cancers can be treated with surgery, chemotherapy, radiotherapy, or a combination of these modalities. For comprehensive recommendations and details of specific therapies, refer to the National Comprehensive Cancer Network (NCCN) clinical practice guidelines in oncology for Uterine Cancer,[29] Ovarian Cancer,[30] and Cervical Cancer.[31]

Uterine Cancer

Uterine malignant epithelial carcinomas are treated with surgery followed by observation or a combination of vaginal brachytherapy, external beam radiation therapy (EBRT), or systemic chemotherapy. Hormone therapy may also be considered. Treatment choice depends on the extent of disease, degree of surgical resection, and tissue pathology.[29]

Treatment for uterine sarcoma includes surgical resection with optimum tumor debulking, which may be followed by observation, estrogen blockade, or chemotherapy with or without a combination of vaginal brachytherapy or EBRT, or vaginal cylinder brachytherapy.[32]

Ovarian Cancer

Surgery is a primary component of treatment. In early-stage disease, total extrafascial hysterectomy with bilateral salpingo-oophorectomy, pelvic and para-aortic lymph node dissection, and infracolic or infragastric omentectomy is the standard procedure used to remove the primary tumor and all visible masses.[33] Fertility-sparing surgery may be an option for some patients. Removing the tissue, as opposed to biopsy, clarifies the origin of the tumor, decreases the potential for metastases to the contralateral side, and decreases postoperative ascites.[34] Complete resection improves survival significantly, although it may be difficult to achieve in advanced cases. Intestinal surgery may be needed in 30% to 50% of advanced cases.[10]

Use of adjuvant therapy depends on the grade of tumor and stage of disease. NCCN guidelines recommend observation alone for resected stage IA or IB disease. Patients with stage IC or higher-grade tumors may receive three to six cycles of intravenous chemotherapy with taxane and carboplatin. Patients with stage II and higher disease receive a taxane- and platinum-containing regimen with or without intraperitoneal chemotherapy.[30] Targeted therapies approved by the US Food and Drug Administration for ovarian epithelial, fallopian-tube, and primary peritoneal cancers include bevacizumab (Avastin), olaparib (Lyn-

Oncology Nutrition for Clinical Practice

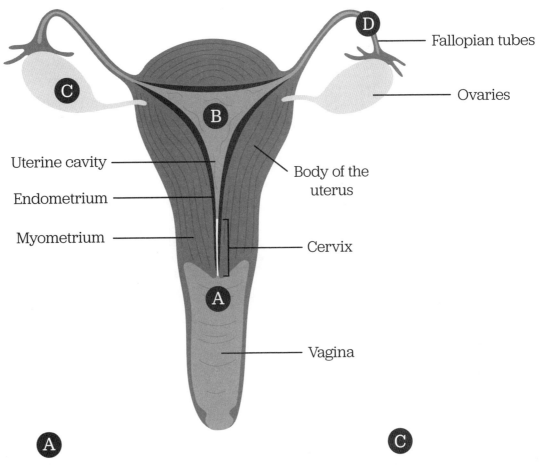

Fallopian tubes

Ovaries

Uterine cavity

Endometrium

Myometrium

Body of the uterus

Cervix

Vagina

(A) Cervical cancer

There are two main types:

- Squamous cell carcinoma begins in the thin, flat cells that line the cervix.
- Adenocarcinoma begins in cervical cells that make mucus and other fluids.

(B) Uterine cancer

Approximately 80% are endometroid adenocarcinoma. Often confined to the uterus, this type is influenced by excess estrogen. It usually has a more favorable prognosis.

Malignant epithelial carcinoma originates in the endometrial mucosa.

Uterine sarcoma is a rare type of uterine cancer that forms in the muscle and tissue that support the uterus.

(C) Ovarian cancer

There are three main types of cells in the ovaries where tumors can occur:

- Epithelial cells cover the ovaries and are the most common site of tumors.
- Germ cells are located inside the ovary and develop into eggs released into the fallopian tubes during reproductive years.
- Stromal cells produce female hormones.

(D)

A range of molecularly distinct cancers may also grow in the ovaries or fallopian tubes, including a high-grade serous ovarian cancer originating in the distal fallopian tube.

Figure 23.1
Sites and types of gynecologic cancers[2,3,5,6]

parza), rucaparib camsylate (Rubraca), and niraparib tosylate monohydrate (Zejula). Bevacizumab or FDA-approved biosimilar may be added to the taxane-carboplatin regimen for ovarian cancer.[30,35]

Radiotherapy is not considered standard treatment for ovarian cancer. Before the advent of platinum-based chemotherapy, radiotherapy was used as adjuvant therapy to sterilize micrometastatic disease. Newer radiotherapy techniques, including intensity-modulated radiotherapy, stereotactic body radiotherapy, and low-dose hyperfractionation, in combination with targeted agents have generated renewed interest in the potential application of radiation therapy to treat ovarian cancer.[36]

Cervical Cancer

Treatment selection depends on the stage of disease, with more advanced disease requiring a total hysterectomy. Procedures such as cryosurgery and laser surgery destroy cervical tissue rather than remove it. Conization is the removal of a cone-shaped piece of tissue from the cervix using either a surgical or laser knife (cold knife cone biopsy) or a thin wire heated by electricity (loop electrosurgical procedure).[28]

For some stages of cervical cancer, the preferred treatment is radiotherapy alone or surgery followed by radiotherapy. Radiotherapies such as EBRT or brachytherapy may be used to treat metastatic or recurrent cervical cancer. Some patients receive concurrent chemoradiation with weekly cisplatin or cisplatin and 5-fluorouracil every 4 weeks. Sometimes, chemotherapy alone is given before or after chemoradiation, or both before and after.[28,31]

Nutrition Assessment

Nutrition considerations vary depending on the stage and treatment of the disease. Because gynecologic cancers are in close proximity to the GI and urinary systems, metastasis to those areas can lead to nutrition-related problems. Because of this and the frequency of malnutrition observed in gynecologic cancers, the diagnosis of gynecologic cancers should trigger a nutrition-risk screening.[37] The role of the registered dietitian nutritionist (RDN) includes early nutrition assessment before treatment to decrease the incidence of malnutrition and the likelihood of associated complications.

Although weight loss is a diagnostic characteristic for malnutrition, ascites and lymphedema (due to para-aortic lymph node dissection performed during surgery) can mask weight loss and skew weight measurement. Nutrition assessment of weight status should consider these phenomena, and conducting a nutrition-focused physical assessment helps clarify the patient's fluid status.[38]

Assessment Tools

A study using the Nutrition Risk Screening (NRS) 2002 system to examine the association between malnutrition and treatment outcomes found a severe risk for malnutrition in 48.9% of women with gynecologic malignancies at the time of hospital admission and before initiation of treatment. This cohort also experienced greater risk of complications and an increase in length of hospital stay from 7 to 10 days. Of the women with gynecologic malignancies, 70.2% of ovarian cancer patients had malnutrition,[39] which is consistent with a study using the patient-generated subjective global assessment (PG-SGA) to identify malnutrition, in which 67% of ovarian cancer patients were malnourished.[40,41] Although the NRS is commonly used in research to identify malnutrition, it has not been identified as a validated tool in this population by the Academy of Nutrition and Dietetics Evidence Analysis Library.[42] Although the PG-SGA is a tool for identifying malnutrition, one study found that the prognostic nutritional index (PNI) was more likely to identify malnutrition in gynecologic cancers than the PG-SGA.[43] The PG-SGA was validated in general surgery patients, while the

PNI was used to examine gynecological patients, who were all women, more malnourished, more obese, and identified as having protein deficiency.[43]

Energy and Nutrient Requirements

Unless otherwise indicated, the energy intake goal for malnourished patients with ovarian cancer is estimated at 30 to 35 kcal/kg/d, reflecting the need for nutrition repletion in a predominantly malnourished population.[44] Energy needs may be closer to 25 to 30 kcal/kg/d for well-nourished patients in whom the disease is diagnosed at an early stage.[45] Protein needs of patients with normal renal function range from 1 to 1.5 g/kg/d, based on stress level.[45] In cases of cancer cachexia, protein needs may increase to 1.5 to 2.5 g/kg/d, depending on renal function and stress level.[44] Micronutrient needs are consistent with Dietary Reference Intakes for the respective age group[46-48] or individualized, as indicated by nutrition assessment. Meal plans customized to address specific treatment side effects can help preserve weight and lean body mass in patients experiencing nutrition impact symptoms. See Chapter 11 for more information on managing side effects of cancer treatment.

Nutrition Problems and Interventions

Malnutrition

Malnutrition is seen in up to 70% of patients with ovarian cancers,[37,39] including metastatic ovarian cancer. A study using the subjective global assessment (SGA) and the PG-SGA to assess the nutritional status of 194 patients with gynecologic cancer showed that 24% of patients were classified as malnourished; and 67% of those had ovarian cancer.[40] The aggressive nature of ovarian cancer treatment is associated with significant morbidity that further contributes to the risk for malnutrition.

Poor nutritional status has been associated with increased postoperative morbidity and mortality in surgical patients.[37]

A retrospective study examining associations between body mass index (BMI) and survival in advanced ovarian cancer found that loss of body weight during chemotherapy is a significant indicator of poor overall survival.[49] Cancer-related weight loss also results in a loss of skeletal muscle and fat stores.

Chemotherapy can cause nutrition impact symptoms. Even when anorexia is not a primary side effect of chemotherapy, nausea, early satiety, and other side effects can lead to reduced dietary intake. Although intraperitoneal chemotherapy has been associated with longer survival,[35] it can also lead to more severe GI side effects and nutrition impact symptoms. See Chapter 9 for a summary of nutrition impact symptoms associated with chemotherapy.

Radiation-Induced Diarrhea

EBRT can lead to significant side effects and nutrition impact symptoms, as the beams are likely directed to the entire pelvic region. More than 70% of patients who receive pelvic radiation develop acute GI symptoms, particularly severe diarrhea.[50] The literature from which pelvic and abdominal radiation therapy statistics and guidelines are derived groups together types of cancers treated with pelvic and abdominal radiation therapy, such as prostate, rectal, and gynecologic cancers. Treatment for radiation-induced diarrhea (RID) might include the following:

- Psyllium fiber supplementation: Fiber supplementation has been recommended for prevention and treatment of RID in clinical guidelines and by clinical experts. Two teaspoons daily were effective in reducing the incidence and severity of diarrhea.[51]

- Probiotics: The use of probiotics shows promise in the prevention and treatment of RID; however, before specific recommendations can be made, more research is needed to determine the timing, dose, and specific strain.[52]

- Loperamide and diphenoxylate: These drugs continue to be recommended as the standard of practice for medication in patients with mild symptoms, based on current clinical practice guidelines.[53]

- Octreotide: This drug has been studied as an intervention for RID in patients with rectal cancer. There are concerns about the cost of octreotide and difficulties in obtaining insurance authorization for its use in RID because the research to support its use is in the early stages.[52]

Postoperative Nutrition Care

Traditional nutrition management of patients undergoing surgery for gynecologic cancer includes withholding oral intake until bowel sounds, flatus, or stool are noted. Once bowel function returns, patients are started on a stepwise diet. Nontraditional postoperative approaches, often as part of "early recovery after surgery" protocols, include early oral postoperative feeding (clear liquid diet, semiliquid diet, and regular diet), enteral feeding, and immune-enhanced enteral feeding. A review of seven clinical trials comparing traditional with nontraditional approaches concluded early oral intake with progressive advancement from a liquid diet to a normal diet was safe and well tolerated following surgery. Length of hospital stay was significantly shorter, postoperative patient satisfaction was higher, and fewer postoperative complications and infections were observed with early feeding. Early intake of a semiliquid diet postoperatively was also found to be safe and well tolerated,

although one of the studies reported significantly higher nausea with this approach. A regular diet as the first postoperative meal was found to be safe following major abdominal surgery. Perioperative immune-enhanced nutrition was found to be safe and effective in increasing postoperative immunologic response. There was reduced length of hospital stay but not improved quality of life (QOL) when enteral feeding, as soon as tolerated, was used to increase caloric and nutritional intake.[54]

In another study, early oral feeding during the first 24-hour period after surgery was defined as clear liquids (water, tea, chamomile tea, or apple juice). In the absence of nausea and vomiting, patients were advanced to a regular diet of boiled or grilled beef, chicken, or fish starting on day 1 and for the duration of hospital stay. Between 78% and 89% of the patients in the early-feeding group resumed solid oral intake on the first postoperative day with no statistically significant difference in the incidence of nausea and vomiting compared with the traditional-feeding group.[55]

Malignant Bowel Obstruction

Malignant bowel obstruction (MBO) is usually a preterminal event in patients with gynecologic cancer, and it occurs in 20% to 50% of patients with ovarian cancer.[56] MBO often results from peritoneal carcinomatosis and may involve the small or large intestine or both. It can be related to the location of the tumor, radiation enteritis, or disease progression. Patients with MBO are unable to tolerate oral intake; they experience severe abdominal pain, intractable nausea, and vomiting, and may have ascites.

Interventions with nutrition implications include surgery and nonsurgical management, such as venting percutaneous endoscopic gastrectostomy (PEG) tubes for drainage or venting, and palliative surgery.[57]

Conservative management measures include nasogastric suction, bowel rest, medication to control symptoms (pain control, antiemetics, steroids, and antisecretory medications), intravenous fluids, or parenteral nutrition (PN).[56,58] Few studies have examined the potential benefits of PN on survival of patients with MBO. One study reported a mean survival rate of 4 to 6 months with PN, with survival of more than 3 months occurring in 30% of patients and a 13% complication rate.[59] PN is not recommended for inoperable cases.

Surgery

If conservative measures are ineffective, surgery for MBO is considered but may not be a viable option. Poor performance status, previous radiotherapy, diffuse carcinomatosis, advanced age, and obstruction of the small bowel have been associated with surgical failure and poor prognosis.[60]

Survival rate is generally low. Reported mean survival is 4 to 5 weeks with inoperable MBO, and the average life expectancy is 6 months in operable cases,[61] with much of this time spent in the hospital. Although some patients can benefit from palliative surgery, it comes at a cost of high mortality (6% to 32%) and substantial hospitalization relative to the patient's remaining survival time. One systematic review found that surgery was able to palliate obstructive symptoms for 32% to 100% of patients, permitted resumption of oral intake for 45% to 75% of patients, and facilitated discharge to home in 34% to 87% of patients. After surgery for MBO, serious complications occurred at a rate of 7% to 44%. Frequent reobstructions (6% to 47%), readmissions (38% to 74%), and reoperations (2% to 15%) occurred. The summary included in this review reported limited survival of 26 to 273 days.[60]

Although there are no defined criteria for selecting surgical candidates, surgery is suggested in patients with good performance status, low-grade histology, and no diffuse carcinomatosis or previous radiotherapy.[56]

Stents and Percutaneous Endoscopic Gastrostomy Tubes

When surgery is not an option for MBO, a venting gastrostomy or PEG tube for decompression or endoscopic stenting may be considered.[62] Both modalities are useful in patients with poor short-term prognosis.[56] PEG tube placement provides a quick and safe method of symptom relief without the risk of a surgical procedure and discomfort of a nasogastric tube.[58] Stents have resolved nausea and vomiting and improved tolerance of oral intake in more than 75% of cases, although this figure is general to all types of cancer, not specific to gynecologic cancer.[56] Gastrostomy tubes have success rates as high as 92% in resolving symptoms, and many patients are able to take in fluids and some softer foods. At minimum, being able to eat for social reasons increases QOL, even though patients may not be able to meet their nutritional needs through oral intake alone.[62] Chapter 12 has further recommendations on nutrition support. Many RDNs consider a low-fiber diet to be best practice for MBO but clinical judgment is recommended to determine the appropriate diet to manage patients' specific symptoms. Patients with small and large bowel obstructions, and postoperative ileus (lack of peristalsis in the bowel not caused by a mechanical obstruction) may benefit from education about a low-fiber diet.[57]

Palliative Care

Although palliative surgery for MBO may help to resolve symptoms, further surgery for recurrent MBO is associated with high morbidity and mortality, and conservative treatment with venting gastrostomy or stenting is preferable in these cases.[60] When a patient's life expectancy is less than 4 months and as short as 4 weeks, care should transition to palliative goals, such as nonsurgical symptom management, to improve QOL.[56,63]

Parenteral Nutrition

Studies examining the use of PN in advanced gynecologic cancers and MBO show conflicting results. In one study, terminally ill patients who received PN survived only 4 weeks longer than patients who did not receive PN.[64] Survival was shorter for patients who received chemotherapy as well as PN.[65] Patients with better performance status and who were able to provide self-care at home benefited from home PN.[59] Patients who may die from starvation rather than their metastatic disease are appropriate for PN, although there is controversy, given the potential discomfort and risks associated with PN.[66] Other issues to consider include cost, QOL, patient and family goals, and clinical judgment, including feedback from a multidisciplinary team.

Performance status may be a key factor when determining the effectiveness of home PN. A small study found that higher performance status (a Karnofsky score of greater than or equal to 50) was associated with a median survival of 6 months compared with a median survival of 3 months for patients with a Karnofsky score of less than 50.[67] Larger studies are needed to confirm these findings. Poor prognosis has prompted researchers to call for inclusion of QOL and symptom benefit as primary endpoints of clinical trials that investigate treatments for ovarian cancer.[68]

Survivorship

Lifestyle changes after treatment for gynecologic cancers can vary, depending on the treatment, disease stage, and future medical treatment plans. For patients in remission, evidence-based recommendations for cancer prevention are appropriate (see Chapter 2) but may need to be modified based on postoperative GI anatomy and function. Symptom- and function-based medical nutrition therapy (MNT) should be provided by RDNs when indicated. RDNs are essential to helping patients decipher the many treatment and curative claims publicized. Providing evidence-based counseling on diets and dietary supplements proposed for cancer treatment can allay fears and help patients make confident decisions regarding a cancer-preventive lifestyle (see Chapter 7).

Long-term survivors who have undergone treatment for ovarian cancer will experience premature menopause and, therefore, have a higher risk for developing heart disease and osteoporosis.[69] It is important for RDNs to emphasize MNT within a nutrition survivorship plan to help decrease the risk for these conditions.

Limited and mixed research exists between dietary intake and ovarian cancer risk and survival. In an observational study of 811 women with invasive ovarian cancer, food frequency records found a survival advantage among women with higher intakes of dietary fiber before diagnosis, while consuming foods with a higher glycemic index was associated with decreased survival.[70] No individual food was associated with improved survival, although there was a suggestion of an advantage for green leafy vegetables and fish, and a higher ratio of polyunsaturated to monounsaturated fatty acids was associated with lower mortality. For women with high-grade serous cancer, there was a trend for reduced mortality risk in those who consumed more cruciferous vegetables and green tea. A separate study showed a survival advantage with prediagnosis vegetable intake and a survival disadvantage for higher intakes of red meat, specifically processed and cured meats.[71]

Summary

Gynecologic cancers often cause complications of the GI tract as a direct result of the proximity of the tumor and the treatment effects on GI tissue. MBO and RID are among the most severe complications. Survivors may transition through many disease phases that pose unique and sometimes difficult nutrition challenges. Nutrition intervention provided by credentialed professionals such as RDNs and board-certified specialists in oncology nutrition may prevent additional barriers to meeting the unique nutritional needs of patients with gynecologic cancers both in and out of treatment.

Sample PES Statements for Gynecologic Cancers

Intake domain: Inadequate oral intake related to early satiety and gastroparesis, as evidenced by a weight loss of more than 5% in the past month and an oral intake of less than 25% of estimated needs.

Clinical domain: Moderate, chronic disease–related or condition-related malnutrition related to partial bowel obstruction, as evidenced by a weight loss of 6% in the past month and a dietary intake of 50% to 75% of estimated needs in the past month.

References

1. Bray F, Ferlay J, Soerjomataram I, Siegel RL, Torre LA, Jemal A. Global cancer statistics 2018: GLOBOCAN estimates of incidence and mortality worldwide for 36 cancers in 185 countries. *CA Cancer J Clin.* 2018 Nov;68(6):394-424.

2. National Cancer Institute Surveillance, Epidemiology, and End Results Program. Cancer stat facts: cervical cancer. Accessed December 7, 2020. https://seer.cancer.gov/statfacts/html/cervix.html

3. National Cancer Institute Surveillance, Epidemiology, and End Results Program. Cancer stat facts: uterine cancer. Accessed December 7, 2020. https://seer.cancer.gov/statfacts/html/corp.html

4. Lortet-Tieulent J, Ferlay J, Bray F, Jemal A. International patterns and trends in endometrial cancer incidence, 1978-2013. *J Natl Cancer Inst.* 2018;110(4):354-361. doi:10.1093/jnci/djx214

5. National Cancer Institute Surveillance, Epidemiology, and End Results Program. Cancer stat facts: ovarian cancer. Accessed December 7, 2020. https://seer.cancer.gov/statfacts/html/ovary.html

6. American Cancer Society. Ovarian cancer. Accessed December 7, 2020. https://cancer.org/cancer/ovarian-cancer.html

7. Ovarian Cancer Research Fund Alliance. Statistics. Accessed December 7, 2020. https://ocrahope.org/patients/about-ovarian-cancer/statistics

8. National Cancer Institute. Ovarian epithelial, fallopian tube, and primary peritoneal cancer prevention (PDQ)–health professional version. Accessed December 8, 2020. https://cancer.gov/types/ovarian/hp/ovarian-prevention-pdq

9. Jammal M, Lima C, Murta E, et al. Is ovarian cancer prevention currently still a recommendation of our grandparents? *Rev Bras Ginecol Obstet.* 2017;39(12):676-685.

10. Burges A, Schmalfeldt B. Ovarian cancer diagnosis and treatment. *Dtsch Ärztebl Int.* 2011;108(38):635-641. doi:10.3238/arztebl.2011.0635

11. American Cancer Society. Cancer facts and figures 2020. Accessed December 7, 2020. www.cancer.org/content/dam/cancer-org/research/cancer-facts-and-statistics/annual-cancer-facts-and-figures/2020/cancer-facts-and-figures-2020.pdf

12. Ricceri F, Giraudo MT, Fasanelli F, et al. Diet and endometrial cancer: a focus on the role of fruit and vegetable intake, Mediterranean diet and dietary inflammatory index in the endometrial cancer risk. *BMC Cancer.* 2017;17:757.

13. Esposito K, Chiodini P, Capuano A, Bellastella G, Maiorino M, Giugliano D. Metabolic syndrome and endometrial cancer: a meta-analysis. *Endocrine.* 2014;45(1)28-36. doi:10.1007/s12020-013-9973-3

14. Chandran U, Bandera E, Williams-King M, et al. Healthy eating index and ovarian cancer risk. *Cancer Causes Control.* 2011;22(4):563-571.

15. Faber M, Jensen A, Søgaard M, et al. Use of dairy products, lactose, and calcium and risk of ovarian cancer—results from a Danish case-control study. *Acta Oncol.* 2012;51(4):454-464.

16. Merritt M, Cramer C, Vitonis A, Titus L, Terry K. Dairy foods and nutrients in relation to risk of ovarian cancer and major histological subtypes. *Int J Cancer.* 2013;132(5):1114-1124.

17. Goodman M, Wu A, Tung K, et al. Association of dairy products, lactose, and calcium with the risk of ovarian cancer. *Am J Epidemiol.* 2002;156(2):148-157.

18. Song X, Li Z, Ji X, Zhang D. Calcium intake and the risk of ovarian cancer: a meta-analysis. *Nutrients.* 2017;9(7). pii: E679.

19. National Cancer Institute. Cervical cancer treatment (PDQ)–health professional version. Accessed February 24, 2021. www.cancer.gov/types/cervical/hp/cervical-treatment-pdq

20. National Cancer Institute. Epidemiology of Endometrial Cancer Consortium E2C2. Accessed December 7, 2020. https://epi.grants.cancer.gov/eecc

21. Centers for Disease Control and Prevention. What are the risk factors. Centers for Disease Control and Prevntion website. Accessed May 10, 2020. https://cdc.gov/cancer/uterine/basic_info/risk_factors.htm

22. South S, Vance H, Farrell C, et al. Consideration of hereditary nonpolyposis colorectal cancer in BRCA mutation-negative familial ovarian cancers. *Cancer.* 2009;115(2):324-333.

23. Rosato V, Zucchetto A, Bosetti C, et al. Metabolic syndrome and endometrial cancer risk."*Ann Oncol.* 2011;22(4):884-889.

24. American Cancer Society. Uterine sarcoma causes, risk factors, and prevention. Accessed May 13, 2020. www.cancer.org/cancer/uterine-sarcoma.html

25. Jelovac D, Armstrong DK. Recent progress in the diagnosis and treatment of ovarian cancer. *CA: Cancer J Clin.* 2011;61(3):183-203.

26. Collaborative Group on Epidemiological Studies of Ovarian Cancer. Ovarian cancer and body size: individual participant meta-analysis including 25,157 women with ovarian cancer from 47 epidemiological studies. *PLoS Med.* 2012;9(4).

27. Russo A, Calò V, Bruno L, Rizzo S, Bazan V, Di Fede G. Hereditary ovarian cancer. *Crit Rev Oncol Hemat.* 2009;69(1):28-44.

28. National Cancer Institute. Cervical cancer. Accessed December 7, 2020. https://cancer.gov/types/cervical

29. National Comprehensive Cancer Network. *NCCN Clinical Practice Guidelines in Oncology (NCCN Guidelines): Uterine Neoplasms.* Version 1.2020. National Comprehensive Cancer Network; 2020. Accessed April 14, 2020. www.nccn.org/professionals/physician_gls/pdf/uterine.pdf

30. National Comprehensive Cancer Network. *NCCN Clinical Practice Guidelines in Oncology (NCCN Guidelines): Ovarian Cancer Including Fallopian Tube Cancer and Primary Peritoneal Cancer.* Version 2.2020. National Comprehensive Cancer Network; 2020. Accessed April 14, 2020. www.nccn.org/professionals/physician_gls/pdf/ovarian.pdf

31. National Comprehensive Cancer Network. *NCCN Clinical Practice Guidelines in Oncology (NCCN Guidelines): Cervical Cancer.* Version 1.2021. National Comprehensive Cancer Network; 2020. Accessed April 14, 2020. www.nccn.org/professionals/physician_gls/pdf/cervical.pdf

32. National Cancer Institute. Uterine sarcoma treatment (PDQ)–health professional version. Accessed December 7, 2020. www.cancer.gov/types/uterine/hp/uterine-sarcoma-treatment-pdq

33. Epithelial carcinoma of the ovary, fallopian tube, and peritoneum: Surgical staging. Uptodate.com. Accessed December 7, 2020. www.uptodate.com/contents/epithelial-carcinoma-of-the-ovary-fallopian-tube-and-peritoneum-surgical-staging

34. Chen L, Berek JS. Epithelial carcinoma of the ovary, fallopian tube, and peritoneum: Clinical features and diagnosis. Uptodate.com. Accessed February 24, 2021. www.uptodate.com/contents/epithelial-carcinoma-of-the-ovary-fallopian-tube-and-peritoneum-clinical-features-and-diagnosis

35. National Cancer Institute. Ovarian, fallopian tube, and primary perintoneal cancer treatment (PDQ)–health professional version. Accessed December 7, 2020. www.cancer.gov/types/ovarian/hp/ovarian-epithelial-treatment-pdq

36. Fields EC, McGuire WP, Lin L, Temkin SM. Radiation treatment in women with ovarian cancer: past, present, and future. *Front Oncol.* 2017;21(7):177.

37. Kathiresan A, Brookfield K, Schuman S, Lucci J. Malnutrition as a predictor of poor postoperative outcomes in gynecologic cancer patients. *Arch Gynecol Obstet.* 2011;284(2):445-451.

38. Hipskind P, American Society for Parenteral and Enteral Nutrition, Galang M, Jevenn A, Pogatschnik C, Hamilton C. *Nutrition-Focused Physical Exam: An Illustrated Handbook.* American Society for Parenteral and Enteral Nutrition; 2016.

39. Hertlein L, Kirschenhofer A, Fürst S, et al. Malnutrition and clinical outcome in gynecologic patients. *Eur J Obstet Gynecol Reprod Biol.* 2014;174:137-140.

40. Laky B, Janda M, Cleghorn J, Obermair A. Comparison of different nutritional assessments and body-composition measurements in detecting malnutrition among gynecologic cancer patients. *Am J Clin Nutr.* 2008;87(6):1678-1685.

41. Laky B, Janda M, Bauer J, Vavra C, Cleghorn G, Obermair A. Malnutrition among gynaecological cancer patients. *Eur J Clin Nutr.* 2007;61(5): 642-646.

42. Thompson J, Elliott L, Fuchs-Talovsky V, Levin R, Voss A, Piemonte T. Oncology evidence-based nutrition practice guideline for adults. *J Acad Nutr Diet.* 2017;117(2):297-310.

43. Santoso JT, Cannada T, O'Farrel B, Alladi K, Coleman RL. Subjective versus objective nutritional assessment study in women with gynaecological cancer: a prospective cohort trial. *Int J Gynecol Cancer.* 2004;14(2):220-223.

44. Dillon E, Volpi E, Wolfe R, et al. Amino acid metabolism and inflammatory burden in ovarian cancer patients undergoing intense oncological therapy. *Clin Nutr.* 2007;26(6):736–743.

45. Russell M, Malone AM. Nutrient requirements. In: Charney P, Malone AM, eds. *Academy of Nutrition and Dietetics Pocket Guide to Nutrition Assessment.* 3rd ed. Academy of Nutrition and Dietetics; 2015.

46. Institute of Medicine. *Dietary Reference Intakes for Vitamin A, Vitamin K, Arsenic, Boron, Chromium, Copper, Iodine, Iron, Manganese, Molybdenum, Nickel, Silicon, Vanadium and Zinc.* The National Academies Press; 2001.

47. Institute of Medicine. *Dietary Reference Intakes for Vitamin C, Vitamin E, Selenium, and Carotenoids.* The National Academies Press; 2000.

48. Institute of Medicine. *Dietary Reference Intakes for Calcium and Vitamin D.* The National Academies Press; 2011.

49. Hess LM, Barakat R, Tian C, Ozols RF, Alberts DS. Weight change during chemotherapy as a potential prognostic factor for stage III epithelial ovarian carcinoma: a gynecologic oncology group study. *Gynecol Oncol.* 2007;107(2):260-265.

50. McGough C, Baldwin C, Frost G, Andreyev H. Role of nutritional intervention in patients treated with radiotherapy for pelvic malignancy. *Brit J Cancer.* 2004;90(12):2278–2287.

51. Murphy J, Stacey D, Crook J, Thompson B, Panetta D. Testing control of radiation-induced diarrhea with a psyllium bulking agent: a pilot study. *Can Oncol Nurs J.* 2000;10(3):96-100.

52. Muehlbauer P, Thorpe D, Davis A, Drabot R, Rawlings B, Kiker E. Putting evidence into practice: evidence-based interventions to prevent, manage, and treat chemotherapy- and radiotherapy-induced diarrhea. *Clin J Oncol Nurs.* 2009;13(3): 336-41.

53. Benson AB, Ajani JA, Catalano RB, et al. Recommended guidelines for the treatment of cancer treatment-induced diarrhea. *J Clin Oncol.* 2004;15;22(14):2918-2926.

54. Obermair A, Simunovic M, Isenring L, Janda M. Nutrition interventions in patients with gynecological cancers requiring surgery. *Gynecol Oncol.* 2017;145(1):192-199.

55. Minig L, Biffi R, Zanagnolo V, et al. Reduction of postoperative complication rate with the use of early oral feeding in gynecologic oncologic patients undergoing a major surgery: a randomized controlled trial. *Ann Surg Oncol.* 2009;16(11):3101-3110.

56. Tuca A, Guell E, Martinez-Losada E, Codorniu N. Malignant bowel obstruction in advanced cancer patients: epidemiology, management, and factors influencing spontaneous resolution. *Cancer Manage Res.* 2012;4:159-169.

57. Dolan E. Malignant bowel obstruction: a review of current treatment strategies. *Am J Hosp Palliat Care.* 2011;28(8):576-582.

58. Rath KS, Loseth D, Muscarella P, et al. Outcomes following percutaneous upper gastrointestinal decompressive tube placement for malignant bowel obstruction in ovarian cancer. *Gynecol Oncol.* 2013;129(1):103-106.

59. Madhok B, Yeluri S, Haigh K, Burton A, Broadhead T, Jayne D. Parenteral nutrition for patients with advanced ovarian malignancy. *J Hum Nutr Diet.* 2011;24(2):187-191.

60. Olson P, Pinkerton C, Brasel K, Schwarze M. Palliative surgery for malignant bowel obstruction from carcinomatosis: a systematic review. *JAMA Surgery.* 2014;149(4):383-392.

61. Santangelo M, Grifasi C, Criscitiello C, et al. Bowel obstruction and peritoneal carcinomatosis in the elderly: a systematic review. *Aging Clin Exp Res.* 2017;29(suppl 1):73-78.

62. Tsahalina E, Woolas RP, Carter PG, et al. Gastrostomy tubes in patients with recurrent gynaecological cancer and intestinal obstruction. *Br J Obstet Gynaecol.* 1999;106(9):964-968.

63. Ripamonti C, Easson A, Gerdes H. Management of malignant bowel obstruction. *Eur J Cancer.* 2008;44(8):1105-1115.

64. Brard L, Weitzen S, Strubel-Lagan S, et al. The effect of total parenteral nutrition on the survival of terminally ill ovarian cancer patients. *Gynecol Oncol.* 2006;103(1):176-180.

65. Abu-Rustum NR, Barakat RR, Venkatraman E, Spriggs D. Chemotherapy and total parenteral nutrition for advanced ovarian cancer with bowel obstruction. *Gynecol Oncol.* 1997;64(3):493-495.

66. Ripamonti C, Bruera E. Palliative management of malignant bowel obstruction. *Intl J Gynecol Cancer.* 2002;12(2):135-143.

67. Soo I, Gramlich L. Use of parenteral nutrition in patients with advanced cancer. *Appl Physiol Nutr Metab.* 2008;33(1):102-106.

68. Vaughan S, Coward J, Bast R, et al. Rethinking ovarian cancer: recommendations for improving outcomes. *Nat Rev Cancer.* 2011;11(10):719-725.

69. Schulz E, Arfai K, Xiaodong L, Sayre J, Gilsanz V. Aortic calcification and the risk of osteoporosis and fractures. *J Clin Endocrinol Metabol.* 2004;89(9):4246-4253.

70. Playdon M, Nagle CM, Ibiebele TI, et al. Pre-diagnosis diet and survival after a diagnosis of ovarian cancer. *Brit J Cancer.* 2017;116(12):1627-1637.

71. Dolucek T, McCarthy B, Joslin C, et al. Prediagnosis food patterns are associated with length of survival from epithelial ovarian cancer. *J Am Diet Assoc.* 2010;110(3):369-82.

Chapter 24
Medical Nutrition Therapy for Prostate Cancer

Greta Macaire, MA, RD, CSO

The prostate, a walnut-sized gland in men that surrounds the top of the urethra, produces seminal fluid. Prostate cancer is the most common type of cancer in men and the second most common cause of cancer deaths in men. Most prostate cancers are slow growing, although a small percentage are aggressive. Metabolically, prostate cancer has been linked to androgen hormones that stimulate prostate cancer growth.[1,2]

More than 95% of prostate cancers are adenocarcinomas, which develop in the mucous-secreting cells of the prostate gland (see Figure 24.1 on page 516). If cancer develops in the fibromuscular tissue of the gland, it is a sarcoma. Increased levels of insulin-like growth factor 1 (IGF-1), overexpression of cyclooxygenase 2 (COX-2), and chronic inflammation also have been implicated in the development of prostate cancer.[1,2] Ongoing research indicates that body fatness, along with dietary and physical activity patterns, likely influences these factors.[3]

Box 24.1 outlines prostate cancer statistics. Metastatic prostate cancer is incurable with current therapies. The 5-year survival rate for men with metastatic prostate cancer is 30%.[4]

> ## Box 24.1
> ### Prostate Cancer in the United States, 2020[4]
>
> Estimated new cases in 2020: 191,930
>
> Estimated deaths in 2020: 33,330
>
> Five-year relative survival rate: 97.8%

Risk Factors

Known risk factors for prostate cancer include age, ethnicity, and heredity.[1,2,5]

Age: Approximately 60% of prostate cancers are diagnosed in men aged 65 years and older.

Ethnicity: Prostate cancer is more prevalent in North America and in northern Europe; in the United States, it is more prevalent in Black men.

Heredity: Approximately 5% to 10% of cases are attributed to family history and genetics. The risk doubles in those who have a first-degree relative with prostate cancer.

Research on gene mutations and molecular subtypes linked with prostate cancer is ongoing. Additional risk factors being researched include diet, obesity, infections, chemical exposures, and vasectomy.[1,2]

Epidemiologic data suggest that differences in diet and lifestyle play a role in the variability of prostate cancer rates worldwide.[5] Observational studies suggest that dietary components may affect prostate cancer risk, progression, and mortality.[6-8] Limited evidence suggests an association between certain diet and lifestyle modifications and increased or decreased risk for recurrent and fatal prostate cancer (see Box 24.2 on page 517).

Diagnosis

Screening recommendations for prostate cancer based on age and risk factors differ among professional health organizations.[9,10] Screening typically involves measuring levels of prostate-specific antigen (PSA), a protein made by the prostate gland and found in the blood. PSA blood levels may

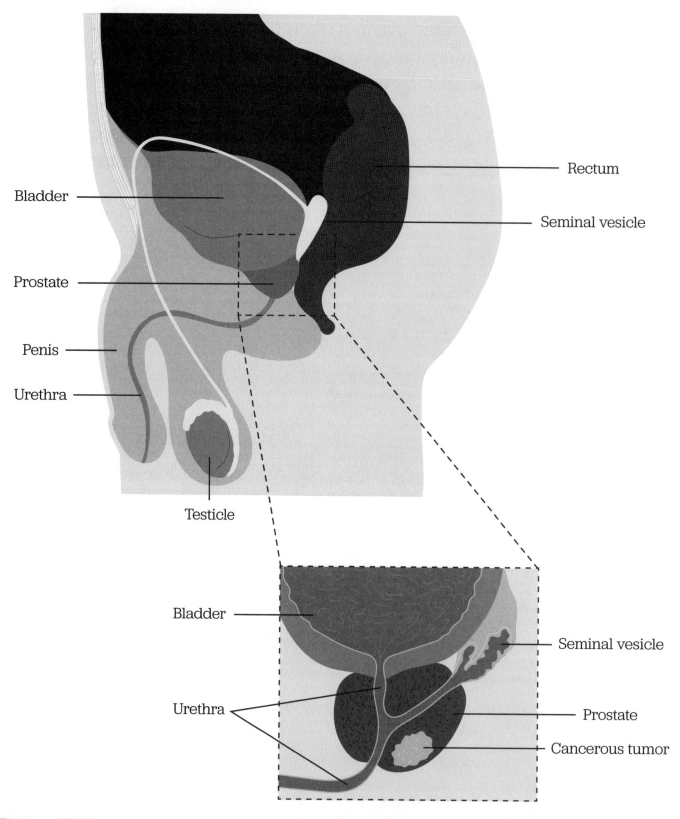

Figure 24.1
Carcinoma of the prostate gland

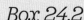

Box 24.2
Diet and Lifestyle Risk Factors and Prostate Cancer Risk[7,8]

Decreases risk	Increases risk
Physical activity	High body mass index
Diet high in lycopene	Smoking
Consumption of the following:	Consumption of the following:
■ cruciferous vegetables	■ dairy (calcium)
■ vegetable fat	■ processed meat
■ fish	■ eggs (choline)
■ soy	■ poultry with skin
■ tea	■ animal fat and other saturated fat
■ coffee	■ selenium supplementation

be higher than normal in men who have prostate cancer, benign prostatic hyperplasia, or infection or inflammation of the prostate gland. Prostate cancer symptoms may include changes in urinary or sexual function and back or pelvic pain. Early stages of prostate cancer are typically asymptomatic.[2]

Prostate cancer usually is diagnosed via biopsy and staged using the American Joint Committee on Cancer's TNM staging system (as described in Chapter 1) and the Gleason score to define the histologic grade of the tumor. Gleason scores range from 2 to 10 and indicate how likely it is that a tumor will spread. A low Gleason score means the cancer tissue is similar to normal prostate tissue and the tumor is less likely to spread. A high Gleason score means the cancer tissue is very different from normal tissue and the tumor is more likely to spread.[2,11]

Treatment

Treatment depends on the cancer stage, life expectancy, and the patient's overall health (see Box 24.3 on page 518). Refer to the *NCCN Clinical Practice Guidelines in Oncology (NCCN Guidelines): Prostate Cancer* regarding details of specific therapies.[12]

Nutrition for Prevention and Recurrence
Plant-Based Diets

A plant-based diet is associated with a decreased risk for prostate cancer and its recurrence.[13-15] Plant-derived foods provide vitamins, minerals, fiber, and phytochemicals that, in experimental studies, have exhibited various anticancer properties.[16,17] Specific foods include cruciferous vegetables, allium vegetables, soy, and tomatoes.

■ Cruciferous vegetables: These have been linked consistently with a decreased risk for prostate cancer, as well as for its recurrence and metastasis. Isothiocyanates and indoles in these foods have been shown to inhibit the growth of prostate cancer cells.[18,19]

■ Allium vegetables: Garlic, onions, and other alliums provide organosulfur compounds that decrease risk for prostate cancer by inducing cell cycle arrest and apoptosis.[20]

■ Soy: Studies suggest that genistein, an isoflavone in soy, may inhibit the synthesis of prostaglandins that promote inflammation, and

Box 24.3
Prostate Cancer Treatment Options and Possible Side Effects[1,2,21-25]

Cancer stage	Treatment options	Possible side effects
Early stages (T1 or T2 disease)	Active surveillance—involves close monitoring without treatment unless there are changes in test results that indicate cancer progression; an appropriate option for older men or men with less aggressive tumors. Certain exams and tests (such as PSA [prostate-specific antigen] levels, prostate ultrasound, and biopsy) are performed on a regular schedule.	None
	Surgery—removes the cancer, the prostate gland, and some surrounding tissue	Infertility; urinary, bowel, and erectile dysfunction
	Radiotherapy—various forms	Infertility; urinary, bowel, and erectile dysfunction
Advanced stages (involvement of regional lymph nodes or distant metastasis)	Androgen deprivation therapy—slows prostate cancer growth by reducing serum levels of androgens or by interfering with the androgen receptors; can be done by removing organs that produce testosterone (eg, orchiectomy) or with medication	Fatigue, hot flashes, sexual changes, mood changes, anemia, weight gain, changes in body composition; increased risk for osteoporosis; potentially increased risk for cardiovascular disease and type 2 diabetes
	Chemotherapy—cabazitaxel (Jevtana), docetaxel (Taxotere), mitoxantrone (Novantrone), and estramustine (Emcyt)	See Chapter 9 for information about the mechanisms of action and side effects of these agents.
	Radiotherapy	Infertility; urinary, bowel, and erectile dysfunction
	Combination therapy	See side effects of individual treatments.
	Immunotherapy—sipuleucel-T (Provenge), an active cellular immunotherapy used to treat hormone-resistant metastatic prostate cancer	Chills, fever, headache, myalgia, sweating, and flu-like symptoms

genistein combined with daidzin and glycitin (also found in soy) may induce cell cycle arrest and apoptosis in prostate cancer cells.[26]

■ Tomatoes: These are a rich source of lycopene, which may convey particular benefit against prostate cancer. The antioxidant activities of this carotenoid, as well as its effects on cell cycles, are believed to inhibit prostate cancer growth and metastasis.[27] Data from the Health Professionals Follow-Up Study showed a 66% decreased risk for metastatic prostate cancer in men consuming two or more servings per week of cooked tomato sauce and a 28% decreased risk for developing lethal prostate cancer in healthy men whose diets contained the most lycopene.[27,28] Lycopene absorption is enhanced when tomatoes are cooked and consumed with oil.[29]

Additional plant-derived foods and compounds being studied for anti–prostate cancer properties include coffee, flaxseed, green tea, milk thistle, pomegranate, and turmeric.[7-9,30] Modes of action include helping prevent DNA mutations that may initiate cancers; promoting cancer cell apoptosis; reducing inflammation; inhibiting angiogenesis; and regulating cell cycles to facilitate cellular repair of DNA mutations.[6-8,30]

Evidence indicates that obtaining plant-derived anticancer compounds from whole foods is more beneficial than obtaining them from supplements. To date, studies examining anticancer benefits of single-nutrient supplementation have produced negative results. Research shows that bioactive compounds in fruits and vegetables work synergistically and on multiple biochemical pathways—benefits difficult to reproduce in trials of single-nutrient supplements.[31]

Fat Consumption

Research suggests that Western diets, characterized by a high intake of sweets and animal fat, are associated with prostate cancer.[32] Western diets tend to increase testosterone levels, a concern for individuals who have sex hormone–dependent prostate cancers.[33] However, it is the types of fatty acids consumed (animal sources vs plant sources) that are of greater importance than total fat intake. Generally, studies have shown a positive association between prostate cancer and the intake of saturated fat from meat and dairy foods.[34,35] Consuming higher amounts of poultry with skin and of processed meats after prostate cancer diagnosis has been linked with an increased risk for disease recurrence.[36] Dairy foods also may promote higher IGF-1 levels, and mutagens in meat cooked at high temperatures also contribute to prostate cancer risk.[36-38]

Although intake of *trans* fatty acids has been correlated with an increased risk for prostate cancer, omega-9 fatty acids and fats from vegetable sources (eg, olive oil and nuts) appear to convey a slightly inverse association.[39,40] Higher than normal blood levels of eicosapentaenoic acid and docosahexaenoic acid—omega-3 fatty acids found in cold-water fish—have been associated with both increased and decreased rates of prostate cancer.[7] Higher fish consumption, however, is correlated with lower risk for prostate cancer and recurrence.[41] Omega-6 fatty acids, linoleic acid, and arachidonic acid may stimulate the growth of prostate cancer cells. Studies suggest a benefit from diets containing a low omega-6 to omega-3 ratio, which may occur through the inhibition of arachidonic acid–derived eicosanoids.[42]

Dairy Products, Calcium, and Vitamin D

The majority of studies in a meta-analysis showed a positive association between a high intake of total and dairy calcium (≥1,500 mg/d) and dairy products and an increased risk for prostate cancer.[43] Although less is known about the influence of calcium and dairy products on prostate cancer after diagnosis, several studies in men with nonmetastatic prostate cancer have linked a higher consumption of whole milk with a higher risk for prostate cancer recurrence and mortality.[44-47] Limited data suggest an association between supplemental calcium and increased risk for fatal prostate cancer.[43]

Biologic plausibility suggests that a higher calcium intake might suppress circulating levels of 1,25-dihydroxyvitamin D.[43] However, most studies examining relationships between vitamin D (intake or circulating levels) and prostate cancer have produced conflicting or null results.[7] Studies suggest that factors such as race, disease stage, and calcium intake may affect the role of vitamin D in men who have prostate cancer.[6]

Dietary Supplements

There is a lack of significant evidence to recommend any single supplement to decrease the risk for prostate cancer.[48] Conversely, there is concern that certain supplements may increase prostate cancer risk. The Selenium and Vitamin E Cancer Prevention Trial (SELECT) showed a slightly increased risk for prostate cancer among men randomly assigned to take vitamin E supplements. In addition, a secondary analysis of the SELECT data found that selenium supplementation in men with higher than normal baseline selenium levels increased the risk for high-grade prostate cancer. Men who reported a selenium intake of 140 mcg/d or more after diagnosis had an increased risk for prostate cancer mortality.[49,50] However, regular multivitamin use is considered safe and was associated with a significant 8% reduction in total cancer incidence in men in the Physicians' Health Study II.[51]

Eggs and Choline

Although a meta-analysis found no association between egg consumption and the risk for prostate cancer, other studies have linked a higher egg intake with an increased risk for fatal prostate cancer.[36,52,53] Choline, found in egg yolks, is highly concentrated in prostate cancer cells, leading researchers to question whether choline may be responsible for the observation. Studies have correlated a high dietary choline intake and higher than normal plasma levels of choline with an increased risk for prostate cancer.[54,55]

Body Weight and Physical Activity

Evidence associating obesity with total or nonadvanced prostate cancer is inconsistent; however, greater body fatness is strongly associated with advanced prostate cancer.[7] Gaining more than 2.2 kg after a prostatectomy has been associated with doubling the risk of recurrence.[56] Weight gain of 5% or more has been associated with a nearly twofold increased risk for prostate cancer–specific mortality,[57] and a 2011 meta-analysis suggested that a high body mass index increased mortality from prostate cancer.[58] Obtaining 3 hours or more per week of vigorous activity is associated with lower mortality in survivors of prostate cancer.[59-61] Aerobic and resistance exercise help mitigate the side effects of androgen deprivation therapy (ADT).[62]

Nutrition Problems and Interventions

See Box 24.4 for a summary of medical nutrition therapy during and after treatment. Few men in whom early-stage prostate cancer is diagnosed are underweight or present with recent weight loss or eating difficulty.[63] Most patients with early-stage prostate cancer complete cancer treatment without major complications; however, it is important for registered dietitian nutritionists (RDNs) to counsel patients on strategies to manage nutrition impact symptoms (NIS) that may occur, as outlined in

Box 24.4
Medical Nutrition Therapy for Prostate Cancer Treatments[21,62,64-69]

Treatments	Suggested medical nutrition therapy
Active surveillance	Not applicable.
Surgery Radical prostatectomy	Prescribe adequate energy, protein, and micronutrient consumption required for healing.
Radiation therapy Directed at the entire prostate, caudal portion of seminal vesicles, and (in advanced cases) the pelvic lymph nodes, which exposes the bladder, rectum, sigmoid colon, and small bowel to radiation	Modify the patient's fiber and fat intake for rectal urgency and loose stools.[a] Confirm use of antidiarrheal medications recommended by the medical team. Consider probiotic supplements (≥10 billion CFUs (colony-forming unit) per day, with lactobacilli or a blend of lactobacilli and bifidobacteria) during pelvic radiation therapy to lessen gas and diarrhea from treatment.

Androgen deprivation therapy (ADT)

Decreases serum testosterone levels by >95% and increases estrogen levels by >80%

Recommended interventions for specific nutrition-related side effects of long-term therapy are as follows:

Bone Loss

Prescribe weight-bearing exercise plus resistance exercise two to three times a week.

Prescribe 1,000 to 1,200 mg of calcium daily (from food or supplements).

Ensure adequate vitamin D level (>30 ng/mL), and prescribe a daily vitamin D supplement (eg, ≥600 IU) to maintain levels in normal range.

Decreased Insulin Sensitivity

Combine weight management interventions with American Heart Association/American College of Cardiology (AHA/ACC) task force, National Lipid Association (NLA), and Academy of Nutrition and Dietetics guidelines for diet and physical activity to reduce cardiovascular disease risk; monitor for need to regulate carbohydrate intake.

Elevated Lipids

Combine weight-management interventions with AHA/ACC, NLA and Academy of Nutrition and Dietetics guidelines for diet and physical activity to reduce cardiovascular disease risk and to promote desired lipid levels.

Hot Flashes

Instruct the patient to maintain a healthy weight, add moderate aerobic exercise, and limit or avoid hot beverages, spicy foods, alcohol, caffeine, and smoking to reduce the severity of vasomotor symptoms.

Sarcopenia

Prescribe resistance exercise two to three times a week.

Consider protein supplementation, as preliminary evidence suggests that supplementation (eg, with whey protein isolate) may assist with muscle protein synthesis, particularly when combined with resistance exercise.

Normochromic, Normocytic Anemia

Provide education on maximizing iron absorption and consuming adequate iron if indicated.

[a] See Chapter 11 for additional suggestions.

Chapter 11. Otherwise, interventions for patients with early-stage prostate cancer should focus on optimizing health and quality of life (QOL). Interventions include strategies to prevent long-term effects of some prostate cancer therapies, such as osteoporosis and cardiovascular disease.[70]

Patients with advanced disease are more likely to present with weight loss and decreased intake, both of which increase the risk for early discontinuation of treatment or treatment breaks and poorer outcomes. These men also have a higher risk for experiencing NIS from systemic therapy and additional weight loss during treatment. Diarrhea is a common NIS resulting from full pelvic radiation, a treatment for advanced disease. In this population, a comprehensive nutrition care plan most often needs to address weight maintenance (to promote full treatment and preserve muscle mass) and diarrhea management (to prevent excess nutrient and fluid loss and to promote weight maintenance).[71] See Chapter 11 for nutrition interventions for diarrhea and other NIS associated with treatment.

Survivorship

Given the increasing evidence showing that weight gain and being overweight or obese may increase the risk for disease recurrence, post-treatment nutrition intervention should address weight maintenance when the patient's weight is within the normal range and promote gradual weight loss while preserving lean body mass when the patient is overweight or obese. Survivors of prostate cancer who are on ADT for advanced disease often gain weight during therapy and seek healthy weight-loss strategies. Guidelines and recommendations from the American Heart Association/American College of Cardiology task force,[64] the National Lipid Association,[65] and the Academy of Nutrition and Dietetics Evidence Analysis Library[66] are appropriate for achieving healthy lipid levels. Nutrition intervention during and after ADT treatment should address calcium needs and sources (emphasizing nondairy food sources), vitamin D status, and physical activity for maintaining bone density.[72] All survivors can benefit from nutrition education targeting foods and dietary intake patterns shown to help prevent disease recurrence. Additionally, physical activity including at least 30 minutes of activity on most days is recommended. If medically appropriate, 3 hours or more of vigorous activity per week is recommended as vigorous activity appears to reduce prostate cancer recurrence and mortality more than moderate-intensity exercise.[59-61] See Box 24.5 for nutrition recommendations for prostate cancer survivors who have completed treatment.

Summary

One in nine men will be diagnosed with prostate cancer in his lifetime. For the majority of these men, their cancer treatment will be curative and without serious complications. With growing scientific evidence that diet and lifestyle habits may slow progression and reduce prostate cancer recurrence, the role of the RDN in early-stage disease is to counsel patients on nutrition habits to optimize their health and QOL. The nutrition care plan for men with advanced-stage disease will also include strategies to manage NIS of treatments and prevent long-term side effects of prostate cancer therapies, such as osteoporosis and cardiovascular disease.

Box 24.5

Evidence for Nutrition and Lifestyle Advice for Prostate Cancer Survivors[2,6,18,19,27,28,30,34-36,40-47,53,64-66]

Food or nutrient	Recommended intake	Comments
Cruciferous vegetables	Include at least one serving daily.	Dietary sources include arugula, broccoli, brussels sprouts, cabbage, cauliflower, collard greens, kale, horseradish, kohlrabi, mustard greens, radishes, rutabaga, turnips, turnip greens, and watercress.
Lycopene-rich fruits and vegetables	Include dietary lycopene daily; lycopene supplements are not recommended.	Dietary sources include tomatoes (raw and cooked forms, such as tomato paste, sauce, juice, and so on), guava, and watermelon. Cooked tomato products or juices contain higher amounts of lycopene. Lycopene is best absorbed when consumed with fat from sources such as olive oil, avocados, or nuts.
Poultry	Choose unprocessed poultry without skin.	Avoid processed, skin on, barbecued, or fried poultry. Substituiting 30 g/day of poultry or fish for total (processed and unprocessed) or unprocessed red meat was associated with a significantly decreased risk for prostate cancer recurrence.
Fis	Include at least two servings per week.	Avoid swordfish, shark, king mackerel, and tilefish due to high mercury levels.
Dairy products	Limit consumption, particularly of whole-milk products. If consuming dairy, low-fat or nonfat products are recommended and should be consumed in moderation (1 serving daily). Combine nondairy sources of calcium with limited dairy selections.	Select reduced-fat or nonfat cheese, milk, yogurt, and similar dairy products. Select leafy green vegetables, fortified nut milks, and soy foods as nondairy sources of calcium and cold-water fish as a nondairy source of vitamin D.
Saturated fat	Limit to <6% of energy intake.	Limit whole-milk dairy foods, red meats, processed meats, poultry skin, and baked goods (unless low in saturated fat and *trans* fat).
Trans fats	Avoid food sources of *trans* fats.	
Eggs	Limit egg-yolk intake to two yolks per week.	Egg whites are acceptable.

(continued)

Box 24.5
Evidence for Nutrition and Lifestyle Advice for Prostate Cancer Survivors[6,18,19,27,28,30,34-36,40-47,53,64-66] *(continued)*

Food or nutrient	Recommended intake	Comments
Omega-6 fatty acids Arachidonic acid and linoleic acid	Limit intake of arachidonic acid by limiting consumption of meat, butter, egg yolks, and whole-milk dairy foods. Limit intake of linoleic acid by limiting vegetable-oil sources to 1 Tbsp daily.	Vegetable oils containing linoleic acid include corn, safflower, sunflower, and cottonseed oils, and processed foods made with these oils.
Omega-3 fats eicosapentaenoic acid (EPA), docosahexaenoic acid (DHA), and α-linolenic acid (ALA)	Consume cold-water fish twice weekly.	Sources of EPA and DHA include salmon, sardines, black cod, trout, herring, and DHA-enriched eggs (within the egg allowance). Sources of ALA include flaxseed, chia seeds, walnuts, hemp seeds, and pumpkin seeds.
Omega-9 fatty acids	Include daily; limit consumption of nuts to ¼ c per meal or snack to keep calorie intake reasonable.	Oleic acid is a primary source of omega-9 fat and is found in olive oil, avocado oil, canola oil, macadamia nut oil, almonds, hazelnuts, pistachios, pecans, and avocados.
Flaxseed	Include 2 Tbsp of ground flaxseed daily.	Ground flaxseed (whole flaxseeds may not be absorbed) is acceptable at intakes of up to 2 Tbsp daily.
Soy	Include soy foods regularly in the diet. Opt for whole soy foods over processed soy products that use soy protein isolate or soy isoflavone extracts.	Whole soy foods include soybeans, edamame, tempeh, tofu, soy milk, soy nuts, and miso. Soy supplements are not recommended.
Green tea	Include 1 c or more daily.	
Calcium	Include the Recommended Dietary Allowance (RDA): 1,000 to 1,200 mg/d (from diet). Do not exceed 1,500 mg/d.	Preferred sources of calcium include reduced-fat or nonfat dairy products (up to one serving daily), canned fish with soft bones, beans, leafy greens, tofu, almonds, calcium-fortified nondairy beverages, and calcium-fortified foods.
Vitamin D	Include the RDA: 600 to 800 IU/d (more if serum 25-hydroxyvitamin D level is below normal). Do not exceed 4,000 IU/d unless prescribed by physician.	Sources of vitamin D include sunlight, fish, and fortified foods.

Sample PES Statements for Prostate Cancer

Behavioral and environmental domain: Food and nutrition–related knowledge deficit related to lack of prior exposure to information, as evidenced by a diet recall revealing an oral intake of more than 18 oz/wk of red meat and consumption of processed meats 10 times in the past month.

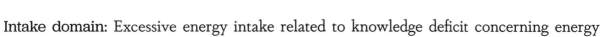

Intake domain: Excessive energy intake related to knowledge deficit concerning energy intake, as evidenced by a 10% weight gain in 6 months.

References

1. American Cancer Society. Detailed Guide: Prostate cancer. Accessed December 20, 2020. http://cancer.org/Cancer /ProstateCancer/DetailedGuide /index

2. National Cancer Institute. Prostate cancer treatment (PDQ)–health professional version. Accessed December 21, 2020. www.cancer .gov/types/prostate/hp/prostate -treatment-pdq#section/all

3. Wilson KM, Mucci LA, Drake BF et al. Meat, fish, poultry, and egg intake at diagnosis and risk of prostate cancer progression. *Cancer Prev Res*. 2016; 9(12): 933-941.

4. National Cancer Institute. Surveillance epidemiology and end results. Seer stat fact sheets: prostate cancer. Accessed May 6, 2020. https://seer.cancer.gov /statfacts/html/prost.html

5. World Cancer Research Fund International, American Institute for Cancer Research. *Diet, Nutrition, Physical Activity, and Prostate Cancer*.3rd ed. World Cancer Research Fund International; 2018. Accessed December 21, 2020. www.wcrf .org/sites/default/files/Prostate -cancer-report.pdf

6. Lin PH, Aronson W, Freedland SJ. An update of research evidence on nutrition and prostate cancer. *Urol Oncol*. 2017 Nov 2. pii: S1078-1439(17)30536-7. doi:10.1016/j .urolonc.2017.10.006

7. Peisch SF, Van Blarigan EL, Chan JM, et al. Prostate cancer progression and mortality: a review of diet and lifestyle factors. *World J Urol*. 2017;35(6):867-874.

8. Ballon-Landa E, Parsons JK. Nutrition, physical activity and lifestyle factors in prostate cancer prevention. *Curr Opin Urol*. 2018;28(1):55-61.

9. US Preventive Services Task Force. *Final Update Summary: Prostate Cancer: Screening*. US Preventive Services Task Force; 2018. Accessed December 21, 2020. https:// uspreventiveservicestaskforce .org/uspstf/recommendation /prostate-cancer-screening

10. American Urological Association. Early Detection of Prostate Cancer (2018). Accessed December 21, 2020. http:// auanet.org/education/guidelines /prostate-cancer-detection.cfm

11. American Joint Committee on Cancer. *AJCC Cancer Staging Manual*. 8th ed. Springer; 2018.

12. National Comprehensive Cancer Network. *NCCN Clinical Practice Guidelines In Oncology (NCCN Guidelines): Prostate Cancer*. Version 1.2020. National Comprehensive Cancer Network; 2020. Accessed December 21, 2020. www.nccn.org /professionals/physician_gls/pdf /prostate.pdf

13. Ornish D, Weidner G, Fair WR, et al. Intensive lifestyle changes may affect the progression of prostate cancer. *J Urology*. 2005:174(3):1065-1070.

14. Saxe GA, Major JM, Nguyen JY, et al. Potential attenuation of disease progression in recurrent prostate cancer with plant-based diet and stress reduction. *Integr Cancer Ther*. 2006;5(3):206-13.

15. Daubenmier JJ, Weidner G, Marlin R, et al. Lifestyle and health-related quality of life of men with prostate cancer managed with active surveillance. *Urology*. 2006;67(1):125-130.

16. Kushi LH, Doyle C, McCullough M., et al. American Cancer Society guidelines on nutrition and physical activity for cancer prevention. *CA Cancer J Clin*. 2012;62(1):30-67.

17. Turati F, Rossi M, Pelucchi C, et al. Fruit and vegetables and cancer risk: a review of southern European studies. *Br J Nutr*. 2015 Apr;113 (suppl 2):S102-10.

18. Higdon JV, Delage B, Williams DE, Dashwood RH. Cruciferous vegetables and human cancer risk: epidemiologic evidence and mechanistic basis. *Pharmacol Res*. 2007;55(3):224-236.

19. Richman EL, Carroll PR, Chan JM. Vegetable and fruit intake after diagnosis and risk of prostate cancer progression. *Int J Cancer*. 2012;131(1): 201-210.

20. Hsing AW, Chokkalingam AP, Gao YT, et al. Allium vegetables and risk of prostate cancer: A population-based study. *J Natl Cancer Inst*. 2002;94(21): 1648-1651.

21. Nguyen PL, Alibhai SM, Basaria S, et al. Adverse effects of androgen deprivation therapy and strategies to mitigate them. *Eur Urol*. 2015;67(5):825-36.

22. Storer TW, Miciek R, Travison TG. Muscle function, physical performance and body composition changes in men with prostate cancer undergoing androgen deprivation therapy. *Asian J Androl.* 2012;14(2):204-221.

23. Bosco C, Bosnyak Z, Malmberg A, et al. Quantifying observational evidence for risk of fatal and nonfatal cardiovascular disease following androgen deprivation therapy for prostate cancer: a meta-analysis. *Eur Urol.* 2015;68(3); 386-96.

24. American Cancer Society. Chemotherapy for prostate cancer. August 2019. Accessed December 21, 2020. www.cancer.org/cancer/prostate-cancer/treating/chemotherapy.html

25. National Cancer Institute. Recurrent or hormone resistant prostate cancer treatment (PDQ)–health professional version. Accessed December 21, 2020. www.cancer.gov/types/prostate/hp/prostate-treatment-pdq#section/_72

26. Yan L and Spitznagel EL. Soy consumption and prostate cancer risk in men: a revisit of a meta-analysis. *Am J Clin Nutr.* 2009;89(4):1155-1163.

27. Zu K, Mucci L, Rosner BA, et al. Dietary lycopene, angiogenesis, and prostate cancer: a prospective study in the prostate-specific antigen era. *J Natl Cancer Inst.* 2014;106(2):djt430. doi:10.1093/jnci/djt430

28. Giovannucci E, Rimm EB Liu Y, Stampfer MJ, Willett WC. A prospective study of tomato products, lycopene, and prostate cancer risk. *J Natl Cancer Inst.* 2002;94(5):391-398.

29. Story EN, Kopec RE, Schwartz SJ, Harris GK. An update on the health effects of tomato lycopene. *Annu Rev Food Sci Technol.* 2010;1:189-210.

30. Azrad M, Vollmer RT, Madden J, et al. Flaxseed-derived enterolactone is inversely associated with tumor cell proliferation in men with localized prostate cancer. *J Med Food.* 2013;16(4):357-60.

31. Liu RH. Health-promoting components of fruits and vegetables in the diet. *Adv Nutr.* 2013;4(3):384S-92S.

32. Fabiani R, Minelli L, Bertarelli G, Bacci S. A western dietary pattern increases prostate cancer risk: a systematic review and meta-analysis. *Nutrients.* 2016;12;8(10).

33. Habito RC, Ball MJ. Postprandial changes in sex hormones after meals of different composition. *Metabolism.* 2001;50(5):505-511.

34. Allott EH, Arab L, Su LJ, et al. Saturated fat intake and prostate cancer aggressiveness: results from the population-based North Carolina-Louisiana Prostate Cancer Project. *Prostate Cancer Prostatic Dis.* 2017;20(1):48-54.

35. Song Y, Chavarro JE, Cao Y, et al. Whole milk intake is associated with prostate cancer-specific mortality among US male physicians. *J Nutr.* 2013;143(2):189-196.

36. Richman EL, Stampfer MJ, Paciorek A, et al. Intakes of meat, fish, poultry, and eggs and risk of prostate cancer progression. *Am J Clin Nutr.* 2010;91(3):712-721.

37. Young NJ, Metcalfe C, Gunnell D, et al. A cross-sectional analysis of the association between diet and insulin-like growth factor (IGF)-I, IGF-II, IGF-binding protein (IGFBP)-2, and IGFBP-3 in men in the United Kingdom. *Cancer Causes Control.* 2012;23(6): 907-917.

38. Key TJ. Nutrition, hormones and prostate cancer risk: results from the European prospective investigation into cancer and nutrition. *Recent Results Cancer Res.* 2014;202:39-46.

39. Hu J, La Vecchia C, de Groh M, et al. Canadian Cancer Registries Epidemiology Research Group. Dietary transfatty acids and cancer risk. *Eur J Cancer Prev.* 2011;20(6):530-538.

40. Richman EL, Kenfield SA, Chavarro JE, et al. Fat intake after diagnosis and risk of lethal prostate cancer and all-cause mortality. *JAMA Internal Medicine.* 2013;173(14):1318-1326.

41. Chan JM, Holick CN, Leitzmann MF, et al. Diet after diagnosis and the risk of prostate cancer progression, recurrence, and death (United States). *Cancer Cause Control.* 2006;17(2):199-208.

42. Apte SA, Cavazos DA, Whelan KA, Degraffenried LA. A low dietary ratio of omega-6 to omega-3 fatty acids may delay progression of prostate cancer. *Nutr Cancer*. 2013;65(4):556-562.

43. Aune D, Navarro Rosenblatt DA, Chan DS, et al. Dairy products, calcium, and prostate cancer risk: a systematic review and meta-analysis of cohort studies. *Am J Clin Nutr*. 2015;101(1):87-117.

44. Tat D, Kenfield SA, Cowan JE, et al. Milk and other dairy foods in relation to prostate cancer recurrence: Data from the cancer of the prostate strategic urologic research endeavor (CaPSUR). *Prostate*. 2018;78(1):32-39.

45. Pettersson A, Kasperzyk JL, Kenfield SA, et al. Milk and dairy consumption among men with prostate cancer and risk of metastases and prostate cancer death. *Cancer Epidemiol Biomarkers Prev*. 2012;21(3):428-436.

46. Yang M, Kenfield SA, Van Blarigan EL, et al. Dairy intake after prostate cancer diagnosis in relation to disease-specific and total mortality. *Int J Cancer*. 2015;137(10):2462-2469.

47. Downer MK, Batista JL, Mucci LA, et al. Dairy intake in relation to prostate cancer survival. *Int J Cancer*. 2017;140(9):2060-2069.

48. National Cancer Institute. Prostate cancer, nutrition, and dietary supplements (PDQ)–health professional version. Accessed December 21, 2020. https://cancer.gov/about-cancer/treatment/cam/hp/prostate-supplements-pdq

49. Kristal AR, Darke AK, Morris JS, et al. Baseline selenium status and effects of selenium and vitamin E supplementation on prostate cancer risk. *J Natl Cancer Inst*. 2014;106(3).

50. Kenfield SA, Van Blarigan EL, DuPre N, et al. Selenium supplementation and prostate cancer mortality. *J Natl Cancer Inst*. 2015;107:360.

51. Gaziano JM, Sesso HD, Christen WG, Bubes V, Smith JP, MacFadyen J, et al. Multivitamins in the prevention of cancer in men: the Physicians' Health Study II randomized controlled trial. *JAMA*. 2012;308:1871-1880.

52. Xie B, He H. No association between egg intake and prostate cancer risk: a meta-analysis. *Asian Pac J Cancer Prev*. 2012;13:4677-4681.

53. Richman EL, Kenfield SA, Stampfer MJ, et al. Egg, red meat, and poultry intake and risk of lethal prostate cancer in the prostate-specific antigen-era: incidence and survival. *Cancer Prev Res (Phila)*. 2011;4:2110-2121.

54. Richman EL, Kenfield SA, Stampfer MJ, et al. Choline intake and risk of lethal prostate cancer: incidence and survival. *Am J Clin Nutr*. 2012;96:855-863.

55. Johansson M, Van Guelpen B, Vollset SE, et al. One-carbon metabolism and prostate cancer risk: prospective investigation of seven circulating B vitamins and metabolites. *Cancer Epidemiol Biomark Prev*. 2009;18:1538-1543.

56. Joshu CE, Mondul AM, Menke A, et al. Weight gain is associated with an increased risk of prostate cancer recurrence after prostatectomy in the PSA era. *Cancer Prev Res (Phila)*. 2011;4:544-551.

57. Bonn SE, Wiklund F, Sjolander A, et al. Body mass index and weight change in men with prostate cancer: progression and mortality. *Cancer Cause Control*. 2014;25:933-943.

58. Cao Y, Ma J. Body mass index, prostate cancer-specific mortality, and biochemical recurrence: a systematic review and meta-analysis. *Cancer Prev Res (Phila)*. 2011;4:486-501.

59. Kenfield SA, Stampfer MJ, Giovannucci E, Chan JM. Physical activity and survival after prostate cancer diagnosis in the health professionals follow-up study. *J Clin Oncol*. 2011;29:726-732.

60. Richman EL, Kenfield SA, Stampfer MJ, et al. Physical activity after diagnosis and risk of prostate cancer progression: data from the cancer of the prostate strategic urologic research endeavor. *Cancer Res*. 2011;71:3889-3895.

61. Bonn SE, Sjolander A, Lagerros YT, et al. Physical activity and survival among men diagnosed with prostate cancer. *Cancer Epidemiol Biomark Prev*. 2015;24:57-64.

62. Moyad MA, Newton RU, Tunn UW, Gruca D. Integrating diet and exercise into care of prostate cancer patients on androgen deprivation therapy. *Res Rep Urol*. 2016;8:133-143.

63. Mehdad A, McBride E, Monteiro Grillo I, Camilo M, Ravasco P. Nutritional status and eating pattern in prostate cancer patients. *Nutrición Hospitalaria.* 2010;25(3):422-427.

64. Arnett DK, Blumenthal RS, Albert MA, et al. 2019 AHA/ACC guideline on primary prevention of cardiovascular disease: a report of the American College of Cardiology/American Heart Association Task Force on Clinical Practice Guidelines. *Circulation.* 2019;140:e596–e646

65. Jacobson TA, Maki KC, Orringer CE, et al; NLA Expert Panel. National Lipid Association Recommendations for Patient-Centered Management of Dyslipidemia: Part 2. *J Clin Lipidol.* 2015;9(6 suppl):S1-122.

66. Academy of Nutrition and Dietetics Evidence Analysis Library. Disorders of lipid metabolism: executive summary of recommendations (2011). Accessed January 6, 2018. www.andeal.org/topic.cfm?menu=5300&cat=4528

67. Meng-Meng Liu, Shu-Ting Li, Yan Shu, He-Qin Zhan. Probiotics for prevention of radiation-induced diarrhea: A meta-analysis of randomized controlled trials. *PLoS One.* 2017;12(6).

68. Ki Y, Kim W, Nam J, et al. Probiotics for rectal volume variation during radiation therapy for prostate cancer. *Int J Radiat Oncol Biol Phys.* 2013;87(4):646-50.

69. Hanson ED, Nelson AR, West DW, et al. Attenuation of resting but not load-mediated protein synthesis in prostate cancer patients on androgen deprivation. *J Clin Endocrinol Metab.* 2017;102(3):1076-1083.

70. Demark-Wahnefried W. Dietary interventions in prostate cancer. *Curr Urol Rep.* 2008;9(3):217-225.

71. Stacey R, Green JT. Radiation-induced small bowel disease: latest developments and clinical guidance. *Ther Adv Chronic Dis.* 2014;5(1):15-29.

72. Owen PJ, Daly RM, Livingston PM, Fraser SF. Lifestyle guidelines for managing adverse effects on bone health and body composition in men treated with androgen deprivation therapy for prostate cancer: an update. *Prostate Cancer Prostatic Dis.* 2017;20(2):137-145.

Chapter 25
Medical Nutrition Therapy for Thyroid Cancer

Megan Schoenfeld, RD

The thyroid is a small gland located in the front part of the neck. It produces thyroid hormone—which helps regulate heart rate, body temperature, and weight—and calcitonin, a hormone that helps maintain normal calcium levels. The lifetime risk for developing thyroid cancer is 1.2%.[1] The incidence of thyroid cancer has nearly tripled since 1975, which can be attributed in part to new technology allowing earlier diagnosis and identification of smaller carcinomas.[2,3] Most thyroid cancers are relatively indolent.[1] Thyroid cancer statistics are shown in Box 25.1.

Box 25.1
Thyroid Cancer Statistics, in the United States, 2020[1,2]

Estimated new cases in 2020: 52,890 (12,720 men, 40,170 women)

Estimated deaths in 2020: 2,180 (1,040 men, 1,140 women)

Five-year relative survival rate: 98.3%

Risk Factors

Although some risk factors are still being investigated, others have been identified. The following have been identified as risk factors for thyroid cancer[4-6]:

- Exposure to high levels of radiation, particularly during infancy or early childhood, is one of the best-established risk factors.

- Genetic mutations have been associated with thyroid cancer, and genetic factors are responsible for 20% to 25% of medullary carcinomas.

- There is increased risk associated with being female. People aged 25 and 65 years old are at greater risk.

- Increased risk is associated with a family and personal medical history of benign thyroid conditions, such as goiters.

- Obesity is a known risk factor for a variety of cancers, including esophageal, colon, kidney, breast, skin, rectal, and gallbladder. It is associated with a higher prevalence of thyroid cancer in women, but the correlation has not been established in males.

Dietary Risk Factors

Much of the research exploring dietary factors and risk for thyroid cancer are limited by the difficulties inherent in measuring diet, which is a multidimensional exposure. It is important to note that much of the evidence is from epidemiological studies, making causality difficult to interpret. Overall, findings are inconsistent across populations, and risk factors appear to vary across different ethnicities, dietary patterns, environmental factors, and lifestyles.

Iodine Intake

This is perhaps the most widely accepted dietary factor associated with thyroid cancer. Research has consistently shown that chronic iodine deficiency is associated with an increased risk for follicular carcinoma, while high iodine intake (such as in iodine supplementation programs) is associated with an increased incidence of papillary carcinoma.[4] Because seafood is a major natural source of dietary iodine, associations between fish intake

---

and thyroid cancer have been examined. Findings have been inconsistent, historically, and reviews show no association between increased thyroid cancer risk and fish intake. Some of these studies suggest fish intake plays a protective role in geographic regions with low iodine content in the soil and ground water. Iodine content of foods varies enormously, based on the iodine content of the soil and ground water, and this variability limits the accuracy of generalized food composition tables for this nutrient.[4,7] Concentrations of iodine in drinking water also vary geographically according to iodine levels in soil and water tables, distance to ocean water, and proximity to agricultural runoff.[8,9]

Cruciferous Vegetable Intake

Cruciferous vegetables contain goitrogens (goiter-producing compounds) that can induce thyroid cancer in animals; however, epidemiology studies show limited support for an association between goitrogens and thyroid cancer in humans.[7] Inverse associations have been found between thyroid cancer risk and noncruciferous vegetable intake. It is hypothesized that any unfavorable effect of goitrogenic substances is outweighed by the protective effect of other vegetable constituents that inhibit carcinogenesis.[4,7]

Other Dietary Components

Some studies suggest potential associations between thyroid cancer risk and intakes of soy, nitrate and nitrite, alcohol, and green tea, but further studies are needed to clarify these associations.[4,7,10-12]

Types of Thyroid Cancer

Thyroid cancers are a heterogeneous group of diseases often distinguished by cellular classification and categorized by clinical features and management. Early thyroid cancer often is asymptomatic, but as the cancer grows, symptoms may develop. Symptoms vary by type of thyroid cancer but may include cough, difficulty swallowing or breathing, enlargement of or lump on the thyroid gland, neck pain, and hoarseness or change in voice.[13] Thyroid cancers develop in the two main cells of the thyroid—follicular cells and parafollicular cells (C cells). For purposes of clinical management, thyroid cancer is identified as either differentiated or undifferentiated.[5,14] Figure 25.1 describes the subtypes of thyroid cancer.

Diagnosis is typically based on blood tests for abnormal levels of thyroid stimulating hormone (TSH) or calcitonin, thyroid ultrasounds, radioactive scans, and biopsies. Staging is based on primary tumor assessment, regional lymph node metastasis, and distant metastasis. Stages range from I to IV for all thyroid cancer types, except for anaplastic carcinoma, which is always stage IV.[14] See Chapter 1 for more information on staging.

Treatment

Surgery

This is frequently the therapy of choice. Often, a total or near-total thyroidectomy is indicated, though in low-risk cases, a lobectomy may be performed. In cases of metastases to lymph nodes, removal of lymph nodes and neck dissection is recommended. For anaplastic thyroid cancer, surgery is rarely indicated, due to advanced disease.[3,13] In all instances of total thyroidectomy, postoperative thyroid hormone replacement should be provided, sometimes at doses sufficient to suppress TSH.[2] Surgery can damage the recurrent laryngeal nerve, which may compromise swallowing function.[14]

Chemotherapy

Use of chemotherapy is rare in differentiated thyroid cancer (DTC), but emerging evidence does support the use of chemotherapy in the case of metastatic DTC that progresses despite radioactive iodine therapy, radiotherapy, and TSH-suppressive therapy. There are limited randomized controlled

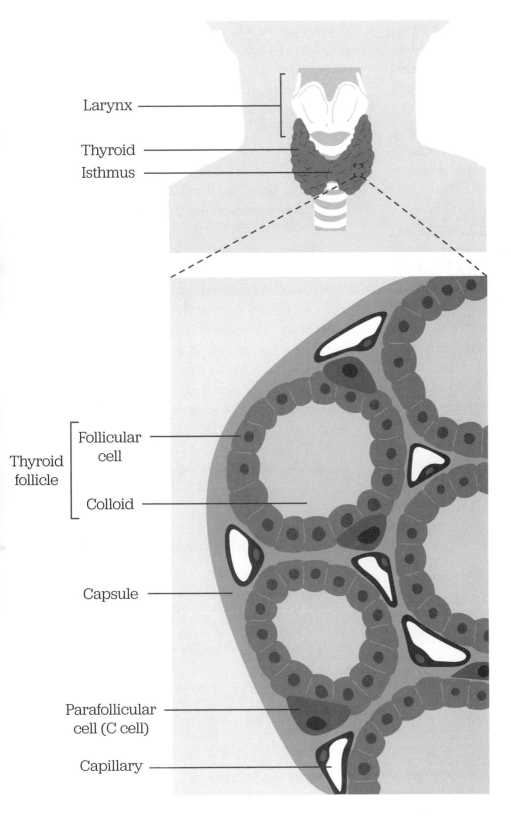

Larynx

Thyroid

Isthmus

Thyroid follicle
- Follicular cell
- Colloid

Capsule

Parafollicular cell (C cell)

Capillary

Anaplastic thyroid carcinoma

- Most undifferentiated type of thyroid cancer
- Originates in the follicular cells
- Very aggressive and usually fatal
- Least common type of thyroid cancer

Follicular thyroid carcinoma

- Differentiated
- Originates in follicular cells
- Generally good outcome
- More aggressive than papillary and can spread to other organs
- More likely to recur than papillary

Medullary thyroid carcinoma

- Less differentiated and somewhat aggressive
- Originates in the C cells
- More likely to spread to lymph nodes and other organs
- Releases high levels of calcitonin and carcinoembryonic antigen

Papillary thyroid carcinoma

- Differentiated
- Originates in follicular cells
- Slow growing
- Curable with early diagnosis
- Most common (~80% of cases) and best prognosis of all thyroid cancers

Figure 25.1
The thyroid gland and subtypes of thyroid cancer

trials examining chemotherapy treatments for medullary thyroid cancer, and available literature shows limited benefit.[15] Use of chemotherapy is also rare in anaplastic thyroid cancer, given the aggressive and fatal nature of that subtype but could be indicated based on the stage of the disease and surgical options.[16] Potential alternative options for treatment, including immunotherapy, vaccine-based therapies, and gene therapies, are being explored.[17,18]

Radiotherapy and Radioactive Iodine Therapy

In high-risk cases of DTC, radioactive iodine (RAI) therapy may be indicated postoperatively to treat persistent disease. RAI is concentrated by thyroid cancer cells and leads to apoptosis; since only thyroid cancer cells take up RAI, no other tissues are harmed. A nondestructive form of RAI can be used to detect residual or recurrent disease.[5] RAI is not used to treat medullary or anaplastic thyroid cancers. In cases of advanced medullary cancer and DTC in which further surgery or RAI is ineffective, radiotherapy could be considered. Radiotherapy also is used along with chemotherapy in combined-modality treatment for anaplastic cancer.[15,16]

Low-Iodine Diet

A low-iodine diet (sometimes abbreviated LID) is used in conjunction with RAI scans and therapy. The rationale is to deplete whole-body iodine stores before scans or therapy and thereby optimize RAI uptake in thyroid cells.[19] A urinary iodine concentration study to assess the patient's iodine status can be used to support initiating a low-iodine diet. In comparison with nonrestricted diets, iodine-restricted diets have been shown to reduce urinary iodine concentrations, with significantly lower concentrations seen in patients after 2 weeks, and 1 week being sufficient in areas where there are low levels of iodine in the soil and groundwater.[19,20] Some research shows that restricting

dietary iodine will increase tumor uptake of RAI, lengthen the half-life of RAI, and improve ablation rates.[19] It is not known whether a low-iodine diet improves long-term outcomes, and although the usual dietary goal is 50 mcg or less of iodine per day, the superiority of this intake level in comparison with less restrictive diets has not been adequately studied.[19,20] In general, research on low-iodine diets is hindered by limited numbers and by the retrospective nature of studies. Nonetheless, the American Thyroid Association management guidelines, which are endorsed by nine international professional organizations, recommend 1 to 2 weeks of adherence to a low-iodine diet before and during treatment with RAI remnant ablation (destruction of residual thyroid tissue), especially in patients with high iodine intakes.[21]

The variability in iodine content of foods, as well as the use of outdated and misinterpreted data, has led to inconsistencies in low-iodine diet guidelines published by various organizations.[22-25] See Box 25.2 for additional explanation. However, key features of most low-iodine diets include avoiding the following:

- iodized salt
- seafood and all sea products
- dairy products
- egg yolks
- erythrosine (FD&C Red No. 3)
- iodate dough conditioners
- chocolate
- any foods or supplements containing significant amounts of these products as ingredients

Guidelines for a Low-Iodine Diet

Patients should be advised to follow these general guidelines to help them implement and adhere to a low-iodine diet[22-25]:

Box 25.2
Explanation for Inconsistencies in Low-Iodine Diet Guidelines[9,26-31]

Confusion regarding low-iodine diets may be attributed to limited and inconsistent data about the iodine content of foods worldwide. Crop-growing conditions, food-production practices related to the use of iodized salt, and laws governing iodine fortification and food labeling vary throughout the world. Thus, guidelines for a low-iodine diet developed for one country may not be valid in another.

In the United States, the Food and Drug Administration (FDA) does not require Nutrition Facts labels to list iodine content, unless the food item is fortified with this nutrient. The amount of iodine in many common foods varies greatly, with one study showing the iodine content of bread ranging from 2.2 to 587.4 mcg per slice. This variability is attributed to inconsistent use of iodate conditioners. However, even the iodine content of less-processed foods, such as fresh produce, varies according to soil, fertilizer, and irrigation practices. This, in turn, affects the iodine content of meat and animal products, as produce may be used for animal feed. Use of iodine-based sanitizing solutions on dairy equipment also contributes to variable iodine content in dairy products, and the variability of iodine in saltwater affects the iodine content of seafood.

The iodine content of foods in the average US diet was examined as part of the FDA's 2008–2012 Total Diet Study. Results showed that dairy contributed a majority of iodine intake, comprising 49% of intake in adults. Grain products and "mixtures" contributed 17% each toward total daily iodine intake in adults. Data also showed high iodine content in eggs, meat, poultry, and fish. Though not examined in the Total Diet Study, iodized salt is recognized as a major dietary source of iodine. Although they are not required to do so, many salt manufacturers in the United States add iodine to table salt, leading to a product that contains approximately 300 mcg of iodine per tsp of salt.

- Check the ingredients on food package labels. Box 25.3 on pages 536 to 538 provides a detailed list of foods allowed and disallowed on a low-iodine diet based on current US data on the iodine content of foods.[31-34] Note that this list may not be appropriate for use outside the United States due to differences in iodine content of foods in other countries.

- Use only non-iodized salts.

- Though avoiding sea salt is often recommended due to presence of iodine in seawater, analysis of sea salt shows only trace levels of iodine.[35] Therefore, the evidence does not support the restriction of sea salt.

- Consult food manufacturers and associated brands to confirm that they use non-iodized salt in their US food production: Most processed or prepared foods made by large food manufacturers in the United States are made with non-iodized salt. If iodized or sea salt is used, it should be specified on the ingredient list. Review manufacturers' websites periodically for the most current information as processing techniques change over time. The most reliable foods for a low-iodine diet are fresh foods.

- Avoid eating out, as it may be impossible to determine the type of salt used for food preparation in restaurants.

- Avoid multivitamins that contain iodine and any supplements (including selenium or fish oil) made from sea-based products, such as oyster shells, kelp, or fish.

- Do not use iodine tablets for water purification.

- Avoid creams or lotions made from seaweed.

- Avoid topical products and antiseptics that contain iodine, such as povidone-iodine (Betadine and other brands).[24,35]

Box 25.3
Low-Iodine Diet[22-25,31-34]

Food category	Foods allowed	Foods *not allowed*
Milk and milk products	Possible milk substitutes: almond milk, rice milk, coconut milk, and hemp milk Nondairy cream substitutes	All milk, including whole, low-fat, and nonfat milk; buttermilk; and powdered milk Cream Lattes and cappuccinos Cream- and milk-based soups and sauces Yogurt and kefir Cheese, cottage cheese Ice cream, sherbet
Eggs	Egg whites, and egg substitutes made from egg whites	Whole eggs Egg yolks Foods made with whole eggs or egg yolks
Seafood	None	All fish, including canned tuna and sardines All shellfish, including lobster, crab, shrimp, and oysters Imitation crab meat Fish sauces, pastes, and spreads Sushi, nori, seaweed, or any sea vegetables, such as kelp and algae
Animal proteins	All fresh red meats, including beef, pork, lamb, and veal All fresh poultry, including turkey and chicken Wild or game meats, including venison and bison	Processed, canned, dried, salted, or cured meats Deli meat (salami, bologna, pastrami) Canned or processed poultry Bacon, sausage, and frankfurters
Nuts and seeds	Any unsalted nuts and seeds Nuts and seeds salted or roasted by large food producers Unsalted nut butters (including peanut, almond, and cashew)	Nuts and seeds salted or roasted by local or small producers Trail mixes that contain any chocolate, yogurt, or other ingredients that are not allowed
Fruits	All fresh, canned, dried, or frozen fruits, and fruit juices	Maraschino cherries containing erythrosine (FD&C Red No. 3) Fruit cocktails with maraschino cherries

(continued)

Oncology Nutrition *for* Clinical Practice

Box 25.3
Low-Iodine Diet[22-25,31-34] *(continued)*

Food category	Foods allowed	Foods *not allowed*
Vegetable proteins and soy	Protein powders made from wheat or nuts and allowed ingredients Meal-replacement bars made from wheat or nuts and allowed ingredients	Protein powders made from soy or whey Meal replacement bars and drinks made from soy or whey Veggie burgers and other imitation meat products[a] Soy milk[a] Tofu[a] Soybeans[a]
Vegetables	Most fresh, frozen, and canned vegetables, including potatoes, peas, lentils, squash, some beans, and corn	Nori, seaweed, or any sea vegetables, such as kelp and algae Cowpeas Navy, lima, kidney, and red beans Commercially prepared potatoes
Breads, grains, and cereals	Homemade breads prepared with allowed ingredients only Commercial breads, including tortillas, that do not contain iodate conditioners Pasta (white and wheat), noodles, rice, bulgur, couscous, oats, quinoa, polenta, cornmeal, and other grains Cold and hot cereals (without milk)	Breads containing iodate conditioners (ie, calcium iodate, potassium iodate) or other ingredients that are not allowed Any grain or cereal prepared with or containing ingredients that are not allowed
Baked goods	Homemade cakes, cookies, and fruit desserts prepared with allowed ingredients only	Cakes, muffins, cookies, or pastries prepared with ingredients that are not allowed
Snack foods	Commercially prepared plain crackers, pretzels, chips (potato and tortilla), and popcorn Fruit ices and popsicles Gelatin desserts Dark chocolate Most nuts and seeds	Snacks made with ingredients that are not allowed Milk chocolate and any chocolate products that contain milk Puddings or custards Cocoa or hot-chocolate mix *(continued)*

[a] US data on iodine content of these foods is lacking; therefore, guidelines are based on food composition data from other countries. It is also possible that soy foods may interfere with uptake of iodine by the thyroid, which would include radioactive iodine. See references 24 and 25. Therefore, it may be safest to avoid all soy-based foods (including tofu), unless following a vegetarian or vegan diet with limited protein sources.

Box 25.3
Low-Iodine Diet[22-25,31-34] *(continued)*

Food category	Foods allowed	Foods *not allowed*
Mixed dishes and soups	Homemade or canned soups, stews, and casseroles prepared with allowed ingredients only Hamburger or meatloaf prepared with allowed ingredients only	Lasagna, pizza, burritos, and other dishes made with cheese Hamburgers or meatloaf prepared with egg yolk or other ingredients that are not allowed
Condiments	Margarine Sugar and sugar substitutes Jelly Catsup and mustard made with non-iodized salt Gravy made without milk Oil and noncreamy salad dressings made with non-iodized salt Vinegar Mayonnaise, soy sauce, and butter in limited amounts (less than 2 Tbsp per day)	Blackstrap molasses Creamy or cream-based sauces and salad dressings Sour cream Fish sauce or anchovy paste
Beverages	Water, coffee, tea, carbonated beverages, and fruit juices and drinks Beer, wine, and other alcohols if permitted by physician	Milk or cream Any beverages containing erythrosine (FD&C Red No. 3) Any beverages containing ingredients that are not allowed
Miscellaneous	Non-iodized salt Fresh and dried herbs and spices	Iodized salt, including any seasoning salts or mixes that contain iodized salt Erythrosine (FD&C Red No. 3) Alginate, agar, carrageenan, and algae (check labels for these additives)

Although rare, it is possible that a low-iodine diet may be required for those dependent on enteral nutrition (EN) or parenteral nutrition (PN). In the United States, PN formulations and trace-element products do not contain iodine.[36] However, there is a recognized lack of commercial EN formulas suitable for a low-iodine diet. Therefore, a low-iodine EN formula should be specially prepared by pureeing food products that are acceptable for a low-iodine diet.[37,38] Avoid iodine-containing medications and antiseptics, which are the primary source of iodine in patients receiving total PN.[38]

Nutrition Problems and Interventions

Although the presenting symptoms of thyroid cancer do not typically include weight loss, and the energy, macronutrient, and micronutrient needs in patients with thyroid cancer are consistent with age and gender, thyroid cancer treatments (surgery, chemotherapy, radiation therapy, and RAI therapy) can result in a range of nutrition impact symptoms (NIS) that may compromise the patient's ability to eat. Registered dietitian nutritionists (RDNs) can identify NIS when conducting a nutrition assessment and provide appropriate education and counseling. See Chapter 11 for additional information on managing nutrition-related side effects of disease and treatment.

Side Effects Related to a Low-Iodine Diet

Few risks are associated with a low-iodine diet, given that the duration of diet is 1 to 2 weeks, though there are case reports of symptomatic hyponatremia while following an iodine-restricted diet. This is likely due to iatrogenic hypothyroidism (thyroid hormone withdrawal), thiazide diuretics, or to the unnecessary restriction of all, including non-iodized, salt.[3,20] Patient feedback has indicated that the diet is challenging, boring, unpalatable, "overwhelming while adapting to a new diagnosis," and difficult to understand.[39,40]

Adherence to a low-iodine diet may be influenced by culture and lifestyle. For example, researchers reported poor adherence among Korean patients due to the cultural prevalence of foods high in iodine, such as kimchi and seafood.[40] RDNs can augment adherence to iodine restriction by working within patients' cultural food preferences and providing individualized counseling to ensure diet adequacy.

Dysphagia

Patients with thyroid cancer may experience dysphagia (see Chapter 11 for management strategies). This usually occurs when the enlarged thyroid compresses on structures involved in swallowing.[41] Conventional management strategies include small, frequent feedings of moist food. A speech-language pathologist consult should be considered when there is concern for safe swallowing function.

Side Effects Related to Radioactive Iodine

The NIS of RAI therapy include transient nausea, dry mouth, change in taste, a low risk of late-onset damage of salivary glands, and dental caries. The RDN should educate and counsel patients receiving RAI on the low-iodine diet (see Box 25.3).

Summary

Although the survival rate for people with thyroid cancer is high, this disease is now recognized as one of the most frequently diagnosed cancers in the United States. Continued research is showing that diet plays a role in the risk for developing thyroid cancer. A low-iodine diet is a necessary component of therapy, as is the management of NIS resulting from treatment. It is essential that RDNs and other health practitioners be aware of the elements involved in the care and management of patients with thyroid cancer.

Sample PES Statements for Thyroid Cancer

Intake domain: Inadequate oral intake related to decreased ability to consume sufficient energy due to side effects of cancer therapy, as evidenced by esophagitis and intake of <75% of estimated needs in the past week.

Behavioral-environmental domain: Food and nutrition–related knowledge deficit related to no prior knowledge of low-iodine foods, as evidenced by the need to follow a low-iodine diet prior to radioactive iodine therapy.

Oncology Nutrition *for* Clinical Practice

References

1. National Cancer Institute. Cancer stat facts: thyroid cancer. Accessed April 16, 2020. https://seer.cancer.gov/statfacts/html/thyro.html

2. American Cancer Society. Thyroid Cancer Survival Rates, by Type and Stage. Accessed April 16, 2020. https://cancer.org/cancer/thyroid-cancer/about/key-statistics.html

3. Davies L, Welch HG. Current thyroid cancer trends in the United States. *JAMA Otolaryngol Head Neck Surg.* 2014;4(140):317-322.

4. Dal Maso L, Bosetti C, La Vecchia C, Franceschi S. Risk factors for thyroid cancer: an epidemiological review focused on nutritional factors. *Cancer Cause Control.* 2009. 20(1):75-86.

5. National Cancer Institute. What you need to know about thyroid cancer. 2012. Accessed April 16, 2020. www.thyca.org/download/document/282/NCI-TCbooklet.pdf

6. Han JM, Kim TY, Jeon MJ, et al. Obesity is a risk factor for thyroid cancer in a large, ultrasonographically screened population. *Eur J Endocrinol.* 2013;168(6):879.

7. Choi WJ, Kim J. Dietary factors and the risk of thyroid cancer: a review. *Clin Nutr Res.* 2014;3(2):75-88.

8. Ershow AG, Skeaff SA, Merkel JM, Pehrsson PA. Development of databases on iodine in foods and dietary supplements. *Nutrients.* 2018;10(1)pii:E100. doi:10.3390/nu10010100

9. Fuge R, Johnson CC. Iodine and human health, the role of environmental geochemistry and diet, a review. *Applied Geochemistry.* 2015;63:282-302.

10. Ward MH, Kilroy BA, Weyer PJ, Anderson KE, Folsom AR, Cerhan JR. Nitrate intake and the risk of thyroid cancer and thyroid disease. *Epidemiology.* 2010;21(3):389-395.

11. Kilroy BA, Zhang Y, Park Y, et al. Dietary nitrate and nitrite and the risk of thyroid cancer in the NIH-AARP diet and health study. *Int J Cancer.* 2011;129(1):160-172.

12. Michikawa T, Inoue M, Shimazu T, et al. Green tea and coffee consumption and its association with thyroid cancer risk: a population-based cohort study in Japan. *Cancer Causes Control.* 2011;22(7):985-993.

13. Randle RW, Balentine CJ, Leverson GE, et al. Trends in the presentation, treatment, and survival of patients with medullary thyroid cancer over the past 30 years. *Surgery.* 2017;161(1):137-146.

14. Zabrodsky M, Boucek J, Kastner J, Kuchar M, Chovanec M, Betka J. Immediate revision in patients with bilateral recurrent laryngeal nerve palsy after thyroid and parathyroid surgery. How worthy is it? *Acta Otorhinolaryngol Ital.* 2012;32(4):222-228.

15. Ball DW. Medullary thyroid cancer: monitoring and therapy. *Endocrinol Metab Clin North Am.* 2007;36(3):823-837,viii.

16. Smallridge RC, Ain KB, Asa AL, et al. American Thyroid Association guidelines for management of patients with anaplastic thyroid cancer. *Thyroid.* 2012;22(11):1104-1139.

17. Pudney D, Lau H, Ruether JD, Falck V. Clinical experience of the multimodality management of anaplastic thyroid cancer and literature review. *Thyroid.* 2007;17(12):1243-50.

18. Wu LS, Roman SA, Sosa JA. Medullary thyroid cancer: an update of new guidelines and recent developments. *Curr Opin Oncol.* 2011;23(1):22-27.

19. Sawka AM, Ibrahim-Zada I, Galacgac P, et al. Dietary iodine restriction in preparation for radioactive iodine treatment or scanning in well-differentiated thyroid cancer: a systematic review. *Thyroid.* 2010;20(10):1129-1138.

20. Li JH, He ZH, Bansal V, Hennessy JV. Low iodine diet in differentiated thyroid cancer: a review. *Clin Endocrinol (Oxf)*. 2016;84(1):3-12.

21. Haugen BR, Alexander EK, Bible KC, et al. 2015 American Thyroid Association Management guidelines for adult patients with thyroid nodules and differentiated thyroid cancer: The American Thyroid Association Guidelines Task Force on Thyroid Nodules and Differentiated Thyroid Cancer. *Thyroid*. 2016;26(1):1-133.

22. Thyroid Cancer Canada. Radioactive iodine treatment (RAI). Accessed April 16, 2020. https://thyroidcancercanada.org /en/treatments/radioactive-iodine -treatment

23. Thyroid Cancer Survivors' Association Inc. Radioactive iodine (RAI). Accessed April 16, 2020. http://thyca.org/pap-fol/rai

24. National Institutes of Health Clinical Center. Low-iodine diet: preparing to receive radioactive iodine. Accessed April 16, 2020. https://thyca.org/pap-fol /lowiodinediet

25. American Thyroid Association. Low Iodine Diet. Accessed April 16, 2020. www.thyroid.org/low -iodine-diet

26. Ju DL, Park YJ, Paik H-Y, Song Y-J. The impact of low adherence to the low-iodine Diet on the efficacy of the radioactive iodine ablation therapy. *Clin Nutr Res*. 2015; 4(4):267-271.

27. Trumbo PR. FDA regulations regarding iodine addition to foods and labeling of foods containing added iodine. *Am J Clin Nutr*. 2016;104 Suppl 3:864s-867s.

28. Pearce EN, Pino S, He X, Bazrafshan HR, Lee SL, Braverman LE. Sources of dietary iodine: bread, cows' milk, and infant formula in the boston area. *J Clin Endocrinol Metab*. 2004;89(7):3421-3424.

29. Pennington JAT, Schoen SA, Salmon GD, Young B, Johnson RD, Marts RW. Composition of core foods of the us food supply, 1982-1991: iii. Copper, manganese, selenium, and iodine. *J Food Compos Anal*. 1995;8(2):171-217.

30. Abt E, Spungen J, Pouillet R, Gamalo-Siebers M, Wirtz M. Update on dietary intake of perchlorate and iodine from U.S. Food and Drug Administration's Total Diet Study: 2008-2012. *J Expo Sci Environ Epidemiol*. 2018;28(1):21-30.

31. Office of Dietary Supplements. Iodine: fact sheet for health professionals. Accessed April 16, 2020. https://ods .od.nih.gov/factsheets/Iodine -HealthProfessional

32. US Food and Drug Administration. Total Diet Study Elements Results summary statistics—Market Baskets 2006 through 2013. Accessed April 16, 2020. www.fda.gov/media/77948 /download

33. USDA Agricultural Research Service. USDA, FDA and ODS-NIH Database for the Iodine Content of Common Foods Release 1.0, 2020. Accessed February 25, 2021. www.ars.usda.gov/northeast -area/beltsville-md-bhnrc /beltsville-human-nutrition -research-center/methods-and -application-of-food-composition -laboratory/mafcl-site-pages /iodine/

34. Haldimann M, Alt A, Blanc A, Blondeau K. Iodine content of food groups. *J Food Compos Anal.* 2005;18(6):461-471.

35. Preedy VR, Burrow GN, Watson RR. *Comprehensive Handbook of Iodine: Nutritional, Biochemical, Pathological and Therapeutic Aspects.* Elsevier Academic Press/Elsevier; 2009.

36. Vanek VW, Borum P, Buchman A, et al. A.S.P.E.N. position paper: recommendations for changes in commercially available parenteral multivitamin and multi-trace element products. *Nutr Clin Pract.* 2012;27(4): 440-491.

37. Ain KB, Dewitt PA, Gardner TG, Berryman SW. Low-iodine tube-feeding diet for iodine-131 scanning and therapy. *Clin Nucl Med.* 1994;19(6): 504-507.

38. Zimmermann MB, Crill CM. Iodine in enteral and parenteral nutrition. *J Clin Endocrinol Metab.* 2010;24(1):143-158.

39. Morris LF, Wilder Ms, Waxman AD, Braunstein GD. Reevaluation of the impact of a stringent low-iodine diet on ablation rates in radioiodine treatment of thyroid carcinoma. *Thyroid.* 2001;11(8):749-755.

40. Lee KJ, Chang SO, Jung KY. Experiences with a low-iodine diet: A qualitative study of patients with thyroid cancer receiving radioactive iodine therapy. *Eur J Oncol Nurs.* 2016;23:43-50.

41. Lindgren S, Janzon L. Prevalence of swallowing complaints and clinical findings among 50-79-year-old men and women in an urban population. *Dysphagia.* 1991;6(4):187-192.

Chapter 26

Nutrition Management of Oncology Patients in Palliative and Hospice Settings

Kelay E. Trentham, MS, RDN, CSO, FAND

Alison Donato, RDN, CSO, CD

Elizabeth A. Huddleston, MS, RDN

Palliative care and hospice are forms of specialized care that are distinct from curative care. Simply defined, to palliate is to lessen or ease symptoms of disease independently of curative efforts.[1] The World Health Organization defines palliative care as "an approach that improves quality of life of patients and their families facing [problems] associated with life-threatening illness, through the prevention and relief of suffering by means of early identification and impeccable assessment and treatment of pain and other problems, physical, psychosocial and spiritual."[2]

Additionally, palliative care activities are characterized as those which, through a team approach, affirm life, incorporate psychological and spiritual aspects of care, provide a support system such that patients may actively live until death, help families cope with a loved one's illness and their grief, enhance quality of life (QOL), and are based on patient needs and not prognosis. Palliative care for oncology patients is as essential to patient care as curative therapy and may be initiated at the time of diagnosis, which may be years before the patient is ready for hospice. Provision of palliative care is appropriate in all care settings, including hospitals, extended-care facilities, home health care, assisted-living facilities, and outpatient clinics, and in the home.[3]

The Hospice Foundation of America defines hospice as "medical care to help someone with a terminal illness live as well as possible for as long as possible, increasing QOL." Hospice care is intended to address symptom management, coordinate care among disciplines, facilitate communication and decision making, clarify goals of care, and attend to QOL.[4] In addition, bereavement and counseling services are offered to families before and for up to 1 year after a patient's death.[5] Hospice care also may be provided in a variety of settings, including the patient's home, hospitals, skilled nursing facilities, and freestanding hospice-care facilities. In the

United States, patients must have a life expectancy of 6 months or less for hospice to be covered by most insurance plans, including Medicare and Medicaid.[6] An estimated 1.49 million Medicare beneficiaries received hospice services in 2017, and 30% had a cancer diagnosis.[5]

Philosophies of Hospice and Palliative Care

There are many similarities in the philosophies of hospice and palliative care. Both seek to palliate symptoms, improve QOL, and incorporate physical, psychological, spiritual, and emotional care for both patients and their families. As symptom palliation is a primary goal of hospice, hospice and palliative care services have often been linked within health care systems.[7] In 2016, the American Society of Clinical Oncology issued a clinical practice guideline update recommending a referral to palliative care services within 8 weeks of an advanced cancer diagnosis and providing palliative services along with standard oncology care.[8] More than half of cancer patients who die do not receive palliative or hospice care,[9] despite early palliative care being associated with less intensive medical care, improved quality outcomes, and cost savings at the end of life for patients with terminal cancer.[10-12] Patients who communicate end-of-life wishes with their physicians are more likely to have care consistent with their desires.[9]

Historically, nourishment has been synonymous with comfort, well-being, and even pleasure. Difficulty eating and malnutrition are significant issues for patients with advanced cancer. Nutrition impact symptoms and the nutritional decline experienced by oncology patients have a negative impact on QOL.[13-15] Many medical nutrition therapy (MNT) interventions that address these issues, such as those designed to manage digestive and oral symptoms in order to improve the enjoyment and tolerance of food intake, are indeed palliative in nature. Depending on the clinical circumstances, enteral and parenteral nutrition may also be considered palliative therapies, though they may be deemed aggressive or contraindicated interventions for patients near the end of life. The registered dietitian nutritionist (RDN) is an integral part of the care team, providing expertise on appropriate nutrition care in palliative and hospice settings. In these settings, the RDN's role is to provide MNT interventions to improve symptom management; educate patients, family members, and the medical team on evidence-based nutrition interventions; and assist with decision-making regarding the use of artificial nutrition and hydration.

Nutrition Impact Symptoms and Quality of Life

Patients with advanced cancer experience a variety of symptoms that affect their nutritional status and QOL. Cancer-induced malnutrition can impair mental and physical health, reduce performance status, and diminish social well-being.[15-17] A study of patients with a variety of cancers (head and neck, esophageal, stomach, and colorectal) found that QOL function scores were significantly lower in patients with weight loss and decreased dietary intake.[13] A large study of patients with oral cancer found that patients who were able to maintain or gain weight had significantly better QOL than those who lost weight.[18] For hospice patients with advanced cancer, nutrition screening scores significantly correlate with QOL, functional well-being, and social-spiritual well-being scores.[16] Malnourished patients with advanced colorectal cancer, as determined by the subjective global assessment (SGA), have diminished physical, role, and cognitive functionality as well as diminished QOL.[19] These same patients also experience more fatigue and appetite loss.

Estimates of the prevalence of malnutrition in patients with advanced cancer vary depending on setting, screening methods used, diagnosis, and severity of disease. The incidence of malnutrition in patients with stage III and IV cancers is significantly greater than in those with stage I or II disease.[20,21] Malnutrition prevalence among patients with advanced cancer ranges from 31% to 69% among hospitalized patients and from 13% to 63% among nonhospitalized patients, with up to 63% being severely malnourished.[16,22-26] Weight loss and malnutrition in patients with advanced disease most commonly occur in those with gastrointestinal, larynx, pancreatic, gynecological, lung, hematological, and prostate cancers.[21,25,27]

In addition to disease processes, factors that affect symptom burden, malnutrition, and QOL include physiologic and psychosocial conditions, treatment modality, and medications.[16] In patients undergoing cancer treatment, typical physiologic symptoms with nutritional impact include oral issues (eg, dysgeusia and parageusia, odynophagia, sore mouth, xerostomia), gastrointestinal issues (eg, nausea, constipation, diarrhea), and anorexia and pain.[28] In a study of patients newly starting chemotherapy, 26% of those screened for palliative care needs were referred to palliative care services for appetite loss, nausea, and constipation.[29] Between 31% and 53% of patients with advanced cancer experience nausea, constipation, xerostomia, weight loss, and anorexia, while 11% to 23%

experience diarrhea, dysphagia, vomiting, sore mouth, dysgeusia, and early satiety.[30] A small study of patients with advanced cancer in hospice care found that 93% had taste and smell abnormalities; taste abnormalities were more prevalent and had a greater impact on food enjoyment and QOL.[31] Symptom prevalence rates from studies of patients with advanced cancer, patients receiving palliative treatment, and medical oncology patients at 1 year of treatment are shown in Table 26.1. In the studies of advanced cancer, prevalent symptoms among patients included appetite loss, constipation, early satiety, weight loss, and xerostomia.[14,28,32-34]

Other causes of distress, including pain and functional and psychosocial factors, also may significantly influence nutritional status, nutritional intake, and QOL.[15,17] The prevalence of pain in patients with advanced cancer varies widely, with 33% of ambulatory patients with newly diagnosed stage IV cancer and 82% of hospitalized patients reporting some degree of pain.[34,35] Pain and its treatment with opioids can result in decreased appetite,

Table 26.1
Prevalence of Specific Nutrition-Related Symptoms in Patients With Cancer[14,28,32-34]

Symptom	Study Population Characteristics[a]				
	Advanced cancer, inpatients and outpatients[32] (n=181)	Palliative treatment, outpatients[14] (n=571)	Advanced cancer (72% of patients), inpatients[33] (n=100)	After 12 months of treatment, outpatients[28] (n=159)	Advanced cancer (82% of patients), inpatients[34] (n=45)
Appetite loss	61%	18%	69%	16%	67%
Constipation	40%	15%	44%	14%	40%
Diarrhea	10%	6%	29%	22%	7%
Dysgeusia	33%	-	44%	13%	11%
Dysphagia	13%	-	15%	6%	7%
Early satiety	50%	-	60%	-	31%
Nausea	28%	14%	65%	21%	22%
Sore mouth	13%	-	22%	5%	13%
Vomiting	12%	6%	32%	4%	18%
Weight loss	56%	-	57%	-	49%
Xerostomia	66%	28%	59%	34%	27%

[a] All percentages are rounded to the nearest whole number.

constipation, and distress.[36,37] Common psychosocial and functional symptoms include anxiety or nervousness, depressed mood, and confusion.[30,32,38] Fatigue, also termed tiredness or weakness, is seen in 45% to 96% of patients with advanced cancer[14,38] and is associated with weight loss, anorexia, and poor performance status.[30]

Symptom management strategies relevant in hospice and palliative care settings include the following:

- For appetite loss, help families understand that it is a normal condition at the end of life, and explain that appetite stimulants only increase the burden of taking medication.

- For constipation, which can cause considerable distress to patients, review the recommendations for constipation management in Chapter 11.

- For oral issues, such as dry mouth, dysgeusia, thrush, and mouth sores, in addition to following previously stated management strategies, ensure that good oral hygiene is provided, as the patient may require assistance with this care.

- For dysphagia, although a swallowing evaluation may be considered an aggressive measure, it may be useful in establishing strategies for safe swallowing and necessary changes in diet consistency.

- For nausea, compounded antiemetics that are administered topically may be prescribed for use when oral medication administration is difficult.

- For weight loss, understand that weighing the patient may result in distress; if anthropometrics are required to monitor nutritional decline, consider more indirect measures, such as arm circumference measurements.

Nutritional Screening and Assessment for Palliative and Hospice Care

Patients in all settings who receive palliative and hospice care should be screened to determine the need for nutrition intervention. The patient-generated subjective global assessment (PG-SGA) is a modified version of the SGA that has been validated for use in the oncology population.[39] The PG-SGA has long been considered a standard for the nutrition screening of cancer patients.[40-42] Several other screening tools, discussed in Chapter 4, have been found to be appropriate for oncology patients and are reviewed in the Evidence Analysis Library of the Academy of Nutrition and Dietetics and reported in a paper by Thompson and colleagues.[43] However, because of the unique needs of patients with advanced cancer, specific screening tools, in addition to the SGA and PG-SGA, have been evaluated for use with this population. These include the Malnutrition Universal Screening Tool (MUST), the Mini Nutritional Assessment (MNA), and a modified version of Nutrition Risk Screening (NRS 2002).[25,26,44,45] Studies comparing the predictive value of the SGA and PG-SGA to anthropometric indicators in patients with advanced cancer found that these tools correlate well with measurements of mid-upper arm circumference, mid upper arm muscle circumference, triceps skinfold, and weight loss.[23,44] The MNA has been found to correlate with baseline history of weight loss but not weight change.[26] Body mass index (BMI) has limited usefulness as an indicator of nutritional status in patients with advanced cancer. In one study, although BMI was correlated with the SGA, malnutrition was not established until BMI values dropped below 20.[44] In other studies, there was no consistent correlation between BMI and subjective screening methods, and patients with BMIs indicative of obesity were screened as malnourished or at risk of malnutrition.[23,26]

Malnutrition is more likely to occur in patients with poorer performance status[46] and is thought to significantly contribute to functional decline.[47] In one cross-sectional study, patients in a home-care hospice setting who were found to have poor nutritional status also scored lower for psychophysiological, functional, and social-spiritual well-being, and for QOL.[16] In addition to indicating nutritional status, PG-SGA scores directly predicted survival of terminal cancer patients in a palliative care center.[48] The French Nutrition Oncology Study Group suggested that nutritional status be used to define cancer patients' clinical condition, as it may more accurately reflect tolerance of treatment than performance status.[47] Thus, functional and QOL assessments performed in palliative- and hospice-care settings may serve as additional tools for identifying patients who would benefit from nutritional intervention.

Goals

Nutrition care and goals for patients under palliative care differ depending on whether palliative care is initiated early in the treatment process or later when treatment options are limited or cure is no longer a goal. Thus, nutrition goals in early palliative care may be as aggressive as early cancer treatment, with a focus on improving treatment outcome, body composition, and physical function, as well as symptom palliation. As the focus of care shifts from curative treatment to end-of-life or hospice care, nutrition goals appropriately become less aggressive and are focused primarily on comfort.

An accurate and unbiased patient assessment may be challenging but is essential. Studies have shown poor agreement between patients receiving palliative care and their providers regarding symptoms and QOL.[49,50] Specifically, anorexia, constipation, nausea, vomiting, and diarrhea have been underestimated by providers.[50] Further, physician assessments have failed to acknowledge three of the most distressing symptoms that patients with advanced cancer face at the end of life: fatigue, cachexia, and anorexia.[51] Differences in symptom estimates were influenced by such factors as cancer diagnosis and previous history of drug abuse.[50] Assessment of malnutrition and other nutrition-related issues by hospice physicians has been found to be inconsistent, and patients may experience inadequate identification and treatment of cancer cachexia due to incomplete provider knowledge of malnutrition characteristics.[52] In a qualitative exploration of patients' experience with cancer cachexia, a dominant theme was "lack of response from health care professionals" regarding their weight loss.[53] Patients wanted their weight loss acknowledged, desired information about its cause, and were interested in interventions to manage weight change. A similar study sought to evaluate emotional distress experienced by family members and the need for improved communication when terminally ill cancer patients are no longer able to take oral nourishment. Of those who experienced a loved one's becoming unable to take daily oral nourishment, 71% reported being distressed or very distressed, and 46% indicated the need for at least some improvement in professional practice.[54] Clearly, assessing the nutritional needs and goals of patients and families is of primary importance in order to provide high-quality care for patients receiving palliative or hospice care in the advanced stages of disease. Nutrition assessment in hospice and palliative-care settings should include evaluation of end-of-life nutrition-related symptoms, the patient's nutrition goals, and patient and caregiver understandings of palliative nutrition interventions. Figure 26.1 on pages 550 to 552 shows an example of an initial nutrition assessment form for use in the hospice setting that includes these elements and utilizes the Nutrition Care Process and terminology.

Patient name: _____ Date of assessment: _____ Medical record #: _____

DOB: _____ Visit location: *Home   LTCF   Other:* _____

Problem or need: _____

Sources of food and preparation ability or needs: _____

Chewing and swallowing abilities: _____

_____

Current daily intake or observation of eating: _____

_____

Patient and caregiver stated goals for nutrition: _____

_____

Problem: Nutrition Diagnosis

Nutrition Intake

☐ NI-1.2 Inadequate energy intake

☐ NI-1.4 Predicted suboptimal energy intake

☐ NI-1.5 Predicted excessive energy intake

☐ NI-2.1 Inadequate oral intake

☐ NI-2.3 Inadequate enteral nutrition infusion

☐ NI-3.1 Inadequate fluid intake

☐ NI-5.2 Inadequate protein-energy intake

☐ NI-5.11.1 Predicted inadequate nutrient intake (specify):

_____

☐ NI-5.11.2 Predicted excessive nutrient intake (specify):

_____

☐ Other: _____

Clinical Signs

☐ NC-1.1 Swallowing difficulty

☐ NC-1.2 Biting or chewing difficulty

☐ NC-1.4 Altered GI function

☐ NC-2.1 Impaired nutrient utilization

☐ NC-2.3 Food-medication interaction (specify):

_____

☐ NC-3.1 Underweight

☐ NC-3.2 Unintended weight loss

☐ NC-3.4 Unintended weight gain

☐ Other: _____

Behavioral/Environmental

☐ NB-1.1 Food- and nutrition-related knowledge deficit
Patient: ____   Caregiver: ____
Family: _____   LTCF: _____

☐ NB-1.2 Unsupported beliefs/attitudes about food- or nutrition-related topics

☐ NB-1.5 Disordered eating pattern

☐ NB-2.4 Impaired ability to prepare foods/meals

☐ NB-2.5 Poor nutrition QOL

☐ NB-2.6 Self-feeding difficulty

☐ NB-3.1 Intake of unsafe food

☐ NB-3.2 Limited access to food

☐ NB-3.3 Limited access to nutrition related supplies

☐ NB-3.4 Limited access to potable water

☐ Other: _____

(continued)

Figure 26.1
Sample hospice initial nutrition assessment

DOB = date of birth

LTCF = long-term care facility

GI = gastronintestinal

QOL = quality of life;

Etiology of Problem

- ☐ Weight loss of >10% in 6 mo, >5% in 1 month
  Usual weight: _____ Current weight: _____ Weight history: _____

- ☐ Previous diets or MNT
- ☐ Poor dentition: _____
- ☐ Early satiety
- ☐ Pancreatic insufficiency
- ☐ Cultural practices that relate to intake: _____
  _____
- ☐ Consistency-altered diet order

- ☐ Neurologic deficit
- ☐ Extreme weakness
- ☐ Pain with eating
- ☐ Malabsorption
- ☐ Constipation, diarrhea
- ☐ Economic constraints
- ☐ Patient entered service with enteral feeding in place
- ☐ Insufficient appetite

- ☐ Belching, gas
- ☐ Disease process: _____
- ☐ Caregiver with knowledge deficit for end-of-life nutrition care
- ☐ Advancing dementia
- ☐ Other: _____
  _____

Signs and Symptoms

- ☐ Weight loss
- ☐ Weight gain
- ☐ Poor skin turgor
- ☐ Open wounds
- ☐ Aspiration
- ☐ BMI <18.5
- ☐ Obvious muscle wasting
- ☐ Growth failure
- ☐ Emesis
- ☐ Unable to recognize food as sustenance

- ☐ Choking on foods, liquids, saliva
- ☐ Altered taste, smell
- ☐ Nutrient intake analysis (3-day food record)
- ☐ Declining ability to self-feed
- ☐ Food safety or sanitation issues
- ☐ Unrealistic expectations
  - ☐ Patient
  - ☐ Caregiver
  - ☐ Family

- ☐ Enteral feeding
  Product: _____
  Rate: _____
  kcals: _____
  Protein: _____
  Additional fluids:
  _____
- ☐ Other:
  _____
  _____

Nutrition Goals

- ☐ Comfort eating/feeding
- ☐ Pleasure eating/feeding
- ☐ Relief of symptoms
  - ☐ Hunger
  - ☐ Thirst
  - ☐ Mouth care

- ☐ MNT for comfort
  - ☐ Low salt for fluid retention
  - ☐ Management of diabetes

- ☐ Wound healing as comfort feeding allows
- ☐ Other:
  _____
  _____

(continued)

MNT = medical nutrition therapy

BMI = body mass index

Interventions

- ☐ Educate patient and caregiver on how to do a 3-day food record for analysis.
- ☐ Educate patient and caregiver on maximizing foods and liquids in the best interest of patient.
- ☐ Educate patient, caregiver, and family on the following principles of comfort feeding:
    - ☐ Offer appropriate and favorite foods.
    - ☐ Assist without force.
    - ☐ Recognize signs of satiety or refusal.
- ☐ Educate patient, caregiver, and family on quality of life at end of life.
- ☐ Educate patient, caregiver, and family on safe feeding techniques:
    - ☐ Manipulated consistency of foods and liquids
    - ☐ Feeding rate and swallow techniques
- ☐ Access community resources for patient.
- ☐ Contact long-term care facility dietary manager as an advocate for hospice care.
- ☐ Educate patient and designated power of attorney of all options concerning nutrition care.
- ☐ Educate patient and caregiver on sanitary food preparation and provision.
- ☐ Recommend adjustments of enteral feeding procedures.
- ☐ Recommend discontinuation of nutrition supplements for patient comfort.
- ☐ Other: _____
  _____
  _____

Follow-Up

_____
_____
_____
_____
_____
_____
_____

Figure 26.1
Sample hospice initial nutrition assessment

Artificial Nutrition and Hydration

Patients, caregivers, and health care professionals often consider the provision of food and fluids to be basic care at the end of life. The use of artificial nutrition and hydration (ANH) for this purpose has long been a complex and controversial topic. Factors that may influence the desire of patients and caregivers to employ ANH at the end of life include cultural and religious practices, a perceived benefit versus burden, the belief that ANH may prolong life or reduce suffering, and the attitudes or advice of health care providers. For some patients, factors such as financial cost, insurance coverage, and increased care needs play a large role in the decision. For others, religion or culture may play the greatest role in decision-making. Religious and cultural traditions vary in regard to the use of ANH at the end of life; some traditions hold that ANH is obligatory, whereas others consider withholding or withdrawing it acceptable.[55-57] Given the prevailing principle of autonomy in the American bioethics culture as well as the increasing diversity of our population, the views of patients and families regarding ANH use at the end of life may conflict with those of health care providers.[58] For those less compelled by religious or cultural factors, lack of knowledge about all nutrition care options during the dying process may lead to unrealistic expectations of medical interventions. An important role for RDNs is to provide objective and evidence-based education for patients, families, and health care providers on the benefits and burdens of ANH at the end of life.

Artificial Nutrition

Between 3% and 53% of patients with end-stage cancer receive artificial nutrition (AN) in the last week of life.[59] AN is most commonly used when bowel obstruction precludes tolerance of an oral diet and most commonly in patients with ovarian cancer.[60] Perceived benefits of AN include its potential ability to prolong life, improve QOL, reduce suffering, maintain weight or body composition, and improve energy levels.[61] In studies, early enteral nutrition decreased weight loss for patients with advanced head and neck cancer who were undergoing concurrent chemoradiation; however, its long-term use resulted in poorer performance status and QOL.[62,63] Home use of parenteral nutrition (PN) in patients with advanced cancer, in contrast with patients without cancer, has been found to positively affect QOL. The benefits of home PN include decreased weight loss and GI symptoms; improved QOL, emotional functioning, energy, activity, performance status, and nutritional status; and increased survival time.[64-70] In patients with intestinal obstruction or limited GI function, PN increased survival time by 4 weeks[67] and improved QOL, performance status, and nutritional status when used for 1 to 3 months.[69] However, PN's effect on survival time was diminished in those patients receiving concurrent chemotherapy.[67] Both performance status and albumin level predict survival in patients with advanced cancer who are using PN,[60,71] and ANH was found to have no influence on survival in an inpatient hospital or palliative care unit when it was initiated in those with end-stage disease.[72] Negative effects of PN, as perceived by patients and caregivers, include sleep interference and restrictions on family activities and social contacts.[64] In summary, the advantage of using AN in the advanced-cancer population varies depending on the diagnosis, whether treatment continues, the prognosis, patient performance scores, and patient and family perceptions. Box 26.1 on pages 554 to 555 summarizes the various published recommendations for the use of AN in this stage of care.

Artificial Hydration

As with AN, a variety of factors influence the views of patients, caregivers, and health care providers

Box 26.1

Guidelines for the Use of Artificial Nutrition in Patients With Advanced Cancer[73-78]

Issuing organization (year of publication) and guideline	Description of use	Summary of recommendations
French National Federation of Cancer Centers (2001)[73] EN (enteral nutrition) and PN (parenteral nutrition) as palliative or terminal nutrition in adults with progressive cancer	EN for palliative care in head and neck cancer	EN may slow nutritional deficiency, prevent dehydration, and improve quality of life (QOL).
	EN for terminal-stage cancer	Gastrostomy is not recommended due to risk of complications.
	PN for malignant bowel obstruction, other food intolerances	PN may slow nutritional deficiency, prevent dehydration, and improve QOL.
	Karnofsky performance status score ≤50 or Eastern Cooperative Oncology Group (ECOG) Performance Status >2	Use of PN is not justified.
Capital Health Home Parenteral Nutrition Program Edmonton (2005)[74] PN for advanced cancer	For when EN is not feasible; intestinal obstruction, short bowel syndrome, malabsorption	Trial of PN should be offered if all of the following criteria are met: ■ death is expected from starvation or malnutrition before disease progression; ■ expected survival time is months and PN will last at least 6 weeks; ■ the patient has a high QOL; ■ the patient has adequate functional status and a home environment supportive of home PN, as determined by the following: ■ problems are manageable at home or with outpatient services; ■ the patient's Karnovsky score is >50; ■ a caregiver is available to assist; ■ clinical and laboratory follow-up are easily accessed; ■ the patient or caregiver is cognitively and psychologically capable of home administration; ■ the home environment is clean, safe, and free of hazards.

(continued)

Box 26.1

Guidelines for the Use of Artificial Nutrition in Patients With Advanced Cancer[73-78] (continued)

Issuing organization (year of publication) and guideline	Description of use	Summary of recommendations
American Society for Parenteral and Enteral Nutrition (2009)[75] EN and PN for adults during anticancer treatment and hematopoietic cell transplantation (HCT)	During palliative care	Use of artificial nutrition is rarely indicated.
German Association for Nutritional Medicine working group for developing guidelines for parenteral nutrition (2009)[76] PN in nonsurgical oncology	For incurable patients with severely impaired intestinal absorption	PN should be initiated if all of the following criteria are met: ■ EN is inadequate to maintain nutritional status; ■ the expected survival time is >4 weeks; ■ PN is expected to stabilize or improve QOL; ■ the patient desires PN for nutrition support.
European Society for Clinical Nutrition and Metabolism (2017)[77] EN and PN for advanced cancer	For patients with advanced cancer who are unable to eat	PN or EN should be offered if all of the following criteria are met: ■ expected survival time is at least several months; ■ the patient has a low tumor burden and no inflammatory response; ■ artificial nutrition and hydration is desired by the patient.
Spanish Society of Medical Oncology (2018)[78] EN and PN for advanced cancer in adults receiving no anticancer treatment	For patients with terminal-stage cancer	Artificial nutrition is unlikely to provide any benefit for most patients.

on the use of artificial hydration (AH) during palliative and end-of-life care. The provision of fluids is often perceived as meeting a basic human need.[79] Patients and families commonly believe that AH will improve quality and length of life, reduce discomfort, and promote a sense of well-being,[60,80] yet beliefs about the use of AH and AN vary globally. In Japan, 38% to 43% of community members believe that AH and AN should continue until death, while 52% to 62% would want AH for the purpose of prolonging life.[60] In Switzerland, 78% of patients with cancer desire AH.[81]

Views of health care providers on including AH in end-of-life care vary considerably; 22% to 100% of health care providers recommend using AH, while up to 75% recommend against it.[60] Persons influencing their support for AH at the end of life include attending physicians or superiors (45%) and patients (38%). Family members deciding on AH for patients elected to provide AH more often (52%) than patients themselves (40%) and reported more confidence in their decision.[82]

Terminal dehydration is thought to cause or contribute to symptoms of confusion, opioid toxicity, constipation, dry mouth, and thirst.[81] Researchers argue that provision of hydration would assist in preventing or relieving these problems while allowing providers a means to maintain the patient relationship and continue attempts to improve QOL.[79] In contrast, other research shows that AH may cause pain, is intrusive, and may increase symptoms such as vomiting, ascites, edema, diarrhea, and pulmonary congestion.[79,83] Studies of the use of AH at the end of life have been inconsistent and have found variable results regarding symptom improvement. Negative aspects of the use of AH at the end of life include that it creates a barrier between patient and family; promotes false hope or denial of the terminal nature of disease; prolongs the dying process; may increase urine output, edema, and ascites; increases the risk of infection; and prevents the production of ketones and other metabolic by-products of dehydration, which can act as natural anesthetics and reduce suffering.[81,84]

When palliative care accompanies chemotherapy, or radiation therapy, addressing hydration needs is crucial. These treatments can cause a variety of side effects that may lead to dehydration and subsequently affect patients' overall well-being. Nausea, vomiting, dysgeusia, diarrhea, dysphagia, and the presence of an ostomy can increase the risk for dehydration. Certain chemotherapies are nephrotoxic, and, therefore, adequate hydration is imperative in order for patients to continue receiving treatment.[85] In addition to morbidity, dehydration increases financial costs due to the unplanned clinic and emergency room visits.[85] For the management of dehydration, palliation allows patients to continue treatment and alleviates symptoms. When the focus of care shifts to comfort, treatment of dehydration should be focused solely on palliation of symptoms.

Decision for Use of Artificial Nutrition or Hydration

Whether or not to use ANH is a complex topic in the setting of palliative and hospice care. Its use may evoke a sense of hope and comfort for patients and caregivers. Health care providers may be hesitant to recommend ANH due to concerns about potential complications. Differing views among patients and their families and health care providers can lead to challenging discussions and the perception of ethical dilemmas regarding use of ANH in end-of-life care. The Academy of Nutrition and Dietetics position and practice paper, "Ethical and Legal Issues in Feeding and Hydration," addresses many of the ethical issues surrounding end-of-life nutrition and hydration.[86] Recommendations for the use of ANH should be individualized to each patient, carefully taking into account the patient's disease and current physical condition, symptoms, care setting, religious and cultural preferences, and the benefit vs burden of the treatment modality. Jonsen and colleagues' *Clinical Ethics: A Practical Approach to Ethical Decisions in Clinical Medicine* is an excellent resource to help guide these discussions.[87] Additional resources are listed in Box 26.2.

Box 26.2
Additional Resources Related to Palliative and Hospice Care

www.nhpco.org/patients-and-caregivers/resources

www.caregiver.org/advanced-illness-feeding-tubes-and-ventilators

www.americanhospice.org/caregiving/artificial-nutrition-and-hydration-at-the-end-of-life-beneficial-or-harmful

www.nia.nih.gov/health/advance-care-planning-healthcare-directives

---

Summary

Palliative care, though once considered synonymous with hospice care, is emerging as a distinct care process for persons with life-threatening illnesses, such as cancer. Patients with advanced cancer often have a significant symptom burden that affects well-being and QOL. Palliative care services are frequently being initiated soon after cancer diagnosis and concurrently with curative treatment to assist patients with maintaining an optimum QOL. As the focus of care shifts from curative intent to the provision of comfort at the end of life, palliative care continues as hospice care. Throughout the continuum of care, RDNs provide MNT that aims to manage symptoms and improve QOL. As part of the palliative and hospice care teams, the RDN can be instrumental in educating patients, caregivers, and health care providers, and in facilitating discussions about nutrition care options, including the use of ANH.

References

1. *Merriam-Webster*. Palliate. Accessed May 23, 2019. www .merriam-webster.com/dictionary /palliate

2. WHO definition of palliative care. World Health Organization website. Accessed May 23, 2019. www.who.int/cancer/palliative /definition/en

3. National Consensus Project for Quality Palliative Care. *Clinical Practice Guidelines for Quality Palliative Care*. 4th ed. National Coalition for Hospice and Palliative Care; 2018. Accessed May 23, 2019. www. nationalcoalitionhpc.org/ncp

4. What is hospice? Hospice Foundation of America website. Accessed May 23, 2019. https:// hospicefoundation.org/Hospice -Care/Hospice-Services

5. National Hospice and Palliative Care Organization. NHPCO Facts and Figures: 2018 Edition. Revised July 2, 2019. Accessed April 25, 2020. www.nhpco.org /wp-content/uploads/2019/07 /2018_NHPCO_Facts_Figures.pdf

6. National Cancer Institute. Advanced Cancer. Choices for care when treatment may not be an option—hospice care. Accessed May 23, 2019. www.cancer.gov/about-cancer /advanced-cancer/care -choices#HC

7. Reville B, Axelrod D, Maury R. Palliative care for the cancer patient. *Prim Care*. 2009;36(4):781-810.

8. Ferrell BR, Temel JS, Temin S, et al. Integration of palliative care into standard oncology care: American Society of Clinical Oncology clinical practice guideline update. *J Clin Oncol*. 2017;35(1):96-112.

9. Goldberg S, Paramanathan D, Khoury R, et al. A patient-reported outcome instrument to assess symptom burden and predict survival in patients with advanced cancer: flipping the paradigm to improve timing of palliative and end-of-life discussions and reduce unwanted health care costs. *Oncologist*. 2019; 24(1):76-85.

10. Hoerger M, Greer J, Jackson V, et al. Defining the elements of early palliative care that are associated with patient-reported outcomes and delivery of end-of-life care. *J Clin Oncol*. 2018;36(11): 1096-1102.

11. Scibetta C, Kerr K, Mcguire J, Rabow MW. The costs of waiting: implications of the timing of palliative care consultation among a cohort of decedents at a comprehensive cancer center. *J Palliat Med*. 2016;19(1):69-75.

12. Haun MW, Estel S, Rücker G, et al. Early palliative care for adults with advanced cancer. *Cochrane Database Syst Rev*. 2017;6.

13. Ravasco P, Monteiro-Grillo I, Vidal PM, Camilo ME. Cancer: disease and nutrition are key determinants of patients' quality of life. *Support Care Cancer*. 2004;12(4):246-252.

14. van den Beuken-van Everdingen MHJ, de Rijke JM, Kessels AG, Schouten HC, van Kleef M, Patijin J. Quality of life and non-pain symptoms in patients with cancer. *J Pain Symptom Manage*. 2009;38(2)216-233.

15. Van Cutsem E, Arends J. The causes and consequences of cancer associated malnutrition. *Eur J Oncol Nurs*. 2005;9(supp 12):S51-S63.

16. Shahmoradi N, Kandiah M, Peng LS. Impact of nutritional status on quality of life of advanced cancer patients in hospice home care. *Asian Pac J Cancer Prev*. 2009;10(6):1003-1010.

17. Caro MMM, Laviano A, Pichard C. Impact of nutrition on quality of life during cancer. *Curr Opin Clin Nutr Metab Care*. 2007;10(4):480-487.

18. Gellrich NC, Handschel J, Holtmann H, et al. Oral cancer malnutrition impacts weight and quality of life. *Nutrients*. 2015;7(4):2145-2160.

19. Thoresen L. *Nutrition care in cancer patients. Nutrition assessment: diagnostic criteria and the association to survival and health-related quality of life in patients with advanced colorectal carcinoma*. Doctoral thesis. Norwegian University of Science and Technology; 2012.

20. Ravasco P, Monteiro-Grillo I, Vidal PM, Camilo ME. Nutritional deterioration in cancer: the role of disease and diet. *Clin Onc*. 2003;15(8):433-450.

21. Muscaritoli M, Lucia S, Farcomeni A, et al. Prevalence of malnutrition in patients at first medical oncology visit: the preMiO study. *Oncotarget*. 2017;8(45):79884-79896.

22. Pirlich M, Schutz T, Norman K, et al. The German hospital malnutrition study. *Clin Nutr*. 2006;25(4):563-572.

23. Kwang AY, Kandiah M. Objective and subjective nutritional assessment of patients with cancer in palliative care. *Amer J Hosp Pall Care*. 2010;27(2): 117-126.

24. Wie G-A, Cho Y-A, Kim S-Y, Kim S-M, Bae J-M, Joung H. Prevalence and risk factors of malnutrition among cancer patients according to tumor location and stage in the National Cancer Center in Korea. *Nutr.* 2010;26(3):263-268.

25. Orrevall Y, Tishelman C, Permert T, Cederholm T. Nutritional support and risk status among cancer patients in palliative home care services. *Supp Care Cancer.* 2009;17(2):153-161.

26. Slaviero K, Read J, Clarke S, Rivory L. A baseline nutrition assessment in advanced cancer patients receiving palliative chemotherapy. *Nutr Cancer.* 2003;46(2):148-157.

27. Segura A, Pardo J, Jara C, et al. An epidemiological evaluation of the prevalence of malnutrition in Spanish patients with locally advanced or metastatic cancer. *Clin Nutr.* 2005;24(5):801-814.

28. Tong H, Isenring E, Yates P. The prevalence of nutrition impact symptoms and their relationship to quality of life and clinical outcomes in medical oncology patients. *Support Care Cancer.* 2009;17(1):83-90.

29. Morita T, Fujimoto K, Namba M, et al. Palliative care needs of cancer outpatients receiving chemotherapy: an audit of a clinical screening project. *Support Care Cancer.* 2008;16(1):101-107.

30. Teunissen SC, Wesker W, Kruitwagen C, de Haes HC, Voest EE, de Graeff A. Symptom prevalence in patients with incurable cancer: a systematic review. *J Pain Symptom Manage.* 2007;34(1):94-104.

31. McGettigan N, Uí Dhuibhir P, Barrett M, et al. Subjective and objective assessment of taste and smell sensation in advanced cancer. *Am J Hosp Palliat Care.* 2019;36(8):688-696.

32. Kirkova J, Walsh D, Rybicki L, et al. Symptom severity and distress in advanced cancer. *Palliat Med.* 2010;24(3):330-339.

33. Halawi R, Aldin ES, Baydoun A, et al. Physical symptom profile for adult cancer inpatients at a Lebanese cancer unit. *Eur J Intenr Med.* 2012;23(8):e185-e189. doi:10.1016/j.ejim.2012.08.018

34. Alshemmari S, Ezzat H, Samir Z, Sajnani K, Alsirafy S. Symptom burden in hospitalized patients with cancer in Kuwait and the need for palliative care. *Am J Hosp Palliat Care.* 2010;27(7):446-449.

35. Isaac T, O Stuver S, Davis RB, et al. Incidence of severe pain in newly diagnosed ambulatory patients with stage IV cancer. *Pain Research & Management.* 2012;17(5):347-352.

36. Dhingra L, Shuk E, Grossman B, et al. A qualitative study to explore psychological distress and illness burden associated with opioid-induced constipation in cancer patients with advanced disease. *Palliat Med.* 2013;27(5):447-456.

37. Rodriguez RF, Bravo LE, Castro F, et al. Incidence of weak opioids adverse events in the management of cancer pain: a double-blind comparative trial. *J Palliat Med.* 2007;10(1):56-60.

38. Cheung WY, Le LW, Zimmermann C. Symptom clusters in patients with advanced cancers. *Support Care Cancer.* 2009;17(9):1223-1230.

39. Ottery F. Definition of standardized nutritional assessment and interventional pathways in oncology. *Nutrition.* 1996;12(1 suppl):S15-19.

40. Wojtaszek CA, Kochis LM, Cunningham RS. Nutritional screening and assessment: an overview. In: Integrating nutrition into your cancer program. *Oncology Issues.* 2002;17(2):S11-12.

41. Bauer J, Capra S, Ferguson F. Use of the patient-generated subjective global assessment (PG-SGA) as a nutrition assessment tool in patients with cancer. *Eur J Clin Nutr.* 2002;56(8):779-785.

42. Jager-Wittenarr H, Ottery FD. Assessing nutritional status in cancer: role of the patient-generated subjective global assessment. *Curr Opin Clin Nutr Metab Care.* 2017;20(5):322-329.

43. Thompson KL, Elliott L, Fuchs-Tarlowsky V, et al. Oncology evidence-based nutrition practice guideline for adults. *J Acad Nutr Diet.* 2017;117(2):297-310.

44. Thoresen L, Fjeldstad I, Krogstad K, Kaasa S, Falkmer UG. Nutritional status of patients with advanced cancer: the value of using the subjective global assessment of nutritional status as a screening tool. *Palliat Med.* 2002;16(1):33-42.

45. Isenring E, Cross G, Daniels L, Kellett E, Koczwara B. Validity of the malnutrition screening tool as an effective predictor of nutritional risk in oncology patients receiving chemotherapy. *Support Care Cancer*. 2006;14(11):1152-1156.

46. Mateus C, Cacheux W, Lemarie E. Relationship between performance status and malnutrition in non-selected cancer patients: A nation-wide one-day survey. *J Clin Oncol*. 2007; ASCO Annual Meeting Proceedings Part 1. 25(18S):9126.

47. Cessot A, Hebuterne X, Coriat R. Defining the clinical condition of cancer patients: it is time to switch from performance status to nutritional status. *Support Care Cancer*. 2011;19(7):869-870.

48. Carvalho CS, Souza DS, Lopes JR, et al. Relationship between patient-generated subjective global assessment and survival in patients in palliative care. *Ann Palliat Med*. 2017;6(1):S4-S12.

49. Petersen MA, Larsen H, Pedersen L, Sonne N, Groenvold M. Assessing health-related quality of life in palliative care: comparing patient and physician assessments. *Eur J Cancer*. 2006;42(8):1159-1166.

50. Laugsand EA, Sprangers MAG, Bjordal K, Skorpen F, Kaasa S, Klepstad P. Health care providers underestimate symptom intensities of cancer patients: a multicenter European study. *Health QOL Outcomes*. 2010;8:104-117. doi:10.1186/1477-7525-8-104

51. Xiao C, Polomano R, Bruner, DW. Comparison between patient-reported and clinician-observed symptoms in oncology. *Cancer Nurs*. 2013;36(6):E1-16. doi:10.1097/NCC.0b013e318269040f

52. Flynn B, Barrett M, Sui J, et al. Nutritional status and interventions in hospice: physician assessment of cancer patients. *J Hum Nutr Diet*. 2018;31(6):781-784.

53. Reid J, Mckenna HP, Fitzsimmons D, McCance TV. An exploration of the experience of cancer cachexia: what patients and their families want from healthcare professionals. *Eur J Cancer Care*. 2010;19(5):682-689.

54. Yamagishi A, Morita T, Miyashita M, Sato K, Tsuneto S, Shima Y. The care strategy for families of terminally ill cancer patients who become unable to take nourishment orally: recommendations from a nationwide survey of bereaved family members' experiences. *J Pain Symptom Manage*. 2010;40(5):671-683.

55. Geppert CMA, Andrews MR, Druyan ME. Ethical issues in artificial nutrition and hydration: a review. *JPEN J Parenter Enteral Nutr*. 2010;34(1):79-88.

56. Hui D, Dev R, Bruera E. The last days of life: symptom burden and impact on nutrition and hydration in cancer patients. *Curr Opin Support Palliat Care*. 2015;9(4):346-354.

57. Druml C, Ballmer PE, Druml W, et al. ESPEN guideline on ethical aspects of nutrition and hydration. *Clin Nutr*. 2016;35(3):545-56.

58. Maillet JO, Potter RL, Heller L. Position of the American Dietetic Association: Ethical and legal issues in nutrition, hydration, and feeding. *J Am Diet Assoc*. 2002;102(5):716-726.

59. Raijmakers NJH, Fradsham S, van Zuylen L, Mayland C, Ellershaw JE, van der Heide A. Variation in attitudes towards artificial hydration at the end of life: a systematic literature review. *Curr Opin Support Palliat Care*. 2011;5(3):265-272.

60. Soo I and Gramlich L. Use of parenteral nutrition in patients with advanced cancer. *Appl Physiol Nutr Metab*. 2008;33(1):102-106.

61. Suter PM, Rogers J, Strack C. Artificial nutrition and hydration for the terminally ill. *Home Healthc Nurse*. 2008;26(1):23-29.

62. Morton RP, Crowder VL, Mawdsley R, Ong E, Izzard M. Elective gastrostomy, nutritional status and quality of life in advanced head and neck cancer patients receiving chemoradiotherapy. *ANZ J Surg*. 2009;79(10):713-718.

63. Wiggenraad RGJ, Flierman L, Goosens A, et al. Prophylactic gastrostomy placement and early tube feeding may limit loss of weight during chemoradiotherapy for advanced head and neck cancer, a preliminary study. *Clin Otolaryngol*. 2007;32(5):384-390.

64. Orrevall Y, Tishelman C, Permert J. Home parenteral nutrition: a qualitative interview study of the experiences of advanced cancer patients and their families. *Clin Nutr*. 2005;24(6):961-970.

65. Winkler MF. Quality of life in adult home parenteral nutrition patients. *JPEN J Parenter Enteral Nutr.* 2005;29(3):162-170.

66. Shang E, Weiss C, Post S, Kaehler G. The influence of early parenteral nutrition on quality of life and body composition in patients with advanced cancer. *JPEN J Parenter Enteral Nutr.* 2006;30(3):222-230.

67. Brard L, Weitzen S, Strubel-Lagan SL, et al. The effect of total parenteral nutrition on the survival of terminally ill ovarian cancer patients. *Gynecol Oncol.* 2006;103(1):176-180.

68. Hasenberg T, Essenbreis M, Herold A, Post S, Shang E. Early supplementation of parenteral nutrition is capable of improving quality of life, chemotherapy-related toxicity and body composition in patients with advanced colorectal carcinoma undergoing palliative treatment: results from a prospective, randomized clinical trial. *Colorectal Dis.* 2010 Oct;12(10 Online):e190-9. doi:10.1111/j.1463-1318.2009.02111.x

69. Vashi PG, Dahlk S, Popiel B, et al. A longitudinal study investigating quality of life and nutritional outcomes in advanced cancer patients receiving home parenteral nutrition. *BMC Cancer.* 2014;14:593. doi:10.1186%2F1471-2407-14-593

70. Cotongni P, De Carli L, Passera R, et al. Longitudinal Study of quality of life in advanced cancer patients on home parental nutrition. *Cancer Med.* 2017;6(7):1799-1806.

71. Dy SM. Enteral and parenteral nutrition in terminally ill cancer patients: a review of the literature. *Am J Hosp Palliat Care.* 2006;23(5):369-377.

72. Chiu T-Y, Hu W-Y, Chuang R-B, Chen C-Y. Nutrition and hydration for terminal cancer patients in Taiwan. *Support Care Cancer.* 2002;10(8):630-636.

73. Bachmann P, Marti-Massoud M, Blanc-Vincent MP, et al. Summary version of the standards, opinions, options and recommendations for palliative or terminal nutrition in adults with progressive cancer (2001). *Br J Cancer.* 2003;89(supp 1):S107-S110.

74. Mirhosseini N, Fainsinger RL, Baracos V. Parenteral nutrition in advanced cancer: indications and clinical practice guidelines. *J Palliat Med.* 2005;8(5):914-918.

75. August DA, Huhmann MB, American Society for Parenteral and Enteral Nutrition (A.S.P.E.N.) Board of Directors. A.S.P.E.N. clinical guidelines: nutrition support therapy during adult anticancer treatment and in hematopoietic cell transplantation. *JPEN J Parent Enteral Nutr.* 2009;33(5):472-500.

76. Arends J, Zuercher G, Dossett A, et al. Non-surgical oncology—guidelines on parenteral nutrition, Chapter 19. *GMS Med Sci.* 2009;7:1612-1625

77. Arends J, Bachmann P, Baracos V, et al. ESPEN guidelines on nutrition in cancer patients. *Clin Nutr.* 2017;36(1):11-48.

78. de las Peñas R, Majem M, Perez-Altozano J, et al. SEOM clinical guidelines on nutrition in cancer patients (2018). *Clin Transl Oncol.* 2019;21(1):87-93.

79. Dev R, Dalal S, Bruera E. Is there a role for parenteral nutrition or hydration at the end of life? *Curr Opin Support Palliat Care.* 2012;6(3):365-370.

80. Cohen MZ, Torres-Vigil I, Burbach BE, de la Rosa A, Bruera E. The meaning of parenteral hydration to family caregivers and patients with advanced cancer receiving hospice care. *J Pain Symptom Manage.* 2012;43(5):855-865.

81. Bavin L. Artificial rehydration in the last days of life: is it beneficial? *Int J Palliat Nurs.* 2007;13(9):445-449.

82. Bukki J, Unterpaul T, Nubling G, et al. Decision making at end of life—cancer patients' and their caregivers' views on artificial nutrition and hydration. *Support Care Cancer.* 2014;22(12):3287-3299.

83. Nakajima N, Satake N, Nakaho T. Indications and practice of artificial hydration for terminally ill cancer patients. *Curr Opin Support Palliat Care.* 2014;8(4):358-363.

84. Bear AJ, Bukowy EA, Patel JJ. Artificial hydration at the end of life. *Nutr Clin Pract.* 2017;32(5):628-632.

85. Price KAR. Hydration in cancer patients. *Curr Opin in Support Palliat Care.* 2010;4(4):276-280.

86. Maillet JOS, Schwartz DB, Posthauer ME. Position of the Academy of Nutrition and Dietetics: ethical and legal issues in feeding and hydration. *J Acad Nutr Diet.* 2013;113(6):828-833.

87. Jonsen A, Siegler M, Winslade W. *Clinical Ethics: A Practical Approach to Ethical Decisions in Clinical Medicine.* 8th ed. Cenveo Publisher Services; 2015.

Chapter 27
Medical Cannabis for Cancer Symptom Management

Kelay E. Trentham, MS, RDN, CSO, CD, FAND

Common conditions or diseases for which cannabis has been used include HIV-related cachexia, nausea caused by cancer or its treatment, seizure disorders, and pain.[1] Registry data from states that have medical cannabis laws show that an estimated 3.5 million people in the United States use medical cannabis.[2] As of November 2020, 36 states, the District of Columbia, and the territories of Guam, Puerto Rico, and the US Virgin Islands have passed comprehensive medical cannabis–related legislation or ballot measures,[3] and 15 states, 3 territories, and the District of Columbia have legalized adult-use cannabis.[4]

Though they do not grant comprehensive access to medical cannabis, laws allowing the use of preparations low in tetrahydrocannabinol (THC) and high in cannabidiol (CBD) have been approved in 11 states for specific medical conditions.[3] As more states seek to legalize the use of cannabis, registered dietitian nutritionists (RDNs) are highly likely to encounter more patients using it to manage their cancer symptoms. In surveys of patients with cancer, 43% to 66% indicated they had previously used cannabis and cited cancer-related pain, nausea, appetite, neuropsychiatric symptoms, and other cancer-related symptoms as reasons for its use.[5,6] Oncology RDNs often discuss integrative approaches to disease and symptom management with their patients, including the use of herbal and botanical products, and thus are in a unique position to provide cannabis education.

The Cannabis Plant and Its Use as Medicine

The cannabis plant is a member of the Cannabaceae family, which also includes hops and hackberry.[7,8] Cannabis contains more than 100 unique phytocannabinoids, the most abundant of which are tetrahydrocannabinolic acid (THCA) and cannabidiolic acid (CBDA).[9,10] Decarboxylation of THCA and CBDA occurs via heating (as in smoking, vaporization, or baking) to yield the better-known cannabinoids tetrahydrocannabinol (THC) and cannabidiol (CBD). The terms *chemical variety* and *chemovar* are used to describe a given plant's concentration of the various cannabinoids and other chemical components that contribute to its unique physiological effects.[10] For simplification, only the terms THC and CBD will be used for the remainder of this chapter.

Cannabis has a long history of medicinal use. The earliest mention is in the medical writings of ancient Egypt, as well as in the world's oldest pharmacopeia, China's *Pen Ts'ao Ching*, which was written in the second century.[7,11] Cannabis was first introduced to modern Western medicine in 1839 by an Irish physician who described the plant's analgesic, anticonvulsant, and antispasmodic effects. Its medical use was described in 1924 and was included in the United States Pharmacopeia (USP); however, by 1937 cannabis was effectively banned in the United States with the passage of the Marihuana Tax Act and was removed from the USP in 1942.[11] In 1970, the Controlled Substances Act classified cannabis as a Schedule I drug, which meant it was considered to be highly addictive with no medicinal value.[12,13] It remains thus classified today.

Interest in medical cannabis resurfaced in the 1990s, when researchers described cannabinoid receptors in the human nervous system.[11] In 1996, California became the first state to legalize cannabis for medical use.[3] Medical cannabis laws in the United States vary widely by state, district, and territory. Some states allow for use of cannabis but have few or no provisions for dispensaries, no hardship provisions for patients who cannot access a dispensary, or no available information about obtaining products.[14] Other limitations include caps or bans on dispensaries, limits on forms of use (smoking is not approved in two states), limits on the ability to grow one's own product, and possession limits set by statute rather than by medical professionals.[3] Thus, understanding local laws and access issues is a critical element of being able to counsel patients on its use.

Endocannabinoid System and Cannabinoids

The human endocannabinoid system consists of endogenous cannabinoids (also known as endocannabinoids), cannabinoid receptors, and related enzymes. Endocannabinoids are lipid mediators found in the brain and peripheral tissues that act on the cannabinoid receptors. The first endocannabinoid was discovered in the porcine brain in 1992 and was termed *anandamide*, or the "happy amide," for the Sanskrit word *ananda*, meaning "happiness" or "bliss." This and other endocannabinoids are released on demand and bind to various cannabinoid receptors. The best-studied of these receptors are type 1 (CB1), found predominantly in the central nervous system, and type 2 (CB2), found primarily in peripheral and immune cells.[15]

The term *phytocannabinoid* refers to plant-derived compounds that have similar chemical composition or bioactivity as the endocannabinoids. THC and CBD are the phytocannabinoids most widely known and studied. THC exhibits analgesic, antiemetic, muscle relaxant, antispasmodic, bronchodilatory, neuroprotective-antioxidant, anti-inflammatory, and antipruritic activities.[16,17] CBD exhibits analgesic, neuroprotective-antioxidant, anticonvulsant, antinausea, antimethicillin-resistant *Staphylococcus aureus* (MRSA), and antianxiety effects, and it also modulates THC-associated adverse effects, such as anxiety, tachycardia, and sedation, which are essential to the effectiveness of an oromucosal cannabis extract—nabiximols—used to treat intractable cancer pain.[16]

Effects of other noted phytocannabinoids include antifungal, anti-inflammatory, anticonvulsant, antibacterial, and analgesic activities, among others. In addition to cannabinoids, cannabis contains terpenoids (essential oil components) which impart characteristic odors and flavors to cannabis as well as to other foods, plants, and herbs that also contain them. Box 27.1 lists some of the terpenoids found in cannabis, examples of other plants in which they are found, and some noted pharmacological effects. When inhaled, terpenoids have pharmacological effects on humans and animals, even when present at very low serum concentrations.[18] It is thought that terpenoid content and the synergistic effects of phytocannabinoids and terpenoids when taken together may explain why cannabis chemovars with similar quantities of THC or CBD exert different effects on the body. This synergistic effect of the various compounds of cannabis is referred to as the "entourage effect."[16]

Cannabinoid Medicines

Cannabinoid medicines can be categorized as single-molecule pharmaceuticals, cannabis-based liquid extracts, and whole cannabis preparations. Dronabinol and nabilone are single-molecule, synthetic THC pharmaceutical products approved by the US Food and Drug Administration and available by prescription,[9] while levonantradol is a synthetic cannabinoid analogue used in

Box 27.1
Terpenoids Found in Cannabis and Their Effects [16]

Terpenoid	Other plants in which commonly found	Pharmacological effects
β-Caryophyllene	Black pepper	Anti-inflammatory
Caryophyllene oxide	Lemon balm	Antifungal
Limonene	Lemon	Anxiolytic
Linalool	Lavender	Antianxiety, analgesic
β-Myrcene	Hops	Sedative, muscle relaxant
Nerolidol	Orange	Sedative
α-Pinene	Pine	Anti-inflammatory, aids memory
Phytol	Green tea	Increases γ-aminobutyric acid (GABA)

research.[19] Dronabinol is approved for treatment of chemotherapy-associated nausea and vomiting that is refractory to standard treatment and for anorexia-associated weight loss in patients with AIDS. Nabilone is also approved for chemotherapy-associated nausea and vomiting in cancer patients.[9] Levonantradol is the only cannabinoid used parenterally and has been studied for its antiemetic properties.[19] Cannabis-based liquid extracts include nabiximols (Sativex) and Epidiolex (both manufactured by GW Pharmaceuticals, United Kingdom). Nabiximols is an oromucosal spray containing THC and CBD that is used for pain and spasticity associated with multiple sclerosis in several countries outside the United States and is approved for treatment of intractable cancer pain in Canada.[9,20] Finally, whole cannabis preparations allow access to the complete complement of cannabinoids and terpenoids rather than single-extracted or synthetic cannabinoid compounds. Although a complete review of the evidence for cannabis use is outside the scope of this chapter, conditions for which patients with cancer commonly use cannabis will be discussed. Available studies may include any combination of the three categories of cannabinoid medicines described.

Efficacy of Use by Cancer Patients and Survivors

Cannabis is used in patients with cancer who are undergoing treatment or seeking palliation of nausea, vomiting, anorexia, and pain. A quantitative systematic review showed the use of orally administered dronabinol or nabilone or intramuscularly administered levanantrodol was more effective for nausea control than prochlorperazine, metoclopramide, chlorpromazine, thiethylperazine, haloperidol, domperidone, or alizapride. However, in this review, cannabinoids were not found to be more effective for patients who received very low or very high emetogenic chemotherapy regimens.[17] A

2008 meta-analysis showed that, compared with an older class of antiemetics, dronabinol use resulted in a significantly lower risk of chemotherapy-induced nausea and vomiting (CINV).[21] A pilot clinical trial of a standardized oromucosally delivered cannabis-based medicine vs placebo for the treatment of CINV found that patients treated with cannabis-based medicine experienced a complete response (no nausea) during the overall observation period, including the 24 to 120 hours following chemotherapy.[22] There was no difference between groups during the acute phase (0 to 24 hours after chemotherapy). Another study showed that cannabinoids were as or more effective at managing nausea than ondansetron, a 5-hydroxytryptamine$_3$ antagonist, with the absence rate of nausea being 71% with dronabinol, 64% with ondansetron, and 15% with placebo.[23] To date, there have been no studies comparing cannabinoids with neurokinin-1 antagonists such as fosaprepitant.

Although cannabis use is commonly thought to increase appetite, clinical evidence for its effectiveness in the setting of cancer is limited. In one study, megestrol acetate improved appetite in 75% of patients with advanced cancer compared to 49% of those patients given dronabinol.[24] In another study comparing a cannabis extract containing THC and CBD, THC only, or placebo, there was no significant difference in appetite among these groups.[25] The THC dose used in this study was quite low at 2.5 mg compared to between 5 and 20 mg used for improving appetite in patients with HIV. In a prospective observational study, patients receiving medical cannabis licenses in Israel were interviewed at baseline (day of receiving license) and 6 to 8 weeks later. For those patients who used cannabis continuously, symptom scores were significantly improved, and the number of people reporting no anorexia increased by 36%, while those reporting minimal anorexia dropped from 65% at baseline to 38% after 6 to 8 weeks.[26] The clinical trial data in patients with cancer may not match the subjective observational data due to more freedom in dosing when patients use whole cannabis ad lib rather than being subject to controlled dosing in a research setting.

Patients with cancer may also experience significant alterations in taste and smell, making it difficult to eat. In a study comparing THC (as dronabinol) to placebo, chemosensory improvement was 36% for THC-treated patients vs 15% for patients in the placebo group. Additionally, 55% of THC-treated patients stated that "food tastes better," compared to only 10% of patients in the placebo group. The premeal appetite score was greater for the treatment group ($P < .05$).[27] It is important to note that this was a pilot study with a total of 21 participants, and more research is needed to establish the chemosensory effects of cannabis.

Using cannabis for pain relief is common in persons with cancer, especially given the side effects of opioid use, such as constipation. Cannabis is increasingly being recognized for its pain-management properties coupled with a lack of overdose risk and low toxicity profile.[28] A 2009 review of the use of various cannabinoids for pain, including cancer pain, found a statistically significant mean difference favoring cannabinoids over placebo. Because this review also pooled results for adverse events and found statistically significant risk for alterations in cognitive and motor function and perception, the authors concluded that the risk of harm may outweigh the benefit of cannabis use for managing pain for conditions studied.[29] In other reviews of cannabinoid use for pain not related to cancer, a majority of studies showed significant analgesic effects without severe adverse effects, and cannabinoids were observed to be well tolerated.[30] In a 2013 review of 38 randomized controlled trials that included studies of cancer-related pain, 71% of studies showed significant pain relief.[28] Another review of cannabis use for chronic pain included six randomized controlled trials, five of which were of high quality and assessed management of neuropathic pain.[31] Statistically significant relief of neuropathic pain with cannabinoid treatment was seen in all six studies, while three of the studies were considered to have "clinically meaningful" benefit: 45%, 52%, and 61% of patients reporting pain relief with cannabis compared to 18%, 24%, and 26% of placebo-treated patients. Noted adverse effects were cognitive, motor function, and neurologic in nature but were not considered severe.[31]

Owing to various website testimonials touting the cancer-curative power of concentrated cannabinoid-containing oils, the belief that cannabis can cure cancer has been growing in popularity.[32] The majority of studies suggesting that cannabinoids can reduce tumor growth are considered preclinical (based on cellular or animal models). In addition, a few studies have found that cannabinoids increase cell proliferation under certain conditions in vitro and may also interfere with tumor suppression mechanisms of the immune system.[33] Several studies suggest that cannabinoids inhibit the growth of glioma; leukemia and lymphoma; melanoma; neuroblastoma; thyroid epithelioma; and breast, colorectal, gastric, hepatocellular, pancreatic, prostate, and skin carcinomas.[32,34] In animal models, cannabinoid administration curbed growth of genetically initiated or xenografted tumors, including breast, colorectal, lung, pancreatic, and skin carcinomas, as well as glioma, lymphoma, melanoma, and thyroid epithelioma.[32] Antitumor effects of cannabinoids include autophagy, apoptosis, and cell cycle arrest; inhibition of angiogenesis; decreased formation of distant tumors in animal models of induced and spontaneous metastases; and inhibition of adhesion, migration, and invasiveness of cells in culture.[33] THC promotes cell death via CB1 and CB2 receptors, while CBD is thought to do so independently of these receptors and at least partly due to enhanced production of reactive oxygen species within tumor cells.[35]

Cannabinoids may work synergistically with standard chemotherapy drugs or radiation. Studies have found some glioma cell lines to be resistant to both temozolamide (the benchmark treatment for glioblastoma multiforme) and THC due to enhanced expression of genes specific to those cell lines. In a series of studies, both in vitro and in vivo, the combination of THC with temozolamide exerted a much stronger antitumor effect than either agent alone.[35] The same researchers found that CBD combined with a lower dose of THC was more effective than either agent alone and was equally as effective as a higher dose of THC. Coadministration of THC and CBD increased radiosensitivity in pretreated glioma cells and, combined with radiation, dramatically reduced tumor volume in a murine model of glioma.[33] In other studies, both synthetic and endogenous cannabinoids increased effectiveness of some standard chemotherapy drugs. Synthetic and endogenous cannabinoids acted synergistically with chemotherapy agents, such as gemcitabine and paclitaxel against pancreatic[36] and gastric cancer cells,[37] suggesting there may be a role for phytocannabinoids alongside traditional chemotherapy.

In what is considered a landmark, pilot, phase 1 study, nine patients with recurrent glioblastoma multiforme were treated with THC. These patients had failed standard treatment consisting of surgery and radiation and showed tumor progression. With the goal of assessing safety, THC was intracranially administered into a surgically created cavity within the tumor. This method of cannabinoid administration was found to be safe, with minimal psychoactive effects, and tumor cell proliferation was inhibited for some patients.[38] Given the size of the study, however, the significance of the effect on cell proliferation is unclear. It is important to note that, though they may appear promising, results of these preclinical studies and a single phase 1 pilot study are not enough to support the use of cannabinoids as a stand-alone cancer treatment. More research is needed to determine which cancers would respond to cannabinoids, whether (and which) cannabinoids may be synergistic with chemo- or radiotherapy, appropriate dosing, and safety.

Pharmacokinetics

In addition to understanding current evidence of cannabis's efficacy, the RDN should have an understanding of its pharmacokinetics. This is a pivotal point when counseling patients, since cannabis-naive patients are often unaware of the differences in onset and duration of effect for the various routes of administration and other issues related to product and dosing. Routes of administration include inhalation, oromucosal, oral, rectal, and topical. Table 27.1 describes the pharmacokinetics of cannabis by route. Inhalation yields the fastest onset and shortest duration.[10] Oral intake has considerably longer onset and duration and has significantly greater first-pass metabolism through the liver, which reduces the bioavailability of THC.[10,39] This first-pass metabolism yields the highly psychoactive metabolite 11-hydroxy-THC,

Table 27.1
Cannabis Pharmacokinetics by Route of Administration[10,39-42]

Route and examples	Time to onset of effect	Duration of effect	Bioavailability	Comments
Inhalation[10,39] ■ Smoking, vaporization	5-10 minutes	2-4 hours	10%-60%; depends on volume inhaled, puff duration, and length of breath hold	N/A
Oromucosal[10,42] ■ Tinctures, sprays, mists	15-45 minutes	6-8 hours	Highly variable; increases with food intake	Limited first-pass metabolism
Oral[10,39] ■ Tablets, capsules, edibles (food, liquid, candy)	60-180 minutes	6-8 hours	10%-30%	Significant first-pass metabolism results in higher 11-hydroxy-tetrahydrocannabinol, decreased THC availability
Rectal[39,40] ■ Suppository	Not described (1-8 hours to "peak concentration")	Not described	Approximately twice that of oral	Lower first-pass metabolism
Topical ■ Creams, salves	Varies	Varies	Not described	Effects are mostly local
Transdermal patches[41]	1.4 hours	48 hours	CBD (cannabidiol) and CBN(cannabinol) concentrations via transdermal patches are 10 times higher than Δ-8-THC (delta-8-THC)	Δ-8-THC in an animal model

a compound that has greater psychoactive effects than THC.[40] Coupled with a highly variable absorption rate, this makes the use of orally ingested cannabis more difficult to titrate.[10,40] Due to lower first-pass metabolism, inhaled, oromucosal, and rectally delivered cannabis are associated with less psychoactivity and often greater tolerance.[39] Less is known about the systemic delivery of THC from topical creams and salves, and there are only pre-clinical data regarding delivery via patches.[41]

Contraindications

Contraindications are another important consideration of cannabinoid use. As with any botanical or drug, a known allergy to cannabis (whole plant), any cannabinoid constituents (eg, THC, CBD), cannabinoid analogues (eg, nabilone), or any delivery vehicle (eg, sesame oil in the case of dronabinol) constitutes a contraindication. Other contraindications may include cannabinoid comorbidity or cannabinoid-drug interactions. Suggested contraindications and precautions for cannabis use are listed in Box 27.2 and pertain primarily to THC. Acutely, cannabis can affect both heart and lung function, causing elevated blood pressure,

tachycardia, increased cardiac labor, systemic vasodilation, and, when inhaled, airway inflammation and resistance, lung tissue damage, increased risk of chronic bronchitis, emphysema, and impaired respiratory function.[43,44] More severe effects, including angina, myocardial infarction, cardiac death, and cardiomyopathy, have been reported in persons with preexisting cardiac conditions.[44] Patients with preexisting lung disease who wish to use medical cannabis should be advised to consume it by means other than inhalation, provided no other contraindications exist. Daily cannabis use was found to be an independent risk factor for steatosis in persons with chronic hepatitis C.[45] In addition, cannabinoids are metabolized by the liver and excreted via the kidneys, so it is thought that their effects could be prolonged or amplified in the setting of liver or renal disease.[46,47]

Acute exposure to THC-predominant cannabis may result in temporary—or when used during adolescence—persistent psychosis.[43,44] Long-term use of THC-predominant cannabis preparations may worsen preexisting symptoms of psychosis and schizophrenia in persons susceptible to mental illness and trigger or amplify manic symptoms in persons diagnosed with bipolar disorder.[44] Known

Box 27.2
Suggested Contraindications and Precautions for Cannabinoid Use[43,44,48]

Contraindications	Diseases: cardiovascular, respiratory (when cannabis is smoked), hepatic, renal
	History: psychiatric disorders, schizophrenia (including family history)
	Pregnancy, planning to become pregnant, breastfeeding
	Cannabis or other substance use disorder (when smoked)
	Age less than 25 years (when smoked)
Precautions	High risk of cardiovascular disease
	Tobacco smoking
	Active mood or anxiety disorder
	Use of higher doses of opioids, benzodiazepines

or suspected personal or family history of mental illness (including schizophrenia, other psychotic illness, severe personality disorder, or other psychiatric disorder, excluding depression) is considered a contraindication for use.[47] Acute anxiety may be exacerbated by cannabis use, although dosage may play a role since lesser amounts of THC can be anxiolytic while greater amounts are anxiogenic. There is evidence that cannabis with high CBD and low THC content may mitigate psychosis and that CBD may mitigate anxiolytic effects of THC.[44] There is also evidence that cannabis use may decrease conception rate, increase risk of miscarriage, and cause long-term developmental problems for children exposed in utero. Cannabinoids are excreted in human milk and may be absorbed through breastfeeding.[48]

Prevalence of cannabis use disorder is noted to be similar among medical and recreational users.[43] Estimates of cannabis dependence range from 9% to 10% overall, to 16% to 17% of those who begin using as adolescents, and 25% to 50% of those who use it daily.[44]

Adverse Effects

As with any botanical product, it is important to be aware of potentially adverse effects. Because most available data regarding adverse effects of cannabinoids are from studies of recreational cannabis or cannabinoid pharmaceuticals and focus on short-term effects, only short-term effects are presented in Box 27.3. Noted cognitive effects include impaired memory, poor concentration, disorientation, confusion, impaired learning, and impaired psychomotor speed.[31] Unlike in the case of opiates, effects such as lethal overdose or organ failure have not been reported with cannabis used for pain.[29] In a 1999 government-commissioned report, the Institute of Medicine (now the Health and Medicine Division of the National Academies of Sciences, Engineering, and Medicine) concluded that "except for the harms associated with smoking,

the adverse effects of marijuana [cannabinoid botanicals] use are within the range of effects tolerated for other medications."[49]

Drug Interactions

Cannabinoids are metabolized in the liver via cytochrome P-450 enzymes, and reported drug-cannabinoid interactions are noted in Box 27.4.[48,50] Most notably, cannabis can increase the effects of central nervous system depressants, such as sedatives or alcohol.[48] High-dose CBD was associated with somnolence in seizure patients concurrently using clobazam.[51] Studies of cannabinoids in patients treated for other conditions suggest that concurrent use of cannabis with a variety of other medications is well tolerated, and typical adverse effects are those psychotropic effects often seen with cannabinoid use.[48]

Other Safety Concerns

The availability of cannabis products depends on state-level medical cannabis laws, which vary widely: Some states allow specialty medical dispensaries; others limit the number or location (or both) of dispensaries; and some do not allow dispensaries at all. Similarly, regulation of medical cannabis products in most jurisdictions is in its infancy. Ideally, patients could someday be confident that medical cannabis products, like other medications, contain no contaminants, are accurately labeled for cannabinoid content, and list all inactive ingredients. However, currently, that is not always the case.

Various types of contaminants are of concern. Like any herb, cannabis plants can carry microorganisms (bacteria, molds), and case reports have described ill effects of *Aspergillus* inhalation from smoked cannabis among immunocompromised patients—including death in some cases. Therefore, whether or not a patient requiring immunosuppressants after stem cell transplantation can safely use cannabis should be carefully considered.

Box 27.3
Commonly Experienced Adverse Effects of Cannabis-Based Medicines by Prevalence[10]

Frequent	Anxiety; cognitive effects; drowsiness and fatigue; dizziness; dry mouth; cough, phlegm, and bronchitis (when cannabis is smoked); nausea
Common	Blurred vision, euphoria, headache
Rare	Ataxia and discoordination; cannabis hyperemesis; diarrhea; depression; orthostatic hypotension; toxic psychosis and paranoia; tachycardia

Box 27.4
Reported Drug-Cannabinoid Interactions[48,50]

Drug	Effect
Ketoconazole	Increases concentration of tetrahydrocannabinol (THC)
	Increases concentration of cannabidiol (CBD)
Rifampin	Decreases concentration of THC
Alcohol and CNS (central nervous system) depressants	Cannabis increases effects

Researchers in Israel have described methods for fully sterilizing cannabis that only reduces THC activity by 12% to 27% compared with nonsterilized samples.[52] Cannabis sterilization may make its use safer and viable in this patient population. Increasingly popular cannabis concentrates are made in various ways, including extraction via solvents and liquid gases, such as naphtha, acetone, hexane, butane, and propane. Raber and colleagues[53] tested medical cannabis concentrates from California and found that more than 80% of samples had some form of contaminant, with the most common contaminants being isopentane and the pesticide paclobutrazol.

Another concern is lack of accuracy in content labeling. Vandrey and colleagues[54] sampled edible medical cannabis products from California and Washington and found that only 17% of products were accurately labeled for cannabinoid content, while 23% of products were underlabeled (ie, had more active constituent than was indicated on the label), and more than 50% of products were overlabeled. Use of an underlabeled product may lead to tolerance issues and difficulty titrating the desired dosage.

Patients should be made aware of all of these issues and encouraged to exercise caution, keeping in mind that, in many locales, cannabis is not currently regulated for purity and quality like traditional medications.

Finally, it is important to consider patients' intent to engage in usual daily activities, such as driving, child care, or safety-sensitive labor, and advise them accordingly. It has been suggested that use of power tools or heavy equipment be avoided until one is familiar with effects of the medicine and that driving be avoided for 4 hours after cannabis inhalation, for 6 hours after cannabis ingestion, and for 8 hours should euphoria be experienced. As with any medication that affects the central nervous system, patients should be counseled to avoid safety-sensitive activities if they feel impaired.

CBD-predominant products with low THC content may be best for daytime activities (ie, while working), whereas THC-predominant products could be employed when safety will not be compromised.[10]

Counseling on Cannabis

For the oncology RDN who elects to provide medical cannabis counseling, there are several things to consider. The primary aim should be to educate patients so that they can make informed decisions about whether to use cannabis for their medical conditions. By federal law, cannabis can be recommended, but not prescribed, by physicians,[55] and the law does not prevent health care providers from giving patients information about the potential benefits and burdens of cannabis use. Though the provision of legal advice is not within the RDN's scope of practice, providing basic and accurate sources of information about local laws and encouraging clients to further educate themselves are commonsense measures the RDN can take. When counseling patients, RDNs should determine for what conditions their patients intend to use cannabis, advise them of evidence for its efficacy, dispel any expectations unsupported by current research (such as that cannabis can "cure" cancer), and recommend they not forgo more effective treatments for serious conditions. Differences in onset time, duration, and psychoactive effects of the various administration methods should be explained, as well as actual or potential concerns, such as cannabis-drug or cannabis-disease interactions, contraindications, adverse effects, and product-safety issues. Patients should be given evidence-based resources (such as those listed in Box 27.5) so that they can further educate themselves. As with any herbal or botanical product, the patient should be encouraged to inform his or her physician and other medical providers of cannabis use.

RDNs should maintain an accurate record with specifics of education and resources given and communicate with the patient's other health care providers as needed. In an institutional setting, RDNs may first want to discuss their intent to provide cannabis education with their manager, risk manager, or legal department. In this author's experience, explaining that patients with cancer may access and use cannabis with limited or inaccurate information and that the goal of medical cannabis counseling is to enhance patient safety can be a compelling rationale for proactively educating patients.

> **Box 27.5**
> ### Additional Resources Related to Cannabis Use
>
> **Americans for Safe Access:**
> www.safeaccessnow.org
>
> **Information for Healthcare Professionals:**
> Cannabis (marihuana, marijuana) and the Cannabinoids (Health Canada 2018)
> www.canada.ca/en/health-canada/services/drugs-health-products/medical-use-marijuana/information-medical-practitioners/information-health-care-professionals-cannabis-marihuana-marijuana-cannabinoids.html
>
> **International Association for Cannabinoid Medicines:**
> www.cannabis-med.org
>
> **National Conference of State Legislatures:**
> State Medical Marijuana Laws: www.ncsl.org/research/health/state-medical-marijuana-laws.aspx

Summary

The cannabis plant has been used medicinally for centuries. Its use was first effectively prohibited in the United States with the Marihuana Tax Act of 1937 and later made federally illegal when it was classified as having no acceptable medical use in 1970. However, a resurgence of public interest is apparent, given that more than half of US states have passed laws allowing its medical use since 1996. In cancer care, cannabis may be useful in the palliation of CINV, cancer and neuropathic pain, anorexia, and weight loss. At present, research does not support claims that it can cure cancer. When educating patients about cannabis, it is important to discuss efficacy for intended use, pharmacokinetics, contraindications, adverse effects, potential drug or disease interactions, and safety concerns. Patients should be directed to reputable resources, including information about local medical cannabis laws. The RDN should record an accurate account of cannabis-related counseling and share appropriate information with the multidisciplinary team. The oncology RDN can serve as a valuable source for evidence-based information about medical cannabis to both patients and other health care providers.

References

1. Procon.org. Should marijuana be a medical option? Accessed December 22, 2020. http://medicalmarijuana.procon.org

2. Procon.org. Number of legal medical marijuana patients (as of May 17, 2018). Accessed December 22, 2020. https://medicalmarijuana.procon.org/number-of-legal-medical-marijuana-patients

3. National Conference of State Legislatures. State medical marijuana laws. Updated November 10, 2020. Accessed December 22, 2020. http://ncsl.org/research/health/state-medical-marijuana-laws.aspx

4. Legislatures NCoS. Marijuana overview. Updated October 17, 2019. Accessed December 22, 2020. http://ncsl.org/research/civil-and-criminal-justice/marijuana-overview.aspx

5. Martell K, Fairchild A, LeGerrier B, et al. Rates of cannabis use in patients with cancer. *Curr Oncol.* 2018;25(3):219-225.

6. Pergam SA, Woodfield MC, Lee CM, et al. Cannabis use among patients at a comprehensive cancer center in a state with legalized medicinal and recreational use. *Cancer.* 2017;123(22):4488-4497.

7. Russo E. History of cannabis and its preparations in saga, science and sobriquet. *Chem Biodivers.* 2007;4(2007):1614-1648.

8. Backes M. *Cannabis Pharmacy.* Black Dog & Leventhal; 2014.

9. Aggarwal SK, Carter GT, Sullivan MD, ZumBrunnen C, Morrill R, Mayer JD. Medicinal use of cannabis in the United States: historical perspectives, current trends, and future directions. *J Opioid Manag.* 2009;5(3):153-168.

10. MacCallum CA, Russo EB. Practical considerations in medical cannabis administration and dosing. *Eur J Intern Med.* 2018;49:12-19.

11. Zuardi AW. History of cannabis as medicine: a review. *Rev Bras Psiquiatr.* 2006;28(2):153-157.

12. Americans for Safe Access. Federal Marijuana Law. Accessed December 22, 2020. http://safeaccessnow.org/federal_marijuana_law

13. Administration USDE. Drug Scheduling. Accessed December 22, 2020. https://dea.gov/drug-scheduling

14. Procon.org. 30 legal medical marijuana states and dc: laws, fees, and possession limits. Updated December 3, 2020. Accessed December 22, 2020. https://medicalmarijuana.procon.org/legal-medical-marijuana-states-and-dc

15. Battista N, Di Tommaso M, Bari M, Maccarrone M. The endocannabinoid system: an overview. *Front Behav Neurosci.* 2012;6:9.

16. Russo EB. Taming THC: potential cannabis synergy and phytocannabinoid-terpenoid entourage effects. *Br J Pharmacol.* 2011;163(7):1344-1364.

17. Tramer MR, Carroll D, Campbell FA, Reynolds DJ, Moore RA, McQuay HJ. Cannabinoids for control of chemotherapy induced nausea and vomiting: quantitative systematic review. *BMJ.* 2001;323(7303):16-21.

18. Russo E, Guy GW. A tale of two cannabinoids: the therapeutic rationale for combining tetrahydrocannabinol and cannabidiol. *Med Hypotheses.* 2006;66(2):234-246.

19. Citron ML, Herman TS, Vreeland F, et al. Antiemetic efficacy of levonantradol compared to delta-9-tetrahydrocannabinol for chemotherapy-induced nausea and vomiting. *Cancer Treat Rep.* 1985;69(1):109-112.

20. GW Pharmaceuticals plc. Sativex prescriber information. Accessed December 22, 2020. https://gwpharm.com/products-pipeline/sativex/prescriber-information-full

21. Machado Rocha FC, Stefano SC, De Cassia Haiek R, Rosa Oliveira LM, Da Silveira DX. Therapeutic use of Cannabis sativa on chemotherapy-induced nausea and vomiting among cancer patients: systematic review and meta-analysis. *Eur J Cancer Care (Engl).* 2008;17(5):431-443.

22. Duran M, Perez E, Abanades S, et al. Preliminary efficacy and safety of an oromucosal standardized cannabis extract in chemotherapy-induced nausea and vomiting. *Br J Clin Pharmacol.* 2010;70(5):656-663.

23. Parker LA, Rock EM, Limebeer CL. Regulation of nausea and vomiting by cannabinoids. *Br J Pharmacol.* 2011;163(7):1411-1422.

24. Jatoi A, Windschitl HE, Loprinzi CL, et al. Dronabinol versus megestrol acetate versus combination therapy for cancer-associated anorexia: a North Central Cancer Treatment Group study. *J Clin Oncol.* 2002;20(2):567-573.

25. Cannabis In Cachexia Study Group, Strasser F, Luftner D, et al. Comparison of orally administered cannabis extract and delta-9-tetrahydrocannabinol in treating patients with cancer-related anorexia-cachexia syndrome: a multicenter, phase III, randomized, double-blind, placebo-controlled clinical trial from the Cannabis-In-Cachexia-Study-Group. *J Clin Oncol.* 2006;24(21):3394-3400.

26. Bar-Sela G, Vorobeichik M, Drawsheh S, Omer A, Goldberg V, Muller E. The medical necessity for medicinal cannabis: prospective, observational study evaluating the treatment in cancer patients on supportive or palliative care. *Evid Based Complement Alternat Med.* 2013;2013:510392.

27. Brisbois TD, de Kock IH, Watanabe SM, et al. Delta-9-tetrahydrocannabinol may palliate altered chemosensory perception in cancer patients: results of a randomized, double-blind, placebo-controlled pilot trial. *Ann Oncol.* 2011;22(9):2086-2093.

28. Aggarwal SK. Cannabinergic pain medicine: a concise clinical primer and survey of randomized-controlled trial results. *Clin J Pain.* 2013;29(2):162-171.

29. Martin-Sanchez E, Furukawa TA, Taylor J, Martin JL. Systematic review and meta-analysis of cannabis treatment for chronic pain. *Pain Med.* 2009;10(8):1353-1368.

30. Lynch ME, Ware MA. Cannabinoids for the treatment of chronic non-cancer pain: an updated systematic review of randomized controlled trials. *J Neuroimmune Pharmacol.* 2015;10(2):293-301.

31. Deshpande A, Mailis-Gagnon A, Zoheiry N, Lakha SF. Efficacy and adverse effects of medical marijuana for chronic noncancer pain: Systematic review of randomized controlled trials. *Can Fam Physician.* 2015;61(8):e372-381.

32. Abrams DI. Integrating cannabis into clinical cancer care. *Curr Oncol.* 2016;23(2):S8-S14.

33. Scott KA, Dalgleish AG, Liu WM. The combination of cannabidiol and Delta9-tetrahydrocannabinol enhances the anticancer effects of radiation in an orthotopic murine glioma model. *Mol Cancer Ther.* 2014;13(12):2955-2967.

34. Velasco G, Sanchez C, Guzman M. Anticancer mechanisms of cannabinoids. *Curr Oncol.* 2016;23(2):S23-32.

35. Torres S, Lorente M, Rodriguez-Fornes F, et al. A combined preclinical therapy of cannabinoids and temozolomide against glioma. *Mol Cancer Ther.* 2011;10(1):90-103.

36. Donadelli M, Dando I, Zaniboni T, et al. Gemcitabine/cannabinoid combination triggers autophagy in pancreatic cancer cells through a ROS-mediated mechanism. *Cell Death Dis.* 2011;2:e152.

37. Miyato H, Kitayama J, Yamashita H, et al. Pharmacological synergism between cannabinoids and paclitaxel in gastric cancer cell lines. *J Surg Res.* 2009;155(1):40-47.

38. Guzman M, Duarte MJ, Blazquez C, et al. A pilot clinical study of Delta9-tetrahydrocannabinol in patients with recurrent glioblastoma multiforme. *Br J Cancer.* 2006;95(2):197-203.

39. Huestis MA. Human cannabinoid pharmacokinetics. *Chem Biodivers.* 2007;4(8):1770-1804.

40. Grotenhermen F. Pharmacokinetics and pharmacodynamics of cannabinoids. *Clin Pharmacokinet.* 2003;42 (4):327-360.

41. Valiveti S, Hammell DC, Earles DC, Stinchcomb AL. Transdermal delivery of the synthetic cannabinoid WIN 55,212-2: in vitro/in vivo correlation. *Pharm Res.* 2004;21(7):1137-1145.

42. Guy GW, Robson PJ. A phase i, open label, four-way crossover study to compare the pharmacokinetic profiles of a single dose of 20 mg of a cannabis based medicine extract (CBME) administered on 3 different areas of the buccal mucosa and to investigate the pharmacokinetics of CBME per oralin healthy male and female volunteers (GWPK0112). *Journal of Cannabis Therapeutics.* 2004;3(4):79-120.

43. Kahan M, Srivastava A, Spithoff S, Bromley L. Prescribing smoked cannabis for chronic noncancer pain: preliminary recommendations. *Can Fam Physician.* 2014;60(12):1083-1090.

44. Sachs J, McGlade E, Yurgelun-Todd D. Safety and toxicology of cannabinoids. *Neurotherapeutics.* 2015;12(4):735-746.

45. Hezode C, Zafrani ES, Roudot-Thoraval F, et al. Daily cannabis use: a novel risk factor of steatosis severity in patients with chronic hepatitis C. *Gastroenterology.* 2008;134(2):432-439.

46. Aggarwal SK, Blinderman CD. Fast facts and concepts #279: cannabis for symptom control Palliative Care Network of Wisconsin. Published 2015. Accessed December 22, 2020. https://mypcnow.org/blank-vg8y7

47. DataPharm electronic Medicines Compendium. Sativex oromucosal spray summary of product characteristics (SPC). Accessed December 22, 2020. www.medicines.org.uk/emc /product/602/smpc#gref

48. Abramovici H. *Information for healthcare professionals: cannabis (marihuana, marijuana) and the cannabinoids.* Health Canada; 2018.

49. Institute of Medicine. In: Joy JE, Watson SJ Jr, Benson JA Jr, eds. *Marijuana and Medicine: Assessing the Science Base.* National Academies Press; 1999.

50. Horn JR, Hansten PD. Drug interactions with marijuana. *Pharmacy Times* website. Accessed December 22, 2020. http://pharmacytimes.com /publications/issue/2014 /december2014/drug-interactions -with-marijuana

51. Devinsky O, Cross JH, Laux L, et al. Trial of cannabidiol for drug-resistant seizures in the dravet syndrome. *N Engl J Med.* 2017;376(21):2011-2020.

52. Ruchlemer R, Amit-Kohn M, Raveh D, Hanus L. Inhaled medicinal cannabis and the immunocompromised patient. *Support Care Cancer.* 2015;23(3):819-822.

53. Raber JC, Elzinga S, Kaplan C. Understanding dabs: contamination concerns of cannabis concentrates and cannabinoid transfer during the act of dabbing. *J Toxicol Sci.* 2015;40(6):797-803.

54. Vandrey R, Raber JC, Raber ME, Douglass B, Miller C, Bonn-Miller MO. Cannabinoid dose and label accuracy in edible medical cannabis products. *JAMA.* 2015;313(24):2491-2493.

55. Americans for Safe Access. State-by-state: recommending cannabis. Accessed April 9, 2017. http://safeaccessnow.org/state_by _state_recommending_cannabis

Appendix A
Evidence-Based Guidelines and Diets for Cancer Prevention and Survival

2020–2025 Dietary Guidelines for Americans, 9th edition

General description	**Key recommendations[1]:** Follow a healthy eating pattern at every life stage. Customize and enjoy nutrient-dense food and beverage choices to reflect personal preferences, cultural traditions, and budgetary considerations. Focus on meeting food group needs with nutrient-dense foods and beverages, and stay within calorie limits. The core elements that make up a healthy dietary pattern include the following: ■ vegetables of all types: dark green, red, and orange; beans, peas, and lentils; starchy; and other vegetables ■ fruits, especially whole fruits ■ grains, at least half of which are whole grains ■ dairy, including fat-free or low-fat milk, yogurt, and cheese, or lactose-free versions and fortified soy beverages and yogurt as alternatives ■ protein foods, including lean meats, poultry, and eggs; seafood; beans, peas, and lentils; and nuts, seeds, and soy products ■ oils, including vegetable oils and oils in food, such as seafood and nuts Limit foods and beverages higher in added sugars, saturated fat, and sodium, and limit alcoholic beverages. ■ Added sugars: Consume <10% of kcal/d starting at age 2. Avoid foods and beverages with added sugars for those younger than age 2. ■ Saturated fat: Consume <10% of kcal/d starting at age 2. ■ Sodium: Consume <2,300 mg/d, and even less for children younger than age 14. ■ Alcoholic beverages: Adults of legal age can choose not to drink or to drink in moderation by limiting intake to two drinks or less in a day for men and one drink or less a day for women. Some adults should not drink alcohol, such as women who are pregnant.
Proposed mechanism or goal	To reduce chronic-disease risk by translating science into food-based guidance
Food groups excluded	None; but the guidelines endorse a greater intake of foods considered beneficial to good health and a reduced intake of foods potentially detrimental to health.
Side effects and nutritional risks	None. Consuming a wide variety of healthful, cancer-fighting foods within a plant-based diet promotes good health.
Dietary supplements recommended or indicated	Not generally indicated. The guidelines provide a wide variety of nutrients associated with good health and a wide range of cancer-preventive bioactive compounds. Registered dietitian nutritionists should provide dietary supplement recommendations when indicated by a nutrition assessment.

Efficacy studied in clinical trials	The Dietary Guidelines Advisory Committee analyzed and reviewed relevant evidence, including "original systematic reviews; existing scientific reviews; meta-analyses; reports by federal agencies or leading scientific organizations; data analyses; and food pattern modeling analyses" before developing and implementing the guidelines.[2]
Comments	These guidelines serve as the evidence-based foundation for nutrition education materials developed for the public by the federal government.
	Appendix 2 of the guidelines includes information on a healthy US-style eating pattern, including recommended amounts of food to consume from each food group at 12 calorie levels.
	This diet is recommended for most Americans and cancer survivors.

References

1. US Department of Health and Human Services, US Department of Agriculture. *2020-2025 Dietary Guidelines for Americans*. 9th ed. US Department of Agriculture; 2020. Accessed January 6, 2021. www .DietaryGuidelines.gov

2. Dietary Guidelines Advisory Committee. *Scientific Report of the 2020 Dietary Guidelines Advisory Committee: Advisory Report to the Secretary of Agriculture and the Secretary of Health and Human Services*. US Department of Agriculture, Agricultural Research Service; 2020. Accessed January 6, 2021. www.dietaryguidelines.gov /2020-advisory-committee-report

American Cancer Society Guideline on Diet and Physical Activity for Cancer Prevention

General description	**Key recommendations[1,2]:**
	Achieve and maintain a healthy body weight throughout life.
	Be physically active.
	▪ Adults should engage in 150 to 300 minutes of moderate-intensity physical activity per week, or 75 to 150 minutes of vigorous-intensity physical activity, or an equivalent combination; achieving or exceeding the upper limit of 300 minutes is optimal.
	▪ Children and adolescents should engage in at least 1 hour of moderate- or vigorous-intensity activity each day.
	▪ Limit sedentary behavior, such as sitting, lying down, and watching television, and other forms of screen-based entertainment.
	Follow a healthy eating pattern at all ages. This includes:
	▪ foods that are high in nutrients in amounts that help achieve and maintain a healthy body weight
	▪ a variety of vegetables—dark green, red, and orange, fiber-rich legumes (beans and peas), and others
	▪ fruits, especially whole fruits with a variety of colors; and whole grains
	A healthy eating pattern limits, or does not include, red and processed meats, sugar-sweetened beverages, and highly processed foods and refined grain products.
	It is best not to drink alcohol. People who do choose to drink alcohol should limit their consumption to no more than 1 drink per day for women and 2 drinks per day for men.
	Recommendation for community action: Public, private, and community organizations should work collaboratively at national, state, and local levels to develop, advocate for, and implement policy and environmental changes that increase access to affordable, nutritious foods; provide safe, enjoyable, and accessible opportunities for physical activity; and limit alcohol for all individuals.
Proposed mechanism or goal	To reduce cancer risk by eating a healthy diet with an emphasis on plant foods
Food groups excluded	None; but the guidelines endorse a greater intake of foods associated with decreased cancer risk and a lower intake of foods associated with greater cancer risk.
Side effects and nutritional risks	None. Consuming a wide variety of healthful, cancer-fighting foods within a plant-based diet promotes good health.
Dietary supplements recommended or indicated	Not generally indicated. The guidelines provide a wide variety of nutrients associated with good health and a wide range of cancer-preventive bioactive compounds.
	Registered dietitian nutritionists should provide dietary supplement recommendations when indicated by a nutrition assessment.

Efficacy studied in clinical trials	Consistent evidence associating certain dietary factors and dietary patterns with cancer provides a strong basis for these guidelines.
Comments	The American Cancer Society website provides resources that support their guidelines on diet and physical activity for cancer prevention.
	These guidelines are also appropriate for cancer survivors.

References

1. Rock CL, Thomson C, Gansler T, et al. American Cancer Society guideline for diet and physical activity for cancer prevention. *CA A Cancer J Clin*. 2020;70:245-271. doi:10.3322/caac.21591

2. American Cancer Society guideline on diet and physical activity. American Cancer Society. Accessed January 6, 2021. www.cancer.org/healthy/eat-healthy-get-active/acs-guidelines-nutrition-physical-activity-cancer-prevention/guidelines.html

World Cancer Research Fund/American Institute for Cancer Research Cancer Prevention Recommendations

General description	**Key recommendations[1]:** Be a healthy weight. Be physically active. Eat a diet rich in whole grains, vegetables, fruits, and beans. Consume at least 30 g of dietary fiber daily from food, and eat at least 400 g or 15 oz of a variety of nonstarchy vegetables and fruit daily. Limit consumption of "fast foods" and other processed foods high in fat, starches, or sugars. Limit consumption of red and processed meats to <350 to 500 g (12 to 18 oz) cooked weight daily, and consume very little, if any, processed meat. Limit consumption of sugar-sweetened drinks (or preferably, do not consume any). Limit alcohol consumption (or preferably, do not drink alcohol). Do not use supplements for cancer prevention; aim to meet nutritional needs through diet alone. For mothers: Breastfeed, if possible. For those with a cancer diagnosis: Follow the above recommendations, if possible; all cancer survivors should receive nutritional care and guidance on physical activity from trained professionals.
Proposed mechanism or goal	To reduce cancer risk and promote cancer survivorship via cancer prevention recommendations based on comprehensive analysis of the research on diet, nutrition, physical activity, and cancer
Food groups excluded	None; but the recommendations endorse a greater intake of foods associated with lower cancer risk and a reduced intake of foods associated with greater cancer risk.
Side effects and nutritional risks	None. Consuming a wide variety of healthful, cancer-fighting foods within a plant-based diet promotes good health.
Dietary supplements recommended or indicated	The use of supplements for cancer prevention is cautioned against. The recommendations provide a wide variety of nutrients and a wide range of cancer-preventive bioactive compounds. Registered dietitian nutritionist should provide dietary supplement recommendations when indicated by a nutrition assessment.
Efficacy studied in clinical trials	The recommendations are based on rigorous and continuous reviews of research examining links between diet, nutrition, cancer risk, and survival.[2]

Comments	To reduce cancer risk, World Cancer Research Fund(WCRF)/American Institute for Cancer Research (AICR) recommends filling two-thirds (or more) of each meal plate with a variety of vegetables, fruits, whole grains, and beans, and one-third (or less) of each meal plate with animal protein.
	WCRF/AICR publishes a variety of nutrition education materials to facilitate implementation of their recommendations, including AICR's New American Plate.[3]
	These recommendations are appropriate for cancer survivors.
	More information about reducing cancer risk through diet and meal plan recommendations are available on these AICR webpages:

- www.aicr.org/reduce-your-cancer-risk/diet
- www.aicr.org/new-american-plate
- www.aicr.org/new-american-plate/cancer-preventive-diet-model-plate.html
- www.aicr.org/new-american-plate/eat-healthy-customize-your-diet-new-american-plate.html
- www.aicr.org/healthyrecipes
- www.aicr.org/healthyrecipes/aicr-recipe-guidelines.html

References

1. Recommendations for cancer prevention. American Institute for Cancer Research. Accessed May 22, 2020. www.aicr.org/cancer-prevention

2. Continuous Update Project: Diet, nutrition, physical activity and the prevention of cancer: Summary of strong evidence. World Cancer Research Fund International/ American Institute for Cancer Research. Accessed May 24, 2020. www.wcrf.org/sites/default/files/Matrix-for-all-cancers-A3.pdf

3. New American plate. American Institute for Cancer Research. Accessed January 6, 2021. www.aicr.org/new-american-plate

2020-2025 Dietary Guidelines for Americans, 9th ed: Healthy Mediterranean-Style Diet

General description

Key recommendations[1-3]:

Include whole grains, legumes, vegetables, nuts, seeds, and fruits.

Include moderate amounts of fish.

Limit red and processed meats and saturated fats.

Use extra virgin olive oil (EVOO) as the primary fat.

Include moderate amounts of low-fat dairy products.

Include moderate amounts of wine (usually red) with meals.

Limit processed foods and refined sugar.

Definitions of the Mediterranean diet vary. Common descriptions and recommendations for adults, including those used in research, include the following[1-3]:

- Vegetable intake: at least two servings at each meal or six servings daily
- Fruit intake: one to two servings at each meal or three servings daily
- Bread and cereal intake: one to two servings at each meal or up to eight servings daily
- Olive oil: at every meal
- Egg intake: two to four servings weekly
- Nut intake: one to two servings daily or three to four servings weekly
- Dairy food intake: two servings daily
- Legume intake: at least two servings weekly or three to four servings weekly
- Red meat intake: fewer than two servings weekly or fewer than four servings monthly
- Fish intake: at least two servings weekly or five to six servings weekly
- Poultry intake: two to four servings weekly
- Sweet food intake: two to three servings weekly
- Red wine: daily and in moderation
- Fiber intake: 31 to 33 g/d
- Mean daily macronutrient distribution as a percentage of energy has been estimated at 14.9% protein, 42.8% carbohydrate, 36.6% fat, 9% saturated fat, and 18.8% monounsaturated fat, with 31 to 33 g of fiber.[1-3]

Several food guides for the Mediterranean diet are available, including one provided by Oldways (https://oldwayspt.org/blog/happy-25-years-mediterranean-diet-pyramid).

Proposed mechanism or goal

Plant-based diets with low energy densities are consistent with established cancer-preventive diet research.[1-3]

Following a healthful eating pattern that provides a wide range of bioactive compounds and nutrients, dietary fibers, omega-3 fats, and monounsaturated fats while limiting added sweets, red meats, and solid fats is associated with reduced risk for chronic disease.[1-4]

Food groups excluded

None. This diet includes a wide variety of food and encourages a greater intake of foods considered beneficial to good health and cancer prevention while limiting red meats and added sugars, which are discouraged on a cancer-fighting diet.

Side effects and nutritional risks	None. Consuming a wide variety of healthful, cancer-fighting foods within a plant-based diet promotes good health.
Dietary supplements recommended or indicated	Not indicated. The diet provides a wide variety of foods and nutrients associated with good health and a wide range of cancer-preventive bioactive compounds.[1-4] Registered dietitian nutritionists should provide dietary supplement recommendations when indicated by a nutrition assessment.
Efficacy studied in clinical trials	Epidemiological studies suggest the Mediterranean diet is a dietary model for primary and secondary prevention of many chronic diseases.[3,4] Incidence of cancer in Mediterranean countries is lower than in the United States, United Kingdom, and Scandinavian countries.[3] The European Prospective Investigation into Cancer and Nutrition study associated lower overall cancer risk with greater adherence to a Mediterranean diet.[4] A meta-analysis associated adherence to a Mediterranean diet with reduced risk of all-cause cancer mortality and colorectal, breast, gastric, prostate, liver, head and neck, and pancreatic cancers.[5] A trial comparing a Mediterranean diet (already high in olive oil) supplemented with additional EVOO (subjects received 1 L of free EVOO weekly for themselves and their families) vs a Mediterranean diet supplemented with nuts vs a control (low-fat) diet found that those on the EVOO-supplemented Mediterranean diet experienced a 62% lower risk of malignant breast cancer than those on the control (low-fat) diet.[6] Higher Mediterranean-diet scores, which suggest greater adherence to a Mediterranean diet, are inversely associated with colorectal cancer risk.[1] A case-control study involving Greek-Cypriot women did not show a reduced breast-cancer risk overall but did show a reduced risk for breast cancer was associated with a greater intake of vegetables, fish, and olive oil.[7]
Comments	Appendix 3 of the Dietary Guidelines for Americans 2020–2025 provides information on a healthy Mediterranean-style eating pattern, including recommended portions to consume from relevant food categories at 12 calorie levels.[8] This diet is appropriate for most Americans and cancer survivors.

References

1. Davis C, Bryan J, Hodgson J, Murphy K. Definition of the Mediterranean diet; a literature review. *Nutrients.* 2015;7(11):9139-9153. doi:10.3390/nu7115459

2. Romagnolo DF, Selmin OI. Mediterranean diet and prevention of chronic diseases. *Nutr Today.* 2017;52(5):208-222.

3. Qaqundah M. Mediterranean diet for cancer prevention: a review of the evidence and a guide to adherence. *Nat Med J.* 2017;9(5). Accessed February 12, 2018. www.naturalmedicinejournal.com/journal/2017-05/mediterranean-diet-cancer-prevention

4. Couto E, Boffeta P, Lagiou BP, et al. Mediterranean dietary pattern and cancer risk in the EPIC cohort. *Br J Cancer.* 2011;104(9):1493-1499.

5. Schwingshaki L, Schwedhelm C, Galbete C, Hoffman G. Adherence to Mediterranean diet and risk of cancer: an updated systematic review and meta-analysis. *Nutrients.* 2017;9(10). doi:10.3390/nu9101063

6. Toledo E, Salas-Salvadó J, Donat-Vargas C, et al. Mediterranean diet and invasive breast cancer risk among women at high cardiovascular risk in the PREDIMED Trial: a randomized clinical trial. *JAMA Intern Med.* 2015;175(11):1752-1760.

7. Demetriou CA, Hadjisavvas A, Loizidou MA. The Mediterranean dietary pattern and breast cancer risk in Greek-Cypriot women: a case control study. *BMC Cancer.* 2012;12:113. doi:10.1186/1471-2407-12-113

8. US Department of Health and Human Services, US Department of Agriculture. *2020-2025 Dietary Guidelines for Americans.* 9th ed. US Department of Agriculture; 2020. Accessed January 6, 2021. www.DietaryGuidelines.gov

2020–2025 Dietary Guidelines for Americans, 9th edition: Healthy Vegetarian Diet

General description	Healthy vegetarian diets exclude flesh foods, may exclude dairy products and eggs, and include a wide variety of vegetables and fruits, whole grains, legumes, soy products, nuts, and seeds.[1,2]
	A lacto-vegetarian diet includes dairy products. An ovo-vegetarian diet includes eggs. A lacto-ovo-vegetarian diet includes dairy and eggs.
	A pescatarian diet includes fish and seafood.[1-4]
Proposed mechanism or goal	Vegetarians avoid meat for health, religious, philosophical, and ethical reasons.[4] Benefits of a healthy vegetarian diet include lower body mass index (BMI) and consumption of a generous amount of phytochemicals, both of which are associated with cancer prevention.[4]
	A meta-analysis of 12 weight-loss studies suggested vegetarian diets promote greater weight loss than other weight-reduction diets.[5] Losing weight via a diet providing a healthy variety of foods helps maintain overall nutritional status while promoting a normal BMI, and maintaining weight within the normal BMI range helps reduce cancer risk.
Food groups excluded	Flesh foods; sometimes dairy products; sometimes eggs; sometimes both dairy products and eggs[1-4]
Side effects and nutritional risks	Vegetarian diets increase the risk for deficiencies of vitamins B12 and D, iron, zinc, calcium, and iodine and possibly increase the risk for protein deficiency.[1,2,6,7]
	Protein intake should be adequate when energy needs are met[1]; regularly consuming legumes and soy foods will help meet protein needs.[1]
	Reported incidence of vitamin B12 deficiency varies[7] but is expected in 50% or more of vegetarians[8]; this also applies to vegans. Reliable supplementation with B12 is essential.[1]
	Calcium intake should be sufficient in lacto-ovo-vegetarians but may be insufficient when dairy products are excluded.[1]
	Iodized salt and sea vegetables are common vegetarian sources of iodine.[1] Vegetarians need to consume adequate iodine; a reliable iodine supplement may be needed.[1]
	For vegetarians, the Dietary Reference Intake for iron is 1.8 times that for nonvegetarians,[1] and iron stores in vegetarians are lower than in nonvegetarians.[1] As iron stores decline, the body adapts to increase absorption of nonheme iron,[9] but deficiency remains a risk.[1] Iron in soy exists in the form of ferritin, and absorption is considered good.[10,11]
	Zinc status of vegetarians is lower than that of nonvegetarians but is usually within the normal range.[1] Nevertheless, it is important to monitor for signs of zinc deficiency.
Dietary supplements recommended or indicated	Supplements may be needed to maintain sufficient stores of vitamins B12 and D, iron, zinc, calcium, and iodine. Registered dietitian nutritionists should provide specific dietary supplement recommendations when indicated by a nutrition assessment.

Efficacy studied in clinical trials	A meta-analysis of seven studies reported an 18% lower overall cancer incidence in vegetarians vs nonvegetarians.[12]
	The Adventist Health Study 2 suggested vegetarians have a reduced risk for colon, rectal, and colorectal cancers when compared with nonvegetarians.[13]
	The California Teachers Study found a lower risk for breast cancer (and, in particular, for estrogen-receptor-negative and progesterone-receptor-negative tumors) among women following a plant-based dietary pattern.[14]
	A prospective study of low-risk men and women in the Adventist Health Study 2 found an inverse association between lacto-ovo-vegetarians (vs meat eaters) and gastrointestinal cancers.[15]
	A small study of Taiwanese women showed an inverse association between breast cancer risk and vegetarian diets; those on vegetarian diets also consumed more soy.[16]
Comments	"It is the position of the Academy of Nutrition and Dietetics that appropriately planned vegetarian, including vegan, diets are healthful, nutritionally adequate, and may provide health benefits for the prevention and treatment of certain diseases."[1]
	Vegetarian diets must be nutritionally balanced and adequate to derive optimal health benefits associated with vegetarianism.[2]
	Appendix 3 of the Dietary Guidelines for Americans 2020–2025 provides information on a healthy vegetarian eating pattern, including recommended portions to consume from relevant food categories at 12 calorie levels.[3]

References

1. Melina V, Craig W, Levin S. Position of the Academy of Nutrition and Dietetics: vegetarian diets. *J Acad Nutr Diet*. 2016;116(12):1970-1980.

2. Rizzo G, Lagana AS, Rapisarda AMC, et al. Vitamin B12 among vegetarians: status, assessment and supplementation. *Nutrients*. 2016;8(12):767. doi:10.3390/nu8120767

3. US Department of Agriculture, US Department of Health and Human Services. *Dietary Guidelines for Americans, 2020-2025*. 9th ed. US Department of Agriculture. December 2020. Accessed January 6, 2021. www.DietaryGuidelines.gov

4. Becoming a vegetarian. Harvard Health Publishing: Harvard Women's Health Watch. Accessed May 20, 2020. www.health.harvard.edu/staying-healthy/becoming-a-vegetarian

5. Tonstad S, Butler T, Yan R, Fraser GE. Type of vegetarian diet, body weight, and prevalence of type 2 diabetes. *Diabetes Care*. 2009;32(5):791-796.

6. Herbert V. Staging vitamin B12 (cobalamin) status in vegetarians. *Am J Clin Nutr*. 1994;59(5 suppl):S1213–S1222.

7. Wantanabe F, Yabuta Y, Bito T, Teng F. Vitamin B12-containing plant food sources for vegetarians. *Nutrients*. 2014;6(5):1861-1873.

8. Pawlak R. RD Resources for consumers: vitamin b12 in vegetarian diets. Vegetarian Nutrition Dietetic Practice Group, Academy of Nutrition and Dietetics. Accessed May 20, 2020. https://vndpg.org/docs/rd-resources/B12-RD.pdf

9. Trost LB, Bergfeld WF, Calogeras E. The diagnosis and treatment of iron deficiency and its potential relationship to hair loss. *J Am Acad Dermatol*. 2006;54(5):824-844.

10. Murray-Kolb LE, Welch R, Theil EC, Beard JL. Women with low iron stores absorb iron from soybeans. *Am J Clin Nutr*. 2003;77(1):180–184.

11. Lonnerdal B, Bryant A, Liu X, Theil E.C. Iron absorption from soybean ferritin in nonanemic women. *Am J Clin Nutr*. 2006;83(1):103–107.

12. Huang T, Zheng YB, G Li, Wahlqvist ML, Li D. Cardiovascular disease mortality and cancer incidence in vegetarians: a meta-analysis and systematic review. *Ann Nutr Metab*. 2012;60(4):233-240.

13. Orlich M, Singh PN, Sabate J, et al. Vegetarian dietary patterns and the risk of colorectal cancers. *JAMA Intern Med*. 2015;175(5):767-776.

14. Link LB, Canchola A, Bernstein L, et al. Dietary patterns and breast cancer risk in the California Teachers Study Cohort. *Am J Clin Nutr*. 2013;98(6):1524-1532.

15. Tantamango-Bartley Y, Jaceldo-Siegl K, Fan J, Fraser G. Vegetarian diets and the incidence of cancer in a low-risk population. *Cancer Epidemiol Biomarkers Prev*. 2013;22(2):286-294.

16. Chang Y-J, Hou Y-C, Chen LJ, et al. Is vegetarian diet associated with a lower risk of breast cancer in Taiwanese women? *BMC Public Health*. 2017;17:800. doi:10.1186/s12889-017-4819-1

Vegan Diet

General description	A healthy vegan diet excludes flesh foods, dairy foods, and eggs and includes a wide variety of vegetables, fruits, whole grains, legumes, soy products, nuts, and seeds.[1-4]
Proposed mechanism or goal	Vegans avoid meat for health, religious, philosophical, and ethical reasons.[3] Benefits of a healthy vegan diet include lower body mass index (BMI) and consumption of a generous amount of phytochemicals, both of which are associated with cancer prevention.[3,4]
	Plant-based dietary patterns are associated with lower BMIs, which in turn are associated with lower cancer risk.[5]
	Gut microbiota of vegans may confer health (eg, anticancer) advantages, partly by reducing inflammation.[6]
	Vegan diets, when compared with other eating patterns, provide higher Healthy Eating Index and Mediterranean diet scores, which suggests the potential for better health outcomes.[7]
Food groups excluded	Flesh foods, dairy products, honey, and eggs[1-4]
Side effects and nutritional risks	Vegan diets increase the risk for deficiencies of vitamins B12 and D, iron, zinc, calcium, and iodine, and possibly increase the risk for protein deficiency.[1-3,7-9]
	Protein intake should be adequate when energy needs are met; regularly consuming legumes and soy foods will help meet protein needs.[1]
	Reported incidence of vitamin B12 deficiency varies[10] but is expected in 50% or more of vegetarians[8]; this also applies to vegans. Reliable supplementation with B12 is essential.[1]
	Calcium intake may be insufficient in vegans. Low-oxalate, vegan sources of calcium (eg, kale, turnip greens, Chinese cabbage, and bok choy), allowed calcium-fortified plant beverages, and calcium-set tofu help vegans consume recommended amounts of calcium.[1] Calcium in soy is absorbed equally as well as calcium in milk.[11]
	Iodized salt and sea vegetables are common vegetarian sources of iodine. It is essential for vegetarians to consume adequate iodine; a reliable iodine supplement may be needed.[1]
	For vegetarians and vegans, the Dietary Reference Intake for iron is 1.8 times that for nonvegetarians.[1] Iron in soy exists in the form of ferritin, and absorption is considered good.[12-13] As iron stores decline, the body adapts to increase absorption of nonheme iron,[14] but deficiency remains a risk.[1]
	Zinc status of vegetarians is lower than that of nonvegetarians but is usually within the normal range.[1] Nevertheless, it is important to monitor for signs of zinc deficiency.
	Cooking food can improve its digestibility and increase micronutrient absorption, so it is important to consume recommended amounts and varieties of foods to ensure adequate nutrient intake.
Dietary supplements recommended or indicated	Supplements may be needed to maintain sufficient stores of vitamins B12 and D, iron, zinc, calcium, and iodine. Registered dietitian nutritionists should provide specific dietary supplement recommendations when indicated by a nutrition assessment.

Efficacy studied in clinical trials	Vegan diets reduce risk of cancer more than any other diet pattern.[9]
	Vegan diets provide lower amounts of essential amino acids than diets that include animal meat. This is associated with the activation of general control nonderepressible 2, which is believed to downregulate insulin-like growth factor 1 and thereby reduce cancer risk.[15] However, it is still important to meet protein needs.
	Among participants in the Adventist Health Study 2 cohort, vegans experienced a 14% reduced all-cancer risk when compared with nonvegetarians but a 73% increased risk for urinary tract cancer.[16]
Comments	"It is the position of the Academy of Nutrition and Dietetics that appropriately planned vegetarian, including vegan, diets are healthful, nutritionally adequate, and may provide health benefits for the prevention and treatment of certain diseases."[1]
	The Vegetarian Nutrition dietetic practice group of the Academy of Nutrition and Dietetics provides resources for healthy vegan diets.[17]
	Vegan diets must be nutritionally balanced and adequate to derive optimal health benefits associated with vegetarianism.[2]

References

1. Melina V, Craig W, Levin S. Position of the Academy of Nutrition and Dietetics: vegetarian diets. *J Acad Nutr Diet.* 2016;116(12):1970-1980.

2. Rizzo G, Lagana AS, Rapisarda AMC, et al. Vitamin B12 among vegetarians: status, assessment and supplementation. *Nutrients.* 2016;8(12):767. doi:10.3390/nu8120767

3. Becoming a vegetarian. Harvard Health Publishing: Harvard Women's Health Watch. Accessed May 20, 2020. www.health.harvard.edu/staying-healthy/becoming-a-vegetarian

4. US Department of Agriculture, US Department of Health and Human Services. *Dietary Guidelines for Americans, 2020-2025.* 9th ed. US Department of Agriculture. December 2020. Accessed January 6, 2021. www.DietaryGuidelines.gov

5. Tonstad S, Butler T, Yan R, Fraser GE. Type of vegetarian diet, body weight, and prevalence of type 2 diabetes. *Diabetes Care.* 2009;32(5):791-796.

6. Glick-Bauer M, Yeh MC. The health advantage of a vegan diet: exploring the gut microbiota connection. *Nutrients.* 2013;6(11):4822-4838.

7. Clarys P, Deliens T, Huybrechts I, et al. Comparison of nutritional quality of the vegan, vegetarian, semi-vegetarian, pesco-vegetarian and omnivorous diet. *Nutrients.* 2014;6(3):1319-1332.

8. Pawlak R. RD Resources for consumers: vitamin b12 in vegetarian diets. Vegetarian Nutrition Dietetic Practice Group, Academy of Nutrition and Dietetics. Accessed May 20, 2020. https://vndpg.org/docs/rd-resources/B12-RD.pdf

9. Herbert V. Staging vitamin B12 (cobalamin) status in vegetarians. *Am J Clin Nutr.* 1994;59(5 suppl):S1213–S1222.

10. Wantanabe F, Yabuta Y, Bito T, Teng F. Vitamin B12-containing plant food sources for vegetarians. *Nutrients.* 2014;6(5):1861-1873.

11. Weaver CM, Heaney RP, Connor L, Martin BR, Smith DL, Nielsen E. Bioavailability of calcium from tofu as compared with milk in premenopausal women. *J Food Sci.* 2006. doi:10.1111/j.1365-2621.2002.tb08873.x

12. Murray- Kolb LE, Welch R, Theil EC, Beard JL. Women with low iron stores absorb iron from soybeans. *Am J Clin Nutr.* 2003;77(1):180–184.

13. Lonnerdal B, Bryant A, Liu X, Theil EC. Iron absorption from soybean ferritin in nonanemic women. *Am J Clin Nutr.* 2006;83(1):103–107.

14. Trost LB, Bergfeld WF, Calogeras E. The diagnosis and treatment of iron deficiency and its potential relationship to hair loss. *J Am Acad Dermatol.* 2006;54(5):824-844.

15. McCarty MF. GCN2 and FGF21 are likely mediators of the protection from cancer, autoimmunity, obesity, and diabetes afforded by vegan diets. *Med Hypotheses.* 2014;83(3):365-371.

16. Le LT, Sabate J. Beyond meatless, the health effects of vegan diets: findings from the Adventist Cohorts. *Nutrients.* 2014;6(6):213-2147. doi:10.3390/nu6062131

17. RD Resources. Vegetarian Nutrition Dietetic Practice Group, Academy of Nutrition and Dietetics. Accessed February 6, 2018. https://vndpg.org/rd-resources

Intermittent Fasting

General description	Intermittent fasting (IF) involves the consumption of little or no food for a specific period of time—from 24 hours to 6 days, though a more common interval is 16 to 48 hours—with intervening periods of normal food intake. IF can result in a significantly reduced energy intake that preclinical studies suggest may extend life span and reduce cancer risk via metabolic alterations such as reduced inflammation, reduced angiogenesis, and lower insulinlike growth factor 1 (IGF-1) levels while also improving insulin sensitivity.[1] IF has also been linked with fewer cancer treatment–related side effects.[2]
	The 5:2 IF protocol consists of 5 days of typical energy consumption with 2 nonconsecutive days of 500 kcal or fewer.[3]
	IF offers health benefits equivalent to prolonged fasting or energy restriction.[4]
Proposed mechanism or goal	IF has demonstrated efficacy for various health issues, resulting in weight loss, improved insulin sensitivity, cardiovascular improvements, and anti-inflammatory benefits.[5-7]
	The metabolic benefits require fasting-mediated increases of vascular endothelial growth factor expression in adipose tissue, which aids the process of thermogenesis.[4]
	The observed anticancer effect is likely due to enhanced oxidative stress and DNA damage during short-term fasting on cancer cells.[1]
	Researchers suggest that some of the beneficial effects are due to the reduction in IGF-1, insulin, and glucose and the increase in insulinlike growth factor–binding protein 1 (IGFBP1) and ketone bodies, which create an environment that forces cancer cells to rely more heavily on metabolites and factors that are limited in the blood, thus resulting in cell death.[7]
Food groups excluded	All, except water, during periods of fasting
Side effects and nutritional risks	Hunger, malnutrition, and potential loss of muscle mass can occur.
	Protocols that allow intermittent energy restriction rather than complete fasting may be preferred for cancer patients; not only would compliance likely improve, but consuming a minimum of 50 g of protein daily would help patients stay in appropriate nitrogen balance and better maintain muscle mass.[8]
	Maintaining appropriate energy intake on nonrestricted days is important, as excess consumption may negate some of the beneficial health effects of intermittent energy restriction (IER).
Dietary supplements recommended or indicated	None
Efficacy studied in clinical trials	During cancer treatment, short-term fasting has improved the efficacy of some chemotherapy agents, including cisplatin, cyclophosphamide, and doxorubicin.[2]
	Short-term weight loss in overweight and obese adults was significantly greater for those following IER and continuous energy restriction than for those following no treatment.[9]
	Short-term fasting improved chemotherapeutic treatment with etoposide,[10] mitoxantrone, oxaliplatin,[11] cisplatin, cyclophosphamide, and doxorubicin[12] in transgenic and transplant mouse models of neuroblastoma, fibrosarcoma, glioma, melanoma, and breast and ovarian cancers.

| Efficacy studied in clinical trials (continued) | Radiosensitivity of mammary tumors in mice improved with alternate-day fasting.[13,14]

Data from animal studies reveal nonsignificant trends toward improved cancer survival with some IF regimens.[15]

Multiple randomized trials are underway to assess the effects of IER in combination with various chemotherapy treatments in cancer patients.

Research suggests that shorter periods of IF (eg, ≥13 h/d), referred to as IER, may also be beneficial.[3]

A review of eating intervals in 2,400 women with breast cancer found that those fasting for fewer than 13 hours per night were at a 36% increased risk for breast cancer recurrence.[16] |
| Comments | Patients with type 2 diabetes taking hypoglycemic medications are advised to use caution with IF due to the increased rate of hypoglycemia.[17]

Cancer survivors wishing to use IF or IER either during or after treatment should meet with a registered dietitian nutritionist to discuss concerns, strategies, and options for maintaining long-term nutritional status.

A published summary of cancer and fasting is available from the Osher Center for Integrative Medicine at the University of California, San Francisco.[3] |

References

1. O'Flanagan CH, Smith LA, McDonell SB, Hursting SD. When less may be more: calorie restriction and response to cancer therapy. *BMC Med*. 2017;15:106. doi:10.1186/s12916-017-0873-x

2. Lee C, Raffaghello L, Brandhorst S, et al. Fasting cycles retard growth of tumors and sensitize a range of cancer cell types of chemotherapy. *Sci Transl Med*. 2012;4(124):124a27. doi:10.1126/scitranslmed.30032933

3. Cancer and fasting/calorie restriction. University of California San Francisco Osher Center for Integrative Medicine. Accessed May 20, 2020. https://osher.ucsf.edu/patient-care/integrative-medicine-resources/cancer-and-nutrition/faq/cancer-and-fasting-calorie-restriction

4. Kim KH, Kim YH, Son JE, et al. Intermittent fasting promotes adipose thermogenesis and metabolic homeostasis via VEGF-mediated alternative activation of macrophage. *Cell Res*. 2017;27(11):1309-1326. Epub 2017 Oct 17. doi:10.1038/cr.2017.126

5. Mattson MP, Longo VD, Harvie M. Impact of intermittent fasting on health and disease processes. *Ageing Res Rev*. 2017;39:46-58. doi:10.1016/j.arr.2016.10.005

6. White E. The role for autophagy in cancer. *J Clin Invest*. 2015;125:42–6.

7. Buono R, Longo VD. Starvation, stress resistance, and cancer. *Trends Endocrinol Metab*. 2018;29(4):271-280. doi:10.1016/j.tem.2018.01.008

8. Harvie MN, Howell T. Could intermittent energy restriction and intermittent fasting reduce rates of cancer in obese, overweight, and normal-weight subjects? A summary of evidence. *Advances in Nutrition*. 2016;7(4):690-705. doi:10.3945/an.115.011767

9. Harris L, Hamilton S, Azevedo LB, et al. Intermittent fasting interventions for treatment of overweight and obesity in adults: a systematic review and meta-analysis. *JBI Database System Rev Implement Rep*. 2018 Feb;16(2):507-547. doi:10.11124/JBISRIR-2016-003248

10. Caderni G, Perrelli MG, Cecchini F, Tessitore L. Enhanced growth of colorectal aberrant crypt foci in fasted/refed rats involves changes in TGFbeta1 and p21CIP expressions. *Carcinogenesis* 2002;23:323–327.

11. Hsieh EA, Chai CM, Hellerstein MK. Effects of caloric restriction on cell proliferation in several tissues in mice: role of intermittent feeding. *Am J Physiol Endocrinol Metab*. 2005;288:E985-972.

12. Varady KA, Roohk DJ, Bruss M, Hellerstein MK. Alternate-day fasting reduces global cell proliferation rates independently of dietary fat content in mice. *Nutrition*. 2009;25(4):486–491.

13. Tomasi C, Laconi E, Laconi S, Greco M, Sarma DS, Pani P. Effect of fasting/refeeding on the incidence of chemically induced hepatocellular carcinoma in the rat. *Carcinogenesis*.1999;20(10):1979–1983.

14. Varady KA, Roohk DJ, Hellerstein MK. Dose effects of modified alternate-day fasting regimens on in vivo cell proliferation and plasma insulin-like growth factor-1 in mice. *J Appl Physiol*. 2007;103(2):547–551.

15. Buschemeyer WC, Klink JC, Mavropoulos JC, et al. Effect of intermittent fasting with or without caloric restriction on prostate cancer growth and survival in SCID mice. *Prostate*. 2010;70(10):1037-1043.

16. Marinac CR, Nelson SH, Breen CI, et al. Prolonged nightly fasting and breast cancer prognosis. *JAMA Oncol*. 2016;2(8):1049-1055.

17. Corley BT, Carroll RW, Hall RM, Weatherall M, Parry-Strong A, Krebs JD. Intermittent fasting in type 2 diabetes mellitus and the risk of hypoglycaemia: a randomized controlled trial. *Diabet Med*. 2018;35(5):588-594. doi:10.1111/dme.13595

Ketogenic Diet

General description	The ketogenic diet (KD) is a high-fat, moderate-protein, very-low-carbohydrate diet.[1,2]
	Common macronutrient distribution (standard version) is 90% fat, 8% protein, 2% carbohydrate.[1,2]
	The modified version consists of approximately 80% fat, 15% protein, and 5% carbohydrate.[3]
	The modified KD may help preserve weight and improve tolerance (as compared to the standard version) while still accomplishing treatment goals.[4]
Proposed mechanism or goal	Cancer cells rely on aerobic glycolysis for energy, which is inefficient and requires large amounts of glucose. This diet and its modified version reduce the amount of glucose available for aerobic glycolysis.[5]
	Gliomas cannot use ketones for energy (as normal brain cells can); therefore, this diet deprives glioma cells of energy and promotes their death.[6]
Food groups excluded	Most carbohydrate-containing foods are avoided, so grains, fruits, milk, sugar, and sweets are severely restricted or avoided.
Side effects and nutritional risks	Side effects include nausea, vomiting, lethargy, gastrointestinal discomfort (including constipation), hypercholesterolemia, renal damage, kidney stones, and bone mineral loss.[1,2,7,8]
	This diet may promote weight loss and cachexia.[8]
	In about 6% of people following this diet, kidney stones occur due to a buildup of calcium in the urine. Research reports some success in preventing this via potassium citrate (appropriate dose taken twice daily).[2]
	Selenium, copper, and zinc deficiencies have been reported[1] but were associated with a specific brand of formula (Ketonformula) used in Japan.[9] Registered dietitian nutritionists (RDNs) should be aware of this potential concern, though it has not been reported in KDs providing whole foods.
	Adverse effects are more prevalent in children than in adults.
Dietary supplements recommended or indicated	The limited variety of foods consumed requires general multivitamin and mineral supplementation.
	The International Ketogenic Diet Study Group states that standard multivitamin and mineral supplements are acceptable as long as they are sugar-free, though additional vitamin D and calcium supplementation may be indicated.[10]
Efficacy studied in clinical trials	Preclinical studies suggest that this diet may enhance the effectiveness of chemotherapy.[1,2,4]
	This diet may reduce tumor growth and improve survival in patients with glioma and neuroblastoma.[8,11,12]
	Research is underway on the role of the KD in cancer treatment. Further research is needed regarding the role of the KD in cancer treatment or prevention.

Comments	This diet can be safely used if dietary intake, nutritional status, and potential side effects are carefully monitored; RDNs must provide ongoing nutrition reassessment and counseling.
	Prior to implementation of the KD, appropriateness should be evaluated by the multidisciplinary care team and patient input should be considered. See Chapter 16 for additional information.

References

1. Allen BG, Bhatia SK, Anderson CM, et al. Ketogenic diets as an adjuvant cancer therapy: history and potential mechanism. *Redox Biol.* 2012;2:963-970 doi:10.1016/j.redox.2014.08.002

2. Oliveira CLP, Mattingly S, Schirrmacher R, Sawyer M, Fine E, Prado CM. A nutritional perspective of ketogenic diet in cancer: a narrative review. *J Acad Nutr Diet.* 2018;118(4):668-688. doi:10.1016/j.jand.2017.02.003

3. Martin K, Jackson CF, Levy RG, Cooper PN. Ketogenic diet and other dietary treatments for epilepsy. *Cochrane Database Syst Rev.* 2016;2:CD001903. doi:10.1002/14651858.CD001903.pub3

4. Ho VW, Leung K, Hsu A, et al. A low carbohydrate, high protein diet slows tumor growth and prevents cancer initiation. *Cancer Res.* 2011;71(13):4484-4493.

5. Block KI, Gyllenhaal C. Nutritional interventions in cancer. In: Abrams DI, Weil AT, eds. *Integrative Oncology.* 2nd ed. Oxford University Press; 2014:120-159.

6. Woolf EC, Syed N, Scheck AC. Tumor metabolism, the ketogenic diet and B-Hydroxybutyrate: novel approaches to adjuvant brain tumor therapy. *Front Mol Neurosci.* 2016;9:122. doi:10.3389/fnmol.2016.00122

7. Wirrell EC. Ketogenic ratio, calories and fluids: do they matter? *Epilepsia.* 2008;49(suppl 8):17-19.

8. Chung H-Y, Park YK. Rationale, feasibility and acceptability of ketogenic diet for cancer treatment. *J Cancer Prev.* 2017;22(3):127-134.

9. Hayashi A, Kumada T, Nozaki F, Hiejima I, Miyajima T, Fujii T. Changes in serum levels of selenium, zinc, and copper in patients on a ketogenic diet using Ketonformula. *No To Hattatsu.* 2013;45(4):288-293.

10. Kossoff EH, Zupec-Kanie BA, Amark PE, et al. Optimal clinical management of children receiving the ketogenic diet: recommendations of the International Ketogenic Diet Study Group. *Epilepsia.* 2009;51(2):304-317.

11. Martin-McGill KJ, Marson AG, Smith CT, Jenkinson MD. Ketogenic diets as an adjuvant therapy in glioblastoma (the KEATING trial): study protocol for a randomized pilot study. *Pilot Feasibility Stud.* 2017;3:67. doi:10.1186/s40814-017-0209-9

12. Aminzadeh-Gohani S, Feichtinger RG, Vidail S, et al. A ketogenic diet supplemented with medium chain triglycerides enhances the anti-tumor and anti-angiogenic efficacy of chemotherapy on neuroblastoma xenografts in a CD1-nu-mouse model. *Oncotarget.* 2017;8(39):64728-64744.

Appendix B
Alternative and Unfounded Diets and Therapies for Cancer Prevention and Treatment

The diets and therapies reviewed here lack sufficient evidence for use in cancer prevention and treatment and may present risks. The reviews are provided for informational purposes because patients may follow or ask about these diets and therapies.

Alkaline Diet

General description	Proponents believe the alkaline diet (also called the acid-alkaline diet) changes the body's pH to the alkaline range needed to fight disease and maintain health.
	Some versions recommend moderate dietary changes, primarily encouraging a plant-based diet that excludes meats, sugars, and processed foods.[1]
	Other versions are part of a strict protocol that changes over time and may include multiple steps that ultimately lead to a very restrictive and unhealthy diet.[2]
	The Acid Alkaline Association (AAA) promotes consuming a diet consisting of 80% alkaline foods (eg, vegetables, low-sugar fruits, legumes) and 20% acid-forming foods (eg, beef, poultry, dairy foods, eggs, coffee, sugar, and alcohol). Other recommendations include[2]:
	■ not eating the following food combinations at the same meal: carbohydrate and acid foods, concentrated sources of protein and carbohydrate, or two concentrated proteins;
	■ not consuming proteins with fats and acids;
	■ eating only one concentrated starch per meal and not consuming starches with sugars;
	■ avoiding melons and not drinking milk with any other foods (if dairy is consumed at all);
	■ drinking 2 or more quarts of water daily; and
	■ using water alkalinizers to raise the pH of water consumed.
	AAA describes 10 levels of the diet, which become more restrictive as the 10th level—a 100% raw food, vegan diet—is approached.[2]
Proposed mechanism or goal	This diet is based on the premise that modern diets cause acidosis and acidosis causes disease.[1-3]
	Proponents claim that:
	■ alkaline foods improve digestion and absorption and that acid in body cells destroys minerals, leading to disease[1-3];
	■ cancer cells thrive in an acidic environment but not an alkaline environment[1-3]; and
	■ cancer can result from improper food combinations.[2]
Food groups excluded	The AAA version of the alkaline diet has 10 levels; dietary restrictions are added as the diet progresses from level 1 to level 10. Level 10 limits intake to raw, vegan foods.[2]
Side effects and nutritional risks	As the diet becomes more restrictive, it becomes difficult to consume adequate energy and protein; regular intake of legumes and soy helps promote adequate protein intake.[4]
	As the diet becomes more restrictive, the risk of multiple nutrient deficiencies increases.
Dietary supplements recommended or indicated	Not routinely recommended.
	Some supplements may be needed. Registered dietitian nutritionists (RDNs) should provide specific dietary supplement recommendations when indicated by a nutrition assessment.

Efficacy studied in clinical trials	One trial demonstrated that the alkaline diet changed systemic pH by only 0.014 pH units, which was insignificant. The diet did change urine pH by 1.02 pH units.[5]

There is no scientific evidence to support the effectiveness or safety of this diet in humans.[1,3]

One observational study revealed no association between diet acid load and bladder cancer.[5] |
| **Comments** | Food consumed does not significantly change the pH of blood. An alkaline diet can change the pH of urine but not pH within the body.[1,3,5]

When kidney function is normal, the body should maintain pH balance regardless of diet.[1,3,5]

Water alkalinizers are expensive, and there is no evidence that drinking alkaline water has any medical value.[6]

Plant-based diets (including vegan and vegetarian diets) that encourage intake of fruits and vegetables and discourage intake of sugar and sweetened foods help promote a healthy weight. These changes alone, in particular when body mass index is in the normal range, may reduce cancer risk and can be made without implementing other unfounded dietary changes recommended by the alkaline diet.

For most people, this diet requires significant and difficult changes.

Preliminary research is exploring the potential of an alkaline extracellular environment to enhance the effects of some chemotherapy drugs. Any claims remain unproven; when asked about this issue, the RDN should investigate current research and consult with the patient's pharmacists and physician.[7]

RDNs should not recommend this diet for cancer treatment or any other medical condition unless significant changes are made to make it healthful and safe.

Because the alkaline diet poses significant nutrient risks, it is essential for RDNs to complete a nutrition assessment and develop a nutrition care plan for each cancer survivor following this diet. |

References

1. Alkaline plan diet review: does it work? WebMD. Accessed May 20, 2020. www.webmd.com/diet/a-z /alkaline-diets

2. The Acid-alkaline diet. Acid Alkaline Association Diet. Accessed May 20, 2020. www.acidalkalinediet.net

3. Does the pH of your diet matter? Berkeley Wellness. February 04, 2016. Accessed May 20, 2020. www .berkeleywellness.com/healthy-eating /food/article/does-ph-your-diet-matter

4. Melina V, Craig W, Levin S. Position of the Academy of Nutrition and Dietetics: vegetarian diets. *J Acad Nutr Diet.* 2016;116(12):1970-1980.

5. Fenton TR, Huang T. Systematic review of the association between dietary acid load, alkaline water and cancer. *BMJ Open.* 2016;6:e010438. doi:10.1136/bmjopen-2015-010438

6. MacGill M. Alkaline water: are there any health benefits? *Medical News Today.* December 6, 2017. Accessed May 20, 2020. www .medicalnewstoday.com/articles /313681.php

7. Longhi A. Manipulating pH in cancer treatment: alkalizing drugs and alkaline diet. *J Complement Med Alt Healthcare.* 2017;2(1):555-580.

Bill Henderson Protocol

General description	First published in 2004, the Bill Henderson protocol is based on the Budwig diet.[1-3] It is sold via books and the internet and promoted via an electronic newsletter.
	Raw fruits and vegetables, gluten-free whole grains, legumes, and a cottage cheese and flaxseed oil mixture form the foundation of this diet.[1-3]
	Meat, dairy, gluten, processed food, sugar, and alcohol are excluded.[1-3]
	The protocol recommends numerous vitamin and herbal "superfood" supplements.[1-3]
	Daily intake of a cottage cheese and flaxseed oil mixture (⅔ to 1 c of reduced- or full-fat cottage cheese blended with 6 to 8 Tbsp of flaxseed oil)[1-3] is part of the protocol. This mixture can be split into two servings daily as needed to improve tolerance.
Proposed mechanism or goal	The protocol is based on a belief that cancer is caused by lack of oxygen to the cells, a weakened immune system, excess acidity, and toxicity secondary to tobacco, alcohol, and asbestos.[1-3]
	The intention is to increase alkaline food intake in order to increase body pH.[1,3]
	The protocol claims to improve cell oxygenation.[1]
	Lignans from flaxseed have antiproliferative, antioxidant, and antiestrogenic activity, but flaxseed oil does not provide lignans. However, high-lignan flax oil is available in capsules as a dietary supplement.[4] Flaxseed oil supplemented with lignans is recommended but not required.[2]
Food groups excluded	Excludes meat, dairy (except for cottage cheese), gluten, processed food, sugar, and alcohol[1-3]
	Certain food combinations are avoided.
Side effects and nutritional risks	Predominantly based on a vegan diet, the protocol may be limited in energy, protein, vitamin B12, iron, zinc, calcium, and iodine.[5]
	The protocol recommends consuming 6 to 8 Tbsp of flaxseed oil daily. More than 2 Tbsp of flaxseed oil daily may cause diarrhea, and more than 4 Tbsp daily may enhance effects of blood-thinning medication.[6-9]
Dietary supplements recommended or indicated	Use of an extensive variety of dietary supplements is recommended by the protocol.[1-3] Up to 46 pills are included in the daily plan, and the range of supplements recommended includes antioxidants, barley grass, nutrient mixtures, and β-glucan. Some micronutrient doses recommended exceed the Tolerable Upper Intake Level set by the US Food and Drug Administration.
	Some supplements may be needed. Registered dietitian nutritionists (RDNs) should provide specific dietary supplement recommendations when indicated by a nutrition assessment.
Efficacy studied in clinical trials	There is no evidence that this diet is safe and effective.[1]
	There is no independent research confirming benefits of the recommended supplements.
	A study that evaluated the potential benefits of a blend of vitamin C and amino acids on (neuroblastoma) tumor growth in mice found that it was ineffective at reducing tumor metastasis.[10]

Efficacy studied in clinical trials (*continued*)	A website that supports the protocol references a "study" that touts patient success on this program. This so-called study is actually a summary of a survey of consumers (66% of whom had declined or discontinued conventional cancer therapy to follow this protocol). Of 11,750 consumers who were sent the survey (via Bill Henderson's electronic database), 630 or 3.6% completed and returned it. The study reports on patient motivations and experiences on the protocol and does not evaluate disease status or changes. Any claims of being cured (50% of respondents stated their cancer was in remission) were based on patient reports and were not validated by a medical professional.[11]
Comments	RDNs should not recommend this diet for cancer treatment or any other medical condition.
	Because of the inherent risk of nutrient deficiency associated with this diet, it is important for an RDN to complete a nutrition assessment for each cancer survivor who follows it. RDNs should also encourage proponents of this diet to seek care from qualified medical practitioners.
	Flaxseed oil will become rancid unless refrigerated and can be destroyed by light, heat, and oxygen.[8]
	Flaxseed oil provides 7 g of α-linolenic acid per tablespoon.[9]

References

1. Mannion C, Page S, Hell LH, Verhoef M. Components of an anticancer diet: dietary recommendations, restrictions and supplements of the Bill Henderson Protocol. *Nutrients*. 2011;3(1):1-26.

2. Henderson Budwig B. The Budwig protocol. Cancer Compass. Accessed May 20, 2020. https://cancercompass alternateroute.com/therapies/bill -henderson-budwig-protocol

3. The full Budwig diet and daily meal plan. The Budwig Diet & Protocol. Accessed May 20, 2020. www.budwig -diet.co.uk/the-full-diet

4. Imran M, Ahmad N, Anjum FM, et al. Potential protective properties of flax lignan secoisolariciresinol diglucoside. *Nutr J*. 2015;14:71. doi:10 .1186/s12937-015-0059-3

5. Melina V, Craig W, Levin S. Position of the Academy of Nutrition and Dietetics: vegetarian diets. *J Acad Nutr Diet*. 2016;116(12):1970-1980.

6. Natural Medicines Comprehensive Database. Flaxseed oil. Web MD. Accessed May 20, 2020. www.webmd .com/vitamins/ai/ingredientmono-990 /flaxseed-oil

7. Flaxseed for healthcare professionals. Memorial Sloan Kettering. Accessed May 20, 2020. www.mskcc.org /cancer-care/integrative-medicine /herbs/flaxseed

8. Flaxseed oil. University of Maryland Medical Center. Accessed May 20, 2020. www.umm.edu/health/medical /altmed/supplement/flaxseed-oil

9. Collins K. Flaxseed and breast cancer. American Institute for Cancer Research. Accessed May 20, 2020. www.aicr.org/resources /blog/healthtalk-flaxseed-and-breast -cancer

10. Lode HN, Heubener N, Strandsby A, Gaedicke G. Nutrient mixture including vitamin C, L-lysine, and epigallocatechin is ineffective against tumor growth and metastasis in a syngeneic neuroblastoma model. *Pediatr Blood Cancer*. 2008;50(2): 284-288.

11. Page S, Mannion C, Heilman L, Verhoef M. The Bill Henderson Protocol: consumer perspectives and practices on an alternative dietary intervention for cancer treatment and cure. *J Evidence-Based Comp Alt Med*. 2011;16(3):226-232.

Budwig Diet

General description	This vegetarian diet promotes eating natural, unrefined foods, including whole grains (eg, wheat, oats, spelt, barley, rye), organic fruits, organic vegetables, juices, nuts, potatoes, certain cheeses from naturally grass-fed herds, oleolux (a spread made from cold-pressed flaxseed oil and coconut oil blended with garlic and onion), green tea, sauerkraut, and sauerkraut juice.[1-5]
	The cornerstone of the diet is a blend of cold-pressed flaxseed oil (45 to 50 g) and quark cheese (a German cottage cheese), which is then used to make "Budwig muesli."[2] This muesli is eaten at breakfast and lunch, for an estimated flaxseed oil intake of up to 100 g (6 to 7 Tbsp) daily.
	Nutritional yeast flakes are allowed, though these are not always reliable sources of vitamin B12.[6,7]
	Prohibited foods include ready-made meals and processed foods, peanuts, animal fats (eg, butter, lard), *trans* fats, hydrogenated fats, margarine, eggs, meat, fish and seafood, poultry, processed meat (eg, sausage, canned meats), sugar, refined foods (eg, white flour, cakes, pastries, and other sweets, except a small amount of honey), unfermented soy products (eg, tofu), and dairy products other than cottage cheese for making Budwig muesli and certain other cheeses.[5]
	Eating eight times a day from allowed foods is recommended.[1-3]
	Dietary recommendations are combined with breathing exercises and enemas if tolerated.[1-4]
	The use of essiac tea[8] is encouraged, and one glass of champagne or wine daily is allowed.[9]
	Kelp and seaweed are allowed.[10]
Proposed mechanism or goal	Johanna Budwig, PhD, proposed that:
	▪ highly unsaturated fatty acids would kill cancer cells by promoting incomplete cell division and cell death[1]; and
	▪ a lack of dietary omega-3 fatty acids reduced cell oxygenation and cottage cheese would improve absorption and availability of flax oil, a source of healthy fat.[11]
Food groups excluded	Dairy (except for cottage cheese and certain other cheeses) and meats[5]
Side effects and nutritional risks	This diet may be low in energy and protein, increasing the risk of weight loss and cachexia.[1,12]
	This is a vegetarian diet with limited dairy (cottage cheese and certain cheeses only), which increases the risk for deficiencies of vitamins B12 and D, iron, zinc, calcium, and iodine.[1,6,12]
	Protein intake should be adequate when energy needs are met[12]; consuming cheeses allowed on the diet helps meet protein needs.
	The amount and type of cheese consumed (and allowed nondairy calcium sources), as well as intake of unfermented soy products, determines calcium intake and the need for supplementation; this should be assessed by a registered dietitian nutritionist (RDN).
	Vitamin B12 deficiency occurs in 50% or more of vegetarians[13]; reliable supplementation is usually needed.[6,12,13]
	Vegan diets can be low in iodine; deficiency can occur when iodized salt and sea vegetables are not regularly consumed.[12]
	For vegetarians and vegans, the Dietary Reference Intake for iron is 1.8 times that for nonvegetarians.[12] Iron in soy exists in the form of ferritin, and absorption is considered good.[14] However, only fermented soy products are allowed on this diet, which may limit soy intake for some individuals. As iron stores decline, the body adapts to increase absorption of nonheme iron[15]; however, iron deficiency remains a risk.[12]

Side effects and nutritional risks (*continued*)	Zinc status of vegetarians is lower than that of nonvegetarians but is usually within the normal range.[12] Nevertheless, it is important to monitor for signs of zinc insufficiency.
	A large intake of flaxseed may result in bloating, gas, diarrhea, and constipation.[1,16-18]
	There is concern that a large intake of flaxseed oil (>4 Tbsp daily) may increase bleeding time and decrease platelet aggregation.[16-18]
Dietary supplements recommended or indicated	Most are excluded; however, vitamin D and supplements that would treat a specific vitamin or mineral deficiency are allowed.[1]
	Budwig believed that synthetic vitamins (found in supplements) do not function well in the body.[5] This belief has since been disproved.
	Some supplements may be needed. RDNs should provide specific dietary supplement recommendations when indicated by a nutrition assessment.
Efficacy studied in clinical trials	There is no scientific evidence to support the effectiveness and safety of this diet in humans; no clinical trials have been published in any peer-reviewed medical journal.[16]
Comments	The discovery of the low-density lipoprotein receptor in 1974 by Michael S. Brown and Joseph L. Goldstein clarified the understanding of fatty-acid metabolism and revealed the faulty science of the Budwig diet.[1]
	This diet poses a significant risk of nutrient deficiencies. It is important for the RDN to complete a nutrition assessment for each cancer survivor who follows this diet to determine its safety. Adherents of this diet must be cautioned about the nutritional risks.

References

1. Mannion C, Page S, Hell LH, Verhoef M. Components of an anticancer diet: dietary recommendations, restrictions and supplements of the Bill Henderson Protocol. *Nutrients*. 2011;3(1):1-26.

2. The full Budwig diet and daily meal plan. The Budwig Diet & Protocol. May 20, 2020. www.budwig-diet.co.uk/the-full-diet

3. These are the foods you must eat on the Budwig diet. The Budwig Diet & Protocol. Accessed May 20, 2020. www.budwig-diet.co.uk/what-you-can-have

4. Quark cottage cheese. The Budwig Diet & Protocol. Accessed May 20, 2020. www.budwig-diet.co.uk/quark-cottage-cheese

5. Foods you must avoid. The Budwig Diet & Protocol. Accessed May 20, 2020. www.budwig-diet.co.uk/what-you-cant-have

6. Rizzo G, Lagana AS, Rapisarda AMC, et al. Vitamin B12 among vegetarians: status, assessment and supplementation. *Nutrients*. 2016;8(12):767. doi:10.3390/nu8120767

7. Paul C, Brady DM. Comparative bioavailability and utilization of particular forms of B12 supplements with potential to mitigate B12-related genetic polymorphisms. *Integr Med (Encinitas)*. 2017;16(1):42-49.

8. Essiac "tea." The Budwig Diet & Protocol. Accessed May 20, 2020. www.budwig-diet.co.uk/essiac-tea

9. Alcohol. The Budwig Diet & Protocol. Accessed May 20, 2020. www.budwig-diet.co.uk/alcohol

10. Antioxidants and supplements. The Budwig Diet & Protocol. Accessed May 20, 2020. www.budwig-diet.co.uk/antioxidants

11. Garcia CM. Budwig diet protocol. Cancer Tutor. Accessed May 20, 2020. www.cancertutor.com/budwig

12. Melina V, Craig W, Levin S. Position of the Academy of Nutrition and Dietetics: Vegetarian diets. *J Acad Nutr Diet*. 2016;116(12):1970-1980.

13. Pawlak R. RD Resources for Consumers: Vitamin B12 in Vegetarian Diets. vegetarian Nutrition Dietetic Practice Group, Academy of Nutrition and Dietetics. https://vndpg.org/docs/rd-resources/B12-RD.pdf

14. Murray-Kolb LE, Welch R, Theil EC, Beard JL. Women with low iron stores absorb iron from soybeans. *Am J Clin Nutr*. 2003;77(1):180-184.

15. Lonnerdal B, Bryant A, Liu X, Theil EC. Iron absorption from soybean ferritin in nonanemic women. *Am J Clin Nutr*. 2006;83(1):103-107.

16. Budwig diet. Memorial Sloan Kettering Cancer Center. Accessed May 20, 2020. www.mskcc.org/cancer-care/integrative-medicine/herbs/budwig-diet-01

17. Collins K. Flaxseed and breast cancer. American Institute for Cancer Research. Accessed May 20, 2020. www.aicr.org/resources/blog/healthtalk-flaxseed-and-breast-cancer

18. Natural Medicines Comprehensive Database. Flaxseed oil. WebMD. Accessed May 20, 2020. www.webmd.com/vitamins/ai/ingredientmono-990/flaxseed-oil

Gerson Therapy

General description

Originally developed to self-treat headaches, this combination of diet and metabolic therapy was recommended by Max Gerson, MD, for tuberculosis in the 1930s before its use was expanded to other medical conditions, including cancer.[1]

The Gerson Institute describes it as a natural treatment utilizing an organic, plant-based diet that includes raw juices and natural supplements. Coffee enemas are recommended as part of this therapy.[2]

This therapy recommends an organic vegetarian diet with no sodium and no fat except for flaxseed oil; restricts soy, beans, and nuts; advises three plant-based meals daily; requires eating 15 to 20 lbs of fruits and vegetables daily; and requires drinking up to 13 glasses of juice daily prepared from raw carrots, apples, and green leafy vegetables.[1-3]

Strict adherence to a meal schedule and meal preparation methods is required.[2]

Multiple dietary supplements, including vitamin B12, thyroid hormone, pancreatic enzymes, potassium, and others, are recommended.[1-3]

Coffee or other approved enemas, vaccines prepared from influenza and *Staphylococcus aureus* bacteria, drugs such as laetrile (illegal in the United States), and injections from liver extract and other products are all recommended.[1-3]

Proposed mechanism or goal

Claims to detoxify the body, return potassium to tissues and cells, reduce sodium in tissues and tumors, and treat the liver to "restore the body's ability to restore itself"[1-4]

Food groups excluded

Fat (except flaxseed oil) and animal protein sources

Side effects and nutritional risks

This diet prohibits animal protein sources and quality plant-based protein sources (eg, soybeans), sodium, fat, and calcium from animal sources. It is high in potassium and carbohydrate.

This diet poses a risk for protein-energy malnutrition and hyponatremia, coma secondary to hyponatremia, dehydration, and colitis from frequent enemas.

This diet may be deficient in several vitamins and minerals, in particular vitamins B12 and D, iron, calcium, zinc, and iodine.

Large amounts of juiced fruits and vegetables may be difficult for those with gastro-intestinal cancers to digest. Patients may also develop mouth sores, which can reduce oral intake and may be particularly challenging for those with head and neck cancers.

The regimen may cause flu-like symptoms, anorexia, weakness and dizziness, cold sores, intestinal cramping, diarrhea, and vomiting.[1,3]

Three deaths possibly related to coffee enemas have been reported.[1,3]

Flaxseed oil is a source of omega-3 fats (via conversion from α-linolenic acid), which can influence bleeding time and decrease platelet aggregation.[5,6] Consuming less than 3 g of eicosapentaenoic acid or docosahexaenoic acid daily does not influence blood clotting,[7] and given the inefficient conversion of α-linolenic acid to omega-3 fats, consuming up to 4 Tbsp of flaxseed oil daily is unlikely to influence blood clotting.[7] Greater intake should be recommended with caution because of potential effects on coagulation, and the patient should be monitored by medical professionals.

Consuming more than 2 Tbsp of flaxseed daily may result in bloating, gas, diarrhea, and constipation.[1,6]

Dietary supplements recommended or indicated	"Natural" supplements are recommended, including pancreatic enzymes; coenzyme Q10; vitamins A, C, B3, and B12; flaxseed oil; pepsin; potassium; pancreatic enzymes; and thyroid hormone.[1] Some supplements may be needed. Registered dietitian nutritionists (RDNs) should provide specific dietary supplement recommendations when indicated by a nutrition assessment.
Efficacy studied in clinical trials	No randomized clinical trials have been conducted with this diet.[1,3] A retrospective review conducted in 1995 by the Gerson Research Organization reported positive results that were later found to be unsubstantiated.[1] The National Cancer Institute reviewed cases of 60 patients treated with this regimen and concluded that available information did not suggest any benefit.[1] There is no evidence of clinical benefit.[1,3]
Comments	The Gerson Institute is a nonprofit organization located in San Diego, CA. The American Cancer Society urges cancer patients to avoid this and other metabolic therapies. This diet is not safe and is not recommended. Should a cancer survivor insist on following this diet, the RDN should complete a nutrition assessment and provide guidance about its risks as well as diet and nutrition changes that would be needed to make this diet safe to follow.

References

1. PDQ Integrative, Alternative, and Complementary Therapies Editorial Board. PDQ Gerson therapy. National Cancer Institute. Accessed May 20, 2020. www.cancer.gov/about-cancer/treatment/cam/hp/gerson-pdq

2. Gerson Institute website. Accessed May 20, 2020. https://gerson.org/gerpress

3. Gerson regimen. Memorial Sloan Kettering Cancer Center. Accessed May 20, 2020. www.mskcc.org/cancer-care/integrative-medicine/herbs/gerson-regimen

4. Cross D. Gerson therapy: Separating fact from fiction. Cancer Tutor. Accessed May 20, 2020. www.cancertutor.com/gerson-therapy

5. Prasad K. Flaxseed and cardiovascular health. *J Cardiovasc Pharmacol.* 2009;54(5):369-377.

6. Natural Medicines Comprehensive Database. Flaxseed oil. Web MD. Accessed May 20, 2020. www.webmd.com/vitamins/ai/ingredientmono-990/flaxseed-oil

7. Collins K. Flaxseed and breast cancer. American Institute for Cancer Research. Accessed May 20, 2020. www.aicr.org/resources/blog/healthtalk-flaxseed-and-breast-cancer

Gonzalez Regimen

General description	Dietary modifications, dietary supplements, extracts of animal organs (as a source of pancreatic enzymes), and detoxification practices, such as coffee enemas twice daily, are components of this regimen.[1-3]
	Dietary patterns are individualized and may range from vegan diets to plans that incorporate red meat several times daily. There are 10 basic diets with 95 variations.[1,4]
	Dietary supplements include vitamins, minerals, amino acids, trace elements, electrolytes, animal extracts, digestive aids (eg, pepsin), and pancreatic enzymes.[1-3]
	Followers may take up to 150 pills daily.[2]
Proposed mechanism or goal	This regimen is considered a metabolic therapy.[2]
	Proponents believe that toxins from processed foods, pesticides, preservatives, and pollutants cause cancer.[3]
Food groups excluded	Specific restrictions vary according to individual recommendations.[1,2,4]
Side effects and nutritional risks	Side effects vary according to individual recommendations.
	Coffee enemas can result in electrolyte imbalances and increase risk for colitis and infection; deaths associated with coffee enemas have occurred.[3,5,6]
Dietary supplements recommended or indicated	Numerous vitamin and mineral supplements are recommended, as well as animal glandular products (primarily for pancreatic enzymes) and food concentrates. Doses and products are individualized to the person.
	Some supplements may be needed. Registered dietitian nutritionists (RDNs) should provide specific dietary supplement recommendations when indicated by a nutrition assessment.
Efficacy studied in clinical trials	In a nonrandomized clinical trial funded by the National Institutes of Health that compared the Gonzalez regimen with conventional chemotherapy for the treatment of pancreatic cancer, quality of life was better and survival time was greater (14 months versus 4.3 months) in patients on conventional chemotherapy rather than the Gonzalez regimen.[7]
	There is no evidence of benefit from this regimen.[3]
Comments	The US Food and Drug Administration has not approved the Gonzalez regimen for cancer treatment.
	The American Cancer Society cautions consumers against using metabolic therapies.
	Because of the inherent risk of nutrient deficiency and toxicity associated with this diet, it is important for an RDN to complete a nutrition assessment for each cancer survivor who follows it and to caution patients on the safe and effective use of dietary supplements, including vitamin and mineral supplements. This diet is not recommended for cancer survivors, and proponents should be counseled about its inherent nutritional risks.
	William Donald Kelly, DDS, originally developed this regimen.[4]

References

1. The Gonzalez Protocol. The Nicholas Gonzalez Foundation. Accessed May 20, 2020. www.dr-gonzalez.com /treatment.htm

2. PDQ Integrative, Alternative, and Complementary Therapies Editorial Board. PDQ Gonzalez regimen. National Cancer Institute. Accessed May 20, 2020. www.cancer.gov/about -cancer/treatment/cam/hp/gonzalez -pdq#section/_4

3. Metabolic therapies. Memorial Sloan Kettering. Accessed May 20, 2020. www.mskcc.org/cancer -care/integrative-medicine/herbs /metabolic-therapies

4. Green S. Nicholas Gonzalez treatment for cancer: gland extracts, coffee enemas, vitamin megadoses, and diets. Quackwatch. Accessed May 20, 2020. www.quackwatch.org /01QuackeryRelatedTopics/Cancer /kg.html

5. Teekachunhatean S, Tosri N, Rojanasthien N, Srichairatanakool S, Sangdee C. Pharmacokinetics of caffeine following a single administration of coffee enema versus oral coffee consumption in healthy male subjects. *ISRN Pharmacology*. 2013. doi:10.1155/2013/147238

6. Margolin KA, Green MR. Polymicrobial enteric septicemia from coffee enemas. *Western J Med*. 1984;140(3):460. PMC 1021723.

7. Chabot JA, Tsai WY, Fine RL, et al. Pancreatic proteolytic enzyme therapy compared with gemcitabine-based chemotherapy for the treatment of pancreatic cancer. *J Clin Oncol*. 2010;28(12):2058-2063. doi:10 .1200/JCO.2009.22.8429

Livingston-Wheeler Therapy

General description	Livingston-Wheeler therapy, developed in the 1970s, is a metabolic treatment.[1,2]
	This therapy combines a vegetarian diet, 75% of which is provided by raw fruits and vegetables, supplemented with megadoses of vitamins and minerals, and digestive enzymes.[1,2]
	Poultry, meat, eggs, milk, sugar, processed foods, food additives, alcohol, caffeine, and fluoridated water are not allowed.[2]
	This therapy also includes a bacille Calmette-Guerin (BCG) vaccine (derived from each patient's own blood or urine); enemas of coffee, lemon juice, or hot water; antibiotics; and vitamin supplements.[1,2]
Proposed mechanism or goal	This therapy is based on the belief that the bacterium *Progenitor cryptocides* (which has not been confirmed to exist) initiates cancer, which grows unless stopped by the immune system.[1,2]
	It is described by its proponents as an immune-boosting cancer prevention program.[1,2]
Food groups excluded	Meat, meat products, and milk products
Side effects and nutritional risks	A healthy vegetarian diet can meet all nutritional needs, but if not planned carefully, it may be deficient in vitamins B12 and D, iron, zinc, calcium, iodine, and protein.[3]
	Protein intake may be acceptable when energy needs are met and if adequate amounts of vegetarian protein sources are consumed; confirming this requires a nutrition assessment conducted by an registered dietitian nutritionist (RDN).
	Megadoses of nutrients may provide amounts more than the recommended Tolerable Upper Intake Level and pose health risks.
	Coffee enemas can result in electrolyte imbalance, electrolyte deficiency, dehydration, malabsorption, and death.[4,5]
	Malaise, aching, and fever have been reported on this therapy.[2]
Dietary supplements recommended or indicated	Megadoses of vitamins and digestive enzymes are advocated.[1,2]
	RDNs should provide specific dietary supplement recommendations when indicated by a nutrition assessment.
Efficacy studied in clinical trials	The link between *Progenitor cryptocides* and cancer has never been confirmed, nor has this bacterium's existence been confirmed.[1]
	There is no scientific evidence supporting the effectiveness or safety of this therapy.[1]
	A prospective comparison of this therapy vs conventional cancer treatment showed lower quality of life among those following the diet than among those receiving conventional treatment and showed no treatment benefits.[6]
	There is no evidence that this therapy extends the life of cancer survivors.[1]

Comments	The rationale for this therapy is faulty. The bacterium identified as causing cancer does not exist, and the recommended BCG vaccine has been found ineffective. This therapy should be avoided.[1]
	In 1990 the California Department of Health Services ordered the clinic that offered this therapy to stop giving the BCG vaccine, and the American Cancer Society advises against using this therapy.[2]
	The clinic that offered this therapy is no longer in operation, but some proponents still follow the diet.
	Because of the inherent risk of nutrient deficiency associated with this therapy, it is important for an RDN to complete a nutrition assessment for each cancer survivor who uses it. Overall, cancer survivors should be cautioned against this therapy.
	Proponents should be advised on the benefits of a vegetarian diet without the other restrictions or program components of this therapy.

References

1. Livingston-Wheeler therapy. Memorial Sloan Kettering Cancer Center. Accessed May 20, 2020. www.mskcc.org/cancer-care/integrative-medicine/herbs/livingston-wheeler-therapy

2. American Cancer Society. Livingston-Wheeler therapy. *CA Cancer J Clin.* 1990;49(2):103-108.

3. Melina V, Craig W, Levin S. Position of the Academy of Nutrition and Dietetics: vegetarian diets. *J Acad Nutr Diet.* 2016;116(12):1970-1980.

4. Teekachunhatean S, Tosri N, Rojanasthien N, Srichairatanakool S, Sangdee C. Pharmacokinetics of caffeine following a single administration of coffee enema versus oral coffee consumption in healthy male subjects. *ISRN Pharmacology.* 2013. doi:10.1155/2013/147238

5. Margolin KA, Green MR. Polymicrobial enteric septicemia from coffee enemas. *West J Med.* 1984;140(3):460. PMC 1021723.

6. Cassileth BR, Lusk EJ, Guerry Du Pont, et al. Survival and quality of life among patients receiving unproven as compared with conventional cancer therapy. *N Engl J Med.* 1991;324:1180-1185. doi:10.1056/NEJM199104253241706

Macrobiotic Diet

General description	A macrobiotic diet is an adaptation of the traditional Japanese diet.[1]
	Several versions exist, from a primarily vegetarian diet (allowing fish on occasion and meat rarely) to a vegan diet.
	Organic, locally grown, primarily vegetarian, and whole foods are recommended in the following proportions[2,3]:
	<ul><li>organically grown whole grains: 40% to 60% of dietary intake</li><li>locally grown vegetables: 20% to 30% of dietary intake</li><li>beans and bean products: 5% to 10% of dietary intake</li><li>soup prepared with beans, miso, and vegetables: 5% of dietary intake</li><li>nuts, seeds, fruits, and fish: on occasion</li></ul>
	Some vegetables (eg, nightshade vegetables, including potatoes, tomatoes, eggplant, and peppers) as well as dairy, eggs, processed foods, refined sugars, and meats are not allowed, though some macrobiotic programs allow some of these foods (eg, meat) on rare occasions.
	Specific cooking methods and utensils are recommended.
	Proponents do not use microwaves or electricity to cook food.
	Food is chewed until fluid (eg, 50 times).
Proposed mechanism or goal	Health is achieved via foods that promote a balance of yin and yang, thus balancing the physical condition, mind, emotions, and spirit.[1,2]
Food groups excluded	Meat, dairy, eggs, and refined sugars are avoided.[1,2]
	The earliest version of this diet advised eating only whole grains and was linked to multiple nutritional deficiencies and death; that version of this diet has since been expanded to allow a greater variety of food.
Side effects and nutritional risks	This diet may be deficient in energy, vitamins B12 and D, iron, zinc, calcium, iodine,[4] and possibly protein.[4]
	Protein intake should be adequate when energy needs are met; regular intake of legumes helps meet protein needs.
	Inadequate energy intake can result in significant weight loss, loss of lean body mass, and cachexia. Patients undergoing cancer treatment should consult with a registered dietitian nutritionist (RDN) to optimize appropriate energy, protein, and nutrient intake.
Dietary supplements recommended or indicated	Not generally recommended.
	Some supplements may be needed. RDNs should provide specific dietary supplement recommendations when indicated by a nutrition assessment.

Efficacy studied in clinical trials	This diet has not been evaluated via a randomized clinical trial.
	Limited research shows no evidence of improved survival in cancer patients on this diet.[5]
	The only reported success stories are testimonials; many people reporting success with this diet also received conventional cancer therapy.[5]
Comments	This diet has evolved since it was first proposed and changes have improved its nutritional adequacy.
	As a low-fat, high-fiber, high–complex carbohydrate, vegan diet, the macrobiotic diet can potentially meet all nutrition needs. RDNs should provide education and counseling to help adopters of this diet meet current cancer-prevention and nutrition guidelines.
	A study comparing nutrient composition and dietary inflammatory indexes for the macrobiotic diet (based on the Kushi Institute's *Way to Health* menu planning guidelines), Recommended Dietary Allowances (RDAs), and National Health and Nutrition Examination Survey (NHANES) 2009–2010 data reported the following results[3]:
	▪ The macrobiotic diet met or exceeded RDAs with the exception of calcium, vitamin D, and vitamin B12.
	▪ Compared with NHANES 2009–2010 data, the macrobiotic diet provided less energy from fat, was higher in dietary fiber, and provided greater amounts of most micronutrients. However, energy intake from the macrobiotic diet averaged 1,444 kcal, which is below the estimated energy needs of most men and many women. Percentages of energy from protein, carbohydrate, and fat were 14.9%, 70.6%, and 14.4%, respectively, and saturated fatty acid intake was 2.9 g/d.
	▪ The dietary inflammatory index for the macrobiotic diet was more anti-inflammatory when compared with the NHANES diet standard.
	This diet may have disease-prevention potential; however, diet prescriptions can vary, which raises questions about the nutritional value of individual diets.
	Vegetarian diets must be nutritionally balanced and adequate to derive the optimal health benefits associated with vegetarianism.[4]

References

1. Natural Medicines Comprehensive Database. Macrobiotic diet. WebMD. Accessed May 20, 2020. www.webmd.com/diet/a-z/macrobiotic-diet

2. What is macrobiotics. Kushi Institute. Accessed May 20, 2020. www.kushiinstitute.org/what-is-macrobiotics

3. Harmon B, Carter M, Hurley TG, Shivappa N, Teas J, Hebert JR. Nutrient composition and anti-inflammatory potential of a prescribed macrobiotic diet. *Nutr Cancer.* 2015;67(6):933-940.

4. Melina V, Craig W, Levin S. Position of the Academy of Nutrition and Dietetics: vegetarian diets. *J Acad Nutr Diet.* 2016;116(12):1970-1980.

5. Horowitz J, Tomita M. The macrobiotic diet as treatment for cancer: review of the evidence. *Perm J.* 2002;6(4):34-37.

Raw Food Plan

General description	A raw food plan includes uncooked food prepared with no animal products, dairy, or eggs.[1] Foods consumed have not been processed in any way from their natural state.[2]
	About 75% of foods consumed are fruits and vegetables.[1]
	Proponents also eat seaweed, sprouts, seeds, beans, whole grains, and nuts.[1]
	Proponents commonly sprout and dehydrate foods.[1]
	Many plans incorporate juice drinks.[3]
	Some plans emphasize carrots, cabbage, green asparagus, broccoli, red beets (ie, beetroot), beet tops, cauliflower, and related vegetables.[3]
	Some plans advise limiting vegetable sources of vitamin K to avoid risk of blood clotting; these plans usually include a list of foods to limit.[3]
Proposed mechanism or goal	Claims that unprocessed foods preserve enzymes in food and provide health benefits[3]
Major food groups avoided	Meat, dairy foods, and eggs
Side effects and nutritional risks	Vegans, whether the foods they consume are raw or cooked, are at risk for deficiencies of vitamins B12 and D, iron, zinc, calcium, iodine, and possibly protein.[4,5]
	Protein intake is more likely to be adequate when energy needs are met; regular intake of legumes helps ensure an adequate protein intake.
	Raw food vegetarian diets have been associated with low bone mass.[2]
	Subjects in a raw foods diet study (N = 18) received 9.1% of energy from protein, 43.2% from fat, and 47.4% from complex carbohydrates. Calcium and vitamin D intakes were below recommended levels. No information was provided about vitamin B12 intake.[2]
	Incidence of B12 deficiency is common (>50%)[6] and expected[7] among vegans and vegetarians; the same percentage would be expected for those following a raw food vegan diet.
Dietary supplements recommended or indicated	Vitamin B12, vitamin D, and calcium
	Registered dietitian nutritionists (RDNs) should provide specific dietary supplement recommendations when indicated by a nutrition assessment.
Efficacy studied in clinical trials	Studies on health and nutrition aspects of raw foods or living food diets are limited.

Comments	There is no evidence that this diet is effective for cancer treatment.
	This diet is difficult to follow and may reduce quality of life.
	Enzyme inhibitors in legumes can reduce the efficacy of pancreatic enzymes, but they are inactivated by cooking; soaking and germinating legumes can also inactivate them.[1]
	Cooking can reduce pesticide levels in foods, though organic foods contain lower levels of pesticides.[1]
	A small study (n = 18) of people who had followed a raw food diet for a mean of 3.6 years found that followers had lower body mass indexes and low bone mass at the hip and lumbar spine, though vitamin D levels and bone turnovers were normal.[2]
	Epidemiologic studies associate plant-based diets (with a higher phytochemical intake) with a reduced risk of certain cancers.[5]
	A meta-analysis of seven studies reported an 18% lower overall cancer incidence in vegetarians versus nonvegetarians.[8]
	Vegetarian diets must be nutritionally balanced and adequate to derive the optimal health benefits associated with vegetarianism.[4]
	Because of the inherent risk of nutrient deficiency associated with this diet, it is important for an RDN to complete a nutrition assessment and develop a nutrition care plan for each cancer survivor who follows it.

References

1. Link LL, Jacobson JS. Factors affecting adherence to a raw vegan diet. *Complent Ther Clin Pract.* 2008;14(1):53-59.

2. Fontana L, Shaw JL, Holloszy JO, Villareal DT. Low bone mass in subjects on a long-term raw vegetarian diet. *Arch Intern Med.* 2005;165(6):684-689.

3. Webster K. Raw food treatment for cancer using vegetables juices. Cancer Tutor. Accessed May 20, 2020. www.cancertutor.com/rawfood

4. Rizzo G, Lagana AS, Rapisarda AMC, et al. Vitamin B12 among vegetarians: status, assessment and supplementation. *Nutrients.* 2016;8(12):767. doi:10.3390 /nu8120767

5. Melina V, Craig W, Levin S. Position of the Academy of Nutrition and Dietetics: vegetarian diets. *J Acad Nutr Diet.* 2016;116(12):1970-1980.

6. Pawlak R. RD Resources for consumers: vitamin B12 in vegetarian diets. Vegetarian Nutrition Dietetic Practice Group, Academy of Nutrition and Dietetics. https://vndpg.org/docs /rd-resources/B12-RD.pdf

7. Pawlak R, Parrott SJ, Raj S, Cullum-Dugan D, Lucus D. How prevalent is vitamin B(12) deficiency among vegetarians? *Nutr Rev.* 2013;71(2):110-117. doi:10.1111/nure.12001

8. Huang T, Zheng YB, G Li, Wahlqvist ML, D Li. Cardiovascular disease mortality and cancer incidence in vegetarians: a meta-analysis and systematic review. *Ann Nutr Metab.* 2012;60(4):233-240.

Appendix C
Select Dietary Supplements and Functional Foods

This information is designed to provide practitioners with available research on select dietary supplements and functional foods and how they relate to cancer. Its purpose is neither to condone nor to discourage use by patients. A patient's health care team can determine which supplements or foods are appropriate, if any.

616
Aloe
(*Aloe barbadensis* miller)

618
α-Lipoic acid

620
Black cohosh
(*Cimicifuga racemosa*)

622
Coenzyme Q10 (CoQ10)

624
Curcumin (*Cucurma longa*)

626
3,3'-Diindolylmethane (DIM)
and indole-3-carbinol (I3C)

628
Flaxseed
(*Linum usitatissimum*)

630
Garlic (*Allium sativum*)

632
Ginger (*Zingiber officinale*)

634
Ginkgo biloba

636
Glutamine

638
Green tea
(*Camellia sinensis*)

640
Melatonin

642
N-acetylcysteine (NAC)

644
Omega-3 fatty acids
eicosapentaenoic acid (EPA)
and docosahexaenoic acid
(DHA)

646
Quercetin

648
Reishi mushroom
(*Ganoderma lucidum*)

650
Resveratrol

652
Selenium

654
Silymarin

656
St. John's wort
(*Hypericum perforatum*)

658
Theanine

660
Turkey tail mushroom or
Yun Zhi (*Coriolus versicolor*,
Trametes versicolor,
Polyporous versicolor)

662
Vitamin D

Aloe (*Aloe barbadensis* miller)

A cactus-like plant, aloe is used predominantly in the form of a gel or a juice.[1-5]

Reported anticancer benefits	May be useful for constipation
Reported anticancer concerns	Well tolerated and good safety data on aloe juice and aloe vera gel Aloe latex used orally may be unsafe and may cause diarrhea
Evidence	Aloe use may delay radiation dermatitis in patients with head and neck cancer.[2] In a randomized study, patients with lung cancer who consumed aloe mixed with honey three times daily during chemotherapy significantly increased response compared with those who had chemotherapy alone.[3] Radiation proctitis significantly improved in patients who used aloe vera 3% ointment in a preliminary randomized controlled clinical trial.[4]
Comments	N/A

References

1. Aloe vera. National Center for Complementary and Integrative Health. Accessed May 27, 2020. www.nccih.nih.gov/health/aloe-vera

2. Rao S, Hegde SK, Baliga-Rao MP, et al. An aloe vera-based cosmeceutical cream delays and mitigates ionizing radiation-induced dermatitis in head and neck cancer patients undergoing curative radiotherapy: a clinical study. *Medicines (Basel)*. 2017 Jun 24;4(3). pii: E44.

3. Lissoni P, Rovelli F, Brivio F, et al. A randomized study of chemotherapy versus biochemotherapy with chemotherapy plus Aloe arborescens in patients with metastatic cancer. *In Vivo*. 2009;23:171-5.

4. Sahebnasagh A, Ghasemi A, Akbari J, et al. Successful treatment of acute radiation proctitis with aloe vera: a preliminary randomized controlled clinical trial. *J Altern Complem Med*. 2017;23(11):858-865.

5. Aloe. Natural Medicines Comprehensive Database. Accessed March 2018. https://naturalmedicines.therapeuticresearch.com/databases/food,-herbs-supplements/professional.aspx?productid=607

α-Lipoic acid

α-Lipoic acid is a cellular antioxidant important for energy production that is naturally synthesized in the body.

Reported anticancer benefits	Improves insulin sensitivity and diabetes management
	Aids with hypertension
	May mitigate radiation damage
	May reduce symptoms of neurotoxicity
	Inhibits growth of breast, colon, lung, liver, and pancreatic cancer cells
Reported anticancer concerns	Generally, very well tolerated
Evidence	α-Lipoic acid used orally or intravenously seems to improve insulin sensitivity and fasting blood glucose levels in patients with type 2 diabetes.[1-4]
	α-Lipoic acid is reported to inhibit tumor cells both in vitro and in vivo.[5]
	α-Lipoic acid has been found to reduce neuropathic symptoms and triglycerides and improve quality of life.[6]
	α-Lipoic acid administration is ineffective at preventing neurotoxicity caused by oxaliplatin or cisplatin.[7] However, Opera (GAMFARMA), a combination product composed of α-lipoic acid, *Boswellia serrata*, methylsulfonylmethane, and bromelain, improved peripheral neuropathy symptoms in a prospective series of patients treated for neurotoxic chemotherapy; no significant toxicity or interaction was observed.[8]
	α-Lipoic acid reduced radiation-induced oral mucositis in rats with head and neck cancer in one study.[9]
Comments	α-Lipoic acid is both fat- and water-soluble and is thus able to function throughout the body.[10]
	Dietary sources rich in α-lipoic acid include spinach, broccoli, and brewer's yeast.
	The evidence for supplemental α-lipoic acid is still to be determined, but there appears to be potential benefit regarding insulin sensitivity, peripheral neuropathy, and mucositis.

References

1. Konrad T, Vicini P, Kusterer K, et al. Alpha-lipoic acid treatment decreases serum lactate and pyruvate concentrations and improves glucose effectiveness in lean and obese patients with Type 2 diabetes. *Diab Care*. 1999;22:280-7.

2. Jacob S, Ruus P, Hermann R, et al. Oral administration of RAC-alpha-lipoic acid modulates insulin sensitivity in patients with type-2 diabetes mellitus: a placebo-controlled, pilot trial. *Free Rad Biol Med*. 1999;27:309-14.

3. Ansar H, Mazloom Z, Kazemi F, Hejazi N. Effect of alpha-lipoic acid on blood glucose, insulin resistance and glutathione peroxidase of type 2 diabetic patients. *Saudi Med J*. 2011;32(6):584-588.

4. Porasuphatana S, Suddee S, Nartnampong A, et al. Glycemic and oxidative status of patients with type 2 diabetes mellitus following oral administration of alpha-lipoic acid: a randomized double-blinded placebo-controlled study. *Asia Pac J Clin Nutr*. 2012;21(1):12-21.

5. Feuerecker B, Pirsig S, Seidl C, et al: Lipoic acid inhibits cell proliferation of tumor cells in vitro and in vivo. *Cancer Biol Ther*. 2012;13(14): 1425-1435.

6. Agathos E, Tentolouris A, Eleftheriadou I, et al. Effect of α-lipoic acid on symptoms and quality of life in patients with painful diabetic neuropathy. *J Int Med Res*. 2018;46(5):1779-1790.

7. Guo Y, Jones D, Palmer JL, et al. Oral alpha-lipoic acid to prevent chemotherapy-induced peripheral neuropathy: a randomized, double-blind, placebo-controlled trial. *Support Care Cancer*. 2014;22(5):1223-1231.

8. Desideri I, Francolini G, Becherini C, et al. Use of an alpha lipoic, methylsulfonylmethane and bromelain dietary supplement (Opera®) for chemotherapy-induced peripheral neuropathy management, a prospective study. *Med Oncol*. 2017 Mar;34(3):46.

9. Kim JH, Jung MH, Kim JP, et al. Alpha lipoic acid attenuates radiation-induced oral mucositis in rats. Oncotarget. 2017;8(42):72739-72747.

10. Shaafi S, Afrooz MR, Hajipour B, et al: Anti-oxidative effect of lipoic acid in spinal cord ischemia/reperfusion. *Med Princ Pract*. 2011;20:19-22.

Black cohosh (*Cimicifuga racemosa*)

The rhizome and roots of this plant are used in herbal treatments. Remifemin (Nature's Way), a commercial preparation, provides 10 mg of root or rhizome per tablet.

Reported anticancer benefits	Suppresses symptoms (eg, hot flashes) associated with menopause and cancer treatment
Reported anticancer concerns	Possibly unsafe during pregnancy and lactation
	While there may be reports of potential liver toxicity,[1] a meta-analysis designed to assess liver safety did not report any liver toxicity in more than 1,000 patients.[2]
	Mild adverse events can include headaches, vomiting, and gastrointestinal irritation.[3]
Evidence	European black cohosh extracts at low doses reduce climacteric complaints (ie, hot flashes) and are devoid of adverse estrogenic effects.[4]
	Though a meta-analysis of nine placebo-controlled studies originally reported no association,[5] a corrective response confirmed the reliable efficacy of black cohosh products for menopausal symptoms.[6,7]
	In a 6-month study, black cohosh was more effective than fluoxetine for treating hot flashes and night sweats associated with menopause.[8]
	German Commission E has found black cohosh to be effective at treating nervous system complaints (eg, tension) associated with menopause.[9]
	In vitro research suggests that black cohosh may interfere with conventional cancer treatments including tamoxifen[10] and may increase toxic effects of doxorubicin and docetaxel.[11]
	A case-control study found that black cohosh was associated with a reduced risk of breast cancer.[12]
Comments	Due to mixed results, more research is needed to assess the relationship between black cohosh and hot flashes and with breast cancer.[3,13]
	There is insufficient evidence to support the use of black cohosh in cancer treatment.
	Black cohosh may interfere with some conventional cancer treatments as well as with the biologic activity of atorvastatin, azathioprine, and cyclosporine.[10,11]

References

1. Mahady GB, Dog TL, Barrett ML, et al. United States Pharmacopeia review of the black cohosh case reports of hepatotoxicity. *Menopause*. 2008;15(4 pt 1):628-638.

2. Naser B, Schnitker J, Minkin MJ, de Arriba SG, Nolte KU, Osmers R. Suspected black cohosh hepatotoxicity: no evidence by meta-analysis of randomized controlled clinical trials for isopropanolic black cohosh extract. *Menopause*. 2011;18(4):366–375.

3. Merchant S, Stebbing J. Black cohosh, hot flushes, and breast cancer. *Lancet Oncol*. 2015;16(2):137-8.

4. Wuttke W, Jarry H, Haunschild J, et al. The non-estrogenic alternative for the treatment of climacteric complaints: Black cohosh (Cimicifuga or Actaea racemosa). *J Steroid Biochem Mol Biol*. 2014;139:302-10.

5. Leach MJ, Moore V. Black cohosh (Cimicifuga spp.) for menopausal symptoms. *Cochrane Database Syst Rev*. 2012 Sep 12;9:CD007244.

6. Beer AM, Osmers R, Schnitker J, Bai W, Mueck AO, Meden H. Efficacy of black cohosh (Cimicifuga racemosa) medicines for treatment of menopausal symptoms—comments on major statements of the Cochrane Collaboration report 2012 "black cohosh (Cimicifuga spp.) for menopausal symptoms (review)." *Gynecol Endocrinol*. 2013;29(12): 1022–1025.

7. Henneicke-von Zepelin HH. 60 years of Cimicifuga racemosa medicinal products: clinical research milestones, current study findings and current development. *Wiener Medizinische Wochenschrift*. 2017;167(7):147-159.

8. Oktem M, Eroglu D, Karahan HB, Taskintuna N, Kuscu E, Zeynelogluy HB. Black cohosh and fluoxetine in the treatment of postmenopausal symptoms: a prospective, randomized trial. *Adv Ther*. 2007;24(2):448-461.

9. Commission E of the German Federal Health Bureau. *Cimicifugae racemosae* rhizoma. Monograph. Bundesanzeiger; 1989.

10. Li J, Gödecke T, Chen SN, et al. In vitro metabolic interactions between black cohosh (Cimifuga racemosa) and tamoxifen via inhibition of cytochromes P450 2D6 and 3A4. *Xenobiotica*. 2011;41(12):1021-1030.

11. Rockwell S, Liu Y, Higgins SA. Alteration of the effects of cancer therapy agents on breast cancer cells by the herbal medicine black cohosh. *Breast Cancer Res Treat*. 2005;90(3):233-239.

12. Obi N, Chang-Claude J, Berger J, et al. The use of herbals preparations to alleviate climacteric disorders and risk of postmenopausal breast cancer in a German case–control study. *Cancer Epidemiol Biomarkers Prev*. 2009;18:2207–2213.

13. Fritz H, Seely D, McGowan J, et al. Black cohosh and breast cancer: a systematic review. *Integr Cancer Ther*. 2014 Jan;13(1):12-29.

Coenzyme Q10 (CoQ10)

This fat-soluble bioactive substance is found in every cell in the body.

Reported anticancer benefits	Endogenous antioxidant involved in cellular energy production
	May reduce renal toxicity and cardiotoxicity of doxorubicin (Adriamycin)[1-3]
Reported anticancer concerns	CoQ10 is structurally similar to menaquinone (vitamin K2) and may have procoagulant effects, thus influencing the efficacy of warfarin.[4]
	Mild gastrointestinal side effects have occurred with CoQ10, including nausea, vomiting, and diarrhea.[5]
Evidence	Preclinical studies suggest that CoQ10 may help prevent cardiotoxic effects of doxorubicin[1,3]; however, others have reported no benefit in breast cancer cell lines.[6]
	An animal study suggested that low and high doses of CoQ10 reduce nephrotoxicity from doxorubicin.[1]
	Low plasma CoQ10 levels are associated with an increased risk of breast cancer[7] and melanoma.[8]
	CoQ10 may reduce radiation-induced nephropathy[9] and renal toxicity of doxorubicin and carboplatin.[3]
	Supplementation with 300 mg/d of CoQ10 significantly increased the antioxidant capacity and reduced the oxidative stress and inflammation levels in patients with hepatocellular carcinoma after surgery.[10]
Comments	CoQ10 may reduce toxicity of some chemotherapy treatments; however, there is insufficient evidence for recommending this supplement for this purpose.[1,2]
	CoQ10 is contraindicated in those who take warfarin.[4]
	As with other antioxidants, there is concern that CoQ10 could interfere with chemotherapy treatments; this interaction has not been confirmed.[5]
	Body levels of CoQ10 decline with aging.

References

1. Colas S, Mahéo K, Denis F, et al. Sensitization by dietary docosahexaenoic acid of rat mammary carcinoma to anthracycline: a role for tumor vascularization. *Clin Cancer Res.* 2006;12(19):5879–5886.

2. Conlin KA. Coenzyme Q10 for prevention of anthracycline-induced cardiotoxicity. *Integr Cancer Ther.* 2005;4(2):110-130.

3. Kabel AM, Elkhoely AA. Ameliorative effect of coenzyme Q10 and/or candesartan on carboplatin-induced nephrotoxicity: roles of apoptosis, transforming growth factor-β1, nuclear factor kappa-B and the Nrf2/Ho-1 pathway. *Asian Pac J Cancer Prev.* 2017 Jun 25;18(6):1629-1636.

4. Heck AM, Dewitt BA, Lukes AL. Potential Interactions between alternative therapies and warfarin. *AM J Health Syst Pharm.* 2000;57(13). Accessed August 11, 2013. www.medscape.com/viewarticle/406896_3

5. Coenzyme Q10. Medline Plus. Last reviewed October 21, 2011. Accessed August 11, 2013. www.nlm.nih.gov/medlineplus/druginfo/natural/938.html

6. Greenlee H, Shaw J, Lau Y-KI, Naini A, Maurer M. Effect of coenzyme Q10 on doxorubicin cytotoxicity in breast cancer cell cultures. *Integr Cancer Ther.* 2012;11(3):10.

7. Cooney RV, Dai Q, Gao YT, et al. Low plasma coenzyme Q10 levels and breast cancer risk in Chinese women. *Cancer Epidemiol Biomarkers Prev.* 2011 Jun;20(6):1124-30.

8. Rusciani L, Proietti I, Rusciani A, et al. Low plasma coenzyme Q10 levels as an independent prognostic factor for melanoma progression. *J Am Acad Dermatol.* 2006 Feb;54(2):234-241. doi:10.1016/j.jaad.2005.08.031

9. Ki Y, Kim W, Kim YH, et al. Effect of coenzyme Q10 on radiation nephropathy in rats. *J Korean Med Sci.* 2017 May;32(5):757-763.

10. Liu H-T, Huang Y-C, Cheng S-B, Huang Y-T, Lin P-T. Effects of coenzyme Q10 supplementation on antioxidant capacity and inflammation in hepatocellular carcinoma patients after surgery: a randomized, placebo-controlled trial. *Nutrition J.* 2016;15:85. doi:10.1186/s12937-016-0205-6

Curcumin (*Curcuma longa*)

Curcumin is a naturally occurring polyphenol found in the turmeric plant (*Curcuma longa*), which naturally grows in India and tropical regions of Asia. It is derived from the plant's rhizomes and is believed to be the active component in turmeric spice.

Reported anticancer benefits	May inhibit growth of cancer cells.[1]
	Has various pharmacological activities, including anti-inflammatory, antioxidant, and anticancer properties.[2,3]
	Has potent anti-inflammatory effects via inhibition of cyclooxygenase 2 (COX-2) enzyme activity.[4]
Reported anticancer concerns	May prolong activated partial thromboplastin time and prothrombin time.[5]
Evidence	Curcumin has been shown to exert therapeutic effects in many types of cancer, including lung, cervical, prostate, breast, osteosarcoma, and liver cancers[6]; esophageal cancer[1]; and gastric cancer.[7]
	Curcumin inhibits proliferation of breast cancer cells, likely by regulating the nuclear factor κB (NF-κB) pathway.[8]
	Curcumin may act to enhance apoptosis, as observed in LNCaP cells,[9] non–small cell lung cancer cells,[10] and pancreatic cancer cells.[11]
	In one study, curcumin inhibited hepatocellular carcinoma proliferation in vitro and in vivo by reducing vascular endothelial growth factor expression.[12]
	Curcumin sensitizes human colon cancer in vitro and in vivo to radiation.[13]
	Curcumin enhances the anticancer effect of 5-fluorouracil (5-FU)[14] and the combination of 5-FU and cisplatin[15] against gastric cancer in vitro and in vivo,[14] possibly by downregulation of COX-2 and NF-κB pathways.
	Curcumin reverses resistance to irinotecan in colon cancer cells.[16]
	Curcumin improves myelosuppression induced by carboplatin.[17]
	Curcumin may sensitize cisplatin-resistant tumor cells to cisplatin, thus improving its efficacy, and it may reduce cisplatin-induced neurotoxicity.
	Liposomal curcumin lessens the resistance of breast cancer cells to doxorubicin.[18]
	Curcumin enhances tumoricidal actions of docetaxel.[19]
	While piperine may help improve the bioavailability of curcumin, it may slow the clearance of several drugs, including phenytoin, propranolol, and theophylline.[20]
	In a phase 1 trial for advanced and metastatic breast cancer, 8,000 mg/d of curcumin was the maximal tolerated dose.[21]
Comments	Curcumin is known to have poor solubility and low bioavailability.
	Some curcumin supplements are combined with piperine, a spice in black pepper to improve absorption, but the addition of piperine slows the clearance of several drugs.[20,22]
	Liposomal curcumin is argued by many to be more bioavailable; this formulation has exhibited greater growth inhibitory and proapoptotic effects on cancer cells.[6]
	Emerging research suggests that curcumin should undergo further study for anticancer effects, but at this time evidence, is insufficient for recommending it for cancer treatment.
	Incorporating turmeric within a varied diet is reasonable and safe.

References

1. Subramaniam D, Ponnurangam S, Ramamoorthy P, et al. Curcumin induces cell death in esophageal cancer cells through modulating notch signaling. *PLoS One.* 2012;7(2):e30590.

2. Turmeric. American Cancer Society. Accessed August 11, 2013. www.cancer.org/treatment /treatmentsandsideeffects /complementaryandalternative medicine /herbsvitaminsandminerals /turmeric

3. Shakeri A, Ward N, Panahi Y, Sahebkar A. Anti-angiogenic activity of curcumin in cancer therapy: a narrative review. *Curr Vasc Pharmacol.* 2019;17(3):262-269.

4. Aggarwal BB, Harikumar K. Potential therapeutic effects of curcumin, the anti-inflammatory agent, against neurodegenerative, cardiovascular, pulmonary, metabolic, autoimmune and neoplastic diseases. *Int J Biochem Cell Biol.* 2009;41(1):40-59.

5. Kim DC, Ku SK, Bae JS. Anticoagulant activities of curcumin and its derivative. *BMB Reports Online.* 2012;45(4):221-226.

6. Feng T, Wei Y, Lee RJ, Zhao L. Liposomal curcumin and its application in cancer. *Int J Nanomedicine.* 2017;12:6027-6044.

7. Li W, Zhou Y, Yang J, Li H, Zhang H, Zheng P. Curcumin induces apoptotic cell death and protective autophagy in human gastric cancer cells. *Oncol Rep.* 2017;37(6):3459-3466.

8. Liu JL, Pan YY, Chen O, et al. Curcumin inhibits MCF-7 cells by modulating the NF-κB signaling pathway. *Oncol Lett.* 2017;14(5):5581-5584.

9. Zhao W, Zhou X, Qi G, Guo Y. Curcumin suppressed the prostate cancer by inhibiting JNK pathways via epigenetic regulation. *J Biochem Mol Toxicol.* 2018;32(5):e22049.

10. Wang A, Wang J, Zhang S, Zhang H, Xu Z, Li X. Curcumin inhibits the development of non-small cell lung cancer by inhibiting autophagy and apoptosis. *Exp Ther Med.* 2017;14(5):5075-5080.

11. Zhu Y, Bu S. Curcumin induces autophagy, apoptosis, and cell cycle arrest in human pancreatic cancer cells. *Evid Based Complem Altern Med.* 2017;2017:5787218.

12. Pan Z, Zhuang J, Ji C, Cai Z, Liao W, Jhengjie H. Curcumin inhibits hepatocellular carcinoma growth by targeting VEGF expression. *Oncol Lett.* 2018;15(4):4821-4826.

13. Yang G, Qiu J, Wang D, et al. Traditional Chinese medicine curcumin sensitizes human colon cancer to radiation by altering the expression of DNA repair-related genes. *Anticancer Res.* 2018;38(1):131-136.

14. Yang H, Huang S, Wei Y, et al. Curcumin enhances the anticancer effect of 5-fluorouracil against gastric cancer through down-regulation of COX-2 and NF-κB signaling pathways. *J Cancer.* 2017;8(18):3697-3706.

15. He B, Wei W, Liu J, Xu Y, Zhao G. Synergistic anticancer effect of curcumin and chemotherapy regimen FP in human gastric cancer MGC-803 cells. *Oncol Lett.* 2017;14(3):3387-3394.

16. Zhang C, Xu Y, Wang H, et al. Curcumin reverses irinotecan resistance in colon cancer cell by regulation of epithelial-mesenchymal transition. *Anticancer Drugs.* 2018;29(4):334-340.

17. Chen X, Wang J, Fu Z, et al. Curcumin activates DNA repair pathway in bone marrow to improve carboplatin-induced myelosuppression. *Sci Rep.* 2017;7(1):17724.

18. Zhou S, Li J, Xu H, et al. Liposomal curcumin alters chemosensitivity of breast cancer cells to Adriamycin via regulating microRNA expression. *Gene.* 2017;622:1-12.

19. Abrams D, Weil A. *Integrative Oncology.* 2nd ed. Oxford University Press; 2014.

20. Velpandian T, Jasuja R, Bhardwaj RK, Jaiswal J, Gupta SK. Piperine in food: interference in the pharmacokinetics of phenytoin. *Eur J Drug Metab Pharmacokinet.* 2001;26(4):241-247.

21. Bayet-Robert M, Kwiatkowski F, Leheurteru M, et al. Phase I dose escalation trial of docetaxel plus curcumin in patients with advanced and metastatic breast cancer. *Cancer Biol Ther.* 2010;9(1):8-14.

22. Bano G, Raina RK, Zutshi U, Bedi KL, Johri RK, Sharma SC. Effect of piperine on bioavailability and pharmacokinetics of propranolol and theophylline in healthy volunteers. *Eur J Clin Pharmacol.* 1991;41(6):615-617.

3,3'-Diindolylmethane (DIM) and indole-3-carbinol (I3C)

3,3'-Diindolylmethane (DIM) is a naturally occurring plant alkaloid bioactive metabolite of indole-3-carbinol (I3C) found in cruciferous vegetables, such as broccoli, cauliflower, brussels sprouts, cabbage, kale, kohlrabi, bok choy, mustard greens, and turnips.[1]

Reported anticancer benefits	Proposed cancer chemoprevention activity for breast cancer[1] and lung squamous cell carcinoma[2]
	DIM and I3C affect multiple signaling pathways and target molecules controlling cell division, apoptosis, or angiogenesis deregulated in cancer cells[3]
Reported anticancer concerns	DIM may interfere with hormone therapy due to potential antiestrogenic effects.[4]
Evidence	In one study, DIM significantly attenuated doxorubicin-induced oxidative stress in the cardiac tissues by reducing the levels of free radicals and lipid peroxidation.[5]
	In a randomized, placebo-controlled trial, DIM promoted favorable changes in estrogen metabolism and circulating levels of sex hormone–binding globulin (SHBG) in women taking tamoxifen for breast cancer.[6]
	DIM increases the efficacy of other drugs or therapeutic chemicals when used in combinatorial treatment for gastrointestinal cancer.[7]
	DIM has been shown to downregulate the androgen receptor in prostate cancer cells.[8]
	In one study, DIM induced apoptosis and inhibited proliferation in nasophyarangeal cancer cells by downregulating telomerase activity.[9]
	DIM enhances the therapeutic efficacy of paclitaxel in gastric cancer.[10]
Comments	DIM is well tolerated.
	DIM may have antiestrogenic activity and so theoretically could interfere with hormone therapy.[4]

References

1. Thomson CA, Ho E, Strom MB. Chemopreventive properties of 3,3'-diindolylmethane in breast cancer: evidence from experimental and human studies. *Nutr Rev.* 2016;74(7):432-443.

2. Song JM, Qian X, Teferi F, Pan J, Wang Y, Fekadu K, et al. Dietary diindolylmethane suppresses inflammation-driven lung squamous cell carcinoma in mice. *Cancer Prev Res (Phila).* 2015;8(1):77-85.

3. Licznerska B, Baer-Dubowska W. Indole-3-carbinol and its role in chronic diseases. *Adv Exp Med Biol.* 2016;928:131-154.

4. Anon. Indole-3-carbinol. Monograph. *Altern Med Rev.* 2005;10(4):337-342.

5. Hajra S, Basu A, Singha Roy S, Patra AR, Bhattacharya S. Attenuation of doxorubicin-induced cardiotoxicity and genotoxicity by an indole-based natural compound 3,3'-diindolylmethane (DIM) through activation of Nrf2/ARE signaling pathways and inhibiting apoptosis. *Free Radic Res.* 2017;51(9-10):812-827.

6. Thomson CA, Chow HHS, Wertheim BC, et al. A randomized, placebo-controlled trial of diindolylmethane for breast cancer biomarker modulation in patients taking tamoxifen. *Breast Cancer Res Treat.* 2017;165(1):97-107.

7. Kim SM. Cellular and molecular mechanisms of 3,3'-diindolylmethane in gastrointestinal cancer. *Int J Mol Sci.* 2016;17(7). pii: E1155.

8. Li Y, Sarkar FH. Role of BioResponse 3,3'-diindolylmethane in the treatment of human prostate cancer: clinical experience. *Med Princ Pract.* 2016;25 (suppl 2):11-7.

9. Li F, Xu Y, Chen C, Chen SM, Xiao BK, Ze-Zhang T. Pro-apoptotic and anti-proliferative effects of 3,3'-diindolylmethane in nasopharyngeal carcinoma cells via downregulation of telomerase activity. *Mol Med Rep.* 2015;12(3):3815-3820.

10. Jin H, Park MH, Kim SM. 3,3'-Diindolylmethane potentiates paclitaxel-induced antitumor effects on gastric cancer cells through the Akt/FOXM1 signaling cascade. *Oncol Rep.* 2015;33(4):2031-2036.

Flaxseed (*Linum usitatissimum*)

Flaxseed is an excellent source of α-linolenic acid (an omega-3 fatty acid) and is also rich in lignans; it provides soluble and insoluble fibers and has phytoestrogenic and antioxidant properties. Secoisolariciresinol diglycoside is considered the major lignan in flaxseed.[1]

Reported anticancer benefits	Provides lignans, fiber, and α-linolenic acid, which are reported to be protective against cancer[2-4]
	Has weak estrogenic activity and may enhance efficacy of tamoxifen, though this is still being studied
Reported anticancer concerns	Side effects, including nausea, gas, and diarrhea
	Possibly contraindicated in those with inflammatory bowel disease
	May affect the absorption of some drugs
	Possible allergic reactions
Evidence	Research suggests that flaxseed increases markers of apoptosis and decreases cancer cell proliferation.[5]
	Cell and animal studies suggest flaxseed, including its lignan and oil fractions, may inhibit growth of breast and prostate cancers.[2,5,6]
	A human study suggested that consuming 25 g of flaxseed daily may reduce tumor growth in women with breast cancer.[7]
	An animal study found that a 10%-flaxseed diet inhibited breast cancer growth to the greatest degree, followed by flaxseed and tamoxifen combined, and then tamoxifen alone.[8]
	Flaxseed may lower prostate-specific antigen levels and slow the growth rate of prostate cancer cells.[3]
	A multisite, randomized, controlled trial found that men who were fed a flaxseed-supplemented diet an average of 30 days before prostactectomy experienced a greater reduction in tumor-cell proliferation rates than men fed a low-fat (<20% of energy) diet, a combined flaxseed and low-fat diet, or a control diet.[9]
Comments	While many flaxseed oils do not contain lignans, unfiltered brands provide both α-linolenic acid and lignans.[4,10]
	Whole flaxseed must be ground to exert its biological effects.
	Medications should be taken 1 to 2 hours before or after consuming flaxseed to reduce its effects on drug absorption.
	Ground flaxseed in the amount of 1 to 2 Tbsp/d is considered acceptable and safe.[4]
	Ground flaxseed can be added to cereals, muffins, yogurt, and salads.

References

1. Collins K. In Depth: Flaxseed and breast cancer. American Institute for Cancer Research. Accessed May 27, 2020. www.aicr.org/wp-content /uploads/2020/05/AICR-InDepth-Issue -01-Flaxseed-and-Breast-Cancer.pdf

2. Flaxseed. Memorial Sloan-Kettering. Accessed May 27, 2020. www.mskcc .org/cancer-care/herb/flaxseed

3. Flaxseed. American Cancer Society. Accessed May 27, 2020. www.cancer .org/treatment/survivorship-during -and-after-treatment/staying-active /nutrition-and-physical-activity -during-and-after-cancer -treatment.html

4. Magee E. The benefits of flaxseed. WebMD. Accessed May 27, 2020. www.webmd.com/diet/features /benefits-of-flaxseed

5. Flower G, Fritz H, Balneaves LG, et al. Flax and breast cancer: a systematic review. *Integr Cancer Ther.* 2014;13(3):181-192.

6. Mason JK, Thompson LU. Flaxseed and its lignan and oil components: can they play a role in reducing the risk of and improving the treatment of breast cancer? *Appl Physiol Nutr Metab.* 2014;39(6):663-678.

7. Thompson LU, Chen JM, Li T, Strasser-Weippl K, Goss PE. Dietary flaxseed alters tumor biological markers in postmenopausal breast cancer. *Clin Cancer Res.* 2005;11(10):3828-3835.

8. Chen J, Hui E, Terence I, Thompson LU. Dietary flaxseed enhances the inhibitory effect of tamoxifen on the growth of estrogen-dependent human breast cancer (mcf-7) in nude mice. *Clin Cancer Res.* 2004;10(22): 7703–7711.

9. Demark-Wahnefried W, Polascit TJ, George SL, et al. Flaxseed supplementation (not dietary fat restriction) reduces prostate cancer proliferation rates in men presurgery. *Cancer Epidemiol Biomarkers Prev.* 2008;17(12):3577-3587.

10. Rodrigues-Leyva D, Bassett C, McCullough R, Pierce G. The cardiovascular effects of flaxseed and its omega-3 fatty acid, alpha-linolenic acid. *Can J Cardio.* 2010;26(9):489-496.87.

Garlic (*Allium sativum*)

This perennial bulb, known for its allium compounds, is often used as a flavor enhancer.

Reported anticancer benefits	May stimulate apoptosis and help regulate cell cycles[1]
Reported anticancer concerns	May interfere with the function of some prescription drugs, including saquinavir and antiplatelet medications[2]
Evidence	A study suggested that 200 mg of synthetic allitridum (an allium compound found in garlic) and 100 mcg of selenium given every other day reduces the risk for all tumors by 33% and for stomach cancer by 52% when compared with placebo.[3]
	Ajoene, a compound found in crushed garlic, has been found to stimulate apoptosis in promyeloleukemic cells.[4]
	Allyl sulfides, which comprise 94% of compounds in garlic, may promote apoptosis and cell cycle arrest and inhibit the growth of tumor cells.[5-7]
	A study examining the effect of crude garlic extract on human breast, prostate, hepatic, and colon cancer cell lines found cell proliferation was reduced by 80% to 90% in all cell types except for colon cancer, which saw a reduction of 40% to 50%.[6]
	Garlic appears to be associated with lower risk for gastric cancer.[8,9]
	An in vitro study reported that sulfide fractions (eg, diallyl sulfide, diallyl disulfide, and diallyl trisulfide) are among the active ingredients that influence the growth of pancreatic cancer cells.[7]
	Meta-analyses examining the effects of a garlic supplement on colorectal cancer risk found no significant risk reduction from garlic use[10,11] and that the use of garlic supplements increased cancer risk.[11]
	Similarly, the VITAL (VITamins And Lifestyle cohort) study found no association between garlic supplements and prostate cancer risk,[12] and use of garlic pills increased colorectal cancer risk by 35%.[13]
Comments	Garlic contains compounds that show potential as anticancer treatments; however, current evidence is insufficient for recommending garlic supplements for this purpose.
	Garlic may interfere with the activity of some medications, particularly anticoagulant drugs.

References

1. Pinto JT, Rivlin RS. Antiproliferative effects of allium derivatives from garlic. *J Nutr.* 2001;131(3):1058S-1060S.

2. Fakhar H, Hashemi Taver A. Effect of the garlic pill in comparison with Plavix on platelet aggregation and bleeding time. *Iran J Ped Hematol Oncol.* 2012;2(4):146-152.

3. Guo-hua Z, Hao L, Wan-ten F, Hui-ging L. Study on the long-time effect on allitridum and selenium in prention of digestive cancers. *Zhonghua Liu Xing Bing Xue Za Zhi.* 2005;26(2):110-112.

4. Li H, Li HQ, Wang Y, et al. An intervention study to prevent gastric cancer by micro-selenium and large dose of allitridum. *Chinese Medical Journal (English).* 2004;117(8):1155-1160.

5. Wang H-C, Pao J, Lin S-Y, Sheen L-Y. Molecular mechanisms of garlic-derived allyl sulfides in the inhibition of skin cancer progression. *Ann NY Acad Sci.* 2012;1271(1):44-52.

6. Bagul M, Kakumanu S, Wilson TA. Crude garlic extract inhibits cell proliferation and induces cell cycle arrest and apoptosis of cancer cells in vitro. *J Med Food.* 2015;18(7):731-737.

7. Lan XY, Sun HY, Liu JJ. Effects of garlic oil on pancreatic cancer cells. *Asian Pac J Cancer Prev.* 2013;14(10):5905-5910.

8. Kodall RT and Eslick GD. Meta-analysis: does garlic reduce risk of gastric cancer? *Nutr Cancer.* 2015;67(1):1-11.

9. Turati F, Pelucchi C, Guercio V, La Vecchia C, Galeone C. Allium vegetable intake and gastric cancer: a case-control study and meta-analysis. *Mol Nutr Food Res.* 2014;59(1):171-179.

10. Hu JY, Hu YW, Zhou JJ, Zhang MW, Li D, Zheng S. Consumption of garlic and risk of colorectal cancer: an updated meta-analysis of prospective studies. *World J Gastroenterol.* 2014;20(41):15413-15422.

11. Zhu B, Zou L, Qi L, Zhong R, Miao X. Allium vegetables and garlic supplements do not reduce risk of colorectal cancer, based on meta-analysis of prospective studies. *Clin Gastroenterol Hepatol.* 2014;12(12):1991-2001.

12. Brasky TM, Kristal AR, Navarro SL, et al. Specialty supplements and prostate cancer risk in the VITamins And Lifestyle (VITAL) cohort. *Nutr Cancer.* 2011;63(4):573-582.

13. Satia JA, Littman A, Slatore CG, Galanko JA, White E. Associations of herbal and specialty supplements with lung and colorectal cancer risk in the VITamins And Lifestyle study. *Cancer Epidemiol Biomarkers Prev.* 2009;18(5):1419-1428.

Ginger (*Zingiber officinale*)

Gingerols are the major bioactive components in fresh ginger (rhizome), whereas shogaols, especially 6-shogaol, are the most abundant polyphenolic constituents of dried ginger. Ginger is available in fresh, dried, pickled, preserved, crystallized, candied, and powdered or ground forms.

Reported anticancer benefits	May help ease nausea, heartburn, anorexia, diarrhea, and gas[1] May help ease nausea associated with chemotherapy May inhibit carcinogenesis Has antioxidant and anti-inflammatory properties.
Reported anticancer concerns	May interfere with the activity of anticoagulant drugs, but evidence is equivocal[1]
Evidence	Ginger promotes apoptosis[2,3] and inhibits vascular endothelial growth factor expression.[1] Ginger extracts have shown promise in inhibiting colorectal, hepatocellular cancer,[2] and prostate cancer.[3] A study of 576 patients suggested that 0.5 to 1.0 g of ginger per day significantly reduced the severity of acute chemotherapy-induced nausea in adults with cancer but not delayed nausea related to chemotherapy.[4] The combination of antiemetic medicine and ginger, at 1 to 2 g daily for 3 days, did not reduce the prevalence or severity of acute or delayed nausea.[5] Ginger has been found to reduce the size of gastric ulcers in rats.[6] Ginger juice and acetone extract of ginger reversed delayed gastric emptying secondary to cisplatin therapy in one study.[7] Pretreatment with 6-shogaol, a phenol extracted from ginger, could sensitize pancreatic cancer cells to gemcitabine-induced apoptosis.[8]
Comments	The US Food and Drug Administration list of supplements generally recognized as safe states that up to 4 g of ginger can be consumed daily; lower amounts are usually used in studies.[9] One report suggested that dried ginger powder provides the highest amount of gingerol products (7 to 14 mg of gingerols per gram of powder), followed by fresh ginger (2.0 to 2.8 mg/g), and powdered ginger tea (0.8 mg/g).[10] Although there is no consensus on the correct dosage of ginger, most clinical studies recommend a safe daily dose of 1,000 mg; less than 1,500 mg is often used for nausea relief.[10] Reported equivalences: 1,000 mg = 1 tsp (5 g) of freshly grated ginger extract, 2 mL of liquid ginger extract, 4 cups (237 mL each) of prepackaged ginger tea, 2 tsp (10 mL) of ginger syrup, or two pieces of crystallized ginger (1 square inch each). Evidence examining the effect of ginger on nausea and vomiting associated with chemotherapy is mixed. Current evidence is insufficient for confidently recommending ginger supplements for antiemetic treatment.

References

1. Janssen PL, Meyboom S, van Staveren WA, et al. Consumption of ginger (*Zingiber officinale* Roscoe) does not affect ex vivo platelet thromboxane production in humans. *Eur J Clin Nutr*. 1996;50:772-774.

2. Prasad S, Tyagi AK. Ginger and its constituents: role in prevention and treatment of gastrointestinal cancer. *Gastroenterol Res Pract*. 2015;2015:1422979.

3. Karna P, Chagani S, Gundala SR, et al. Benefits of whole ginger extract in prostate cancer. *Br J Nutr*. 2012;107(4):473-484.

4. Ryan JL, Heckler CE, Roscoe JA, Dakhil SR, Kirshner J, Flynn PJ. Ginger (*Zingiber officinale*) reduces acute chemotherapy-induced nausea: A URCC CCOP study of 576 patients. *Support Care Cancer*. 2012;20(7): 1479-1489.

5. Zick SM, Ruffin MT, Lee J, et al. Phase II trial of encapsulated ginger as a treatment for chemotherapy-induced nausea and vomiting. *Support Care Cancer*. 2009;17(5):563-572.

6. Ko JK, Leung CC. Ginger extract and polaprezinc exert gastroprotective actions by anti-oxidant and growth factor modulating effects in rats. *J Gastroenterol Hepatol*. 2010;25(12):1861-1868.

7. Sharma SS, Gupta YK. Reversal of cisplatin-induced delay in gastric emptying in rats by ginger (*Zingiber officinale*). *J Ethnopharmacol*. 1998;62(1):49-55.

8. Zhou L, Qi L, Jiang L, et al. Antitumor activity of gemcitabine can be potentiated in pancreatic cancer through modulation of TLR4/NF-κB signaling by 6-shogaol. *AAPS J*. 2014;16(2):246-257.

9. Ryan JL, Morrow GR. Ginger. *Oncol Nurse Ed*. 2010;24(2):46-49.

10. Lete I, Allue J. The effectiveness of ginger in the prevention of nausea and vomiting during pregnancy and chemotherapy. *Integr Med Insights*. 2016;11:11-17.

Ginkgo biloba

The seeds and leaves of the slow-growing *Ginkgo biloba* tree are a source of many bioactive compounds. Current interest primarily focuses on triterpene, lactones, and flavonoids within the *G biloba* leaf.[1]

Reported anticancer benefits	May inhibit proliferation of cancer cells.
Reported anticancer concerns	Though side effects are uncommon, there is concern that *G biloba* may increase bleeding risk, but evidence is inconclusive.[2]
Evidence	The Ginkgo Evaluation of Memory study found that those who received *G biloba* (as opposed to a placebo) were not less likely to develop cancer over a 6-year period.[3]
	Treatment of pancreatic cell lines with 70-micromolar kaempferol (an active component of ginkgo) for 4 days significantly inhibited cell proliferation.[4]
	The addition of *G biloba* (100 mg/kg of body weight) to tamoxifen treatment resulted in a slightly enhanced tumor reduction in a study in rats.[5]
	G biloba may reduce the toxicity of cisplatin.[6]
	A study reported no differences in toxicity and tolerance between treatment with hormone therapy only and treatment with hormone therapy plus 120 mg of *G biloba* twice daily for 3 weeks.[7]
	In one study, *G biloba* extract induced apoptosis of melanoma cells.[8] Conversely, another study reported that the rate of metastasis to the liver was higher in mice injected with *G biloba* extract (35 mg/kg of body weight).[9] And another group of researchers found notable increases in incidences of multiple hepatocellular adenomas, hepatocellular carcinomas, and hepatoblastomas in mice injected with *G biloba* extract.[10]
Comments	Cell studies suggest that researchers should explore the anticancer potential of *G biloba*, but at this time evidence is insufficient for recommending this supplement for cancer treatment.
	G biloba may interfere with the activity of some medications, in particular anticoagulant drugs[2] and antiseizure medications.[11]
	Discourage the use of *G biloba* with alkylating agents, antitumor antibiotics, and platinum analogues because of free radical scavenging effects.[12]
	G biloba extract is generally dried to a powder and formulated into pills, tablets, or capsules for ingestion.[3]
	The standardized extract administered in Europe is a clinical daily dosage of 120 to 240 mg for at least 8 weeks and is composed of at least 24% *G biloba* flavone glycosides and 6% terpene lactones.[1]

References

1. Isah T. Rethinking *Ginkgo biloba* L: medicinal uses and conservation. *Pharmacogn Rev.* 2015;9(18):140-148.

2. Roland PD, Nergard CS. *Ginkgo biloba*–effect, adverse events and drug interactions. *Tidsskr Nor Laegeforen.* 2012;143(8):956-959.

3. Biggs ML, Sorkin BC, Nahin RL, Kuller LH, Fitzpatrick AL. *Ginkgo biloba* and risk of cancer: secondary analysis of the ginkgo evaluation of memory (GEM) study. *Pharmacoepidemiol Drug Saf.* 2010;19(7):694-698.

4. Zhang Y, Chen AY, Chen C, Yao Q. *Ginkgo biloba* extract kaempferol inhibits cell proliferation and induces apoptosis in pancreatic cancer cells. *J Surg Res.* 2008;148(1):17-23.

5. Dias MC, Furtado KS, Rodrigues MAM, Barbisan LF. Effects of *Ginkgo biloba* on chemically-induced mammary tumors in rats receiving tamoxifen. *BMC Complement Altern Med.* 2013;13:93.

6. Abrams D, Weil A. *Integrative Oncology.* 2nd ed. Oxford University Press; 2014.

7. Vardy J, Dhillon HM, Clarke SJ, et al. Investigation of herb-drug interactions with *Ginkgo biloba* in women receiving hormonal treatment for early breast cancer. *Springerplus.* 2013;2(1):126.

8. Wang Y, Lv J, Cheneg Y, et al. Apoptosis induced by *Ginkgo biloba* (EGb761) in melanoma cells is Mcl-1-dependent. *PLoS One.* 2015;10(4):e-124812.

9. Wang H, Wu W, Lezmi S, et al. Extract of *Ginkgo biloba* exacerbates liver metastasis in a mouse colon cancer xenograft model. *BMC Complement Altern Med.* 2017;17:56.

10. Rider CV, Nyska A, Cora MC, et al. Toxicity and carcinogenicity studies of *Ginkgo biloba* extract in rat and mouse: liver, thyroid, and nose are targets. *Toxicol Pathol.* 2014;42(5)830-843.

11. Avoiding drug interactions. US Food and Drug Administration. Developed November 10, 2008. Accessed May 28, 2020. www.fda.gov/ForConsumers/ConsumerUpdates/ucm096386.htm

12. Sparreboom A, Baker SD. Botanical-drug interactions in oncology—what is known? In: Abrams DI and Weil AT. *Integrative Oncology.* 2nd ed. Oxford University Press; 2014:285-316.

Glutamine

Glutamine is the most abundant nonessential amino acid in the human body; it is involved in cell replication for rapid cell turnover, primarily in the gastrointestinal mucosa and immune system.[1]

Reported anticancer benefits	May reduce inflammatory side effects of cancer treatment (ie, may reduce degree of mucositis, stomatitis, esophagitis, and diarrhea)[2]
	Plays a role in maintaining the intestinal mucosal barrier: glutamine-enriched nutritional support can reduce intestinal damage from chemotherapy[2]
Reported anticancer concerns	Is converted to ammonia and may decrease the effectiveness of lactulose when glutamine and lactulose are taken at the same time.[3]
	May interact with seizure medication and should be avoided by individuals taking such medication.[4]
Evidence	Oral glutamine appears to reduce the severity of stomatitis occurring secondary to cytotoxic chemotherapy[5] and chemoradiotherapy for head and neck cancer, and appears to reduce pain in patients receiving radiation.[6,7]
	Glutamine (15 g twice daily for 7 days following infusion) significantly reduces oxaliplatin-induced peripheral neuropathy incidence and severity without affecting chemotherapy response and survival.[8]
	Glutamine may help decrease mucus membrane injury induced by radiation by altering the inflammatory response.[9]
	The immunologic tolerance of enteral nutrition supplemented with glutamine is favorable, which provides a protective effect on the intestinal mucosal barrier in patients with gastric carcinoma undergoing intraoperative peritoneal hyperthermic chemotherapy.[10]
	Glutamine provided slight clinical benefits compared with placebo in terms of reducing oral mucositis induced by radiation therapy or chemoradiation therapy in patients with head and neck cancers at the week 6; the results of this study, however, were not statistically significant.[1]
	Oral glutamine may reduce severity of radiation-induced esophagitis.[11]
	The administration of glutamine in patients undergoing pelvic radiation correlates to a reduced incidence of radiation enteritis, higher response rate, as well as improved symptoms, though the results were not statistically significant.[12]
	While there is some concern that glutamine might be preferentially used by rapidly growing tumors and, hence, possibly stimulate tumor growth, preliminary research shows that glutamine supplementation does not increase tumor growth[13-15] and might actually reduce tumor growth, particularly for tumors of the gastrointestinal tract.[14] Oral glutamine was not found to be beneficial when used in autologous transplant patients.[16]
	Certain types of cancers, however, such as those driven by MYC oncogene, appear to depend on glutamine, while others do not depend on circulating glutamine to maintain cancer growth.[17]
Comments	Glutamine is essential for gut health, and some evidence suggests it can reduce inflammation secondary to chemotherapy. However, its effectiveness remains equivocal, and use should be evaluated by the medical team with consideration of individual factors and potential contraindications.
	Glutamine supplementation is well tolerated and associated with improvements in sensory function and self-reported overall quality of life.[18]
	Glutamine is depleted with stress, such as major surgery, sepsis, and cancer.[19]
	Glutamine is contraindicated in those taking antiseizure medication[4] and lactulose.[3]

References

1. Lopez-Vaquero D, Gutierrez-Bayard L, Rodriguez-Ruiz J-A, Saldaña-Valderas M, Infante-Cossio P. Double-blind randomized study of oral glutamine on the management of radio/chemotherapy-induced mucositis and dermatitis in head and neck cancer. *Molec and Clin Oncol.* 2017;6(6):931-936.

2. Wang J, Li Y, Qi Y. Effect of glutamine-enriched nutritional support on intestinal mucosal barrier function, MMP-2, MMP-9 and immune function in patients with advanced gastric cancer during perioperative chemotherapy. *Oncol Lett.* 2017;14(3):3606-3610.

3. Natural Medicines Comprehensive Database. Glutamine. WebMD. Accessed May 27, 2020. www.webmd.com/vitamins/ai/ingredientmono-878/glutamine

4. Chapman AG. Glutamate and epilepsy. *J Nutr.* 2000;130(4S suppl):1043S-1045S.

5. Anderson PM, Schroeder G, Skubitz. Oral glutamine reduces the severity and duration of stomatitis after cytotoxic cancer chemotherapy. *Cancer.* 1998;83(7):1433-1439.

6. Tsujimoto T, Yamamoto Y, Wasa M, Takenaka Y, Nakahara S, et al. L-glutamine decreases the severity of mucositis induced by chemoradiotherapy in patients with locally advanced head and neck cancer: A double-blind, randomized, placebo-controlled trial. *Oncol Rep.* 2015;33(1):33–39.

7. Chattopadhyay S, Saha A, Azam M, Mukherjee A, Sur PK. Role of oral glutamine in alleviation and prevention of radiation-induced oral mucositis: a prospective randomized study. *South Asian J Cancer.* 2014;3(1):8–12.

8. Wang WS, Lin JK, Lin TC, et al. Oral glutamine is effective for preventing oxaliplatin-induced neuropathy in colorectal cancer patients. *Oncologist.* 2007;12(3):312-319.

9. de Urbina JJO, San-Miguel B, Vidal-Casariego A, et al. Effects of oral glutamine on inflammatory and autophagy responses in cancer patients treated with abdominal radiotherapy: a pilot randomized trial. *Int J Med Sci.* 2017;14(11):1065-1071.

10. Xu XD, Sun YS, Shao QS, et al. Effect of early enteral nutrition supplemented with glutamine on postoperative intestinal mucosal barrier function in patients with gastric carcinoma. *Zhonghua Wei Chang Wai Ke Za Zhi.* 2011;14(6):436–439.

11. Topkan E, Yavuz MN, Onal C, Yavuzz AA. Prevention of acute radiation-induced esophagitis with glutamine in non-small cell lung cancer patients treated with radiotherapy: evaluation of clinical and dosimetric parameters. *Lung Cancer.* 2008;63(3):393-399.

12. Cao D, Xu H, Xu M, Qian X, Yin Z, Ge W. Therapeutic role of glutamine in management of radiation enteritis: a meta-analysis of 13 randomized controlled trials. *Oncotarget.* 2017;8(18):30595-30605.

13. Bozzetti F, Biganzoli L, Gavazzi C, et al. Glutamine supplementation in cancer patients receiving chemotherapy: a double-blind randomized study. *Nutrition.* 1997;13(7-8):748-51.

14. Miller AL. Therapeutic considerations of L-glutamine: a review of the literature. *Altern Med Rev.* 1999;4(4):239-248.

15. Ziegler TR. Glutamine supplementation in cancer patients receiving bone marrow transplantation and high dose chemotherapy. *J Nutr.* 2001;131(9 suppl):2578S-2584S.

16. Pytlik R, Benes P, Patorkova M, et al. Standardized parenteral alanyl-glutamine dipeptide supplementation is not beneficial in autologous transplant patients: a randomized, double-blind, placebo-controlled study. *Bone Marrow Transplant.* 2002;30(12):953-961.

17. Altman BJ, Stine ZE, Dang CV. From Krebs to clinic: glutamine metabolism to cancer therapy. *Nat Rev Cancer.* 2016;16(10):619–634. doi:10.1038/nrc.2016.71

18. Sands S, Ladas EJ, Kelly KM, et al. Glutamine for the treatment of vincristine-induced neuropathy in children and adolescents with cancer. *Support Care in Cancer.* 2017;25(3):701-708.

19. Brami C, Bao T, Deng G. Natural products and complementary therapies for chemotherapy-induced peripheral neuropathy: a systematic review. *Crit Rev Onc Hemat.* 2016;98:325-334.

Green tea (*Camellia sinensis*)

Green tea is produced from the fresh leaves of *Camellia sinensis* by steaming or drying without fermenting. Polyphenols, mainly composed of catechins, are the main functional extracts from green tea, and the major polyphenol is epigallocatechin-3-gallate (EGCG), accounting for more than 50% of total polyphenols.[1]

Reported anticancer benefits	The pharmacologically active constituents of this plant have been shown to possess hepatoprotective,[2] cardioprotective,[3] neuroprotective,[4,5] anticancer,[6] antiobesity,[7,8] antidiabetic,[9] antibacterial and antiviral,[10] and hypoglycemic effects.[11]
Reported anticancer concerns	Green tea has been reported to inhibit several drug-metabolizing enzymes, but clinical testing of some of these predicted interactions showed no effects.
	Nervousness, anxiety, heart irregularities, headache, tremors, hypotension, restlessness, insomnia, irritation of the gastrointestinal mucosa, diuresis, and daytime irritability are some possible side effects of consumption.[12]
	Theoretically, green tea might increase the risk of bleeding when used with antiplatelet or anticoagulant drugs, though this interaction has not been reported in humans.[13]
Evidence	Green tea and EGCG have been demonstrated to inhibit tumorigenesis in many animal models for different organ sites, including lung, oral cavity, esophagus, stomach, small intestine, colon, skin, liver, pancreas, bladder, prostate, and mammary glands.[14]
	According to animal studies, green tea and its components have a variety of drug interactions due to inhibitory effects on cytochrome P-450 isozymes.[15]
	A systematic review and meta-analysis found that, although there was no statistical significance in the comparison of the highest vs lowest category, there was a trend of reduced incidence of prostate cancer with each 1-cup increase of green tea per day; this demonstrated that higher tea consumption linearly reduced prostate cancer risk with more than 7c daily, and green-tea catechins were effective for preventing prostate cancer.[1]
	Green tea enhances tumoricidal actions of doxorubicin, idarubicin, paclitaxel, tamoxifen, fluorouracils, and interleukin-2.[16]
	Among 11 meta-analyses, 7 studies reported an inverse association between green tea consumption and cancer risk from the summarized results of case-control studies. However, a meta-analysis of only prospective cohort studies found no statistically significant association between green tea and cancer risk.[17]
	Green tea reduces the toxicity of doxorubicin and idarubicin.[16]
Comments	Studies of green tea and cancer in animals have shown consistently positive results, but studies in humans are much less consistent and have even shown conflicting results.[14]
	Studies from numerous countries indicate that, even at the maximum consumption level (13 g of green tea daily) and the maximum brewing rate for green tea catechins calculated with the highest extracting rate (20%), the greatest intake of catechins was 2.6 g/d; this is 11.5 to 58.4 times lower than the safety dosage (maximum daily intake of 150 g of green tea extracts[18] or 30 g of EGCG[17]). Thus, it is impossible to damage the human liver under traditional tea-drinking conditions.[14]
	Hepatotoxicity and gastrointestinal disturbances (vomiting and diarrhea) are considered to be the harsh side effects of green tea and its constituents in acute, subacute, subchronic, and chronic tests.[15]
	The use of green tea is discouraged with erlotinib and pazopanib because of possible effects on cytochrome P-450 1A2 isozyme induction.[19]

References

1. Guo Y, Zhi F, Chen P, et al. Green tea and the risk of prostate cancer: A systematic review and meta-analysis. *Medicine*. 2017;96(13):e6426.

2. Sugiyama K, He P, Wada S, Tamaki F, Saeki S. Green tea suppresses D-galactosamine-induced liver injury in rats. *Biosci Biotech Biochem*. 1998;63(3):570-572.

3. Kuriyama S, Shimazu T, Ohmori K, et al. Green tea consumption and mortality due to cardiovascular disease, cancer, and all causes in Japan: the Ohsaki study. *JAMA*. 2006;296(10):1255–1265.

4. Schmidt HL, Garcia A, Martins A, Mello-Carpes PB, Carpes FP. Green tea supplementation produces better neuroprotectiv effects than red and black tea in Alzheimer-like rat model. *Food Res Int*. 2017;100(pt 1):442-448.

5. Esmaeelpanah E, Razavi BM, Vahdati Hasani F, Hosseinzadeh H. Evaluation of epigallocatechin gallate and epicatechin gallate effects on acrylamide-induced neurotoxicity in rats and cytotoxicity in PC^{12} cells. *Drug Chem Toxicol*. 2018;41(4):441-448.

6. Khan N, Mukhtar H. Cancer and metastasis: prevention and treatment by green tea. *Cancer Metastasis Rev*. 2010;29(3):435–445.

7. Rains TM, Agarwal S, Maki KC. Antiobesity effects of green tea catechins: amechanistic review. *J Nutr Biochem*. 2011;22(1):1–7.

8. Thavanesan N. The putative effects of green tea on body fat: An evaluation of the evidence and a review of the potential mechanisms. *Brit J Nutr*. 2011;106(9):1297–1309.

9. Sabu MC, Smitha K, Kuttan R. Anti-diabetic activity of green tea polyphenols and their role in reducing oxidative stress in experimental diabetes. *J Ethnopharmacol*. 2002;83(1-2):109–116.

10. Suzuki Y, Miyoshi N, Isemura M. Health-promoting effects of green tea. *Proc Jpn Acad Ser B Phys Biol Sci*. 2012;88(3):88–101.

11. Mohan T, Velusamy P, Chakrapani Narasunhab L, et al. Impact of EGCG supplementation on the progression of diabetic nephropathy in rats: an insight into fibrosis and apoptosis. *J Agric Food Chem*. 2017;65(36):8028-8036.

12. Brinckmann J, Wollschlaeger B. *The ABC Clinical Guide to Herbs*. American Botanical Council; 2003.

13. Natural Medicines Comprehensive Database. Green tea. Accessed May 28, 2020. https://naturalmedicines.therapeuticresearch.com/databases/food,-herbs-supplements/professional.aspx?productid=960

14. Chen Z, Lin Z. Tea and human health: biomedical functions of tea active components and current issues. *J Zhejiang Univ Sci B*. 2015;16(2):87-102.

15. Bedrood Z, Rameshrad M, Hosseinzadeh H. Toxicological effects of *Camellia sinensis* (green tea): A review. *Phytother Res*. 2018;32(7):1163-1168.

16. Abrams D, Weil A. *Integrative Oncology*. 2nd ed. Oxford University Press; 2014.

17. Yu F, Jin Z, Jiang H, et al. Tea consumption and the risk of five major cancers: a dose–response meta-analysis of prospective studies. *BMC Cancer*. 2014;14:197.

18. Saleh IG, Ali Z, Abe N, et al. Effect of green tea and its polyphenols on mouse liver. *Fitoterapia*. 2013;90:151-159.

19. Avoiding drug interactions. U.S. Food and Drug Administration. Developed November 10, 2008. Accessed May 28, 2020. www.fda.gov/ForConsumers/ConsumerUpdates/ucm096386.htm

Melatonin

Melatonin is a natural indolamine produced by the pineal gland that has many functions, including regulation of the circadian rhythm.[1]

Reported anticancer benefits	Anticancer effects for multiple cancer types, possibly including antiproliferative and proapoptotic effects[2,3] as well as sustained proliferation, evading growth suppressors, metastasis, replicative immortality, angiogenesis, resisting cell death, altered cellular energetics, and immune evasion[1]
Reported anticancer concerns	May be unsafe for use during pregnancy[4]
	May increase the effects of herbs with anticoagulant products so could, theoretically, increase the risk of bleeding[4]
Evidence	Several prospective studies have demonstrated the inverse correlation between melatonin metabolites and the risk of breast cancer; melatonin disrupts estrogen-dependent cell signaling, resulting in a reduction of estrogen-stimulated cells.[3,5]
	Clinical studies have shown that circadian disruption of melatonin synthesis, specifically night-shift work, is linked to increased breast cancer risk.[5]
	Melatonin inhibits the enhanced aromatase expression in obese women, increases adiponectin secretion, counteracts the oncogenic effects of elevated concentrations of leptin, and decreases blood glucose levels and insulin resistance.[6]
	Cotreatment with oxaliplatin and melatonin increases endoplasmic reticulum stress and apoptosis of colon cancer cells.[7]
	Melatonin may enhance sorafenib cytotoxicity and overcome the hypoxia-mediated resistance mechanisms in hepatocellular carcinoma.[8]
	Melatonin enhances the antiproliferative and apoptotic responses to low doses of docetaxel in breast cancer cells.[9]
	Melatonin increases the sensitivity of colon cancer cells to 5-fluorouracil treatment.[10,11]
	Melatonin enhances the chemotherapeutic effect of cisplatin in ovarian cells and improves human cervical cancer cell apoptosis induced by cisplatin.[12,13]
	The cytotoxicity of gemcitabine is enhanced by melatonin in pancreatic ductal adenocarcinoma cells.[14]
	Melatonin may limit the development of neuropathic pain in patients undergoing chemotherapy.[15]
	In a randomized, double-blind, double-dummy, placebo-controlled clinical trial, patients with head and neck cancer receiving concurrent chemoradiation therapy experienced less mucositis when therapy was combined with the use of melatonin.[16]
	When simultaneously administered with tamoxifen, melatonin may improve the anticancer response of women with metastatic breast cancer who have not responded to tamoxifen alone.[17]
	Melatonin is being investigated as a potential treatment for limiting oxidative damage to normal tissue during radiotherapy.
Comments	Melatonin is generally safe and well tolerated.
	Melatonin taken at doses of 1 to 5 mg/d is common for managing insomnia, and up to 20 mg/d is often suggested for anticancer effects.

References

1. Talib WH. Melatonin and cancer hallmarks. *Molecules*. 2018;23(3):518.

2. Chen CQ, Fichna J, Bashashati M, Li YY, Stor M. Distribution, function and physiological role of melatonin in the lower gut. *World J Gastroenterol*. 2011;17(34):3888-3898.

3. Nooshinfar E, Safaroghli-Azar A, Bashash D, Akbari ME. Melatonin, an inhibitory agent in breast cancer. *Breast Cancer*. 2017;24(1):42-51.

4. Natural Medicines Comprehensive Database. Melatonin. Accessed May 28, 2020. https://naturalmedicines .therapeuticresearch.com /databases/food,-herbs-supplements /professional.aspx?productid=940

5. Kubatka P, Zubor P, Busselberg D, et al. Melatonin and breast cancer: evidences from preclinical and human studies. *Crit Rev Oncol Hematol*. 2018;122:133-143.

6. González-González A, Mediavilla MD, Sánchez-Barceló EJ. Melatonin: a molecule for reducing breast cancer risk. *Molecules*. 2018 Feb 6;23(2):336.

7. Lee JH, Yoon YM, Han YS, Yun CW, Lee SH. Melatonin promotes apoptosis of oxaliplatin-resistant colorectal cancer cells through inhibition of cellular prion protein. *Anticancer Res*. 2018;38(4):1993-2000.

8. Prieto-Domínguez N, Méndez-Blanco C, Carbajo-Pescador S, et al. Melatonin enhances sorafenib actions in human hepatocarcinoma cells by inhibiting mTORC1/p70S6K/HIF-1α and hypoxia-mediated mitophagy. *Oncotarget*. 2017;8(53):91402-91414.

9. Alonso-González C, Menéndez-Menéndez J, González-González A, et al. Melatonin enhances the apoptotic effects and modulates the changes in gene expression induced by docetaxel in MCF-7 human breast cancer cells. *Int J Oncol*. 2018;52(2):560-570.

10. Pariente R, Bejarano I, Rodríguez AB, Pariente JA, Espino J. Melatonin increases the effect of 5-fluorouracil-based chemotherapy in human colorectal adenocarcinoma cells in vitro. *Mol Cell Biochem*. 2018;440(1-2):43-51.

11. Gao Y, Xiao X, Zhang C, et al. Melatonin synergizes the chemotherapeutic effect of 5-fluorouracil in colon cancer by suppressing PI3K/AKT and NF-κB/iNOS signaling pathways. *J Pineal Res*. 2017;62(2).

12. Zemla A, Grzegorek I, Dziegiel P, Jablonska K. Melatonin synergizes the chemotherapeutic effect of cisplatin in ovarian cancer cells independently of MT1 melatonin receptors. *In Vivo*. 2017;31(5):801-809.

13. Chen L, Liu L, Li Y, Gao J. Melatonin increases human cervical cancer HeLa cells apoptosis induced by cisplatin via inhibition of JNK/Parkin/mitophagy axis. *In Vitro Cell Dev Biol Anim*. 2018;54(1):1-10.

14. Ju HQ, Li H, Tian T, et al. Melatonin overcomes gemcitabine resistance in pancreatic ductal adenocarcinoma by abrogating nuclear factor-κB activation. *J Pineal Res*. 2016;60(1):27-38.

15. Galley HF, McCormick B, Wilson KL, Lowes DA, Colvin L, Torsney C. Melatonin limits paclitaxel-induced mitochondrial dysfunction in vitro and protects against paclitaxel-induced neuropathic pain in the rat. *J Pineal Res*. 2017;63(4):e12444.

16. Onseng K, Johns NP, Khuayjarernpanishk T, et al. Beneficial effects of adjuvant melatonin in minimizing oral mucositis complications in head and neck cancer patients receiving concurrent chemoradiation. *J Altern Complem Med*. 2017;23(12):957-963.

17. Sabzichi M, Samadi N, Mohammadian J, Hamishehkar H, Akbarzadeh M, Molavi O. Sustained release of melatonin: a novel approach in elevating efficacy of tamoxifen in breast cancer treatment. *Colloids Surf B Biointerfaces*. 2016;145:64-71.

N-acetylcysteine (NAC)

N-acetylcysteine (NAC) is an antioxidant that contains thiol groups; it stimulates glutathione synthesis and scavenges free radicals.

Reported anticancer benefits	Has antioxidant properties Prevents nuclear factor κB activation, which increases the inflammatory response Has been used as a mucolytic and as an antidote for overdosed drugs in the emergency department[1]
Reported anticancer concerns	None
Evidence	NAC improves the utility of chemotherapy by enhancing the cytotoxic effects of chemotherapeutic agents and by protecting the host tissues against their toxic effects.[2] NAC attenuated the cardiotoxic side effects of combination doxorubicin and trastuzumab in an animal model of chemotherapy-induced cardiac dysfunction by decreasing oxidative stress and apoptosis.[3] However, in another prospective randomized controlled trial, NAC did not prevent anthracycline-induced cardiotoxicity, though the authors note that the study was underpowered.[1] NAC significantly reduced severe oral mucositis incidence in a double-blind, randomized, placebo-controlled trial.[4] A combination treatment of bromelain and NAC resulted in a reduction of approximately 50% in gastrointestinal tumor growth, where NAC markedly enhanced tumor apoptosis.[2] As a chemoprotectant, NAC has been shown to provide protection against the toxic effects of a variety of chemotherapeutic agents, including cisplatin, 5-fluorouracil, cyclophosphamide, ifosfamide, methotrexate, oxaliplatin, doxorubicin, and combined carboplatin, melphalan, and etoposide phosphate.[2] In one study, though NAC did not increase glutathione levels at 20 hours after treatment, it did protect the tumor cells from apoptosis and mitochondrial damage.[5] NAC has a recognized hepatoprotective effect and may help with the management of trabectedin-induced hepatotoxicity.[6]
Comments	NAC is generally well tolerated and has a very safe profile with minimal side effects.[1] Dosages frequently range from 600 to 1,800 mg daily.[7] Most side effects of NAC result when single doses of greater than 9 g daily are used.[7]

References

1. Jo SH, Kim LS, Kim SA, et al. Evaluation of short-term use of N-acetylcysteine as a strategy for prevention of anthracycline-induced cardiomyopathy: EPOCH Trial—a prospective randomized study. *Korean Circ J.* 2013;43(3):174-181.

2. Amini A, Masoumi-Moghaddam S, Ehteda A, Liauw W, Morris DL. Potentiation of chemotherapeutics by bromelain and N-acetylcysteine: sequential and combination therapy of gastrointestinal cancer cells. *Amer J Cancer Res.* 2016;6(2):350-369.

3. Goyal V, Bews H, Cheung D, et al. The cardioprotective role of N-acetyl cysteine amide in the prevention of doxorubicin and trastuzumab-mediated cardiac dysfunction. *Can J Cardiol.* 2016;32(12):1513-1519.

4. Moslehi A, Taghizadeh-Ghehi M, Gholami K, et al. N-acetyl cysteine for prevention of oral mucositis in hematopoietic SCT: a double-blind, randomized, placebo-controlled trial. *Bone Marrow Transplant.* 2014;49(6):818-23.

5. Neuwelt AJ, Nguyen T, Wu YJ, et al. Preclinical high-dose acetaminophen with N-acetylcysteine rescue enhances the efficacy of cisplatin chemotherapy in atypical teratoid rhabdoid tumors. *Pediatr Blood Cancer.* 2014;61(1):120-127.

6. Grisanti S, Cosentini D, Tovazzi V, et al. Hepatoprotective effect of N-acetylcysteine in trabectedin-induced liver toxicity in patients with advanced soft tissue sarcoma. *Support Care Cancer.* 2018;26(8):2929-2935.

7. Natural Medicines Comprehensive Database. N-acetyl cysteine. Accessed May 28, 2020. https://naturalmedicines .therapeuticresearch.com /databases/food,-herbs-supplements /professional.aspx?productid=1018

Omega-3 fatty acids—eicosapentaenoic acid (EPA) and docosahexaenoic acid (DHA)

These long-chain polyunsaturated fatty acids are found in fatty fish and in dietary supplements (eg, fish oil). They influence a wide range of chronic diseases through their ability to direct eicosanoid metabolism toward anti-inflammatory pathways.

Reported anticancer benefits	Offer cardioprotective, anti-inflammatory, and immunomodulatory effects May reduce inflammation[1]
Reported anticancer concerns	Eicosapentaenoic acid (EPA) and docosahexaenoic acid (DHA) may increase bleeding risk if taken in high doses (≥4 g EPA and DHA daily)
Evidence	Omega-3 fatty acids influence genes that modulate inflammation.[1] Preclinical studies suggest that omega-3 fatty acid supplements may increase apoptosis.[2] A meta-analysis of prospective cohort studies did not show an association between omega-3 fatty acid intake and colorectal risk,[3] and results of efforts to associate omega-3 fatty acid intake with prostate cancer risk are mixed.[4] The Women's Health Initiative Observational Study found that the risk of endometrial cancer was significantly reduced in women with a body mass index <25 who had a greater intake of omega-3 fatty acids (EPA, DHA, and docosapentaenoic acid).[5] Data from the Women's Healthy Eating and Living (WHEL) study suggested that consuming more than 73 mg/d of EPA and DHA from food reduced breast cancer events and all-cause mortality.[6] A randomized, double-blind, placebo-controlled trial demonstrated that EPA and DHA supplements reduced incidence of peripheral neuropathy from paclitaxel.[7] Omega-3 fatty acids may enhance the clinical benefit of doxorubicin, cisplatin, and vincristine.[8] EPA enhances the apoptotic and cancer-cell inhibiting effects of combination oxaliplatin and 5-fluorouracil.[9] Omega-3 fatty acids may reduce the severity of chemotherapy-induced oral mucositis[10] and esophageal mucositis.[11] Patients with breast cancer who underwent paclitaxel therapy had a 70% lower risk of peripheral neuropathy with the use of 640 mg of EPA and DHA three times daily, in a randomized, double-blind, placebo-controlled trial.[12]
Comments	Inclusion of food sources of omega-3 fatty acids in the diet is appropriate as recommended in the *2020–2025 Dietary Guidelines for Americans*.[13] EPA and DHA up to 3 g daily are considered safe[14]; and if monitored by a physician for bleeding risk, up to 4 g daily can be safely used.[15]

References

1. Vedin I, Cederholm T, Freund-Levi Y, et al. Effects of DHA- rich n-3 fatty acid supplementation on gene expression in blood mononuclear leukocytes: the OmegAD study. *PLoS One.* 2012;7(4):e35425.

2. Shaikh IA, Brown I, Wahle KW, Heys SD. Enhancing cytotoxic therapies for breast and prostate cancers with polyunsaturated fatty acids. *Nutr Cancer.* 2010;62(3):284-296.

3. Shen XJ, Zhou JD, Ding WQ, Wu JC. Dietary intake of n-3 fatty acids and colorectal cancer risk: a meta-analysis of data from 489,000 individuals. *Br J Nutr.* 2012;108(9):1550-1556.

4. Brasky TM, Darke AK, Song X, et al. Plasma phospholipid fatty acids and prostate cancer risk in the SELECT trial. *J Natl Cancer Inst.* 2013;105(15):1132-1141. doi:10.1093/jnci/djt174

5. Brasky TM, Rodabouh RJ, Liu J, et al. Long-chain omega-3 fatty acid intake and endometrial cancer risk in the Women's Health Initiative. *Am J Clin Nutr.* 2015;101(4):824-834. doi:10.3945/ajcn.114.098988

6. Patterson RE, Flatt SW, Newman VA, et al. Marine fatty acid intake is associated with breast cancer prognosis. *J Nutr.* 2011;141(2):201-206.

7. Ghoreishi Z, Esfahani A, Djazayeri A. Omega-3 fatty acids are protective against paclitaxel-induced peripheral neuropathy: A randomized double-blind placebo-controlled trial. *BMC Cancer.* 2012;12:355.

8. Pardini R. Nutritional intervention with omega-3 fatty acids enhances tumor response to anti-neoplastic agents. *Chem Biol Interact.* 2006;162(2):89-105.

9. Vasudevan A, Yu Y, Banerjee S, et al. Omega-3 fatty acid is a potential preventive agent for recurrent colon cancer. *Cancer Prev Res (Phila).* 2014;7(11):1138-1148.

10. Hashemipour MA, Barzegari S, Kakoie S, Aghahi RH. Effects of omega-3 fatty acids against chemotherapy-induced mucositis: a double-blind randomized clinical trial. *Wounds.* 2017;29(12):360-366.

11. Miyata H, Yano M, Yasuda T, et al. Randomized study of the clinical effects of ω-3 fatty acid-containing enteral nutrition support during neoadjuvant chemotherapy on chemotherapy-related toxicity in patients with esophageal cancer. *Nutrition.* 2017;33:204-210.

12. Ghoreishi Z, Esfahani A, Djazayeri A, et al. Omega-3 fatty acids are protective against paclitaxel-induced peripheral neuropathy: a randomized double-blind placebo-controlled trial. *BMC Cancer.* 2012;12:355.

13. US Department of Health and Human Services, US Department of Agriculture. *2020–2025 Dietary Guidelines for Americans.* 9th ed. US Department of Agriculture; 2020. Accessed May 28, 2020. https://health.gov/our-work/food-and-nutrition/2015-2020-dietary-guidelines/

14. Department of Health and Human Services, US Food and Drug Administration. Substances affirmed as generally recognized as safe: menhaden oil. *Federal Register.* 1997;62(108):30751-30757. 21 CFR Part 184 (Docket No. 86G-0289).

15. Kris-Etherton PM, Harris WS, Appel LJ, American Heart Association. Nutrition Committee. Fish consumption, fish oil, omega-3 fatty acids, and cardiovascular disease. *Circulation.* 2002;106(21):2747-2457.

Quercetin

Quercetin is a flavonoid found in a variety of foods, including citrus fruits, apples, onions, parsley, and tea; it is also sold as a dietary supplement.[1-3]

Reported anticancer benefits	Provides anti-inflammatory effects and induces apoptosis in breast cancer cells[2]
Reported anticancer concerns	More studies are necessary to assess safety and tolerability when used intravenously, as side effects such as flushing, sweating, nausea, vomiting, and dyspnea have been reported.[4]
Evidence	Quercetin can bind with iron and thereby decrease iron bioavailability, potentially increasing the risk of iron deficiency in vulnerable individuals undergoing cancer treatment.[3] Due to quercetin's effects on limiting intestinal iron absorption, it may be beneficial to patients at risk for hemachromatosis.[1]
Comments	As a common food component, quercetin taken orally is generally safe and well tolerated.

References

1. Lesjak M, Hoque R, Balesaria S, et al. Quercetin inhibits intestinal iron absorption and ferroportin transporter expression in vivo and in vitro. *PLoS One*. 2014 Jul 24;9(7):e102900.

2. Khorsandi L, Orazizadeh M, Niazvand F, Abbaspour MR, Mansouri El. Quercetin induces apoptosis and necroptosis in MCF-7 breast cancer cells. *Bratisl Lek Listy*. 2017;118(2):123-128.

3. Guo M, Perez C, Wei Y, et al. Iron-binding properties of plant phenolics and cranberry's bio-effects. *Dalton Trans*. 2007;43:4951-4961.

4. Ferry DR, Smith A, Malkhandi J, et al. Phase 1 clinical trial of the flavonoid quercetin: pharmacokinetics and evidence for in vivo tyrosine kinase inhibition. *Clin Cancer Res*. 1996;2(4):659-668.

Reishi mushroom (*Ganoderma lucidum*)

The reishi mushroom is a bitter fungus with a glossy exterior and a woody texture; its spore powder has many effective components, including bioactive compounds, such as polysaccharides, triterpenoids, alkaloids, enzymes, and proteins.[1]

Reported anticancer benefits	Used to prevent aging, to enhance the immune system, and for the treatment of hypertension, hyperlipidemia, viral infections such as influenza (including swine and avian), cancer, colorectal adenoma, inflammatory disease, cardiovascular disease, diabetes, and asthma and bronchial diseases[2]
Reported anticancer concerns	Possibly unsafe when used in powdered form for more than 1 month[2] May increase the risk of bleeding when combined in high doses (≥3 g daily) with anticoagulant medication
Evidence	Evidence from in vitro and in vivo studies has demonstrated that reishi possesses potential anticancer activity through immunomodulatory, antiproliferative, proapoptotic, antimetastatic, and antiangiogenic effects.[3] Results from a small clinical study show that taking 1,000 mg of reishi mushroom powder orally three times daily for 4 weeks can improve cancer-related fatigue, compared to placebo, in breast cancer patients undergoing endocrine therapy.[4] Research indicates the possible use of reishi mushroom extract for the therapeutic management of melanoma and triple-negative breast cancer.[5] Data from in vitro and animal studies indicate that reishi extracts, mainly polysaccharides or triterpenoids, exhibit protective activities against liver injury induced by toxic chemicals.[1]
Comments	Reishi is a type of mushroom that grows on live trees.[6] It is usually dried and taken as an extract in the form of a liquid, capsule, or powder. While there is no sufficient evidence to justify the use of reishi mushroom as a first-line treatment for cancer, it could be administered as an adjunct to conventional treatment in consideration of its potential for enhancing tumor response and stimulating host immunity.[7] It is the most studied mushroom with respect to hepatoprotective effects.

References

1. Soares AA, de Sá-Nakanishi AB, Bracht A, et al. Hepatoprotective effects of mushrooms. *Molecules*. 2013;18(7):7609-7630.

2. Natural Medicines Comprehensive Database. Reishi mushroom. Accessed May 28, 2020. https://naturalmedicines .therapeuticresearch.com /databases/food,-herbs-supplements /professional.aspx?productid=905

3. Sohretoglu D, Huang S. Ganoderma lucidum polysaccharides as an anti-cancer agent. *Anticancer Agents Med Chem*. 2018;(5):667-674.

4. Zhao H, Zhang Q, Zhao L, Huang X, Wang J, Kang X. Spore powder of ganoderma lucidum improves cancer-related fatigue in breast cancer patients undergoing endocrine therapy: a pilot clinical trial. *Evid Base Complement Alternat Med*. 2012;2012:809614.

5. Barbieri A, Quagliariello V, Del Vecchio V, et al. Anticancer and anti-inflammatory properties of Ganoderma lucidum extract effects on melanoma and triple-negative breast cancer treatment. *Nutrients*. 2017;9(3):210.

6. PDQ Integrative, Alternative, and Complementary Therapies Editorial Board. PDQ Medicinal Mushrooms. National Cancer Institute. www .cancer.gov/about-cancer/treatment /cam/hp/mushrooms-pdq

7. Jin X, Ruiz Beguerie J, Sze DM, Chan GC. Ganoderma lucidum (Reishi mushroom) for cancer treatment. *Cochrane Database Syst Rev*. 2016;4(4):CD007731. doi:10.1002 /14651858.CD007731.pub3

Resveratrol

Resveratrol (*trans*-3,5,4′-trihydroxystilbene) is a naturally occurring stilbenoid, a polyphenol compound, and is considered to be a phytoestrogen with multifaceted biological activities.[1]

Reported anticancer benefits	Has anticancer properties arising from antioxidative, anti-inflammatory, antimutagenic, anticarcinogenic, and antiproliferative characteristics[1]
	Has been reported to cause cell cycle arrest, promote apoptosis, and inhibit cancer cell proliferation[2]
Reported anticancer concerns	Has antiplatelet effects, so could cause excessive bleeding in persons taking blood-thinning medications[3]
Evidence	Animal experiments, along with clinical studies, have shown the anticarcinogenic action of resveratrol in the following cancers: colon, prostate, lung, breast, and ovaries,[1,4] as well as oral squamous carcinoma, glioblastoma, liver carcinoma, nonmelanoma skin cancers, and thyroid cancer.[2]
	Resveratrol exerts inhibitory effects on many types of cancers by inducing redifferentiation and apoptosis and by inactivating cancer-associated signaling pathways.[5]
	Resveratrol has been shown to inhibit the growth of human gastric carcinoma cells via apoptosis.[6]
	Resveratrol has been reported to exhibit both nontoxic properties in normal cells[5] and minor cytotoxic effects on normal cells.[7]
	Experimental studies suggest that resveratrol may reduce cisplatin renal toxicity.[8]
	Resveratrol is a potential radiosensitizer of breast cancer cells.[9]
	The coadministration of resveratrol during doxorubicin treatment was sufficient to normalize molecular markers of cardiotoxicity and restore the ability of the heart to undergo adaptive remodeling in response to hypertension later in life in mice.[10]
	Resveratrol supplementation at 1 mg/kg of body weight may potentially prevent bone loss caused by methotrexate.[11]
	Research suggests a potential therapeutic application in the treatment or prevention of insulin-resistance–related metabolic symptoms.[12]
Comments	The root of the knotweed (polygunum) is a rich source of resveratrol. Another dietary source is grapes, with black grapes having greater concentrations than red and green; grape skins are particularly rich in resveratrol.[1]

References

1. Dybkowska E, Sadowska A, Świderski F, Rakowska R, Wysocka K. The occurrence of resveratrol in foodstuffs and its potential for supporting cancer prevention and treatment: a review. *Rocz Panstw Zakl Hig*. 2018;69(1):5-14.

2. Angulo P, Kaushik G, Subramaniam D, et al. Natural compounds targeting major cell signaling pathways: a novel paradigm for osteosarcoma therapy. *J Hematol Oncol*. 2017;10(1):10.

3. Natural Medicines Comprehensive Database. Resveratrol. Accessed May 28, 2020. https://naturalmedicines.therapeuticresearch.com/databases/food,-herbs-supplements/professional.aspx?productid=307

4. Huang CY, Ju DT, Chang CF, Muralidhar Reddy P, Velmurugan BK. A review on the effects of current chemotherapy drugs and natural agents in treating non–small cell lung cancer. *BioMedicine (Taipei)*. 2017;7(4):23.

5. Li YT, Tian XT, Wu ML, et al. Resveratrol suppresses the growth and enhances retinoic acid sensitivity of anaplastic thyroid cancer cells. *Int J Mol Sci*. 2018;19(4). pii: E1030.

6. Yang Y, Huang X, Chen S, et al. Resveratrol induced apoptosis in human gastric carcinoma SGC-7901 cells via activation of mitochondrial pathway. *Asia Pac J Clin Oncol*. 2018;14(5):e317-e324.

7. Zhong LX, Zhang Y, Wu ML, et al. Resveratrol and STAT inhibitor enhance autophagy in ovarian cancer cells. *Cell Death Discov*. 2016;2:15071.

8. Valentovic MA. Evaluation of resveratrol in cancer patients and experimental models. *Adv Cancer Res*. 2018;137:171-188.

9. da Costa Araldi IC, Bordin FPR, et al. The in vitro radiosensitizer potential of resveratrol on MCF-7 breast cancer cells. *Chem Biol Interact*. 2018;282:85-92.

10. Matsumura N, Zordoky BN, Robertson IM, et al. Co-administration of resveratrol with doxorubicin in young mice attenuates detrimental late-occurring cardiovascular changes. *Cardiovasc Res*. 2018;114(10):1350-1359.

11. Lee AMC, Shandala T, Soo PP, et al. Effects of resveratrol supplementation on methotrexate chemotherapy-induced bone loss. *Nutrients*. 2017;9(3):255.

12. Chen S, Zhao Z, Ke L, et al. Resveratrol improves glucose uptake in insulin-resistant adipocytes via Sirt1. *J Nutr Biochem*. 2018;55:209-218.

Selenium

Selenium is an essential trace mineral found in a variety of foods.[1-8]

Reported anticancer benefits	Serves as a cofactor for glutathione peroxidase, an enzyme of the antioxidant defense system
Reported anticancer concerns	When consumed in excessive amounts, can cause symptoms of acute toxicity including nausea, vomiting, abdominal pain, dermatitis, nail changes, fatigue, irritability, alopecia, impaired endocrine function, neurotoxicity, and weight loss
Evidence	Most research suggests that selenium supplementation does not reduce the risk of cancer.[2]
	While data from the Selenium and Vitamin E Cancer Prevention Trial (SELECT) suggested no effect of selenium supplementation on prostate cancer risk,[1] other data indicate a greater risk of prostate cancer mortality in men who consume 140 mcg or more of selenium daily.[3]
	Selenium enhances the anticancer effects of cisplatin on breast cancer cells.[3]
	Selenium may enhance apoptosis from taxol and etoposide and improve treatment efficacy of taxol.[5,6]
	The combination of selenium and docetaxel has resulted in greater inhibition of cell growth via apoptosis in breast cancer cells.[7]
	Selenium may mitigate potential for 5-fluorouracil–induced mucositis.[8]
Comments	Orally, selenium is safe and well tolerated at dosages of up to the Tolerable Upper Intake Level (400 mcg/d).
	Selenomethionine is a more bioavailable and preferred form of selenium.

References

1. Lippman SM, Klein EA, Goodman PJ, et al. Effect of selenium and vitamin E on risk of prostate cancer and other cancers: the Selenium and Vitamin E Cancer Prevention Trial (SELECT). *JAMA*. 2009;301(1):39-51.

2. Vinceti M, Filippini T, Del Giovane C, et al. Selenium for preventing cancer. *Cochrane Database Syst Rev*. 2018;1(1):CD005195. Accessed May 28, 2020. doi:10.1002/14651858.CD005195.pub4

3. Kenfield SA, Van Blarigan EL, DuPre N, Stampfer M, Giovannucci E, Chan J. Selenium supplementation and prostate cancer mortality. *J Natl Cancer Inst*. 2015;107(1):360.

4. Sakallı Çetin E, Nazıroğlu M, Çiğ B, Övey İS, Aslan Koşar P. Selenium potentiates the anticancer effect of cisplatin against oxidative stress and calcium ion signaling-induced intracellular toxicity in MCF-7 breast cancer cells: involvement of the TRPV1 channel. *J Recept Signal Transduct Res*. 2017;37(1):84-93.

5. Hu H, Jiang C, Ip C, Rustum YM, Lu J. Methylseleninic acid potentiates apoptosis induced by chemotherapeutic drugs in androgen-independent prostate cancer cells. *Clin Cancer Res*. 2005;11(6):2379-2388.

6. Qi Y, Fu X, Xiong Z. Methylseleninic acid enhances paclitaxel efficacy for the treatment of triple-negative breast cancer. *PLoS One*. 2012;7(2):2379-2388.

7. Park SO, Yoo YB, Kim YH, et al. Effects of combination therapy of docetaxel with selenium on the human breast cancer cell lines MDA-MB-231 and MCF-7. *Ann Surg Treat Res*. 2015;88(2):55-62.

8. Lee JM, Chun HJ, Choi HS, et al. Selenium administration attenuates 5-flurouracil-induced intestinal mucositis. *Nutr Cancer*. 2017;69(4):616-622.

Silymarin

Silymarin is an extract of the milk thistle (*Silybum marianum*) plant. Silymarin contains various compounds, such as silybin, isosilybin, silychristin, isosilychristin, silydianin, and taxifolin. Most studies have been done in silymarin or silybin, instead of the whole plant.

Reported anticancer benefits	Acts as an antioxidant[1,2]; reveals immunomodulatory effects with both immunostimulatory and immunosuppressive activities[3]; and has anti-inflammatory effects[2,3] and liver-protective and anticancer effects[1]
Reported anticancer concerns	Allergic reactions at intakes >1,500 mg/d[4] Should be used cautiously in patients taking tamoxifen[5]
Evidence	Human studies of silymarin have been done in acute lymphoblastic leukemia (ALL), prostate cancer, breast cancer, and head and neck cancer.[6] Silymarin may regulate cell cycles, induce apoptosis, and reduce angiogenesis.[7] Silymarin may reduce inflammation and oxidative stress and may protect DNA.[8] Silymarin may reduce the side effects of cisplatin (rat study),[9] while silybin may reduce its toxicity.[10] Preliminary clinical research shows that taking a specific product containing silybin (Siliphos, Thorne Research) at a dosage of 80 to 320 mg (depending on patient weight) orally daily for 28 days concurrently with chemotherapy does not improve liver function test (LFT) results or bilirubin levels compared to placebo in children and adults up to 21 years of age with ALL and higher than normal LFT results.[11] Prophylactic administration of a silymarin topical formulation may significantly reduce the severity of capecitabine-induced hand-foot syndrome and delays its occurrence in patients with gastrointestinal cancer after 9 weeks of application.[12] Results from a small clinical study show that, compared to placebo, taking a milk thistle extract standardized to 70% to 80% silymarin (Liverherb, Amin Pharmaceutical Company) at a dosage of 140 mg orally three times daily with meals, starting 24 to 48 hours before cisplatin and continuing until the end of three 21-day cycles, does not prevent cisplatin-induced acute kidney injury.[13] Preliminary clinical research shows that applying a specific topical product containing an extract of silymarin (Leviaderm, Madaus GmbH) significantly reduces the incidence and prolongs the time to onset of radiation-induced skin toxicity compared to a panthenol-containing cream in women with breast cancer.[14] Prophylactic administration of a conventional form of silymarin tablets may significantly reduce the severity of radiotherapy-induced mucositis and delay its occurrence in patients with head and neck cancer.[15]
Comments	Research suggests that silymarin may have some anticancer activity, but research is inadequate to support recommending it for patients undergoing cancer treatment. Silymarin is generally well tolerated. Silybin has poor absorbance and bioavailability due to low water solubility, thereby limiting its clinical applications and therapeutic efficiency. To overcome this problem, the combination of silybin with phosphatidylcholine (PC) as a formulation was used in a study to enhance solubility and bioavailability. The results indicated that silibinin-PC taken orally had markedly enhanced bioavailability and therapeutic efficiency.[1]

References

1. PDQ Integrative, Alternative, and Complementary Therapies Editorial Board. PDQ Milk Thistle. National Cancer Institute. Accessed May 28, 2020. www.cancer.gov/about-cancer/treatment/cam/patient/milk-thistle-pdq

2. Polachi N, Bai G, Li T, et al. Modulatory effects of silibinin in various cell signaling pathways against liver disorders and cancer—a comprehensive review. *Eur J Med Chem.* 2016;123:577-595.

3. Esmaeil N, Anaraki SB, Gharagozloo M, Moayedi B. Silymarin impacts on immune system as an immunomodulator: one key for many locks. *Int Immunopharmacol.* 2017;50:194-201.

4. Natural Medicines Comprehenisve Database. Milk thistle: benefits and side effects. WebMD. Accessed May 28, 2020. www.webmd.com/heart-disease/milk-thistle-benefits-and-side-effects

5. Milk thistle. Natural Medicines Comprehensive Database. Accessed May 28, 2020. https://naturalmedicines.therapeuticresearch.com/databases/food,-herbs-supplements/professional.aspx?productid=138

6. PDQ Integrative, Alternative, and Complementary Therapies Editorial Board. Milk Thistle: Patient Version. PDQ Cancer Information Summaries. National Cancer Institute. Accessed May 28, 2020. www.ncbi.nlm.nih.gov/books/NBK65841/

7. Ramasamy K, Agarwal R. Multitargeted therapy of cancer by silymarin. *Cancer Letter.* 2008;269(2):352-362.

8. Feher J, Lengyel G. Silymarin in the prevention and treatment of liver diseases and primary liver cancer. *Curr Pharm Biotechnol.* 2012;13(1):210-217.

9. Abdelmeguide NE. Silymarin ameliorates cisplatin-induced hepatotoxicity in rats: histopathological and ultrastructural studies. *Pak J Biol Sci.* 2010;13(10):463-479.

10. Abrams D, Weil A. *Integrative Oncology.* 2nd ed. Oxford University Press; 2014.

11. Ladas E, Kroll D, Oberlies N, et al. A randomized controlled, double-blind pilot study of milk thistle for the treatment of hepatotoxicity in childhood acute lymphoblastic leukemia (ALL). *Cancer.* 2010;116(2):506-513.

12. Elyasi S, Shojaee FSR, Allahyari A, Karimi G. Topical silymarin administration for prevention of capecitabine-induced hand-foot syndrome: a randomized, double-blinded, placebo-controlled clinical trial. *Phytother Res.* 2017;31(9):1323-1329.

13. Shahbazi F, Sadighi S, Dashti-Khavidaki S, et al. Effect of silymarin administration on cisplatin nephrotoxicity: report from a pilot, randomized, double-blinded, placebo-controlled clinical trial. *Phytother Res.* 2015;29(7):1046-53.

14. Becker-Schiebe M, Mengs U, Schaefer M, Bulitta M, Hoffmann W. Topical use of a silymarin-based preparation to prevent radiodermatitis: results of a prospective study in breast cancer patients. *Strahlenther Onkol.* 2011;187(8):485-91.

15. Elyasi S, Hosseini S, Niazi Moghadam MR, Aledavood SA, Karimi G. Effect of oral silymarin administration on prevention of radiotherapy induced mucositis: a randomized, double-blinded, placebo-controlled clinical trial. *Phytother Res.* 2016;30(11):1879-1885.

St. John's wort (*Hypericum perforatum*)

St. John's wort is a bush that usually blooms around June 24 (the birthday of John the Baptist). Yellow flowers from this bush are used as herbal remedies.

Reported anticancer benefits	May make cancer cells more sensitive to photodynamic therapies[1]
	Has antinociceptive and analgesic properties that validate the traditional uses of the plant for pain conditions[2]
Reported anticancer concerns	May interact with many medications, including warfarin[3]
Evidence	In the VITamins And Lifestyle cohort (VITAL) study, the use of St. John's wort was inversely associated with the risk of colorectal cancer.[4]
	Cell and animal studies suggest that St. John's wort may make cancer cells more sensitive to photodynamic therapies and, therefore, may have the potential to improve the anticancer effects of these modalities.[1]
	Studies demonstrate that hypericin, a bioactive component of St. John's wort, may have a cytotoxic effect on malignant cell lines.[5]
	Preclinical studies indicate a potential use of St. John's wort for medical pain management.[2]
Comments	Current evidence is insufficient for recommending St. John's wort for cancer treatment.
	St. John's wort induces cytochrome P-450 (CYP) 3A4, resulting in lower plasma levels of drugs that are CYP 3A4 substrates, including cyclosporine, simvastatin, warfarin, and amitriptyline.[3]
	Products that contain a daily dose of less than 1 mg of hyperforin (bioactive component of St. John's wort) are less likely to be associated with major interactions with drugs that were CYP 3A4 or P-glycoprotein substrates. Although a risk of interactions cannot be excluded even for low-dose-hyperforin extracts of St. John's wort, the use of products that result in a dose of 1 mg or less of hyperforin per day is recommended to minimize the risk of interactions.[6]
	Taking St. John's wort induces CYP 2C19, which may clinically affect warfarin.[7]
	St. John's wort, ginseng, Korean red ginseng, *Gingko biloba*, ginger, garlic, aged garlic, and echinacea did not significantly alter the pharmacodynamic parameters of warfarin.[8]
	Avoid St. John's wort with all concurrent chemotherapy due to possible effects on enzyme induction for multiple enzymes (CYP 2B6, CYP 2C9, and others).[9]

References

1. Wessels JT, Busse AC, Rave-Fränk M, et al. Photosensitizing and radiosensitizing effects of hypericin on human renal carcinoma cells in vitro. *Photochem Photobiol*. 2008;84(1): 228-235.

2. Galeotti N. Hypericum perforatum (St John's wort) beyond depression: A therapeutic perspective for pain conditions. *J Ethnopharmacol*. 2017;200:136-146.

3. Roby CA, Anderson GD, Kantor E, Dryer DA, Burstein AH. St John's Wort: effect on CYP3A4 activity. *Clin Pharmacol Ther*. 200;67(5):451-457.

4. Satia JA, Littman A, Slatore CG, Galanko JA, White E. Associations of herbal and specialty supplements with lung and colorectal cancer risk in the VITamins And Lifestyle study. *Cancer Epidemiol Biomarkers Prev*. 2009;18(5):1419-1428.

5. Mirmalek SA, Azizi MA, Jangholi E, et al. Cytotoxic and apoptogenic effect of hypericin, the bioactive component of Hypericum perforatum on the MCF-7 human breast cancer cell line. *Cancer Cell Intl*. 2016;16:3.

6. Chrubasik-Hausmann S, Vlachojannis J, McLachlan AJ. Understanding drug interactions with St John's wort (*Hypericum perforatum* L.): impact of hyperforin content. *J Pharm Pharmacol*. 2019;17(1):129-138.

7. Fan Y, Adam TJ, McEwan R, Pakhomov SV, Melton GB, Zhang R. Detecting signals of interactions between warfarin and dietary supplements in electronic health records. *Studies Health Technoll Inform*. 2017;245: 370-374.

8. Choi S, Oh DS, Jerng UM. A systematic review of the pharmacokinetic and pharmacodynamic interactions of herbal medicine with warfarin. *PLoS ONE*. 2017;12(8):e0182794.

9. Sparreboom A, Baker SD. Botanical-drug interactions in oncology—what is known? In: Abrams DI and Weil AT. *Integrative Oncology*. 2nd ed. Oxford University Press; 2014:285-316.

Theanine

Theanine is an amino acid found in tea and mushrooms.

Reported anticancer benefits	Has antioxidant benefits
	May enhance efficacy of doxorubicin and idarubicin and reduce their adverse side effects[1,2]
Reported anticancer concerns	Few side effects reported; may reduce blood pressure and, therefore, interact with antihypertensive medications[3]
Evidence	Cell studies suggest that theanine suppresses the growth of non–small cell lung cancer cells.[1]
	At 0 to 125µM concentrations, theanine suppresses the migration of tumor cells.[4]
	Studies have shown that theanine can improve memory and learning ability by activating relative central neurotransmitters.[5]
	Theanine has the potential to reduce blood pressure, maintain stability, and promote relaxation and concentration by inhibiting the negative effects of caffeine.[6,7]
	Theanine enhances antitumor activity, preventing vascular diseases and offering neuroprotection.[4,8,9]
	Theanine attenuates doxorubicin-induced adverse reactions involved in oxidative damage.[1]
Comments	Studies suggest theanine may enhance some chemotherapies, but there is no evidence that taking theanine supplements is superior to drinking theanine in tea.
	Theanine may interact with antihypertensive medications.[3]
	Common dosage is 200 to 400 mg daily or twice daily, with a maximum daily dose of 1,200 mg.[3]

References

1. Sugiyama T, Sadzuka Y. Combination of L-theanine with doxorubicin inhibits hepatic metastasis of M5076 ovarian sarcoma. *Clin Cancer Res.* 1999;5(2):413-416.

2. Sadzuka Y, Sugiyama T, Sonobe T. Improvement of idarubicin induced antitumor activity and bone marrow suppression by L-theanine, a component of tea. *Cancer Lett.* 2000;158(2):119-124.

3. Cleveland Clinic Wellness. L-Theanine Supplement Review. www.cleveland clinicwellness.com/Features/Pages/l -theanine-pro-con.aspx

4. Liu Q, Duan H, Luan J, Yagasaki K, Zhang G. Effect of theanine on growth of human lung cancer and leukemia cells as well as migration and invasion of human lung cancer cells. *Cytotechnology.* 2009;59(3):211-217.

5. Haskell CF, Kennedy DO, Milne AL, Wesnes KA, Scholey AB. The effects of L-theanine, caffeine and their combination on cognition and mood. *Biol Psychol.* 2008 Feb;77(2):113-122.

6. Yokogoshi H, Kato Y, Sagesaka YM, Takihara-Matsuura T, Kakuda T, et al. Reduction effect of theanine on blood pressure and brain 5-hydroxyindoles in spontaneously hypertensive rats. *Biosci Biotechnol Biochem.* 1995;59(4):615-618.

7. Kakuda T, Nozawa A, Unno T, Okamura N, Okai O. Inhibiting effects of theanine on caffeine stimulation evaluated by EEG in the rat. *Biosci Biotechnol Biochem.* 2000;64(2):287-293.

8. Rogers PJ, Smith JE, Heatherley SV, Pleydell-Pearce CW. Time for tea: mood, blood pressure and cognitive performance effects of caffeine and theanine administered alone and together. *Psychopharmacology (Berl).* 2008;195(4):569-577.

9. Zhao Y, Zhao B. Natural antioxidants in prevention and management of Alzheimer's disease. *Front Biosci (Elite Ed).* 2012;4:794-808.

Turkey tail mushroom or Yun Zhi (*Coriolus versicolor*, *Trametes versicolor*, *Polyporous versicolor*)

The bioactive components obtained from the cultured mycelia of this mushroom include the protein-bound polysaccharide-K (PSK) and polysaccharopeptide (PSP).

Reported anticancer benefits	Has demonstrated antimicrobial, antiviral, immunomodulatory, and antitumor properties[1]
	Ancient Chinese formulations of this mushroom have long been believed to promote health, strength, and longevity[2]
Reported anticancer concerns	Generally low incidence of mild and tolerable side effects.[3]
Evidence	The results of numerous studies and clinical trials confirm that *C versicolor* inhibits the growth of cancer cells in both in vitro and in vivo settings as well as decreases cancer treatment-related adverse side effects, such as fatigue, loss of appetite, nausea, vomiting, and pain.[4]
	C versicolor has a potent effect on the in vivo and in vitro expression of tumor necrosis factor.[2]
	A meta-analysis has provided strong evidence that *C versicolor* would have survival benefit in cancer patients, particularly in breast, gastric, and colorectal carcinomas.[5]
	PSK may improve immune function, reduce tumor-associated symptoms, and extend survival in patients with lung cancer.[6]
	PSP appears to protect against the adverse effects of radiation.[2]
Comments	This type of mushroom grows on dead logs worldwide.
	It is generally safe and very well tolerated.
	Products using *C versicolor* extracts are currently approved as adjunct therapies in China and Japan for patients with cancer who are already receiving chemotherapy or radiotherapy.[2]
	A common dosage used in many cancer studies is 3 g of extract daily.[1,3]
	Strong studies are needed to standardize preparation methods and optimize the kinetics, biodistribution, and activity of *C versicolor*—and of PSK and PSP specifically—to better determine specific immunomodulatory effects.[2]

References

1. PDQ Integrative, Alternative, and Complementary Therapies Editorial Board. PDQ medicinal mushrooms. National Cancer Institute. www.cancer.gov/about-cancer/treatment/cam/hp/mushrooms-pdq

2. Saleh MH, Rashedi I, Keating A. Immunomodulatory properties of *Coriolus versicolor*: the role of polysaccharopeptide. *Frontiers Immun.* 2017;8:1087.

3. Coriolus mushroom. Natural Medicines Comprehensive Database. Accessed April 15, 2018. https://naturalmedicines.therapeuticresearch.com/databases/food,-herbs-supplements/professional.aspx?productid=648

4. Piotrowski J, Jedrzejewski T, Kozak W. Immunomodulatory and antitumor properties of polysaccharide peptide (PSP). *Postepy Hig Med Dosw.* 2015 Jan 21;69:91-97.

5. Eliza WL, Fai CK, Chung LP. Efficacy of Yun Zhi (*Coriolus versicolor*) on survival in cancer patients: systematic review and meta-analysis. *Recent Pat Inflamm Allergy Drug Discov.* 2012 Jan;6(1):78-87.

6. Fritz H, Kennedy DA, Ishii M, et al. Polysaccharide K and *Coriolus versicolor* extracts for lung cancer: a systematic review. *Integr Cancer Ther.* 2015 May;14(3):201-11.

Vitamin D

Vitamin D is a fat-soluble vitamin with anti-inflammatory, immunomodulatory, bone protective, and anticancer effects.

Reported anticancer benefits	Regulates genes that influence cell proliferation and apoptosis[1]
Reported anticancer concerns	Toxicity, which can result in hypercalcemia[1]
Evidence	People living in geographic areas with greater sun exposure (which triggers vitamin D synthesis in the human body) have lower cancer rates.[2]
	Vitamin D helps regulate genes that influence cell proliferation, differentiation, and apoptosis.[1]
	Vitamin D controls immune cell regulation and differentiation, gut barrier function, and antimicrobial peptide synthesis, all of which may serve as protective factors against colon cancer.[3]
	An inverse association between cancer and 25-hydroxyvitamin D levels is strongest for colon cancer.[3-5]
	Several observational studies have supported an inverse association between vitamin D intake or 25-hydroxyvitamin D level and breast cancer,[6,7] while others have not.[8,9]
	A meta-analysis reported a significant inverse association between vitamin D and breast cancer in postmenopausal women[10] but not in premenopausal women.[11]
	Researchers reported a consistent prognostic association between 25-hydroxyvitamin D levels and survival in patients with colorectal cancer.[12]
	Most observational studies have found that vitamin D consumption is not associated with a risk for prostate[13,14] and ovarian cancers.[15]
	There may be an inverse association between vitamin D supplementation and overall mortality.[16] In a large prospective trial (1,260 cases vs 1,331 controls), men in the highest quartile for plasma 25-hydroxyvitamin D levels had a significantly lower risk for lethal prostate cancer than men in the lowest quartile.[17]
Comments	Vitamin D sufficiency is important for overall health, including cancer prevention.
	Because 25-hydroxyvitamin D has a longer half-life than 1,25 dihydroxyvitamin D (15 days vs 15 hours, respectively), 25-hydroxyvitamin D is used to assess vitamin D status.[1]
	The bioavailability of vitamin D3 (cholecalciferol) is significantly greater than that of vitamin D-2 (ergocalciferol).[18]
	The Dietary Reference Intakes for vitamin D were revised in 2010 and the Tolerable Upper Intake Level of vitamin D increased to 4,000 IU/d.[1]
	The Endocrine Society has suggested that maintenance of a 25-hydroxyvitamin D blood level of 40 to 60 ng/mL is ideal (this takes into account assay variability) and that up to 100 ng/mL is safe.[19]

References

1. Institute of Medicine, Food and Nutrition Board. *Dietary Reference Intakes for Calcium and Vitamin D.* National Academy Press, 2010.

2. Garland FC, Garland CF, Gorham ED, Young JF. Geographic variation in breast cancer mortality in the United States: a hypothesis involving exposure to solar radiation. *Prev Med.* 1990;19(6):614–622.

3. Meeker S, Seamons A, Maggio-Price L, Paik J. Protective links between vitamin D, inflammatory bowel disease and colon cancer. *World J Gastroenterol.* 2016;22(3):933-948.

4. Feskanich D, Ma J, Fuchs CS, et al. Plasma vitamin D metabolites and risk of colorectal cancer in women. *Cancer Epidemiol Biomarkers Prev.* 2004;13(9):1502–1508.

5. Ma Y, Zhang P, Wang F, Yang J, Liu Z, Qin H. Association between vitamin D and risk of colorectal cancer: a systematic review of prospective studies. *J Clin Oncol.* 2011;29(28): 3775-3582.

6. Robien K, Cutler GJ, Lazovich D. Vitamin D intake and breast cancer risk in postmenopausal women: the Iowa Women's Health Study. *Cancer Causes & Control.* 2007;18(7):775-782.

7. Yousef FM, Jacobs ET, Kang PT, et al. Vitamin D status and breast cancer in Saudi Arabian women: case-control study. *Am J Clin Nutr.* 2013;98(1): 105-110.

8. Chlebowski RT, Johnson KC, Kooperberg C. Calcium plus vitamin D supplementation and the risk of breast cancer. *J Natl Cancer Inst.* 2008;100(22):1581-1591.

9. Gissel T, Rejnmark L, Mosekilde L, Vestergaard P. Intake of vitamin D and risk of breast cancer—a meta-analysis. *J Ster Biochem Molec Biol.* 2008;111(3-5):195-199.

10. Bauer SR, Hankinson SE, Bertone-Johnson ER, Ding EL. Plasma vitamin D levels, menopause, and risk of breast cancer: dose-response meta-analysis of prospective studies. *Medicine (Baltimore).* 2013;92(3):123-131.

11. Wang D, Vélez de-la-Paz O, Zhai JX, Liu DW. Serum 25-hydroxyvitamin D and breast cancer risk: a meta-analysis of prospective studies. *Tumour Biol.* 2013;34(6):3509-3517.

12. Dou R, Ng K, Giovannucci EL, Manson JE, Qian ZR, Ogino S. Vitamin D and colorectal cancer: molecular, epidemiological, and clinical evidence. *Brit J Nutr.* 2016;115(9):1643-1660.

13. Tseng M, Breslow RA, Graubard BI, Ziegler RG. Dairy, calcium, and vitamin D intakes and prostate cancer risk in the National Health and Nutrition Examination Epidemiologic Follow-up Study cohort. *Am J Clin Nutr.* 2005;81(5):1147-1154.

14. Kristal AR, Arnold KB, Neuhouser ML, et al. Diet, Supplement use, and prostate cancer risk: results from the Prostate Cancer Prevention Trial. *Am J Epidemiol.* 2010;172(5):566-577.

15. Qin B, Moorman PG, Alberg AJ, et al. Dairy, calcium, vitamin D and ovarian cancer risk in African–American women. *Br J Cancer.* 2016;115(9): 1122-1130.

16. Christakos S, Dhawan P, Verstuyf A, Verlinden L, Carmeliet G. Vitamin D: metabolism, molecular mechanism of action, and pleiotropic effects. *Physiol Rev.* 2016;96(1):365-408.

17. Shui IM, Mucci LA, Kraft P, et al. Vitamin D–related genetic variation, plasma vitamin D, and risk of lethal prostate cancer: a prospective nested case–control study. *J Natl Cancer Inst.* 2012;104(9):690-699.

18. Binkley N, Gemar D, Engelke J, et al. Evaluation of ergocalciferol or cholecalciferol dosing, 1,600 IU daily or 50,000 IU monthly in older adults. *J Clin Endocrinol Metab.* 2011;96(4):981-988.

19. Bischoff-Ferrari HA. Optimal serum 25-hydroxyvitamin D levels for multiple health outcomes. *Adv Exp Med Biol.* 2014;810:500-525.

Continuing Professional Education

This second edition of *Oncology Nutrition for Clincal Practice* offers readers 12.5 hours of Continuing Professional Education (CPE) credit. Readers may earn credit by completing the interactive online quiz at: https://publications.webauthor.com/oncology_nutrition_clinical_practice_2nd

Index

Page numbers followed by *t* indicate a table, page numbers followed by *b* indicate a box, and page numbers followed by *f* indicate a figure.

A

Americans for Safe Access, cannabis use, 572*b*

American Society for Parenteral and Enteral Nutrition, 60, 62, 67, 84, 196, 219, 225, 555*b*
  hematopoietic cell transplantation and, 316
  recommendations, 239–240
  Safe Practices for Enteral Nutrition Therapy, 230

American Society of Clinical Oncology, 135, 354, 545
  cancer survivorship, 148*b*
  pancreatic cancer, 437

American Thyroid Association, 534

amino acids
  glutamine, 636
  parenteral nutrition, 235–236, 237*b*
  theanine, 658

Amin Pharmaceutical Company, 654

amputations
  children with, 262, 262*t*
  equations for adjusting body weight for, 265*b*

amyloidosis, hematologic malignancies, 282, 290–291

anal cancer, risk factors, 410–411*t*

anal carcinoma, 405, 425–426. *See also* gastrointestinal cancers
  characteristics, 406*f*
  interventions for nutrition problems, 412–413*b*, 426
  surgery, 426
  treatment, 426
  United States statistics, 407*t*

Anandamide, endocannabinoid, 564

anaplastic thyroid carcinoma, 533*f*

anastrozole (Arimidex), hormonal agents, 178–179*b*

androgen deprivation therapy, prostate cancer, 521*b*

anorexia and early satiety, 196
  considerations, 197*b*
  definition, 196*b*
  interventions, 197*b*
  pharmacotherapy, 197*b*
  severity grades, 197*b*

ANS. *See* autonomic nervous system

anthracycline antitumor antibiotics, chemotherapy, 167–168*b*

anthropometric measurements, 40, 63*b*

antiandrogens, hormonal agents, 178–179*b*

antibiotics, enteral nutrition, 231*b*

antidiarrheals, enteral nutrition, 231*b*

antiemetics, enteral nutrition, 231*b*

antiestrogens, hormonal agents, 178–179*b*

anti-inflammatory foods
  antioxidant nutrients, 25
  nutrition, 25–26
  supplying omega-3 fatty acids, 26
  supporting protective microbiome, 25–26

antimetabolites, chemotherapy, 165–166*b*

antioxidant supplements
  breast cancer, 360, 362
  chemotherapy and, 118–119
  dietary, 118–119
  radiotherapy and, 118–119

antitumor antibiotics, chemotherapy, 167*b*

Anusara, yoga lineage, 98*b*

appetite loss, prevalence in cancer patients, 547*t*

appetite stimulants
  enteral nutrition, 231*b*
  pediatric oncology, 269*b*

aromatase inhibitor-induced musculoskeletal symptoms, breast cancer, 351

aromatase inhibitors, hormonal agents, 178–179*b*

artificial hydration
  decision for use, 556–557
  palliative care, 553, 556

artificial nutrition
  decision for use, 556–557
  guidelines for patients with advanced cancer, 554–555*b*
  palliative care, 553, 554–555*b*

ascites, medical nutrition therapy, 453–454

ascitic fluid, patients with hepatic compromise, 417*b*

Ashtanga, yoga lineage, 98*b*

ASPEN. *See* American Society for Parenteral and Enteral Nutrition

Aspergillus inhalation, 570

Aspiration, enteral nutrition therapy, 228*b*

assessment parameters, pediatric oncology patients, 263–264*b*

assessment tools, gynecologic cancers, 504–505

astrocytoma, category and nutrition, 255*b*

atypical teratoid/rhabdoid tumor, category and nutrition, 255*b*

autonomic nervous system, 92, 93*f*, 99

axillary lymph node dissection, breast cancer, 349

Ayurveda, 91, 102*b*

azacitidine (Vidaza), chemotherapy agent, 165*b*

azotemia, parenteral nutrition, 243*b*

B

Bacteroides fragilis, colorectal cancer, 421

basal energy expenditure, 81*b*

basal metabolic rate, 81*b*

BEE. *See* basal energy expenditure

bendamustine (Treanda), chemotherapy agent, 162*b*

β carotene, dietary supplement, 22, 116

bevacizumab (Avastin), angiogenesis inhibitors, 175*b*

beverages
  alcoholic, 21–22
  sugar-sweetened, 20–21

Bhajan, Yogi, 98*b*

bicalutamide (Casodex), hormonal agents, 178–179*b*

Bikram, yoga lineage, 98*b*

bile duct, 442*f*, 443*f*, 444*f*, 445*f*
  cholangiocarcinoma, 436
  obstructed, 446
  sample PES statements of cancers, 462
  symptoms of blocked, 447*b*

bile reflux gastritis, postgastrectomy, 393*b*

Bill Henderson protocol, 600–601

Billroth I/II, gastrectomy, 384, 385*f*, 386

breast-conserving surgery, breast cancer, 349

breastfeeding
 lactation and, 23
 practice points for, 23*b*

Brown, Michael S., 603

Budwig, Johanna, 602

Budwig diet, 600, 602–603

busulfan (Busulfex), chemotherapy agent, 162*b*

busulfan (Myleran), chemotherapy agent, 162*b*

C

cachexia
 identifying cancer, 61–62
 inflammation, 75
 lung cancer, 494
 sarcopenic obesity and, 44–46
 stages of cancer, 45*f*

calcium
 breast cancer, 351–352
 dietary supplement, 22
 osteoporosis, 292–293
 ovarian cancer, 500
 pediatric cancer patients, 267, 268*t*
 prostate cancer, 519–520, 524*b*

California Department of Health Services, 609

California Teachers Study, 589

Camellia sinensis (green tea), 638

Canadian Foundation for Dietetic Research, functional foods, 115*b*

cancer. *See also* childhood cancer; hematologic malignancies
 alcoholic beverages, 21–22
 body composition changes with, 76
 common types in US, 1*t*
 cost of care, 1–2
 dietary supplements and, 114–119
 functional foods and, 111–114
 metabolic changes in, 75
 nutrition concerns and outcomes, 8*b*, 9*b*
 nutrition-related side effects and interventions, 128–131*b*

screening, 2–3
staging, 3–4
survival rates by race, 2*f*
survivorship, 148*b*
term, 1

cancer cachexia
 definition, 61
 identifying, 61–62
 stages of, 45*f*

Cancer Council of Australia, 479

Cancer Exercise Trainer, 51

cancer patients
 efficacy of cannabis use by, 565–568
 functional foods in care process, 114
 malnutrition and, 59
 navigating dietary supplements, 119
 palliative care, 546–548
 prevalence of nutrition-related symptoms, 547*t*
 refeeding syndrome, 85

cancer prevention
 adiposity and weight gain, 13, 15–16
 alcoholic beverages, 21–22
 American Cancer Society on diet and physical activity, 582–583
 anti-inflammatory foods, 25–26
 dietary supplements, 22–23
 flaxseed, 27–28
 foods promoting weight gain, 19
 genetically engineered foods, 25
 lactation and breastfeeding, 23
 organic foods, 24–25
 physical activity, 16–17
 physical activity guidelines, 41–43*b*
 predominantly plant-based diet, 17–19
 recommendations for, 13, 14–15*b*
 red and processed meats, 19–20
 soy foods, 26–27
 sugar-sweetened beverages, 20–21
 World Cancer Research Fund/American Institute for Cancer Research recommendations, 584–585

Cancer Prevention Study II, 279, 354

cancer risk
 energy restriction and, 39–40
 evidence for body fatness and, 38*f*
 intentional weight loss and, 39
 obesity, weight gain and, 37, 39
 physical activity and, 40

Cancer Survival Through Lifestyle Change (CASTLE), 138–139*t*

cancer survivors
 breast cancer, 23–24, 27–28
 clinically-based supervised programs, 136–137*t*
 commercial programs, 140–141*t*
 community-based programs, 140–141*t*
 dietary intervention and physical activity, 136–143*t*
 dietary intervention trials, 144–145*t*
 dietary patterns and quality, 135, 146–147
 efficacy of cannabis use by, 565–568
 excess adiposity during, 46–47
 flaxseed and, 27–28
 home-based programs, 142–143*t*
 lifestyle interventions, 134*f*
 managing symptoms early posttreatment, 127, 132
 medical nutrition therapy (MNT), 133, 135
 mixed-modality programs, 138–139*t*
 nutritional assessment of, 132–135
 nutritional resources for, 147, 148–149*b*
 nutrition-related side effects and interventions, 128–131*b*
 physical activity guidelines, 41–43*b*
 post-symptom diet therapy, 133
 practice points for, 24*b*
 role of physical activity and lean mass, 147
 soy and breast cancer, 26–27
 technology-based programs, 142–143*t*

chronic myeloid leukemia, 284
conditioning regimens, 306, 307f
epipodophyllotoxins, 168b
Hodgkin lymphoma, 285
lung cancer, 489–490
modes of action, 160
nausea and vomiting induced by, 287
non-Hodgkin lymphoma, 284–285
nutritional implications, 160–161, 162–169b
pancreatic adenocarcinoma, 438b
side effects of, 7, 160–161, 162–169b
taxanes for, 169b
vinca alkaloids, 169b
chemotherapy-induced nausea and vomiting, 287, 352
medical cannabis and, 566
chemotherapy-induced peripheral neuropathy, 50, 352
chemovar, cannabis, 563
chicory root, functional foods, 113
childhood cancer. *See also* nutrition assessment in childhood cancer
acute lymphoblastic leukemia, 253, 254b
acute myeloid leukemia, 253
central nervous system tumors, 253, 255–256b
children with amputations, 262, 262t, 265b
chimeric antigen receptor (CAR) T-cell therapy, 258
distribution of diagnoses in US, 251f
Ewing sarcoma, 258
hepatoblastoma, 258
Hodgkin lymphoma, 253, 256
hyperthermic intraperitoneal chemotherapy (HIPEC), 258
malnutrition prevalence and outcomes, 259, 259b, 260t
neuroblastoma, 257
non-Hodgkin lymphoma, 256–257
nutrition assessment, 262, 266–268
nutrition impact symptoms and, 252–258

nutrition interventions and support, 268–270
nutrition screening, 260–261, 261f
osteosarcoma, 258
resources, 253b
rhabdomyosarcoma, 257
survival by diagnosis, 252f
survivors of, 252
Wilms tumor, 257
Children's Oncology Group, 252, 253b
chimeric antigen receptor (CAR) T-cell therapy, 177, 258, 285
hematologic malignancies, 323
non-Hodgkin lymphoma, 285
China's *Pen Ts'ao Ching*, 563
chlorambucil (Leukeran), chemotherapy agent, 163b
CHOICE Study, 136–137t
cholangiocarcinoma, 405. *See also* gastrointestinal cancers
biliary system, 417f
characteristics, 406f
distal cholangiocarcinoma (dCCA), 417f
interventions and nutrition, 415, 418
interventions for nutrition problems, 412–413b
intrahepatic cholangiocarcinoma (iCCA), 417f
palliative interventions, 415
perihilar cholangiocarcinoma (pCCA), 417f
risk factors, 408–409t
surgery, 415
treatment, 415
types, 417f
United States statistics, 407t
cholestasis, parenteral nutrition, 244b
choline, prostate cancer, 520
Choudhury, Bikram, 98b
chronic kidney disease, 290
chronic lymphocytic leukemia
hematologic malignancy, 281f
treatment, 284
chronic myeloid leukemia
hematologic malignancy, 281f
treatment, 284

chyle leak, medical nutrition therapy, 458
Cimicifuga racemosa (black cohosh), 620
CIPN. *See* chemotherapy-induced peripheral neuropathy
cisplatin (Platinol, CDDP), chemotherapy agent, 163b
classification system, tumor, lymph node, metastasis (TNM), 3b
Clinical Oncological Society of Australia, 196
Clostridium difficile, 268
colorectal cancer, 421
hematopoietic cell transplantation, 315
Cochrane Collaboration, 96, 99, 101
Cocinar Para Su Salud, 140–141t
coenzyme Q10 (CoQ10), 362, 622
colorectal cancer, 405
animal foods, 20
bowel management, 424
characteristics, 406f
cytoreductive surgery, 421
hyperthermic intraperitoneal chemotherapy, 421
incidence, 420
interventions for nutrition problems, 412–413b, 421, 424–425
low anterior resection syndrome, 424–425
neorectal reservoirs, 425
nutrition-related side effects and interventions, 129b
ostomy management, 424
red and processed meat, 19–20
risk factors, 410–411t
surgery, 421, 422–423f
treatment, 421
United States statistics, 407t
vitamin and mineral malabsorption, 425
colorectal cancers. *See* gastrointestinal cancers
Common Terminology Criteria for Adverse Events, 195
anorexia and early satiety, 196, 196–197b
constipation, 196, 200–201b
diarrhea, 196, 202–203b
dysphagia, 196, 204–205b

postoperative nutrition
complications, 380–381
prevalence and risk factors,
376*b*
sample PES statements, 395
squamous cell carcinomas, 375,
376*b*
surgery, 375, 377
survivorship and, 381–382
treatment, 375, 376*b*, 377
types of, 375
weight loss and sarcopenia, 379
esophagitis
considerations, 212–213*b*
definition, 212*b*
interventions, 213*b*
pharmacotherapy, 213*b*
severity grades, 212*b*
ESPEN. *See* European Society
for Clinical Nutrition and
Metabolism
essential fatty acid deficiency,
parenteral nutrition, 242*b*
estimated energy expenditure, 81*b*
estimated energy requirement, 81*b*
estrogen, obesity and cancer, 44
etoposide (Vepesid, VP-16),
chemotherapy agent, 168*b*
European Prospective Investigation
into Cancer and Nutrition, 331,
354, 355
European Society for Clinical
Nutrition and Metabolism, 60, 75,
76, 288, 380
guidelines for patients with
advanced cancer, 555*b*
Guidelines on Nutrition for
Cancer Patients, 76, 77
hematopoietic cell
transplantation and, 316
nutrition support, 454
everolimus (Affinitor), protein-
targeted agent, 174*b*
Evidence Analysis Library
Oncology Workgroup, 61
Ewing sarcoma, nutrition side
effects, 258
exemestane (Aromasin), hormonal
agents, 178–179*b*
Exercise and Nutrition to Enhance
Recovery and Good Health for
You (ENERGY) study, 138–139t,
360

exocrine pancreatic insufficiency,
380–381, 439
external beam radiation therapy,
183
dosage, 185
image-guided radiation therapy
(IGRT), 184
intensity-modulated radiation
therapy (IMRT), 184
intraoperative radiation therapy
(IORT), 184–185
side effects, 185, 186*f*, 187*b*,
188*b*
stereotactic radiation therapy
(SRT), 184
stereotactic radiosurgery (SRS),
184
three-dimensional conformal
radiation therapy (3D-CRT),
184
total body irradiation (TBI),
184
uterine cancer, 502

F

fasting, breast cancer treatment and,
353
fat consumption, prostate cancer,
519
fatigue
breast cancer, 350
considerations, 206*b*
definition, 206*b*
interventions, 207*b*
pharmacotherapy, 207*b*
severity grades, 206*b*
fat malabsorption, after gastrectomy,
395*b*
fats
Dietary Reference Intake
(DRI), 77–78, 78*t*
requirements during
hematopoietic cell
transplantation, 311*b*
FDA. *See* US Food and Drug
Administration
Federal Trade Commission, 116
fish
consumption, 20
prostate cancer, 523*b*

Fit4Life, 142–143*t*
FITT (frequency, intensity, time
and type) principle, 51
flaxseed (*Linum usitatissimum*),
628
breast cancer, 356
cancer survivors and, 27–28
functional foods, 113
nutrition, 27
prostate cancer, 524*b*
fludarabine (Fludara),
chemotherapy agent, 165*b*
fluid requirements, 78, 79*t*
estimating needs for pediatric
cancer patients, 267, 267*b*
hematopoietic cell
transplantation, 312*b*
fluorouracil (5-FU), chemotherapy
agent, 5, 161, 165*b*
flutamide (Eulexin), hormonal
agents, 178–179*b*
focused attention, 96
folate deficiency, after gastrectomy,
394*b*
follicular thyroid carcinoma, 533*f*
food advice, breast cancer, 354–358,
361*b*
Food and Agriculture Organization
of the United Nations, 491
Frankenfield, David, 84
French National Federation of
Cancer Centers, 554*b*
French Nutrition Oncology Study
Group, 549
FRESH START, 144–145*t*
functional foods. *See also* dietary
supplements/functional foods
cancer and, 111–114
definition of, 111–112
effects on carcinogenesis, 112
examples and evidence for,
112–114
incorporating in cancer
Nutrition Care Process, 114
regulation of, 114
resources, 115*b*

G

gallbladder carcinoma, 405. *See also*
gastrointestinal cancers

Index

Iowa Women's Health Study, 39, 113
ipilimumab (Yervoy), monoclonal antibodies, 170, 173*b*
iron, pancreatic cancer survivors, 461*b*
iron deficiency, after gastrectomy, 394*b*
iron overload, hematopoietic cell transplantation, 323
isoflavones, soy foods, 26, 27
Iyengar, yoga lineage, 97, 98*b*
Iyengar, B. K. S., 98*b*

J

Journal of Developments in Sustainable Agriculture, 115*b*
Journal of Parenteral and Enteral Nutrition, 62
Journal of the Academy of Nutrition and Dietetics, 62

K

Kabat-Zinn, Jon, 90*b*
Kelly, William Donald, 606
ketogenic diet, 594–595, *See also* brain tumor
    brain tumor, 335–337
    implementing, 336–337, 337*b*
    managing potential side effects of, 338–339*b*
    resources for professionals, 338*b*
    screening and monitoring, 335*b*
    types of, 336
kidney cancer, nutrition-related side effects and interventions, 130*b*
Kripalu, yoga lineage, 98*b*, 100
Krishnamacharya, T., 98*b*
Kundalini, yoga lineage, 98*b*
Kushi Institute, 611

L

lactation
    breastfeeding and, 23

    practice points for, 23*b*
lactose intolerance, surgeries for pancreatic cancer, 441*b*
large cell carcinoma, lung cancer, 487, 488*f*
Lasater, Judith, 98*b*
laxatives, enteral nutrition, 231*b*
lenalidomide (Revlimide), angiogenesis inhibitors, 175*b*
leptin, obesity and cancer, 44
letrozole (Femara), hormonal agents, 178–179*b*
leukemia, 279
    distribution of childhood cancer, 251*f*
    hematologic malignancies, 280, 281*f*
    nutrition-related side effects and interventions, 131*b*
leuprolide acetate (Lupron), hormonal agents, 178–179*b*
levonantradol, cannabinoids, 564–565
Life After Cancer Epidemiology Study, 117, 357
Lifestyle, Exercise, and Nutrition (LEAN), 138–139*t*
Lifestyle Intervention for Ovarian Cancer Enhanced Survival (LIVES), 144–145*t*
lifestyle interventions
    breast cancer, 354, 361*b*
    cancer survivors, 134*f*
lignans, breast cancer, 356
Linum usitatissimum (flaxseed), 628. *See also* flaxseed
Linus Pauling Institute, 115*b*
    dietary supplements, 120*b*
    functional foods, 115*b*
lipids
    metabolism 75*b*
    parenteral nutrition, 235–236, 237*b*
    prostate cancer, 521*b*
LISA Trial, 140–141*t*
LiverTox, 116
Livingston-Wheeler therapy, 608–609
low anterior resection syndrome, colorectal cancer, 424–425
low-iodine diet
    guidelines for, 534–535, 538

    inconsistencies in guidelines, 535*b*
    radioactive iodine, 534
    side effects related to, 539
    thyroid cancer, 534–535, 536–538*b*, 538
Lugano Classification System, 283
lung and bronchus cancer, side effects and interventions, 128*b*
lung cancer
    adenocarcinoma, 487, 488*f*
    chemotherapy, 489–490
    diagnosis, 489
    identifying patients at high nutritional risk, 493*b*
    immunotherapy, 490
    incidence, 487
    interventions for nutrition problems, 491–493
    large cell carcinoma, 487, 488*f*
    malnutrition and weight loss, 492
    nutrition assessment, 490–491
    radiotherapy, 490
    risk factors, 487
    sample PES statements, 494
    sarcopenia and muscle loss, 492–493
    sarcopenic obesity, 493
    small cell carcinoma, 487, 488*f*
    squamous cell carcinoma, 487, 488*f*
    surgery, 489
    survivorship, 494
    targeted therapies, 489–490
    treatment, 489–490
    types, 487, 488*f*
luteinizing hormone-releasing hormone (LHRH) agonists, hormonal agents, 178–179*b*
lycopene-rich fruits and vegetables, prostate cancer, 523*b*
lymphedema, breast cancer, 350–351
lymphoma, hematologic malignancy, 279, 280, 281*f*

M

macrobiotic diet, 610–611
macronutrient metabolism, systemic inflammation, 75*b*

qigong, 96
resources, 102*b*
selected popular, 90*b*
tai chi, 96
yoga, 97, 99–100
mindfulness-based cancer recovery, 97
mindfulness-based stress reduction (MBSR), mind-body intervention, 90*b*, 96–97
mineral intake. *See also* vitamin(s)
colorectal cancer, 425
parenteral nutrition, 244*b*
patients with hepatic compromise, 416*b*
Mini Nutritional Assessment, 548
mitomycin-C (Mutamycin), chemotherapy agent, 167*b*
MNT. *See* medical nutrition therapy (MNT)
Modified-Atkins, 136–137*t*
modified radical mastectomy, breast cancer, 349
monoclonal antibodies, targeted therapy, 170–171, 172–173*b*
monoclonal gammopathy of undetermined significance, hematologic malignancies, 281*f*, 282
mREE. *See* measured resting energy expenditure
MRI. *See* magnetic resonance imaging (MRI)
mucositis
chemotherapy-induced, and breast cancer, 352–353
head and neck cancers, 480
hematopoietic cell transplantation, 314
Multiethnic Cohort Study, 118
multiple myeloma, 279, 281*f*
diagnosis of, 282
treatment, 284
multivitamin and mineral (MVM) supplement, 117–118

N

nabilone, cannabinoids, 564–565
nabiximols, cannabinoids, 565
N-acetylcysteine (NAC), 642

National Academies of Science, Engineering, and Medicine, 76, 268, 288
National Cancer Institute, 1, 252, 253*b*, 412, 605
cancer survivorship, 148*b*
Common Terminology Criteria for Adverse Events (CTCAE), 195, 196*b*
lung cancer, 487
National Coalition for Cancer Survivorship, cancer survivorship, 149*b*
National Comprehensive Cancer Network, 135, 157, 333, 405
breast cancer treatments, 349
Clinical Practice Guidelines in Oncology for Uterine Cancer, Ovarian Cancer and Cervical Cancer, 502
esophageal cancer, 375
head and neck cancers, 474, 477*b*, 482
lung cancer, 489
multiple myeloma, 284
pancreatic cancer, 437
physical activity guidelines and cancer, 43*b*
practice points for cancer survivors, 24*b*
prostate cancer, 517, 518*b*
website, 283
National Conference of State Legislatures, State Medical Marijuana Laws, 572*b*
National Health and Nutrition Examination Survey (NHANES), 360, 611
National Health Interview Survey, 89, 91, 92
National Institute of Diabetes and Digestive and Kidney Diseases, 116, 290
National Institutes of Health, 116, 606
National Center for Complementary and Integrative Health, 89
Office of Dietary Supplements, 120*b*
National Kidney Foundation, 290, 292

National Library of Medicine, 116
National Lipid Association, 522
National Osteoporosis Foundation, 288
nausea and vomiting
chemotherapy-induced, 287
chemotherapy-induced, and breast cancer, 352
considerations, 210*b*
definition, 210*b*
enteral nutrition therapy, 228*b*
interventions, 211*b*
pharmacotherapy, 211*b*
prevalence in cancer patients, 547*t*
severity grades, 210*b*
NCCN. *See* National Comprehensive Cancer Network
NCI. *See* National Cancer Institute
NCI-Designated Cancer Centers, 91, 94–95
neck cancers. *See* head and neck cancers
neorectal reservoirs, colorectal cancer, 425
NETSBs. *See* neuroendocrine tumors of small bowel
neuroblastoma
distribution of childhood cancer, 251*f*
nutrition side effects, 257
survival percentage in children, 252*f*
neuroendocrine tumors of small bowel, 405. *See also* gastrointestinal cancers
carcinoid syndrome, 419–420
characteristics, 406*f*
diagnostic testing, 418–419
interventions for nutrition problems, 412–413*b*, 419–420
niacin deficiency, 420
radiopharmaceuticals, 419
risk factors, 410–411*t*
secretory diarrhea, 420
somatostatin analogue therapy, 419
surgery, 419
treatment, 419
United States statistics, 407*t*
neuropathy, breast cancer, 352

O

physical activity, 37, 51
  breast cancer, 360
  cancer prevention, 16–17
  cancer risk and, 40
  cancer survivorship and, 49–51
  guidelines for cancer
    prevention and survivorship,
    41–43b
  levels, 81b
  long-term survivorship, 50–51,
    147
  mechanisms of energetics and
    cancer, 44
  practice points, 17b
  prescriptions and referrals, 51
  prostate cancer, 520
Physicians' Health Study II, 118
phytochemicals
  anti-inflammatory foods, 25
  foods containing, 25
  predominantly plant-based diet,
    17–19
  resveratrol, 21b
phytoestrogens
  safety, 116
  soy and, 26
pineal gland, 332f
pituitary gland, 332f
plant-based diet. *See also* diets
  cancer and predominantly,
    17–19
  practice points, 18b
  prostate cancer, 517, 519
plants, dietary supplements, 117
plasma cell neoplasms, hematologic
  malignancy, 280, 281f, 282
plasmacytomas, hematologic
  malignancies, 281f, 282
Polyporous versicolor, 660
Pooling Project, breast cancer, 355
positron emission tomography
  (PET), 282, 375, 489
postgastrectomy
  complications, 387–388
  syndromes, 390–393b
postoperative nutrition
  esophageal cancer, 379–381
  gynecologic cancers, 506
  pancreaticoduodenectomy, 455
postoperative pancreatic fistula,
  medical nutrition therapy, 457
postvagotomy diarrhea,
  postgastrectomy, 392–393b

poultry, 20
  prostate cancer, 523b
prebiotics, functional foods, 113
precision medicine, 161, 170
predicted resting energy
  expenditure, 76, 80
predictive equations
  decision tree for, 82f
  energy needs, 81, 83–85
pREE. *See* predicted resting energy
  expenditure
primary brain tumor, 331. *See also*
  brain tumor
    nutrition impact symptoms for
    medications for, 334b
processed meats. *See also* red meat
  cancer prevention, 19–20
  practice points, 20b
  recommendations, 14b
  term, 19
Progenitor cryptocides, 608
progesterones, hormonal agents,
  178–179b
prostate cancer, 515
  animal foods, 20
  body weight and physical
    activity, 520
  carcinoma of prostate gland,
    516f
  cases in United States, 515b
  dairy products, calcium and
    vitamin D, 519–520
  diagnosis, 515, 517
  dietary supplements, 520
  eggs and choline, 520
  fat consumption, 519
  interventions for nutrition
    problems, 520, 522
  medical nutrition therapy, 521b
  nutrition recommendations for
    survivors, 523–524b
  nutrition-related side effects
    and interventions, 128b
  plant-based diets, 517, 519
  prostate-specific antigen (PSA),
    515
  risk factors, 515, 517b
  sample PES statements, 525
  survivorship, 522, 523–524b
  treatment, 517, 518b
protein
  Dietary Reference Intake
    (DRI), 77, 77t

estimating needs for pediatric
  cancer patients, 262, 266–
  267, 267t
lung cancer, 491
metabolism, 75b
patients with hepatic
  compromise, 416b
requirements during
  hematopoietic cell
  transplantation, 311b
Pulling Through Study, 353
pylorus-preserving
  pancreaticoduodenectomy, 440.
  See also pancreatic cancer
    anatomical reconstruction,
    444f
    nutrition impact symptoms,
    441b

Q

qigong, 89
  mind-body intervention, 90b,
    96
  resources, 102b
QOL. *See* quality of life
quality of life, 89, 185
  nutrition impact symptoms and,
    546–548
  palliative care and hospice, 545
  pancreatic cancer, 440
  yoga, 100
quercetin, 646

R

race, cancer survival rates by, 2f
radiation
  Hodgkin lymphoma, 285
  multiple myeloma, 284
  non-Hodgkin lymphoma,
    284–285
radiation-induced diarrhea,
  gynecologic cancers, 505–506
radiation oncology, 158f, 183
  brachytherapy, 183, 185, 188b,
    189b, 190b
  direct effects of, 183

small-molecule drugs
    angiogenesis inhibitors, 171, 175*b*
    protein-targeted agents, 171, 174*b*
    targeted therapy, 171, 174–175*b*
smell. *See* taste and smell changes
SNS. *See* sympathetic nervous system
Society for Integrative Oncology
    acupuncture, 95
    evidence grades, 94*b*
    meditation, 96
    qigong, 96
    yoga, 100
Society of Critical Care Medicine, 84, 85, 225
somatostatin analogue therapy, neuroendocrine tumors of small bowel, 419
sorafenib (Nexavar), protein-targeted agent, 174*b*
soy foods
    breast cancer, 356–357
    breast cancer survivors and, 26–27
    dietary soy amounts, 27
    human data on consumption, 26
    isoflavone content of, 357*t*
    nutrition, 26–27
    phytoestrogens, 26
    prostate cancer, 517, 519, 524*b*
Spanish Society of Medical Oncology, 555*b*
spinal cord, 332*f*
squamous cell carcinoma, lung cancer, 487, 488*f*
SRS. *See* stereotactic radiosurgery
SRT. *See* stereotactic radiation therapy
staging, cancer, 3–4
Staphylococcus aureus, 268, 604
    anti-methicillin-resistant, 564
steatosis, parenteral nutrition, 244*b*
Stepping Stone, 138–139*t*
stereotactic radiation therapy, 184
stereotactic radiosurgery, 184
stomach, normal anatomy of, 383*f*.
    See also gastric cancer
stress, mind-body interventions and, 92, 94

strontium 89 (Metastron), 191
    possible side effects for metastatic bone pain, 192*b*
subjective global assessment, 505
    categories, 333
    patient-generated, 286, 504–505, 548
SUCCEED. *See* Survivors of Uterine Cancer Empowered by Exercise and Healthy Diet (SUCCEED) trial
sugar-sweetened beverages
    cancer and, 20–21
    practice points, 21*b*
    recommendations, 14*b*
sunitinib (Sutent), 171
    protein-targeted agent, 174*b*
surgical oncology, 158*f*
Surveillance, Epidemiology, and End Results Program, National Cancer Institute (NCI), 1
Survivors of Uterine Cancer Empowered by Exercise and Healthy Diet (SUCCEED) trial, 133, 136–137*t*
sympathetic nervous system, 92, 93*f*, 100
systemic inflammation
    cancer and, 75
    macronutrient metabolism, 75*b*
systemic therapy, breast cancer, 349

T

tai chi, 89
    mind-body intervention, 90*b*, 96
    resources, 102*b*
talimogene laherparepvec (Imlygic) (T-VEC), oncolytic viral therapy, 176–177
tamoxifen citrate (Novaldex), hormonal agents, 178–179*b*
targeted therapy, 158*f*
    cancer treatment, 170–171
    lung cancer, 489–490
    monoclonal antibodies, 170–171, 172–173*b*
    side effects of, 170
    small-molecule drugs, 171, 174–175*b*

taste and smell changes
    considerations, 198*b*
    definition, 198*b*
    head and neck cancers, 480
    interventions, 199*b*
    pharmacotherapy, 198*b*
    severity grades, 198*b*
taxanes, chemotherapy, 169*b*
TBI. *See* total body irradiation
TCM. *See* traditional Chinese medicine
telephone counseling, cancer survivors, 138–141*t*
temozolomide (Temodar), chemotherapy agent, 164*b*
temsirolimus (Torisel), protein-targeted agent, 174*b*
teniposide (Vumon, VM-26), chemotherapy agent, 168*b*
terpenoids, cannabis, 565*b*
tetrahydrocannabinol, cannabis, 563, 564–567
tetrahydrocannabinolic acid, 563
Text4Diet, 142–143*t*
thalidomide (Thalomid), angiogenesis inhibitors, 175*b*
THC. *See* tetrahydrocannabinol
THCA. *See* tetrahydrocannabinolic acid
theanine, 658
Therapeutic Research Center, dietary supplements, 120*b*
thiamine supplementation, 85
thioguanine (6-TG), chemotherapy agent, 166*b*
thiotepa (Thioplex), chemotherapy agent, 164*b*
Thorne Research, 654
three-dimensional conformal radiation therapy (3D-CRT), 184
thrush, head and neck cancers, 480
thyroid cancer
    anaplastic thyroid carcinoma, 533*f*
    chemotherapy, 532, 534
    cruciferous vegetable intake, 532
    dietary risk factors, 531–532
    distribution of childhood cancer, 251*f*
    dysphagia, 539
    follicular thyroid carcinoma, 533*f*

vitamin C, 18, 25
vitamin D, 132
  breast cancer, 351–352
  breast cancer and supplements, 362–363
  dietary supplement, 22, 662
  hematologic malignancies, 288–290
  hematopoietic cell transplantation, 321
  osteoporosis, 292
  pancreatic cancer survivors, 460b
  pediatric cancer patients, 267–268, 268t
  prostate cancer, 519–520, 524b
  Recommended Dietary Allowance, 268t
VITamin D and OmegA-3 TriaL (VITAL), 22
vitamin E, 18, 25, 116, 132
  antioxidants, 119
  dietary supplement, 22
  pancreatic cancer survivors, 461b
vomiting. *See also* nausea and vomiting
  chemotherapy-induced, 287, 352, 566
  prevalence in cancer patients, 547t
vulvar cancer. *See also* gynecologic cancers
  United States statistics, 499t

W

Warburg, Otto, 335
Way to Health (Kushi Institute), 611
WCRF. *See* World Cancer Research Fund (WCRF)
weight gain
  adiposity and, 13, 15–16
  breast cancer treatment and, 353–354
  evaluating weight-related risk, 15–16
  foods promoting, 19, 19b
weight loss
  breast cancer risk and, 359–360

cancer risk and intentional, 39
  esophageal cancer, 379
  lung cancer, 492
  prevalence in cancer patients, 547t
weight management
  breast cancer risk and, 358–359
  cancer survivors, 47, 48–49b
  medical nutrition therapy (MNT), 133, 135
weight method, hydration, 78
Weight Watchers (WW), 140–141t, 360
Weir formula, 81
WHEL. *See* Women's Healthy Eating and Living (WHEL)
Wilms tumor
  distribution of childhood cancer, 251f
  nutrition side effects, 257
  survival percentage in children, 252f
WINS. *See* Women's Intervention Nutrition Study (WINS)
women, cancer types common in US, 1t
Women's Health Initiative, 117, 146, 351
Women's Health Initiative Observational Study, 644
Women's Healthy Eating and Living, breast cancer, 355, 356
Women's Healthy Eating and Living (WHEL), 144–145t, 146
Women's Intervention Nutrition Study (WINS), 144–145t, 146
World Bank, functional foods, 115b
World Cancer Research Fund (WCRF), 13, 111
  alcoholic beverages, 21
  animal foods, 20
  cancer risk and body fatness, 37, 38f
  cancer survivors, 23–24, 26
  cancer survivorship, 149b
  dietary supplements, 22
  physical activity, 40
  predominantly plant-based diet, 17, 18b
  prevention recommendations, 14–15b
  red and processed meats, 19

World Cancer Research Fund/ American Institute for Cancer Research (WCRF/ AICR), Cancer Prevention Recommendations, 584–585
World Cancer Research Fund International, 135, 279
World Health Organization, 262, 331, 491
World Health Research Fund, physical activity guidelines and cancer, 42b

X

xerostomia
  considerations, 215b
  definition, 215b
  interventions, 215b
  pharmacotherapy, 215b
  prevalence in cancer patients, 547t
  severity grades, 215b

Y

Yin Yoga, 99b
yoga, 89
  lineages, 98–99b
  mind-body intervention, 90b, 97, 99–100
  resources, 102b
Yoga for Cancer Survivors, 97
Yoga in America study, 97
Yoga nidra, 99b
Yoga of Awareness, 97
Yoga therapy, 99b
Yoga Thrive, 97
Yun Zhi (*Coriolus versicolor, Trametes versicolor, Polyporous versicolor*), 660

Z

zinc, pancreatic cancer survivors, 461b
Zingiber officinale (ginger), 632
Zink, Paulie, 99b